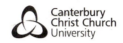 Canterbury
Christ Church
University

- LIBRARY SERVICES -

This item must be returned (or renewed) on
or before the last date indicated below.

Issue Desk: 01227 782352

NB: A fine will be charged for late return

CLARK'S
POSITIONING IN
RADIOGRAPHY

CLARK'S POSITIONING IN RADIOGRAPHY

12TH EDITION

A. STEWART WHITLEY · CHARLES SLOANE · GRAHAM HOADLEY
ADRIAN D. MOORE · CHRISSIE W. ALSOP

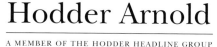

Hodder Arnold

A MEMBER OF THE HODDER HEADLINE GROUP

London

First published in Great Britain in 2005 by
Arnold, a member of the Hodder Headline Group,
338 Euston Road, London NW1 3BH

http://www.arnoldpublishers.com

Distributed in the United States of America by
Oxford University Press Inc.,
198 Madison Avenue, New York, NY10016
Oxford is a registered trademark of Oxford University Press

Whilst the advice and information in this book are believed to be true and
accurate at the date of going to press, neither the authors nor the publisher
can accept any legal responsibility or liability for any errors or omissions
that may be made. In particular (but without limiting the generality of the
preceding disclaimer) every effort has been made to check drug dosages;
however it is still possible that errors have been missed. Furthermore,
dosage schedules are constantly being revised and new side effects
recognized. For these reasons the reader is strongly urged to consult the
drug companies' printed instructions before administering any of the drugs
recommended in this book.

British Library Cataloguing in Publication Data
A catalogue record for this book is available from the British Library

Library of Congress Cataloging-in-Publication Data
A catalog record for this book is available from the Library of Congress

ISBN   0 340 76390 6

1 2 3 4 5 6 7 8 9 10

Commissioning Editor: Joanna Koster
Development Editor: Sarah Burrows
Project Editor: Anke Ueberberg
Production Controller: Joanna Walker
Indexer: Lawrence Errington
Cover Design: Sarah Rees

Typeset in 9.5/12 Berling Roman by Charon Tec Pvt. Ltd, Chennai, India
www.charontec.com
Printed and bound in India by Replika Press Pvt. Limited.

What do you think about this book? Or any other Arnold title?
Please send your comments to **feedback.arnold@hodder.co.uk**

Dedication

This volume is dedicated to our wives, partners and families, without whose unstinting support this work could not have taken place. They have endured countless nights and weekends as 'book windows', and we thank them for their tolerance and forebearance.

We also wish to acknowledge the professional support and advice of a huge number of colleagues who have given of their own time to offer advice and help in the preparation of the twelfth edition. This has truly been a team effort.

Contents

Contributors   ix

Preface   xi

Acknowledgements to the Twelfth Edition   xiii

1   Basic Principles of Radiography and Digital Technology   1

2   The Upper Limb   37

3   The Shoulder   77

4   The Lower Limb   105

5   The Hip, Pelvis and Sacro-iliac Joints   141

6   The Vertebral Column   163

7   The Thorax and Upper Airways   193

8   The Skull   229

9   The Facial Bones and Sinuses   259

10   Dental Radiography   279
     Vivian Rushton

11   The Abdomen and Pelvic Cavity   331

12   Ward Radiography   351

13   Theatre Radiography   367

14   Paediatric Radiography   381
     J. Valmai Cook and Kaye Shah

15   Mammography   435
     Gill Marshall

16   Miscellaneous   465
     With a contribution by Gail Jefferson – Forensic section

Index   505

Contributors

Chrissie Alsop Superintendent Radiographer, Department of Diagnostic Radiology, Manchester Medical School and Manchester Royal Infirmary, Manchester, UK

J. Valmai Cook Consultant Radiologist, Queen Mary's Hospital for Children, Epsom and St Helier University NHS Trust, Carshalton, UK

Sue Field Advanced Practitioner in Radiography Reporting, Blackpool, Fylde and Wyre Hospitals NHS Trust, Blackpool, Lancashire, UK

Graham Hoadley Consultant Radiologist, Directorate of Radiology and Physiotherapy Services, Blackpool, Fylde and Wyre Hospitals NHS Trust, Blackpool, Lancashire, UK

Gail Jefferson Clinical Tutor, Radiography Department, Carlisle Infirmary, Carlisle, UK

Gill Marshall Chair of Faculty Academic Standards/Principal Lecturer, Division of Medical Imaging Sciences, St Martin's College, Lancaster, UK

Adrian Moore Dean, Faculty of Science and Technology, Anglia Polytechnic University, Cambridge, UK

Vivian E. Rushton Senior Lecturer in Dental and Maxillofacial Radiology, School of Dentistry, University of Manchester, Manchester, UK

Kaye Shah Superintendent Radiographer, Queen Mary's Hospital for Children, Epsom and St Helier University NHS Trust, Carshalton, UK

Charles Sloane Senior Lecturer, Division of Medical Imaging Sciences, St Martin's College, Lancaster, UK

A. Stewart Whitley Directorate Manager, Directorate of Radiology and Physiotherapy Services, Blackpool, Fylde and Wyre Hospitals NHS Trust, Blackpool, Lancashire, UK

Preface

This new edition builds on the achievements of the previous editions in containing all current plain radiographic imaging techniques in a single volume. The companion volume 'Clark's Special Procedures in Diagnostic Imaging' contains details of imaging techniques by other modalities commonly available in a modern imaging department. Techniques that are no longer undertaken, or are associated with high radiation patient doses, have been removed or reference made to the best alternative modern technique.

This fully-revised 12th edition will ensure that the title retains its pre-eminence in the field, with hundreds of new positioning photographs and radiographic images. Specialist authors have been commissioned to contribute in their own fields, such as the Dental and Mammography chapters. New Paediatric and Forensic sections reflect the changing demands on a modern department. The book has also been expanded to include a Trauma section with reference to Advance Trauma Life Support. The Miscellaneous chapter includes trauma, foreign bodies, tomography, macroradiography, skeletal survey and soft tissue sections that have all been extensively revised, as well as a brand new forensic radiography section.

The authors have remained aware throughout that this edition is being published at a time when digital imaging is on the ascendancy, and have made reference to this. In the context of computed radiography the expression 'film' has been replaced by 'cassette' or 'image receptor' whilst recognizing that using direct digital radiography the term 'image receptor' should be exclusively used to reflect this developing situation. Equally it should be recognized that the words 'film' and 'image' are interchangeable in the context of viewing an acquired image by conventional film/screen technology. The Introduction chapter will allow the reader to understand basic digital imaging concepts, enabling them to undertake further study and learn how to adapt techniques to ensure that optimum image acquisition is made with the relevant imaging dose.

This edition also reflects the developing role of the radiographer/technologist with the introduction of 'Radiological Considerations' subheadings across all chapters, to give the reader a better understanding of image interpretation requirements and the clinical context in which imaging is undertaken. It recognizes the increasing role allied health professionals play in image interpretation, and the improved quality of imaging that results from radiographer/technologists having a clear understanding of the reason for any examination.

The layout is further refined by introducing other subheadings such as 'Essential Image Characteristics' and 'Common Faults and Remedies' to guide and assist the reader as to what to look for, as well as the general guide as to how to undertake each radiographic projection.

We hope that these changes will improve the usefulness of the book and its relevance to current radiographic practice, and provide a lasting tribute to the originator, Miss K.C. Clark.

Acknowledgements to the Twelfth Edition

We are indebted to the help and advice given by a vast range of colleagues throughout the radiological community with contributions enthusiastically given by radiographers, radiologists, physicists; lecturers from many learning institutions and colleagues in the imaging industry.

Particular thanks go to AGFA Health Care, Bracco and Siemens Medical Solutions for their financial support in sponsoring much of the artwork of the book.

We would particularly like to thank all of our partners and families who patiently endured the long process and for Mrs Sue Field at Blackpool Victoria Hospital for overseeing the text as it developed and for her valuable advice and support in updating many of the technical and clinical applications. We would like to thank Louise Tracy for her sterling secretarial and administration support and for many helpers with the Department at Blackpool Victoria Hospital who never lost patience in assisting with the location of images and helping with the photographic sessions. In particular, special thanks go to Sue Field for assisting with photography and to Gail Miller who helped on many occasions. Our thanks goes to Anne Marie Hodgkinson and Steven Farley of the Medical Illustration Department for their valuable contribution and helpful advice and to Vida Docherty at Anglia Polytechnic University who assisted with chapter preparation and to Professor David Manning who checked the content of Chapter 1 for scientific accuracy.

There were many models used, drawn mainly from Blackpool Victoria Hospital and St. Martins College Lancaster representing both members of staff and students alike. We would therefore like to thank: Amanda Spence, Simon Wilsdon, Mark Jackson and Ann Falcomer (née Holmes) who featured in many of the photographs and others including Nick Cantlay, Louise Perry, Denise Green, Gill Beavan, Nick Holt, Aidan McNicholl, Baby Joseph Legg, John Entwistle, Hayley Leadbetter, Nicola Thistlethwaite, Justine Bracewell, Leanne Chesters, Julie Mawson, Anita Sloane, Katherine Harvey, Fiona Zirmer, Rachel Cocker, Helen Pritchard, Caroline Stott and Chris Nicoll.

We are particularly indebted for advice and illustrations to the following: Alistair Mackenzie, KCARE; Andy Shaw, NWMP; Angela Meadows, Sue Field, Lesley Stanney, Dr Tom Kane, Mrs K Hughes, Mrs R Child, Mrs Sue Chandler, Miss Caroline Blower, Mr Nigel Kidner, Mr Sampath and Dr Vellore Govindarajan Chandrasekar and Sister Kathy Fraser, Blackpool Victoria Hospital; Dr JR Drummond, Dental School, University of Dundee; Sue Carter, Furness General Hospital, Barrow-in-Furness; Sheila Doyle, Clare Davies and staff, Alder Hey Hospital; Major John Beamer and Mark Viner of the Association of Forensic Radiographers St Bartholomew's & The Royal London Hospitals, London; Peter Hobson IGE; Clive West, Siemens; Keith Taylor, St Martin's College, Lancaster; Sue Simmons, Blackburn Royal Infirmary, Blackburn.

In updating the chest radiography section we wish to acknowledge the work undertaken by Elizabeth M Carver (née Unett) and Barry Carver, lecturers at the School of Radiography, University of Wales Bangor and that published in Synergy, November 2001. We have also incorporated recommendations referred to in the European guidelines on quality criteria for diagnostic radiographic images. EUR 16260-EN. Office for Official Publications of the European Communities. Luxembourg, June 1996.

Acknowledgements to previous editions

Miss K.C. Clark was Principal of the ILFORD Department of Radiography and Medical Photography at Tavistock House, from 1935 to 1958. She had an intense interest in the teaching and development of radiographic positioning and procedure, which resulted in an invitation by Ilford Limited to produce Positioning in Radiography.

Her enthusiasm in all matters pertaining to this subject was infectious. Ably assisted by her colleagues, she was responsible for many innovations in radiography, playing a notable part in the development of mass miniature radiography. Her ability and ever active endeavour to cement teamwork between radiologist and radiographer gained worldwide respect.

At the conclusion of her term of office as President of the Society of Radiographers in 1936 she was elected to Honorary Fellowship. In 1959 she was elected to Honorary Membership of the Faculty of Radiologists and Honorary Fellowship of the Australasian Institute of Radiography.

Miss Clark died in 1968 and the Kathleen Clark Memorial Library was established by the Society of Radiographers at their then premises in Upper Wimpole Street, London, as a tribute to her contribution to Radiography. Today the library is located in the library at the British Institute of Radiology, Portland Place, London.

The ninth edition was published in two volumes, edited and revised by James McInnes FSR, TE, FRPS, whose involvement with Positioning in Radiography began in 1946 when he joined Miss Clark's team at Tavistock House. He originated many techniques in radiography and in 1958 became Principal of Lecture and Technical Services at Tavistock House, which enabled him to travel as lecturer to the Radiographic Societies of Britain, Canada, America, South and West Africa.

The tenth edition, also published in two volumes, was revised and edited by Louis Kreel MD, FRCP, FRCR, a radiologist of international repute and wide experience of new imaging technologies.

The eleventh edition, totally devoted to plain radiographic imaging, was edited by Alan Swallow FCR, TE and Eric Naylor FCR, TE and assisted by Dr E J Roebuck MB, BS, DMRD, FRCR and Steward Whitley FCR, TDCR. Eric and Alan were both principals of Schools of Radiography and well respected in the radiography world and champions in developing and extending radiography education to a wide radiographer and radiological community.

We are indebted to these editors and the many radiographers and radiologists who contributed to previous editions for providing us with the foundations of the current edition and we hope that we have not failed to maintain their high standards.

Section 1

Basic Principles of Radiography and Digital Technology

CONTENTS

TERMINOLOGY	2
Anatomical terminology	2
Positioning terminology	3
Projection terminology	7
THE RADIOGRAPHIC IMAGE	12
Image formation	12
Projection and view	12
Density and contrast	13
Magnification and distortion	17
Image sharpness	18
Image acquisition and display	21
DIGITAL IMAGING	22
Introduction	22
Image acquisition	22
Factors affecting image quality	24
Networking	25
Image processing	26
Typical PACS components and workflow	27

EXPOSURE FACTORS	28
Milliampere seconds	28
Kilovoltage	28
Focus-to-film distance	29
Intensifying screens	30
Digital image capture	30
Secondary radiation grid	31
Choice of exposure factors	31
SUMMARY OF FACTORS CONTRIBUTING TO RADIOGRAPHIC IMAGE QUALITY	32
RADIATION PROTECTION	33
Dose quantities	33
Radiation risks	33
Medical exposure legislation	34
Practical protection measures	35

1 Terminology

The human body is a complicated structure, and errors in radiographic positioning or diagnosis can easily occur unless practitioners have a common set of rules that are used to describe the body and its movements.

This section describes terminology pertinent to radiography. It is vital that a good understanding of the terminology is attained to allow the reader to fully understand and practise the various techniques described in this text.

All the basic terminology descriptions below refer to the patient in the standard reference position, known as the anatomical position (see opposite).

Anatomical terminology

Patient aspect

- **Anterior aspect:** that seen when viewing the patient from the front.
- **Posterior (dorsal) aspect:** that seen when viewing the patient from the back.
- **Lateral aspect:** refers to any view of the patient from the side. The side of the head would therefore be the lateral aspect of the cranium.
- **Medial aspect:** refers to the side of a body part closest to the midline, e.g. the inner side of a limb is the medial aspect of that limb.

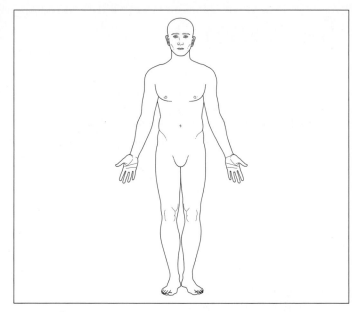

Anatomical position

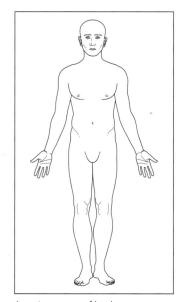

Anterior aspect of body

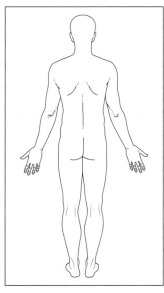

Posterior aspect of body

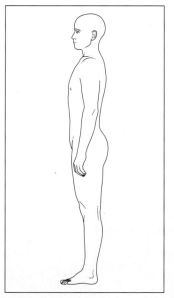

Lateral aspect of body

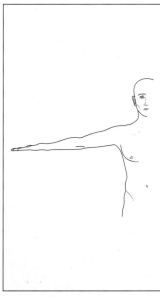

Medial aspect of arm

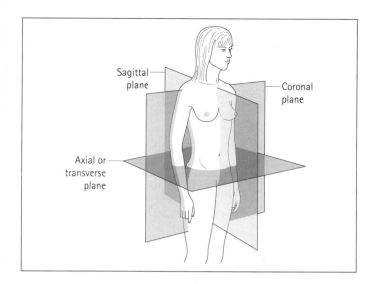

Sagittal plane

Coronal plane

Axial or transverse plane

Positioning terminology

Planes of the body

Three planes of the body are used extensively for descriptions of positioning both in plain-film imaging and in cross-sectional imaging techniques. The planes described are mutually at right-angles to each other:

- **Median sagittal plane:** divides the body into right and left halves. Any plane that is parallel to this but divides the body into unequal right and left portions is known simply as a sagittal plane or parasagittal plane.
- **Coronal plane:** divides the body into an anterior part and a posterior part.
- **Transverse or axial plane:** divides the body into a superior part and an inferior part.

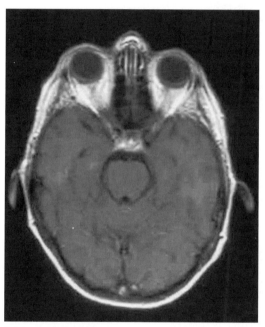

Axial or transverse plane

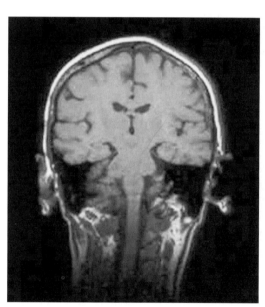

Coronal plane

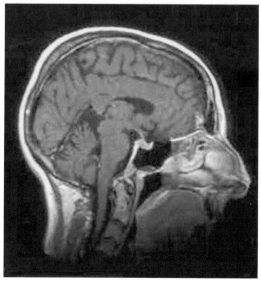

Sagittal plane

Positioning terminology (*contd*)

This section describes how the patient is positioned for the various radiographic projections described in this text:

Erect: the projection is taken with the patient sitting or standing. In the erect position, the patient may be standing or sitting:

- with the posterior aspect against the cassette; or
- with the anterior aspect against the cassette; or
- with the right or left side against the cassette.

Decubitus: the patient is lying down. In the decubitus position, the patient may be lying in any of the following positions:

- **Supine (dorsal decubitus):** lying on the back.
- **Prone (ventral decubitus):** lying face-down.
- **Lateral decubitus:** lying on the side. Right lateral decubitus – lying on the right side. Left lateral decubitus – lying on the left side.
- **Semi-recumbent:** reclining, part way between supine and sitting erect, with the posterior aspect of the trunk against the cassette.

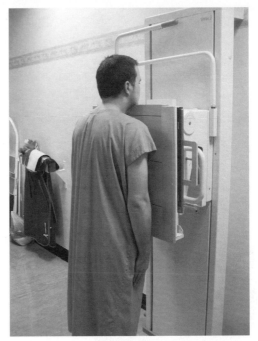

Erect: standing with the anterior aspect of the thorax against a vertical Bucky

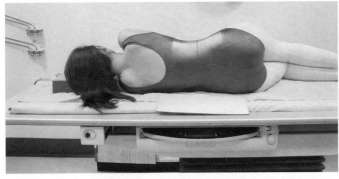

Left lateral decubitus: the median sagittal plane is parallel to the table and the coronal plane is perpendicular to the table

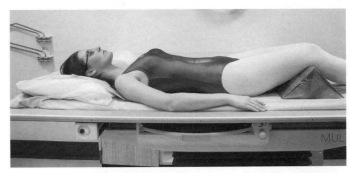

Supine: the median sagittal plane is at right-angles to the table and the coronal plane is parallel to the table

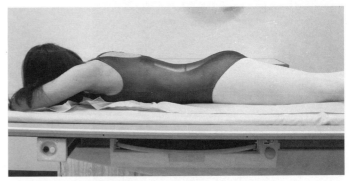

Prone: the median sagittal plane is at right-angles to the table and the coronal plane is parallel to the table

Positioning terminology

All the positions may be described more precisely by reference to the planes of the body. For example, 'the patient is supine with the median sagittal plane at right-angles to the tabletop' or 'the patient is erect with the left side in contact with the cassette and the coronal plane perpendicular to the cassette'.

When describing positioning for upper-limb projections, the patient will often be 'seated by the table'. The photograph below shows the correct position to be used for upper-limb radiography, with the coronal plane approximately perpendicular to the short axis of the tabletop. The patient's legs will not be under the table, therefore avoiding exposure of the gonads to any primary radiation not attenuated by the cassette or the table.

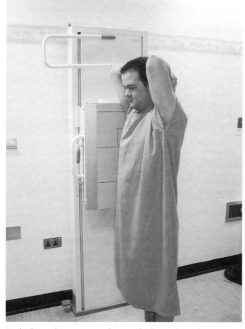

Right lateral erect: standing with the right side against a vertical Bucky

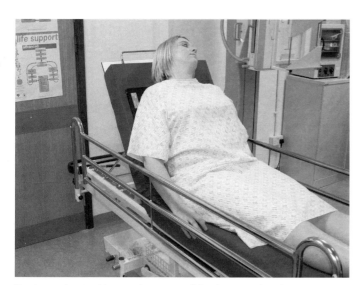

Semi-recumbent, with posterior aspect of the thorax against the cassette and median sagittal plane perpendicular to the cassette

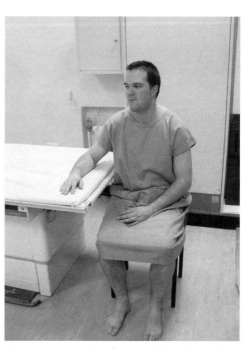

Correct patient position for upper-limb radiography with the patient seated

Positioning terminology (*contd*)

Terminology used to describe the limb position

Positioning for limb radiography may include:

- a description of the aspect of the limb in contact with the cassette;
- the direction of rotation of the limb in relation to the anatomical position, e.g. medial (internal) rotation towards the midline, or lateral (external) rotation away from the midline;
- the final angle to the cassette of a line joining two imaginary landmarks;
- the movements, and degree of movement, of the various joints concerned.

- **Extension:** when the angle of the joint increases.
- **Flexion:** when the angle of the joint decreases.
- **Abduction:** refers to a movement away from the midline.
- **Adduction:** refers to a movement towards the midline.
- **Rotation:** movement of the body part around its own axis, e.g. medial (internal) rotation towards the midline, or lateral (external) rotation away from the midline.
- **Pronation:** movement of the hand and forearm in which the palm is moved from facing anteriorly (as per anatomical position) to posteriorly. **Supination** is the reverse of this. Other movement terms applied to specific body parts are described in the diagrams.

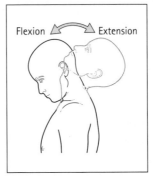

Flexion and extension of neck

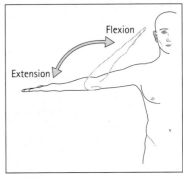

Flexion and extension of elbow

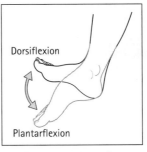

Dorsiflexion and plantarflexion of foot

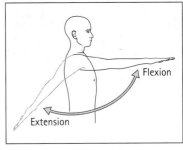

Flexion and extension of shoulder

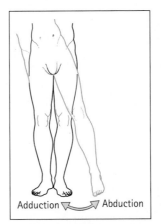

Abduction and adduction of hip

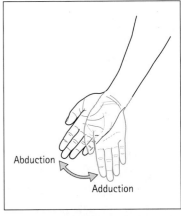

Abduction and adduction of wrist

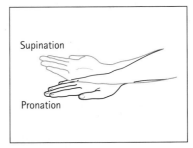

Pronation and supination of hand/forearm

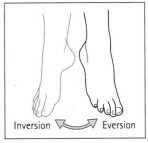

Inversion and eversion of foot

A **projection** is described by the direction of the central ray relative to aspects and planes of the body.

Antero-posterior

The central ray is incident on the anterior aspect, passes along or parallel to the median sagittal plane, and emerges from the posterior aspect of the body.

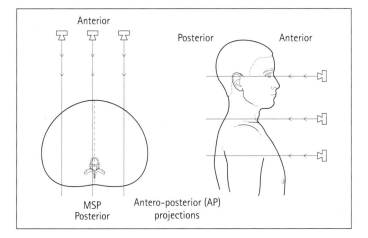

Antero-posterior (AP) projections

Postero-anterior

The central ray is incident on the posterior aspect, passes along or parallel to the median sagittal plane, and emerges from the anterior aspect of the body.

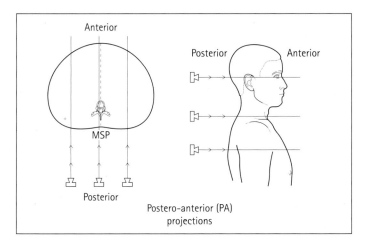

Postero-anterior (PA) projections

Lateral

The central ray passes from one side of the body to the other along a coronal and transverse plane. The projection is called a right lateral if the central ray enters the body on the left side and passes through to the image receptor positioned on the right side. A left lateral is achieved if the central ray enters the body on the right side and passes through to the image receptor, which will be positioned parallel to the median sagittal plane on the left side of the body.

In the case of a limb, the central ray either is incident on the lateral aspect and emerges from the medial aspect (lateromedial), or is incident on the medial aspect and emerges from the lateral aspect of the limb (medio-lateral). The terms 'lateromedial' and 'medio-lateral' are used where necessary to differentiate between the two projections.

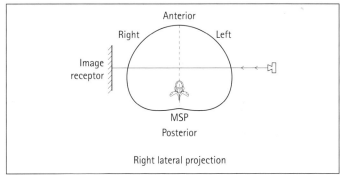

Right lateral projection

Beam angulation

Radiographic projections are often modified by directing the central ray at some angle to a transverse plane, i.e. either caudally (angled towards the feet) or cranially/cephalic angulation (angled towards the head). The projection is then described as, for example, a lateral 20-degree caudad or a lateral 15-degree cephalad.

Projection terminology (*contd*)

Oblique

The central ray passes through the body along a transverse plane at some angle between the median sagittal and coronal planes. For this projection, the patient is usually positioned with the median sagittal plane at some angle between zero and 90 degrees to the cassette, with the central ray at right-angles to the cassette. If the patient is positioned with the median sagittal plane at right-angles to or parallel to the cassette, then the projection is obtained by directing the central ray at some angle to the median sagittal plane.

Anterior oblique

The central ray enters the posterior aspect, passes along a transverse plane at some angle to the median sagittal plane, and emerges from the anterior aspect. The projection is also described by the side of the torso closest to the cassette. In the diagram below, the left side is closest to the cassette, and therefore the projection is a described as a left anterior oblique.

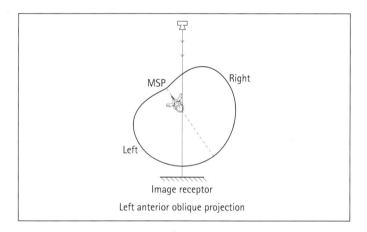

Left anterior oblique projection

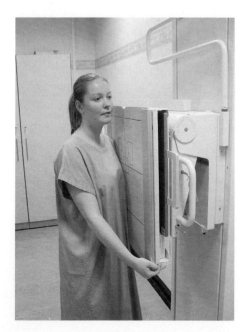

Posterior oblique

The central ray enters the anterior aspect, passes along a transverse plane at some angle to the median sagittal plane, and emerges from the posterior aspect. Again, the projection is described by the side of the torso closest to the cassette. The diagram below shows a left posterior oblique.

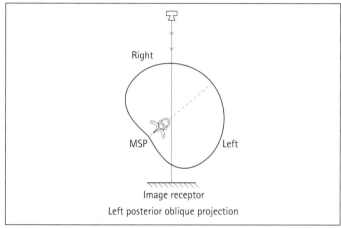

Left posterior oblique projection

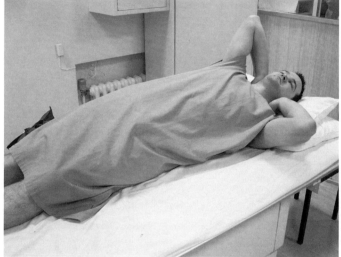

Oblique using beam angulation

When the median sagittal plane is at right-angles to the cassette, right and left anterior or posterior oblique projections may be obtained by angling the central ray to the median sagittal plane. (NB: this cannot be done if using a grid, unless the grid lines are parallel to the central ray.)

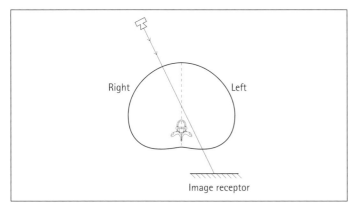

Example of left posterior oblique obtained using a beam angulation

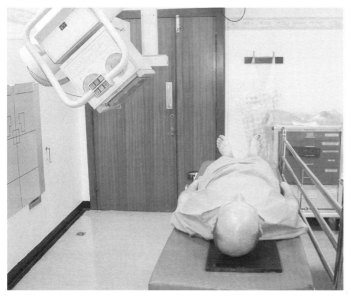

Example of the position for a right posterior oblique

Lateral oblique

The central ray enters one lateral aspect, passes along a transverse plane at an angle to the coronal plane, and emerges from the opposite lateral aspect.

With the coronal plane at right-angles to the cassette, lateral oblique projections can also be obtained by angling the central ray to the coronal plane. (NB: this cannot be done if using a grid, unless the grid lines are parallel to the central ray.)

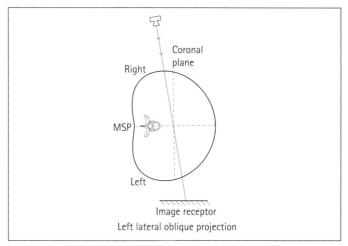

Example of lateral oblique obtained using a beam angulation

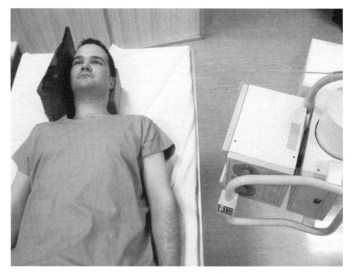

Example of the position for a right lateral oblique

Terminology

Projection terminology (*contd*)

The chapters that follow describe radiographic projections by reference to the following criteria:

- The position of the patient relative to the cassette.
- The direction and centring of the X-ray beam: this is given by reference to an imaginary central ray of the X-ray beam.
- Beam angulation relative to horizontal or vertical.

Examples of these are given below:

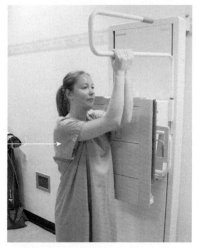

Projection: left lateral
Position: erect; left side against the cassette and median sagittal plane parallel to the cassette
Direction and centring of X-ray beam: the central ray is directed horizontally (at right-angles to the median sagittal plane) to a point 5 cm anterior to the spinous process of the seventh thoracic vertebra

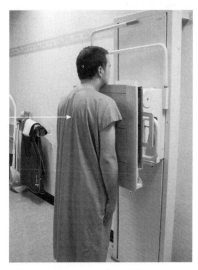

Projection: postero-anterior (PA)
Position: erect; anterior aspect facing the cassette and median sagittal plane at right-angles to the film
Direction and centring of X-ray beam: the central ray is directed horizontally (along the median sagittal plane) and centred to the spinous process of the sixth thoracic vertebra

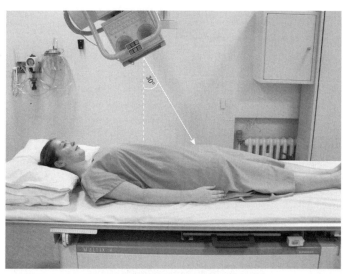

Projection: antero-posterior 30 degrees caudad
Position: supine; median sagittal plane at right-angles to the table
Direction and centring of X-ray beam: from the vertical, the central ray is angled 30 degrees caudally and directed to a point 2.5 cm superior to the symphysis pubis

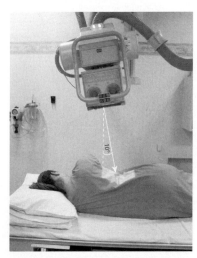

Projection: left lateral 10 degrees caudad
Position: left lateral decubitus; median sagittal plane parallel to the cassette
Direction and centring of X-ray beam: from the vertical, the central ray is angled 10 degrees caudally and directed (along a coronal plane) to a point in the mid-axillary line 7.5 cm anterior to the posterior aspect of the patient, at the level of the lower costal margin

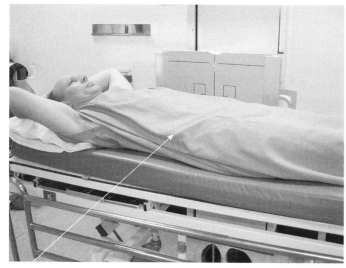

Projection: left lateral
Position: supine; median sagittal plane parallel to the cassette placed
in a vertical Bucky against the patient's left side
Direction and centring of X-ray beam: the horizontal central ray is directed
(at right-angles to the median sagittal plane) to the lower costal margin in
the mid-axillary line

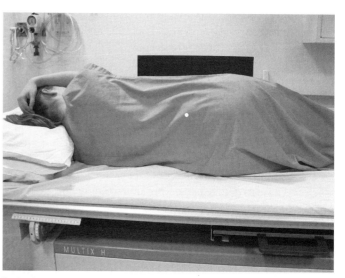

Projection: postero-anterior
Position: left lateral decubitus; median sagittal plane parallel to the
table and at right-angles to a cassette supported vertically against the
patient's anterior aspect
Direction and centring of X-ray beam: the horizontal central ray is at right-
angles to the posterior aspect of the patient in the midline (and passes along
the median sagittal plane) at the level of the third lumbar vertebra

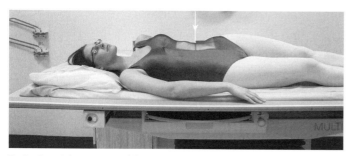

Projection: right posterior oblique
Position: supine and then rotated so that the left side is moved away from the
table to bring the median sagittal plane at 45 degrees to the table
Direction and centring of X-ray beam: the vertical central ray is
directed to a point 2.5 cm to the right of the midline at the level of the third
lumbar vertebra

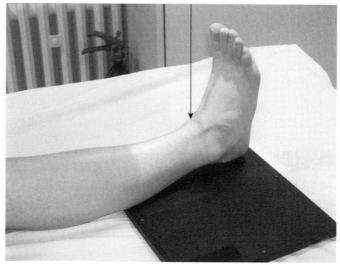

Projection: antero-posterior
Position: semi-recumbent or supine; leg extended fully; posterior
aspect of the ankle in contact with cassette; lateral and medial malleoli
equidistant from the cassette
Direction and centring of X-ray beam: vertical central ray directed
to a point midway between the malleoli

1 The radiographic image

Image formation

The X-rays used in medical diagnosis are produced from a small area within the X-ray tube when an exposure is made. They diverge outwards from this area, travel in straight lines, and can be detected by a variety of devices used for medical imaging.

As the X-rays pass through the body, some will be absorbed by the organs and structures within the body whilst others will pass through to the equipment used to form the image.

The term 'density' is often used in radiography. It can have different meanings depending on the context. In the diagram opposite, the X-ray beam enters the body and then encounters various structures. The bone has a high density because it has a relatively high mass per unit volume and consequently will absorb more X-rays than the adjacent area of lung. The lung contains air, which has a relatively low mass per unit volume and therefore can be said to have a low density. When the beam emerges from the body, there will be more X-rays directly under the area of lung compared with the area directly under the bone.

The image is then captured using an image-acquisition device. When a relatively large number of X-rays are incident upon the detector (e.g. the area under the lung), the image will appear to be quite dark and may be described as having a high image density. The area under the bone will appear lighter, since fewer X-rays will come into contact with the detector. This area therefore has a lower image density.

When examining an image for disease, the diagnostician may refer to a small focal area of disease as a density within the image. Rather confusingly, this could be of a higher or lower image density compared with the surrounding tissues, depending on the organ or tissue involved, e.g. a tumour in the lung (higher density) or bone (lower density, depending on tumour type).

In summary, the term 'density' can be used in the following ways:

- **Patient or physical density:** relates to the mass per unit volume of the structures within the patient and their absorption characteristics.
- **Image density:** the amount of signal detected in the image receptor or, put crudely, 'blackening' within the image. If measured on film using a densitometer, this will be **optical density**.
- **In diagnosis:** refers to a small defined area of pathology.

Projection and view

It is important to note that X-ray images are formed by projection, i.e. images of objects in the path of X-rays are projected on to a device for capturing the image, e.g. photographic material. This differs from the way in which images are formed on the retina of the eye or on the photographic film in a camera, where light travels from the object to the recording median to produce an image that is a **view** of the object; a radiographic image is a **projection** of the object.

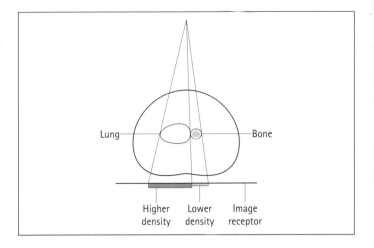

Lung — Bone

Higher density | Lower density | Image receptor

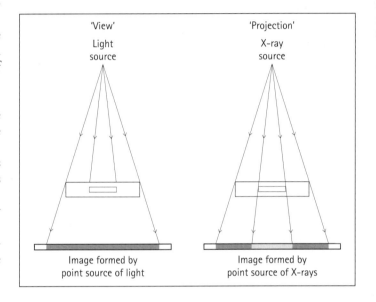

'View'
Light source

'Projection'
X-ray source

Image formed by point source of light

Image formed by point source of X-rays

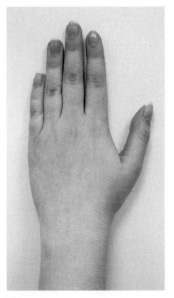

View

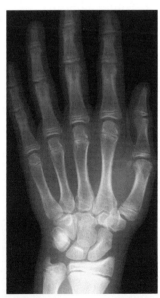

Projection

Density

The various uses of the term 'density' were discussed briefly in the previous section. When considering the radiographic image, the term 'density', as stated previously, can be defined crudely as the degree of 'blackening' within the image. The greater the amount of radiation that is incident upon the image detector, the greater will be the density within the image.

The general term 'density' can be defined more accurately when the type of image receptor is considered:

Photographic film

If the image is captured on a photographic emulsion, then the term 'photographic density' or 'optical density' should be used. Higher densities will be produced by greater exposures of radiation, which in turn leads to a form of silver being liberated from the photographic emulsion. This remains on the film after processing and produces the 'blackening' within the image. Photographic or optical density can be measured by determining the degree of opacity, i.e. the proportion of light absorbed by the processed film.

Radiograph produced on film, showing three different densities. The highest density is on the right of the image

Digital image capture

If the image was captured by a digital system such as computed radiography (CR) or direct radiography (DR), then the term 'image density' refers to the greyscale displayed on the monitor used to display the image. Put simply, it is the computer screen brightness.

The image-processing software will analyse the range of exposures that were captured by the image receptor (e.g. the CR phosphor screen). It will then assign the highest computer screen brightness to areas that have received relatively low exposures (low image density). Conversely, the lowest computer screen brightness (darkest areas) will be assigned to areas that have received a relatively high radiation exposure (high image density).

Contrast

In order to detect pathology, an imaging system must be able to detect the differences in the density (patient density) of the pathology compared with that of the surrounding tissues. This must then be translated into differences in density within the final image (image or film density) that are visible to the observer. **Contrast** is the difference in density between structures of interest within the image. A low-contrast image will show little difference in density between structures of interest, whereas a high-contrast image will show a larger difference in density between structures.

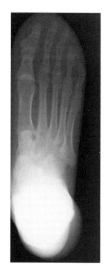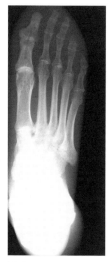

Lower contrast   Higher contrast

The contrast seen on a radiograph is built up in three main stages:

- **Subject contrast** is a feature of the object (subject) under examination. The differences in radiation intensities emerging from the object result from the spatial distribution of linear attenuation coefficients within the object. At a given beam energy, the degree of beam attenuation between anatomical structures is determined by the physical density and atomic number of those structures. Subject contrast will change if the beam energy (kVp) is varied or via the use of a contrast agent, which will change atomic number within an area of the object.
- **Radiographic contrast** is the difference in optical density on different parts of the processed film or differences in computer screen brightness recorded as a result of the range of emergent beam intensities.
- **Subjective contrast** is the personal appreciation of the differences in optical density or computer screen brightness when the image is viewed.

Some of the factors that influence each of the above will now be considered.

Density and contrast (*contd*)

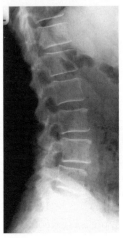

Subject contrast

X-Radiation passing through the body is attenuated by different amounts by the different thicknesses, densities and atomic numbers of the structures in the body. The beam emerging from the patient varies in intensity: more will emerge if the beam encounters only a small thickness of soft tissue. The difference in intensities in the emergent beam is called subject contrast or radiation contrast.

Radiograph showing the effect of high subject contrast between the bodies and spinous processes of the lumbar spine

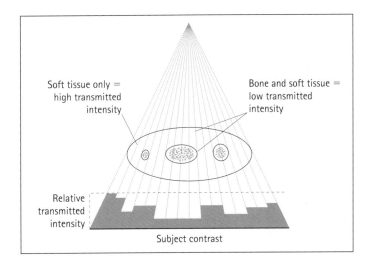

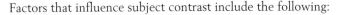

Subject contrast

Factors that influence subject contrast include the following:

- **The region of the body under examination:** there is less subject contrast if all parts of the region have a similar linear attenuation coefficient. Soft-tissue structures such as the breast have a low subject contrast, whereas the subject contrast increases if the region includes bone or large differences in the thickness of tissue. A good example of an area of the body that demonstrates high subject contrast is the body and spinous process of a lumbar vertebra on a lateral projection of the spine and the lateral cervicothoracic junction.
- **Contrast media:** if high- or low-density/atomic number substances are introduced into cavities in a region, then there will be a greater difference in absorption of X-rays by different parts of that region and thus an increase in subject contrast.
- **Pathology:** if the density of a structure is changed due to pathology, then there will be a change in subject contrast; for instance, it will be reduced if the bone density reduces, as in osteoporosis.

- **Kilovoltage:** at lower kilovoltage, there is a greater difference in attenuation by structures of different density and atomic number than at higher kilovoltage. Therefore, at lower kilovoltage, there is a greater subject contrast. This can be used to advantage when examining areas of low subject contrast, such as the breast. Conversely, there is a high subject contrast within the chest (marked differences in patient density when comparing the lungs and the heart). A higher kilovoltage will therefore reduce this subject contrast and produce a more even image density.

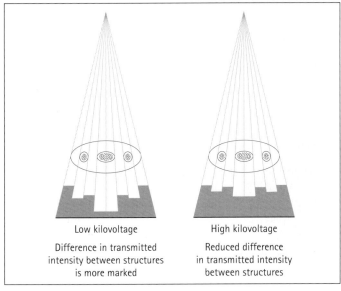

| Low kilovoltage | High kilovoltage |
| Difference in transmitted intensity between structures is more marked | Reduced difference in transmitted intensity between structures |

Low and high kilovoltage

Density and contrast

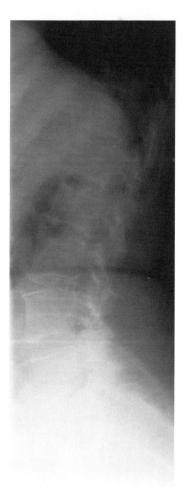

Low contrast due to osteoporosis

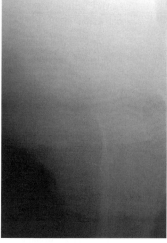

Low contrast due to poor collimation

Subjective contrast

When a radiograph is viewed, the observer sees an image made up of different densities or brightnesses. However, different observers might have a different appreciation of the image contrast. The personal appreciation of the contrast in the image is called **subjective contrast**. Subjective contrast depends not only on the person but also on the viewing conditions. For example, if an image is viewed on a computer monitor and that monitor is placed near a window, then the sunlight incident upon the screen will severely impair the observer's ability to appreciate the density differences within the image. There may be good radiographic contrast but the observer cannot appreciate this because of the sunlight on the screen, so the subjective contrast will be low.

Subjective contrast depends on:

- **the observer:** visual perception, fatigue, etc.;
- **viewing conditions:** e.g. ambient lighting.

Radiographic contrast

After leaving the patient, the X-radiation passes to an image-capture device. As it passes through the body, some of the radiation will be scattered. Scatter reduces the differences in X-ray intensity emerging from different areas of the body and thus reduces contrast. The production of scattered radiation can be reduced by collimating the beam or by the use of compression devices. In each of these cases, this reduces the volume of tissue irradiated. In a large proportion of examinations, a secondary radiation grid is placed between the patient and the image-capture device to intercept a large proportion of the scattered radiation, which, if it were to reach the image detector, would reduce image contrast. Once the image has been captured, it can be viewed either on photographic film or by some electronic means such as a computer monitor. The different patient densities are recorded either as varying photographic densities or as differences in computer screen brightness. These different densities can be measured either using a densitometer or image-analysis software to give an objective measurement of contrast. Thus, differences in measured image density between specified parts of the radiographic image are known as **radiographic** or **objective contrast**.

Density and contrast (*contd*)

Radiographic (objective contrast) depends upon the following:

- **Subject contrast.**
- **Scattered radiation reaching the image receptor:** the use of a secondary radiation grid between the patient and the cassette to reduce the scatter reaching image receptor improves radiographic contrast. Lead-backed cassettes or lead rubber under cassettes may reduce back-scatter, which may also improve radiographic contrast. If the cassette is some distance away from the patient, then scatter crossing the intervening gap might not reach the image receptor.
- **Image-acquisition device:** the design and function of the device used to acquire the image can have a profound effect on contrast. For example, certain types of film emulsion, intensifying screen and phosphor plate may be designed to give inherently greater contrast. In digital systems, the contrast is also influenced profoundly by the software used to process the initial image captured by the device.
- **Film fog:** if the image is viewed using a photographic-based system, then film fogging due to incorrect film handling or storage may reduce radiographic contrast.
- **Exposure:** if too much or too little radiation is used, then the image-acquisition device may be unable to respond or may be saturated to the point that it is unable to function properly. In these examples, there may be a reduced range of densities or no difference in density visible on the image, thus radiographic contrast will be reduced or non-existent.
- **Development:** if a photographic emulsion is used to capture the image, then optimum radiographic contrast can be attained only if the film is developed to the correct film contrast. This is achieved by careful control of factors such as developer temperature, development time and processing chemical activity. To ensure this, the film processor must be subject to a rigid quality-control regime.

Subjective contrast depends upon the following:

- **Radiographic contrast.**
- **The observer:** poor eyesight, fatigue.
- **Viewing box:** brightness, evenness and colour of illumination.
- **Computer monitor:** many factors related to the quality of construction and design of the monitor will influence the contrast visible to the observer.
- **Ambient lighting:** if the room lighting is low and there is a reduction in extraneous light reaching the eye, then subjective contrast will improve. Radiographs are often viewed under poor conditions in hospital, especially in the ward environment. Radiographers have an important role in educating all hospital staff as to the benefits of viewing radiographs under proper lighting conditions.

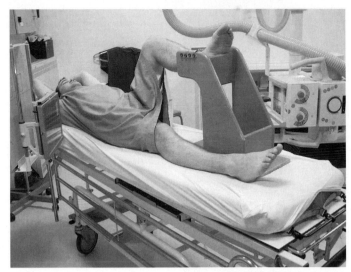

Scatter reduction in lateral hip radiography using an air-gap technique and a secondary radiation grid

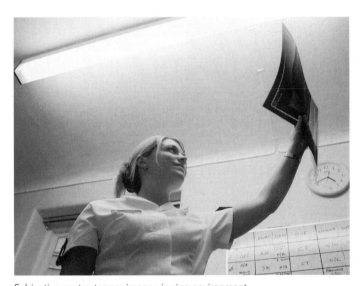

Subjective contrast: poor image-viewing environment

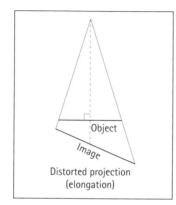

Magnification and distortion

Magnification

In a projected image, magnification will always be present because the X-rays continue to diverge as they pass from the object to the image-acquisition device (henceforth referred to as a film for simplicity). The source of the X-rays is the X-ray tube focal spot. For a given focus-to-film distance (FFD), the greater the distance between the object and the film, the greater will be the magnification of the image. To minimize magnification, the object under examination should be positioned as close to the film as is reasonable to do so.

$$\text{Magnification} = \frac{\text{image size}}{\text{object size}} = \frac{\text{FFD}}{\text{FOD}}$$

where FOD is the focus-to-object distance.

If the object-to-film distance has to be increased, e.g. in the case of a patient on a trolley, then the FFD can also be increased. This will then reduce the magnification caused by the above. (NB: an increase in exposure will be needed in this case due to the effect of the inverse square law on the beam intensity).

Image distortion

A distorted image will be produced if not all parts of the image are magnified by the same amount. Considering a thin, flat object, there will be constant magnification and thus no distortion when the film is parallel to the object. When possible, the part being radiographed should be placed parallel to the film to avoid distortion. If the object and film are not parallel to each other, then there is a difference in magnification of different parts of the object, leading to a distorted image.

In the diagrams opposite, the object and film are not parallel to each other. It can be seen that if the centre of the X-ray beam is directed at right-angles to the object but the object is not parallel to the image receptor, then a distorted, elongated image is produced. If the centre of the beam is directed at right-angles to the image receptor but is angled in relation to the object, then a distorted, foreshortened image will be produced.

In cases when the object and film cannot be parallel to each other, a compromise can be made by directing the central ray at right-angles to an imaginary line bisecting the angle between the object and the film. Although distortion does occur, the net effect is neither elongation nor foreshortening of the image. This technique may be required if a patient is unable to straighten a limb to bring it parallel to the film when imaging a long bone.

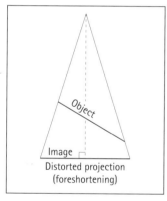

Undistorted image

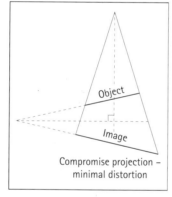

Distortion: elongation

Distortion: foreshortening

Compromise projection: minimal distortion

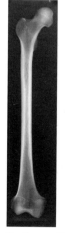

Undistorted long bone

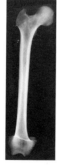

Foreshortened long bone

1 The radiographic image

Image sharpness

In radiography, the aim is to produce an image that is as sharp as possible in order to resolve fine detail within the image. This is particularly important when looking for subtle fractures or changes in bone architecture.

Unfortunately, there are several factors that lead to image unsharpness. These are unsharpness due to:

- geometry (Ug);
- movement (Um);
- absorption (inherent factors) (Ua);
- photographic/acquisition factors (Up).

Geometric unsharpness

If X-rays originated from a point source, then a perfectly sharp image would always be obtained. In an X-ray tube, however, the X-rays are produced from the small area of the focal spot on the anode. As can be seen from the diagram opposite, this leads to the formation of penumbra or 'partial shadows' at the edge of the object; it is this that gives rise to geometric unsharpness.

The degree of geometric unsharpness increases with an increased focal spot size and increased object-to-film distance:

$$\text{Geometric unsharpness (Ug)} = \frac{\text{object-to-film distance}}{\text{object-to-focus distance}}$$
$$\times \text{ focal spot size.}$$

Geometric unsharpness can be a small, insignificant quantity if the object is close to the film and a small focal spot is used. For instance, with a postero-anterior projection of the wrist, where the maximum object film distance is about 5 cm, and if a normal FFD of 100 cm is used, then geometric unsharpness is only 0.05 mm using a 1-mm focal spot and only 0.1 mm with a 2-mm focal spot. When thicker parts of the body are being examined, which might require the use of a larger (broad) focal spot, then geometric unsharpness can make a significant contribution to total image unsharpness owing to the greater object-to-film distance.

Movement unsharpness

This type of unsharpness is due to patient, equipment or film movement during the exposure. Patient movement may be involuntary, e.g. owing to heartbeat or peristalsis, or it may the type of movement that may be controlled by immobilization. It is important to note that any patient movement is magnified on the image because of the space between the moving object and the film. Sharpness can be increased by using a shorter exposure time (achieved by a lower mAs with higher kVp, higher mA, or greater tube loading), by a small object-to-film distance and particularly by immobilization.

Various accessories can be used for immobilization, including non-opaque pads and sandbags to immobilize the extremities.

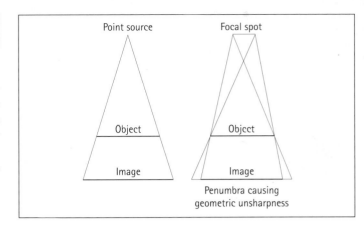

Penumbra causing geometric unsharpness

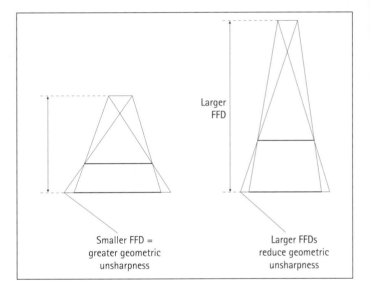

Smaller FFD = greater geometric unsharpness

Larger FFDs reduce geometric unsharpness

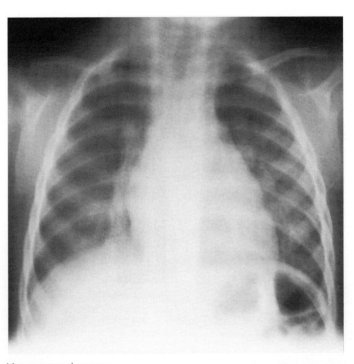

Movement unsharpness

Image sharpness

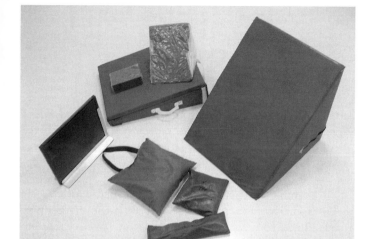

Immobilization devices

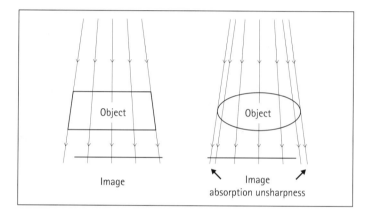

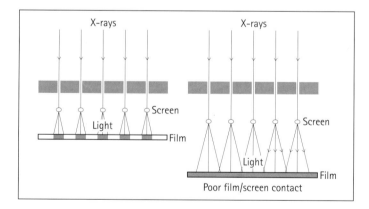

Poor film/screen contact

Binders and Velcro straps may be used for the trunk and head. These accessories should be available in all examination rooms and should be used routinely. It is equally important to make the patient as comfortable as possible and to explain the procedure fully. The radiographer can also invite questions about the procedure, thus increasing the likelihood of achieving full cooperation from the patient. It may be worthwhile rehearsing respiratory manoeuvres prior to an actual exposure being made.

Absorption unsharpness

This is due to the shape of the structures in the body. As illustrated, unless the structure has a particular shape, with its edges parallel to the diverging beam, then absorption of the X-ray beam will vary across the object. Considering a spherical object of uniform density, then absorption will be greatest at the centre and least at the periphery due to the difference in thickness. This gradual fall-off in absorption towards the edges leads to the image having an ill-defined boundary called absorption unsharpness, particularly as most structures in the body have a round edge. Little can be done to reduce this type of unsharpness, apart from increasing image contrast or using digital edge-enhancement techniques.

Photographic unsharpness

An X-ray image could be formed by the direct action of X-rays on a photographic emulsion, but more usually the X-ray image is first converted into a light image by intensifying screens. This increases the photographic effect of the X-rays and thus allows exposure to be greatly reduced. The intensifying screens contain crystals that fluoresce when irradiated by X-rays. Photographic unsharpness is the spread of light between the crystals and the photographic emulsion. The spread of light will be greater with larger crystals (regular or fast screens) and will also be greater with increasing distance between the crystal and the film (poor film/screen contact). Duplitized film with the emulsion on both sides of the film base is commonly used to decrease the exposure given to the patient, but the unsharpness will be greater than if a single-sided emulsion is employed. This is caused by the image on one side of the emulsion crossing over to the other side. As it does so, the light diverges and produces an image slightly larger than the image on the opposite side. Another possible cause of unsharpness in duplitized films occurs when the final image is viewed. If the observer is in such a position that the images on each side of the emulsion are not exactly superimposed, this introduces further unsharpness known as parallax.

Photographic unsharpness is reduced by ensuring that all cassettes maintain good film/screen contact and by using fine-grained screens or single-sided emulsions when appropriate. The least photographic unsharpness occurs when intensifying screens are not used, but this is unjustifiable for the majority of radiographic examinations.

Image sharpness (*contd*)

Complex formulae have been given to calculate the total unsharpness due to several contributory factors. These show that if any one type of unsharpness is much greater than the others, then only by reducing that type will any significant improvement be made in image sharpness. For example, when dealing with a restless patient, the greatest source of unsharpness will be the patient movement, and image sharpness will not be improved visibly by reducing other sources of unsharpness.

A summary of the methods used to reduce different types of unsharpness is shown in the table below.

Unfortunately, the factors in group A are interrelated, and attempts to reduce one form of unsharpness will tend to increase another. For example, if one chooses to use fine-grained screens to reduce photographic unsharpness, then an increase in mAs may be required, which could lead to a longer exposure time, thus increasing the possibility of movement unsharpness. This increase in mAs may in turn require an increase in focal spot size due to the additional thermal stresses on the anode, and there will be an increase in geometric unsharpness as a consequence of this. Choice of factors in group A is part of the radiographer's skill. If movement unsharpness will be a predominant factor, e.g. with a restless patient, then it must be reduced, perhaps by using a higher tube loading on the broad focus or by the use of the faster intensifying screen to reduce exposure time. In the former situation the geometric unsharpness will increase, and in the latter situation photographic unsharpness will increase. If the patient can be fully immobilized, then the above strategies may not have to be used and an image with a greater degree of sharpness will be obtained.

If we examine the factors in group B, we find that reducing any type of unsharpness with these does not cause another type of unsharpness to increase. For example, by having good/film screen contact, then neither movement nor geometrical unsharpness is increased. There is no increase in geometrical unsharpness or photographic unsharpness if the patient is immobilized.

To obtain the sharpest image possible, we must make a judgement about the factors in group A. We have to decide whether we will use the broad or fine focus, fine-grain or regular/fast screens. But there are no decisions to make about the factors in the group B. We should always strive to position the part under examination as near as possible to the cassette, to immobilize the patient in as comfortable position as possible, and to give the patient clear instructions and check their understanding of these instructions. All film cassettes should be maintained to ensure good film/screen contact, and other imaging equipment should be maintained regularly.

	Geometric	Movement	Photographic
A	Use fine focus, standardized (large) FFD	Use short exposure time with high tube loading	Use fine-grained screens, single-sided emulsion or non-screen film (if appropriate)
B	Use small OFD, avoid equipment vibration	Use small OFD; immobilization; make patient comfortable; give clear instructions to patient about keeping still; if necessary, rehearse the patient; eliminate equipment vibration	Ensure all cassettes maintain good film/screen contact

FFD, focus-to-film distance; OFD, object-to-film distance.

Image acquisition and display

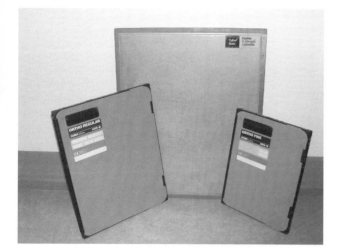

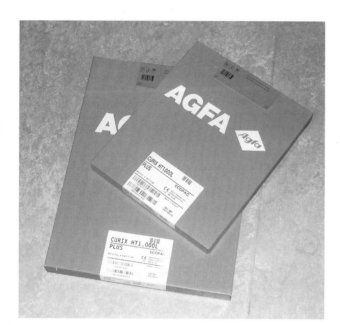

Images can be acquired in several different ways depending on the equipment used by any particular imaging department. These are:

- conventional film/screen technology;
- fluoroscopy/fluorography;
- digital imaging:
  - computed radiography (CR);
  - direct digital radiography (DDR).

Each of the above will be considered briefly.

Conventional film/screen technology

At the time of writing, this is the cheapest and most versatile method of image capture. Photographic film is capable of storing an image alone, but the exposure required can be reduced considerably if the film is placed between intensifying screens that convert the X-ray energy into light, which in turn exposes the film. The film and cassettes are widely available in a variety of sizes and can be used with almost any piece of imaging equipment.

An image captured on photographic film will have high resolution, although it has narrower exposure latitude compared with other image-capture systems. This means that the radiographer has much less margin for error when selecting exposure factors before making an exposure. It is relatively easy to overexpose or underexpose an image compared with other image-acquisition devices.

A variety of systems are available in which the screen and film can be varied to suit a particular task. Thus, the speed and resolution can be changed in any given clinical situation by selecting a different film and screen. Graduated or asymmetric systems have been used to enhance spine and chest radiography, where the subject contrast is high.

X-ray film is highly portable, although a considerable amount of space is required to store the film bags.

A series of X-ray film processors are required in a department using conventional imaging technology. These must be regularly cleaned, serviced and subjected to a rigorous quality-control programme in order to ensure consistency of performance.

Fluoroscopy/fluorography

This method of image acquisition employs an image intensifier to capture images, which are then displayed in real time or as static images on a monitor. Fluoroscopy is very useful for following the progress of contrast agent around the body, but its resolution is poor compared with that of other image-acquisition methods so it is not currently used for plain radiographic imaging. Fluorography employs photographic film to capture the image from the image intensifier. This method has now been largely superseded by digital image-capture methods.

1 Digital imaging

Introduction

Film/screen imaging in radiography is gradually being replaced by digital imaging. There are many advantages to digital imaging; the workflow should be faster, and it allows image processing to optimize the clinical information from an image.

Advantages of digital systems

Digital imaging exhibits a number of advantages when compared with conventional film/screen imaging:

- increased latitude and dynamic range;
- acquisition and display are separate processes;
- images can be accessed simultaneously at any workstation;
- viewing stations can be set up in any location;
- ability to use digital image archives rather than film libraries;
- images will generally be quicker to retrieve and less likely to be lost;
- ability to post-process images to aid visualization of anatomy and pathology;
- availability of soft-copy reporting;
- no manual handling of cassettes for direct digital radiography (DDR) systems;
- potential patient dose reduction;
- potential lower running costs, providing only soft-copy reporting is used;
- no handling of processing chemicals.

Uses

CR is used in all areas where film/screen systems are currently used, including mammography. DDR can be used in general radiography and mobile radiography. DDR is very popular in small-field mammography and is being introduced into full-field mammography. DDR detectors are now being used instead of image intensifiers in fluoroscopy.

Image acquisition

Technology overview

There are a number of technologies used for digital imaging in planar radiography. They can be divided into CR and DDR.

CR is, in first appearance, similar to the use of a film/screen system. The CR plate is in a cassette, which will fit the table and vertical Bucky trays and can be used with mobile equipment. The plate is then scanned in a reading system similar in size to a daylight processor. This therefore makes the change to digital radiography easier.

A DDR system entails more changes in X-ray couch and vertical Bucky design and often changes to the X-ray tube assembly. Unlike the removable CR cassette, the DR plate or detector is fully integrated into the exposure equipment. The patient is radiographed and the image appears on the acquisition workstation in a few seconds. Here, the image can be optimized and then sent for reporting or repeated if necessary.

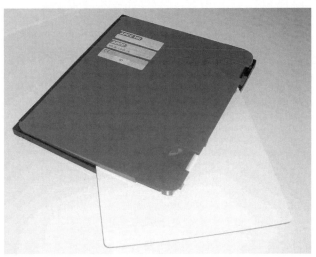

An example of a computed radiography plate and cassette

Computed radiography technology

The active phosphor layer of a CR plate usually comprises a layer of europium-doped barium fluorobromide, which is coated on to a semi-rigid or flexible polyester base. X-ray photons are absorbed by the phosphor layer, and the phosphor electrons become 'excited' and are raised to a higher energy level, where they can stay trapped in a semi-stable higher-energy state. The trapped electrons represent a latent image in the phosphor plate in the form of 'stored energy'. The stored energy can be released by adding energy to the trapped electrons. This is done by stimulation with a laser beam. The trapped electrons then 'escape' from the traps to fall back to their equilibrium state. As they fall back, the electrons release energy in the form of light. This phenomenon is otherwise known as photostimulable luminescence (PSL). The emitted light intensity is proportional to the original X-ray intensity. The light energy is detected and the signal is digitized. These data are processed digitally to produce a visible diagnostic image on a monitor. The phosphor plate is then 'erased' with a bright white light to remove any remaining trapped electrons, and the plate is then ready for the next examination.

Digital radiography technologies

The main detector technologies used in digital radiography are:

- X-ray scintillator bonded to a read-out array (amorphous silicon photodiode/thin-film transistor (TFT) array) or coupled to a charge-coupled device (CCD);
- X-ray detector of amorphous selenium bonded to a TFT read-out array.

Both types can be constructed in the form of a flat panel.

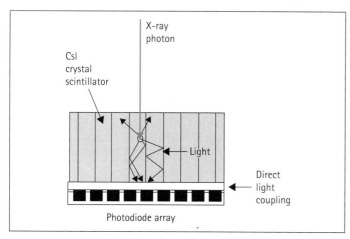

Schematic diagram of flat-panel detector with a scintillator and an amorphous silicon photodiode thin-film transistor array

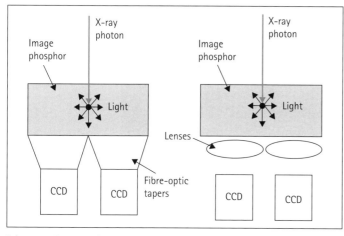

Schematic diagrams showing a charge-coupled device coupled to a phosphor scintillator by lenses and fibre-optics

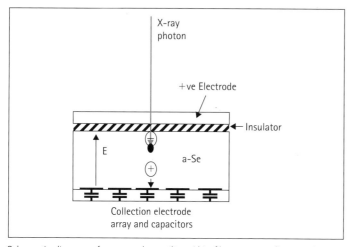

Schematic diagram of an amorphous silicon/thin-film transistor flat-panel detector

Scintillator detector

The X-ray detector is normally a scintillator of thallium-doped CsI(Tl) crystals, although other phosphors such as Gd_2O_2S are also used. The scintillator converts the X-rays into a light output. The CsI has a columnar crystal structure that guides the light to the read-out device, which allows the CsI to be thicker than a phosphor powder without significantly increasing unsharpness. As with phosphors in film cassettes, thinner powder phosphors (such as Gd_2O_2S) will have lower unsharpness. Gd_2O_2S phosphors are thinner than CsI scintillators, but they have higher conversion efficiency.

Scintillators are usually coupled directly to an amorphous silicon photodiode TFT flat-panel read-out array. The light from the scintillator is converted into electrical charge in a photodiode array, which stores the charge until it is read out from each of the pixels. These are commonly referred to as amorphous silicon systems.

Charge-coupled device

The light output from the scintillator detector can be read out by a CCD camera. The CCD is generally smaller than the phosphor, and so it is usually coupled using a lens or fibre-optic bundles. Demagnification may be necessary, and this can result in a loss of sensitivity if the demagnification is high.

Amorphous selenium/thin-film transistor flat-panel detector

The detector consists of a layer of amorphous selenium with a matrix of electrodes on each face. The X-ray energy produces electron-hole pairs in the selenium layer, which are attracted towards the electrodes by an electric field. The charge is collected and read out using a TFT array. The resolution of this type of detector is better than that using a phosphor due to the absence of light scattering.

Scanning technology

An alternative detection method for covering the full image area is to use slot-scanning technology. A linear array of detectors scans across the patient in conjunction with a narrow-fan X-ray beam. This method may result in good scatter rejection and contrast differentiation, but it has a number of disadvantages, including a long exposure time and high tube loading. Also, the alignment of the scanning radiation beam and the detectors requires tight mechanical tolerances and mechanical stability of the scanning mechanism.

1 Digital imaging

Factors affecting image quality

There are a number of factors, both inherent in equipment design and external, that affect image quality. The following are important examples:

Fill factor

For flat-panel detectors, a proportion of the detector contains the read-out circuitry and will be insensitive to the incoming light photons or electrons. This leads to the concept of the fill factor (see equation below), which is the ratio of the sensitive area of the pixel to the effective area of the detector element itself.

Any improvements in resolution will require a reduced pixel pitch. The fill factor will decrease with improved resolution, as the read-out electronics will take up a larger proportion of the detector element and decrease the detector sensitivity.

$$\text{Fill factor} = \frac{\text{area}_{\text{sensitive}}}{\text{area}_{\text{pixel}}}$$

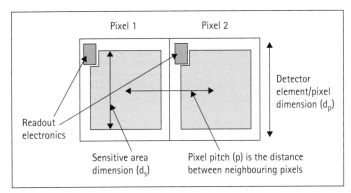

Diagram of fill factor

Tiling

A tiled array consists of a number of detectors abutted together to sample the whole image. However, there may be small areas on read-out devices that are not sensitive; these are caused by gaps between the detectors (typically about $100\,\mu\text{m}$). There may be some image processing to compensate for this, although this may give some stitching artefacts.

Grids

Low grid strip densities can cause interference patterns in the image called Moiré patterns. This can be solved by using moving grids or high-density grids of over 60 lines/cm. When using CR, ideally the grid lines should also be perpendicular to the scan lines in the reader.

Radiation exposure (image optimization)

Image quality is related to the radiation exposure received by the detector. Although a relatively low exposure will result in a noisy image, it may still contain sufficient information to be diagnostically acceptable. A high exposure will result in improved image quality, since quantum noise is reduced. However, image-quality improvement is not linear: it will eventually level off as the quantum noise becomes less dominant and decrease as the plate becomes overexposed. Ideally, a system should be set up to obtain adequate image quality for the lowest possible dose (optimization).

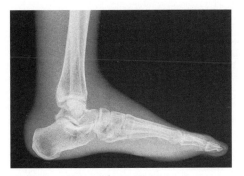

Underexposed lateral foot image

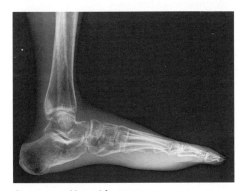

Overexposed lateral foot image

Automatic exposure control response

An automatic exposure control (AEC) for a film/screen system is set up by ensuring that the correct optical density is achieved across a range of kilovoltages. This method is not practical for digital imaging, as the image will be displayed according to pre-set parameters, irrespective of the exposure used. The AEC will need to be set up in collaboration with the radiology and medical physics departments and the supplier. The level of exposure must be optimized for the selected examination and the receptor dose measured.

One other consideration is that sometimes when film/screen systems are replaced by a CR system, then for simplicity the AEC is kept at the same settings. This may not be the optimal working level, because the sensitivity and energy response of the digital system are different from those of the film/screen system it replaces. A DDR system can use the detector itself as an AEC, although currently most use a conventional AEC chamber system.

Bit depth/image size

A pixel is the smallest element of a digitized picture. A smaller pixel size will generally give an improved spatial resolution in the image. The pixel pitch is the distance between the centres of adjacent pixels.

The matrix size is the number of pixels or memory locations into which the image is divided. Thus, the total number of pixels in a 1024×1024 matrix is $1\,048\,576$, defined as one megapixel.

The bit depth of the image determines the contrast resolution. The analogue value of the output from each pixel is converted to digital form, and the results are stored at a separate location in a matrix. The number of grey levels available equals two to the power of the number of bits, e.g. $2^8 = 256$.

Number of grey levels per bit depth

Number of bits	Grey levels
1	2
2	4
4	16
8	256
10	1024
12	4096

Clinical images require good contrast resolution, which is difficult to achieve due to the noise inherent in a radiographic image. In order to achieve good contrast resolution, high bit depths are required. The number of bits required depends on the noise level: the lower the level of noise, the higher the number of bits that can be used.

Networking

So far, the digital-acquisition technology has been discussed. However, the great advantage of digital imaging is to be able to integrate it into a health community-wide system. Linking the digital X-ray into the hospital information system (HIS) and radiology information system (RIS) and storing the images on a Picture Archive and Communications Systems (PACS) system enables images to be reviewed at various reporting rooms, consultants' offices, wards, etc. Images can also be reported off site using teleradiology (see p. 27 for summary of components and workflow).

Hospital information systems and radiology information systems

HIS and RIS contain patient details and examination information. If the digital acquisition system and PACS is connected to a HIS/RIS, then the workflow of a department can be increased by using the RIS data to control workflow, thereby delivering improved patient throughput. For instance, by automatically attaching patient demographic and examination details from the RIS to the image, images can be delivered to the correct destination much faster. Reporting, storage and retrieval can also be made more efficient. HIS/RIS systems typically use the Health Level 7 (HL7) standard to transfer patient details.

Digital Imaging and Communications in Medicine (DICOM)

Digital Imaging and Communications in Medicine (DICOM) Version 3.0 is a protocol-based standard to facilitate the transfer of digital images and associated information between devices manufactured by a range of vendors and to aid in the development of PACS.

When purchasing a system, a DICOM conformance statement should be received, which will inform how the device and software conform to the standard for its particular function. If a modality does not produce images in DICOM format and it cannot be upgraded to DICOM, then a DICOM secondary capture device will be needed to convert the image to a DICOM-conformant image (secondary capture only) and allow the system to be connected to the PACS.

Picture Archive and Communications System

PACS is an image-management and communication system. It stores and distributes images and information around the system. It is connected to each of the digital acquisition systems and other modalities in order that images and information can be transmitted to their appropriate destinations. Patient data from the HIS/RIS system are used to correctly route and retrieve images, and printers are used to produce hard copy if needed.

A PACS can range from so-called 'mini-PACS' systems serving just one or two imaging modalities with perhaps only one reporting workstation to enterprise-wide PACS handling all image data with multiple reporting and speciality workstations and image distribution to all necessary locations throughout the hospital and beyond. There are many PACS models; a simple schematic diagram for a typical radiology department is shown on the next page.

Images will be viewed at various points in the system. The extent to which these images can be manipulated will depend on the type and function of the equipment. Typical viewing components include:

- acquisition, reporting and viewing workstations;
- monitors;
- laser printers.

Acquisition and reporting workstations

The acquisition workstation is where the data are initially received and pre-processing will be undertaken. This is true for some manufacturers, but with others this happens within the CR reader. Ideally, if the CR system has been calibrated and operated correctly, the image that appears should not require further processing.

Reporting workstations can be a component of the PACS or can be dedicated to a digital unit. In either case, these will be high-specification workstations with a comprehensive range of post-processing facilities.

Networking (*contd*)

Monitors

At the time of writing, the maximum light out of a video monitor is limited, so that it is advisable to specify the ambient light when measuring performance. In order to perceive two adjacent areas as black and white respectively, it is necessary for the areas to have a difference in brightness of the order of 30 : 1.

The blackest area in the picture should have a brightness that is approximately the same as the light reflected back to the observer from the unilluminated cathode ray tube (CRT) face. This will depend on the ambient light level, the colour of the phosphor, and the filtration of the glass.

The ambient light level can be measured by standing in the normal viewing position and pointing a spot photometer at the centre of the CRT screen with the monitor turned off. The reading should fall between 1 and 10 Cd/m^2. The idea value would be 3.3 Cd/m^2, but it would be difficult to adjust the ambient light level with this degree of accuracy.

The limiting resolution of the monitor is dependent upon the CRT cathode current and, therefore, brightness. As a rough guide, a good-quality monitor should be capable of generating a high-quality image when the maximum large area brightness is about 100 Cd/m^2.

Laser printers

The image can be printed on a laser printer for remote departments. However, to get the full benefits of a digital system, images should be reported on soft copy. It should be noted that laser film is more expensive than standard radiography film.

Image processing

Ideally, the acquisition workstation should enable the following:

- addition of anatomical markers;
- demographics correction;
- image annotation;
- window and level adjustment;
- electronic collimation;
- magnification;
- application of different look-up tables (LUTs).

The reporting workstation will be a high-specification workstation with a comprehensive range of post-processing facilities, which include most of those listed previously (not addition of markers and LUTs), plus other functions, including:

- edge enhancement;
- noise reduction;
- tools for measuring pixel values, distances and angles;
- zoom and roam.

Look-up table

An LUT converts each pixel value into a new value. An LUT has two main uses:

- A digital detector generally has a much wider dynamic range than the range of intensities in a clinical image, and therefore an LUT is used to compress the data to cover only the clinically useful data.
- An LUT may be a curved rather than a linear relationship to enhance the contrast in the clinically useful densities. There may be a range of curves suitable for different clinical examinations.

The graph below shows an example LUT compressing a 12-bit image to a 10-bit image and applying a characteristic curve.

Compression

Compression of the image dataset is achieved using a processing algorithm. Compression of images is useful because the smaller an image, the more that can be stored for a given archive and the faster the transmission. Compression can either be lossless or lossy. Reconstruction of the image from a lossless compression will be the same as the original image, while a lossy image will have some changes. Some systems, although lossy, will claim to be 'visually lossless', i.e. there is no perceptible difference between the original and the reconstructed image. Compression ratio is defined as the ratio of the image size to the compressed image size, such that a 4 : 1 compression has reduced the image size by a factor of four.

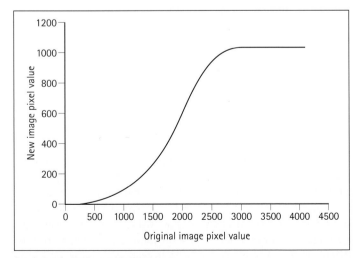

Example of a look-up table (LUT)

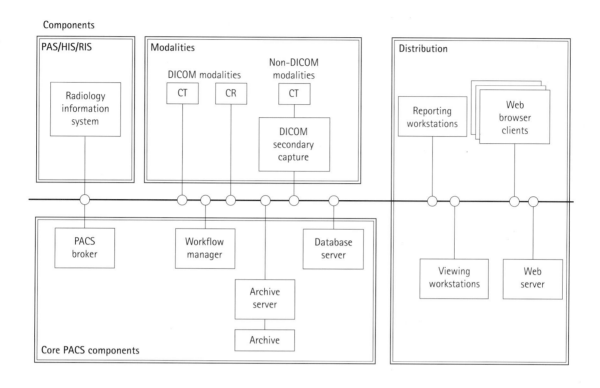

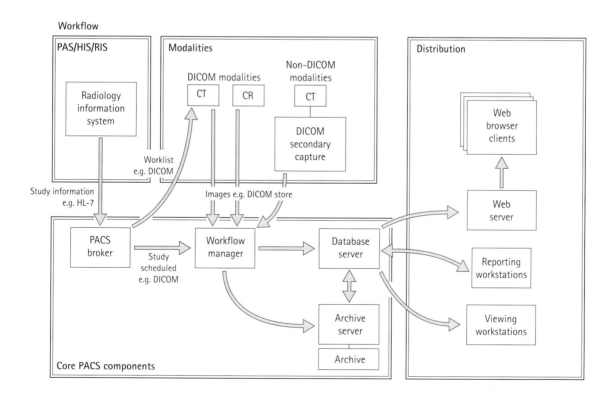

1 Exposure factors

Each time a radiograph is to be produced, a set of exposure factors has to be chosen to give the type of image required. The choice of these factors will depend on the region being examined, including its thickness, density, pathology, etc. The exposure factors to be selected are:

- the milliampere seconds (mAs);
- the kilovoltage;
- the FFD.

The exposure factors chosen will differ for different types of image-acquisition device and will depend on whether a grid is being used.

Milliampere seconds

This indicates the intensity or, put simply, the amount of radiation being used. If the radiation has enough energy to penetrate the body, then it will be detected by the image-acquisition device and will determine the image density or, again put simply, the image 'blackening'.

mAs is a product of the X-ray tube current (mA) and exposure time (seconds). As a general rule, the mA should be as high as possible with a short time, to reduce the risk of movement unsharpness. The X-ray generator will automatically select the highest mA and lowest time that is consistent with an acceptable amount of thermal stress upon the tube. The radiographer does, however, have the option of increasing this tube loading to give a shorter time and higher mA should the clinical situation demand this, e.g. in the case of a restless patient.

If insufficient mA is used, then a photographic film will be underexposed and will lack photographic density and therefore will show reduced contrast. If an electronic image-acquisition device is used, then an insufficient mAs will manifest itself as noise or mottle, even though the image-processing software will have produced a computer screen brightness (image) density that appears adequate. A mAs level that is too high will result in an overexposed film with excessive density and, again, a lack of contrast. In the case of a digitized electronic image-acquisition system, an increasing mAs will produce images that are of increasing quality with progressively less noise and improved signal-to-noise ratio.

Kilovoltage

This indicates how the X-ray beam will penetrate the body. The range of kilovoltages used in diagnostic radiography is normally between 50 and 120 kVp, although a kilovoltage as low as 25 kVp may be used for certain soft-tissue examinations, such as mammography. High-kVp techniques, such as those used in chest radiography, employ a kilovoltage in excess of 120 kVp.

The kilovoltage will have a profound effect on the image density.

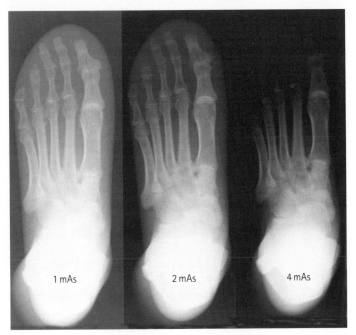

Effect of changing mAs on film density for the same kV

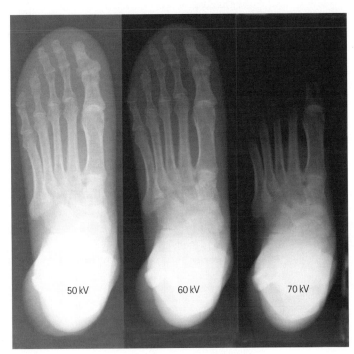

Effect of changing kV on film density for the same mAs

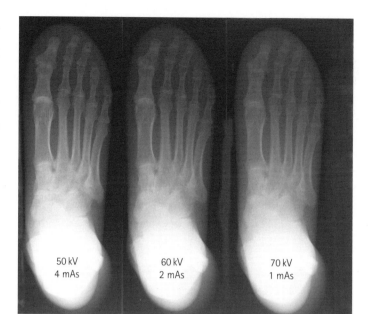

Effect of increasing kV and reducing mAs on film density

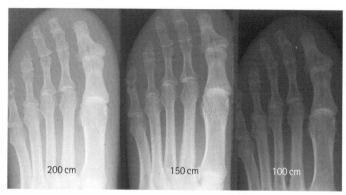

Effect on image density when FFD is varied but kV and mAs remain the same

Kilovoltage

As the kilovoltage increases, the X-rays produced have a higher energy and more will be able to penetrate the body. This will be detected by the image-acquisition device.

Kilovoltage is also the most important factor in the control of contrast of the radiographic image and should therefore be chosen carefully.

The kilovoltage should be such that the radiation has enough energy to penetrate the body part and reach the image-acquisition device. Maximum contrast will be achieved if the lowest possible kVp is used which will allow a reasonable proportion of the radiation to penetrate the body part. Dense structures within the body (e.g. bone) will absorb these low-energy X-rays, but structures of lower density (e.g. soft tissue) will absorb relatively few X-rays. This leads to a large difference in image density between these structures, i.e. high contrast. As the kilovoltage increases, proportionately more radiation will be able to penetrate the denser body part compared with the less dense part. The resulting difference in density between the two images will be reduced, giving a lower-contrast image.

If there is a very wide range of patient densities within the region being examined (e.g. the chest), then the image may show excessive contrast and it might be necessary to reduce the contrast within the image to allow a diagnostic image density to be attained throughout the region of interest. This can be achieved by increasing the kVp and, as mentioned previously, is commonly undertaken in chest radiography.

Another reason for increasing the kVp is to allow the mAs, and therefore the exposure time, to be reduced. As kilovoltage is increased, not only does the radiation have more energy but also more radiation is produced, thus allowing the reduction in mAs. This reduction in exposure time will, however, be at the expense of image contrast.

Focus-to-film distance

For a given kVp and mAs, the greater the FFD, the lower the intensity of radiation reaching the film. Therefore, to obtain the same film blackening, if the FFD is increased the mAs must also be increased.

When choosing the FFD, the following factors are taken into consideration:

- The X-ray tube must not be too close to the patient's skin, otherwise radiation damage could be caused.
- Short FFDs could give unacceptable geometric unsharpness.
- The FFD must not be excessive, otherwise the large increase in mAs required would mean high tube loading.

Most radiographic examinations are carried out with an FFD of 100 cm, which gives acceptable focus-to-skin distance and geometrical unsharpness but does not put unnecessary thermal stress on the X-ray tube. If this is the customary FFD used, then the department will require grids focused at 100 cm.

Exposure factors

Focus-to-film distance (*contd*)

If there is a large object-to-film distance, FFD is sometimes increased to reduce geometrical unsharpness and magnification.

To calculate the new exposure at the changed distance, the following formula can be used:

$$\text{New mAs} = \frac{\text{new distance}^2}{\text{old distance}^2} \times \text{original mAs.}$$

For example, if at 100 cm FFD an exposure of 65 kVp and 20 mAs produced a satisfactory result, then at 200 cm FFD, the new mAs would be calculated as follows:

$$\text{New mAs} = \frac{200^2}{100^2} \times 20 = 4 \times 20 = 80 \text{ mAs.}$$

Therefore, the exposure factors required at an FFD of 200 cm will be 65 kVp and 80 mAs.

Intensifying screens

Intensifying screens used in conjunction with photographic film are usually in pairs, with the film sandwiched between them and contained in a rigid, light-tight container, i.e. a cassette.

Different types of intensifying screen emit different intensities and different colours of light when irradiated by X-rays. It is important to ensure that the type of film used with a particular type of screen is matched in terms of the colour of light it is most sensitive to.

'Fast' or regular screens require less radiation to produce the same film blackening than the 'slow' screens used for extremity radiography. When changing from slow to fast screens, the exposure must be reduced. This has the advantage that a lower radiation dose is received by the patient; however, greater screen speed will result in greater photographic unsharpness, with a resultant decrease in image quality. It is important to consult the screen manufacturers' guidelines to become aware of the difference in speed of the particular screens used in a particular department.

Digital image capture

If a digital method of image acquisition is being used, such as CR, then a wide range of exposures will produce an image. If the equipment does not receive an optimal exposure, then the image will show noise or mottle and will not be suitable for diagnosis. Exposures over a given optimum will still produce an acceptable image up to a point, but the patient will have been exposed to a radiation dose that is unjustifiable.

The equipment used for digital image acquisition should have some indication of how much exposure was used in for a particular examination. The radiographer should consult this and compare the value with the optimal range of values recommended by the manufacturer.

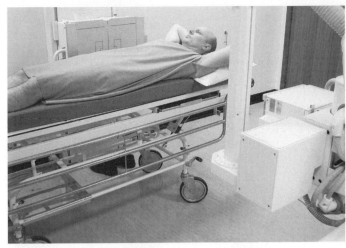

FFD increased to reduce increased geometric unsharpness from a large OFD

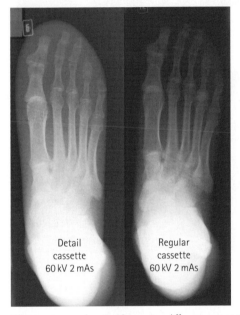

Effect on image density when using different screen types

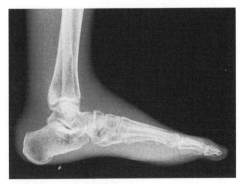

Underexposed digital image

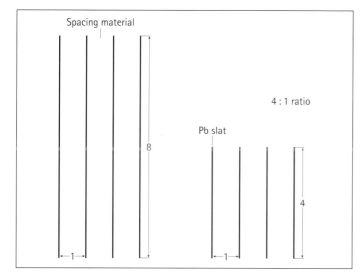

Grid ratio

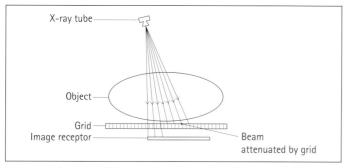

One cause of grid cut-off: beam angulation across grid lines

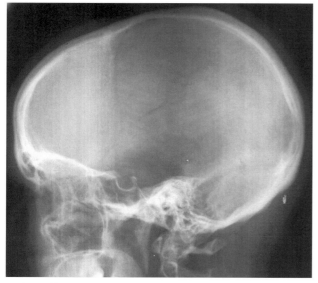

Grid cut-off due to focused grid being upside down

Secondary radiation grid

Grids are used when the thicker or denser parts of the body are being examined, where scattered radiation is likely to reduce significantly the contrast of the image. A grid, either stationary or moving, is placed between that patient and the cassette. Its design allows a high percentage of primary radiation to pass to the film while absorbing a high percentage of scattered radiation.

Because the grid stops both primary and secondary radiation, mAs must be increased when a grid is used. The increase required is generally by a factor of two to four, but this may vary considerably with the type of grid used.

Grids are usually focused (e.g. at 100 cm), which means that the X-ray tube should be at this distance (e.g. 100 cm) above the grid for maximum transmission of primary radiation through all parts of the grid.

With a low-ratio grid (the ratio between the height of lead strips to the width of the strips) and a small field size, this distance is not critical and the tube could be some 20–30 cm above or below the grid focus without any noticeable effect on the radiographic image. If, however, a high-ratio grid is used (14:1 or 16:1) with a large field size, then the X-ray tube must be within a few centimetres of the grid focus, otherwise there will be a loss of image density at the two edges of the film that were parallel with the grid slats.

The central ray of the X-ray beam can be angled along the line of the grid slats but not across it, otherwise there will be a loss of transmission by the grid, resulting in reduced image density over part or the whole of the image (a grid 'cut-off').

If the grid remains stationary during the exposure, then the grid pattern will be seen on the radiograph. This is usually the case when a stationary grid is used, e.g. for ward and some trauma radiography. In the imaging department, the grid is attached to a mechanism that gives it some kind of oscillatory movement, so that the grid pattern is not seen. If the grid has a lattice of 50 lines or more per centimetre, then it can be used stationary without the grid lines being obvious on the radiograph.

Choice of exposure factors

Kilovoltage is selected to give the required penetration and subject contrast. mAs is selected to give the correct image density. Its value depends on:

- the type of image-acquisition device, e.g. the relative speed of intensifying screens;
- the FFD;
- the grid factor (if a grid is used).

Measures used to reduce the exposure time, e.g. increasing tube loading to 100%, should be considered if movement unsharpness is likely to be a problem.

1 Summary of factors contributing to radiographic image quality

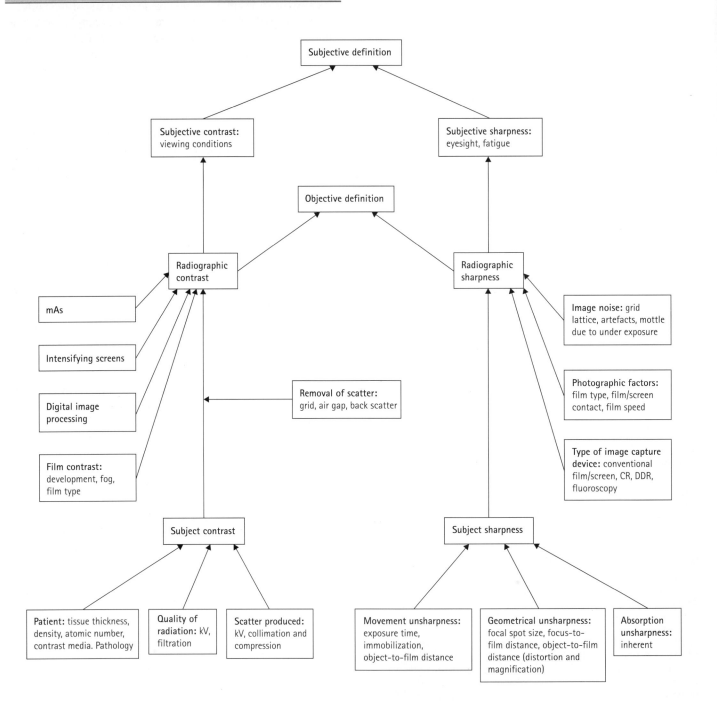

Radiation dose quantities

Dose quantity	Unit	Definition
Absorbed dose	Gy	Energy absorbed in known mass of tissue
Organ dose	mGy	Average dose to specific tissue
Effective dose	mSv	Overall dose weighted for sensitivity of different organs; indicates risk
Entrance surface dose	mGy	Dose measured at entrance surface; used to monitor doses and set DRLs for radiographs
Dose–area product	Gy.cm2	Product of dose (in air) and beam area; used to monitor doses and set DRLs for examinations

DRL, dose reference level.

Dose reference levels proposed by National Radiological Protection Board (NRPB)*

Radiograph	Entrance surface dose (mGy)	Dose–area product (Gy.cm^2)
Skull AP/PA	3	–
Skull lateral	1.5	–
Chest PA	0.2	0.12
Chest lateral	1.0	–
Thoracic spine AP	3.5	–
Thoracic spine lateral	10	–
Lumbar spine AP	6	1.6
Lumbar spine lateral	14	3
Lumbar spine lumbar-sacral junction	26	3
Abdomen AP	6	3
Pelvis AP	4	3

Examination	Fluoroscopy time (min)	Dose–area product (Gy.cm^2)
Barium (or water-soluble) swallow	2.3	11
Barium meal	2.3	13
Barium follow-through	2.2	14
Barium (or water-soluble) enema	2.7	31
Small-bowel enema	11.0	50
Intravenous urogram	–	16
Micturating cystogram	2.7	17

* Based on 2000 review of NRPB national patient dose database. The Department of Health (DoH) is likely to adopt some of these as national diagnostic reference levels.
AP, antero-posterior; PA, postero-anterior.

Dose quantities

X-ray examinations provide significant benefits to patients as a diagnostic tool, but the use of ionizing radiation also carries a small risk of causing harm.

The likelihood and severity of harm depends on the amount of X-ray energy absorbed in the patient. Radiation dose (expressed in joules/kilogram (J/kg) or Gray (Gy)) is used to quantify the amount of energy absorbed within a known mass of tissue. Some types of radiation cause more harm than others for the same absorbed dose. The equivalent dose (expressed in Sieverts (Sv)) is found by multiplying the absorbed dose by the quality factor assigned to specific types of radiation. For diagnostic X-rays, the quality factor is one, so that absorbed dose and equivalent dose have the same value. The risk also depends on which organs and tissues are irradiated. To take account of this, the tissues are given a weighting factor according to their susceptibility to harm from radiation. Organ dose multiplied by the tissue-weighting factor gives the weighted equivalent dose for that organ. The effective dose for an examination (expressed in Sv) is found by adding up the weighted equivalent doses for tissues or organs that have been irradiated. Effective dose indicates the detriment to health of an X-ray, allowing for the site of the examination and the exposure conditions.

For most tissues, it is not feasible to measure organ doses directly. However, they can be derived using mathematical models of the dose distributions within simulated patients, for different examinations and exposure conditions. The models are used to convert patient dose–area product readings (expressed in Gy.cm^2) or entrance skin dose measurements (expressed in mGy) into organ doses. Combining the weighted organ doses gives the effective dose for the given examination conditions. Skin doses are usually measured using thermoluminescent dosimeters (TLDs) or are calculated indirectly from tube output and back-scatter data.

For monitoring the relative patient dose levels for different types of examination performed using a variety of equipment, it is usually sufficient to analyse dose–area product readings or skin dose data without deriving effective doses. National and local diagnostic reference levels (DRLs) will also be set in terms of these quantities. Some proposed values are shown in the table here.

Radiation risks

Radiation can cause several forms of harm. The doses for radiographic examinations are substantially lower than the threshold needed to cause immediate harmful effects due to cell-killing, such as radiation sickness. Other threshold or deterministic effects such as skin burns or damage to the lens of the eye occur only after prolonged or repeated X-ray exposures giving doses in excess of 1–2 Gy. Occasionally, skin damage has been seen after complex interventional investigations. For these procedures, it is necessary to manage this type of risk. Irradiation of a fetus during organogenesis could also lead to deterministic effects such as malformations and mental retardation when doses exceed 100–200 mGy.

Radiation risks

However, even low X-ray doses can cause changes to cell DNA, resulting in a slight increase in the probability of cancer occurring in the years following exposure. The additional risk of a fatal cancer ranges from less than one in 1 000 000 for chest, extremity and dental examinations to typically one in 30 000 for abdominal radiographs and more than one in 10 000 for abdominal computed tomography (CT) and barium examinations. Typically, risks for children are two or three times greater than those for average adults, while risks for elderly people are five times lower than those for average adults. Radiation protection measures reduce this stochastic risk to patients by minimizing the X-ray dose used to obtain diagnostic information.

In addition to the risk of causing somatic harm to the patient, there is also the possibility of causing genetic harm to future offspring. Irradiating the gonads of patients could potentially harm their children through the risk of heritable disease. The risk is small compared with the natural risks, but using techniques and protective measures to minimize gonad doses is a sensible and simple precaution.

Medical exposure legislation

The basic measures for the radiation protection of people undergoing medical exposures were contained in the 1990 Recommendations of the International Commission on Radiological Protection. In 1997, the European Council set out these measures in the Medical Exposure Directive (Council Directive 97/43/Euratom) for adoption by member states. Great Britain implemented most of the provisions in the directive in the Ionising Radiations (Medical Exposure) Regulations (IRMER) 2000.

IRMER provides a comprehensive framework for protecting patients and others undergoing medical exposures and keeping their doses as low as reasonably practicable (ALARP). The requirements of IRMER follow the fundamental principles for radiation protection: all medical exposures must be justified before they take place. Possible alternatives must be considered and the benefits weighed against possible harm. Once an exposure is justified, then the equipment and protocols used for the examination must be optimized to keep doses ALARP.

Patient dose information is recorded to enable periodic dose auditing against established diagnostic reference levels.

IRMER addresses all stages of the examination process, from initial referral to evaluation of the images produced. All members of staff involved in medical exposures have clear responsibilities for protecting patients. The duty holders are the referrer, the practitioner who justifies the examination and the operators who carry out practical aspects of the examination from identification of the patient to using equipment to make the exposures.

Responsibility for implementing IRMER falls on employers. They must put in place written procedures that clearly identify the duty holders, and set out their responsibilities and the steps they must follow to ensure that the patients are properly protected through the various stages of the examination. Implementation includes the need to use written protocols, which should define standard imaging projections for a specific medical condition for each anatomical area, e.g. skull and exposure charts, to improve the consistency of standard techniques.

Procedures must also focus on issues that need special consideration by duty holders because the potential risks may be greater or the benefits less clear. These include the exposure of children, high-dose examinations, exposure of women who may be pregnant, and exposure for medical research or medicolegal purposes.

Employers must ensure that the duty holders are adequately trained to perform their duties and to meet their responsibilities to protect patients. For example, an operator carrying out a medical exposure needs to know how to optimize all aspects of that exposure in order to obtain the necessary information with the lowest practicable dose. In this case, qualified radiographers are the appropriate operators because they have the adequate training to perform these duties. To maintain their competency, practitioners and operators are required to keep up to date with the latest developments in patient protection and improved techniques through continuing education.

Radiation risk for X-ray examinations to an average adult

Examination	Typical effective dose (mSv)	Risk*
Chest	0.02	1 in 1000 000
Mammography	0.06	1 in 300 000
Abdomen	0.7	1 in 30 000
Lumbar spine	1.3	1 in 15 000
CT head	2	1 in 10 000
Barium enema	7.2	1 in 2800
CT body	9	1 in 2200

*Additional lifetime risk of fatal cancer.

Example list of Ionising Radiation (Medical Exposure) Regulations (IRMER) employers' procedures for X-ray examinations

Patient identification
Identification of referrers, practitioners and operators
Medical exposure justification
Females of childbearing age
Examination evaluation and dose recording
Patient dose assessment
Use of diagnostic reference levels
Quality assurance of IRMER operation
Medicolegal exposures
Exposures for medical research
Reducing unintended doses
Investigation of unintended exposures

ADULT EXPOSURE GUIDE ROOM :-						

Blackpool Victoria Hospital **NHS**
NHS Trust

PROJECTION	kV$_p$	mAs	AEC	FFD	GRID	F/S
SKULL						
OF/FO						
OF 30/FO 30						
LAT						
SCALP F.B.						
FACIAL BONES						
OM						
OM 30						
OF 30 (ORBITS FB)						
MANDIBLE – PA						
LAT MAND.						
LAT OBL MAND.						
LAT NOSE						

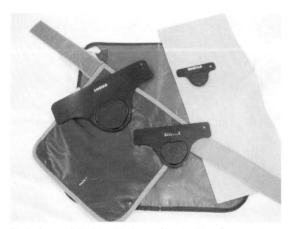

Typical gonad shields with sheet of lead rubber for gonad protection

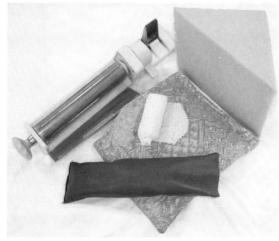

Examples of immobilization devices

Practical protection measures

It is the duty of the operators carrying out medical exposures to take practical steps to protect the patient. These may involve:

- patient preparation;
- patient identification;
- special patient issues, e.g. paediatrics, females;
- selection of imaging equipment;
- type of image receptor;
- patient positioning;
- exposure technique;
- image projection;
- beam collimation;
- exposure parameters;
- patient protective equipment and shielding.

Protection of the patient from any unnecessary primary and scatter radiation should be employed. The gonads should not be in the line of the primary beam for projections other than the abdomen, and therefore careful radiographic technique is essential, e.g. radiography of the hand (see p. 5).

Special care must be taken to collimate the beam to the area of interest, thus avoiding the unnecessary irradiation of tissue and reducing scatter radiation. When more radiation-sensitive tissues are located in the image-acquisition field, these should be excluded whenever possible, e.g. the use of gonad shields and the modification of projections to reduce irradiation of the lens of the eye or the thyroid gland.

Protection from scattered radiation is employed by the intelligent use of lead protective materials protecting the gonads and should be employed regularly in extremity radiography.

In order to reduce repeat images, the use of foam pads, sandbags and other immobilizing devices should be used to ensure that the patient is immobilized and in a position that is as comfortable as possible. The shortest exposure time should be selected to avoid movement unsharpness.

The fastest imaging system (film/screen combination or fastest CR phosphor plates) should be selected appropriate to the diagnostic information required, thus ensuring that the dose is ALARP.

Pregnancy rule

To avoid irradiating a fetus, a 'pregnancy rule' should be observed carefully. IRMER requires employers to have a written procedure for this. If a woman of childbearing age is, or cannot be certain that she is not, pregnant, then direct irradiation of the abdomen and pelvis should be avoided. The only exception to this rule is when those justifying the procedure in conjunction with the referring clinician can state that there are overriding clinical reasons for the requested examination to proceed. In such cases, all steps must be taken to minimize the number of exposures and the absorbed dose per exposure. Examinations of regions other than the abdomen and pelvis may proceed, provided there is good beam collimation and lead protection of the abdomen and pelvis.

Reference

Manaster BJ (1997). *Handbook of Skeletal Radiology*, 2nd edn. St Louis: Mosby.

Section 2

The Upper Limb

CONTENTS

RECOMMENDED PROJECTIONS	38
POSITION OF PATIENT IN RELATION TO TABLE	39
HAND	40
Basic projections	40
Postero-anterior – dorsi-palmar	40
Radiographic anatomy	41
Anterior oblique – dorsi-palmar oblique	42
Postero-anterior – both hands	43
Posterior oblique – both hands (ball catcher's or Nørgaard projection)	44
Lateral	45
FINGERS	46
Basic projections	46
Postero-anterior	46
Lateral – index and middle fingers	46
Lateral – ring and little fingers	47
THUMB	48
Lateral	48
Antero-posterior	48
Postero-anterior – foreign body	49
SCAPHOID	50
Postero-anterior – ulnar deviation	50
Anterior oblique – ulnar deviation	51
Posterior oblique	52
Lateral	53
CARPAL TUNNEL	54
Axial – method 1	54
Axial – method 2	54
WRIST	55
Basic projection	55
Postero-anterior	56
Lateral – method 1	56
Lateral – method 2	57
Oblique (anterior oblique)	58

FOREARM	59
Antero-posterior – basic	59
Lateral – basic	60
ELBOW	61
Lateral	61
Antero-posterior	62
Antero-posterior – partial flexion	62
Antero-posterior – forearm in contact	63
Antero-posterior – upper arm in contact	63
Full flexion	64
Axial – upper arm in contact	64
Axial – forearm in contact	65
Lateral head of radius	66
Proximal radio-ulnar joint – oblique	67
Ulnar groove – axial	67
Radiological considerations	68
HUMERUS – SUPRACONDYLAR FRACTURE	69
Lateral	69
Antero-posterior	70
HUMERUS – SHAFT	71
Antero-posterior – supine	71
Lateral – supine	71
Antero-posterior – erect	72
Lateral – erect	72
HUMERUS – INTERTUBEROUS SULCUS (BICIPITAL GROOVE)	73
Axial	73
Alternative axial projection	73
HUMERUS – NECK	74
Antero-posterior	74
Axial projection	75
Lateral – supero-inferior	75
Lateral – infero-superior	76
Lateral oblique	76

Area	Indication	Projection
Hand	Fractures and dislocation of metacarpals	Postero-anterior (basic) Anterior oblique (basic)
	Serious injury or foreign bodies	Lateral (basic) Antero-posterior (alternate)
	Pathology e.g. rheumatoid arthritis	Postero-anterior – both hands Postero-oblique – both hands (ball catcher's)
Fingers	Fractures and dislocation/foreign bodies	Postero-anterior (basic) Lateral (basic)
Thumb	Fractures and dislocation of phalanges	Antero-posterior (basic) Lateral (basic)
	Injury to base of first metacarpal e.g. Bennett's fracture	Antero-posterior (basic) Lateral (basic)
Carpal bones	e.g. Scaphoid	Postero-anterior with hand adducted (ulnar deviation) Anterior oblique (basic) Posterior oblique Lateral (basic)
Carpal tunnel syndrome		Axial Postero-anterior
Distal end radius and ulna	Trauma or pathology	Postero-anterior (basic) Lateral (basic) Oblique
Forearm	Trauma or pathology	Antero-posterior (basic) Lateral (basic)
	Serious injury	Antero-posterior (modified) Lateral (modified)
Elbow joint	Trauma or pathology	Lateral (basic) Antero-posterior (basic)
	Elbow cannot be extended	Lateral (basic) Antero-posterior Axial
	Trauma or pathology head of radius	Antero-posterior (basic) Lateral with rotation of radius Axial (2)
	Proximal radio-ulnar joint	Lateral (basic) Antero-posterior – oblique
	Ulnar groove	Antero-posterior (basic) Axial
	Supracondylar fracture	Antero-posterior (modified) Lateral (modified)
Humerus	Trauma or pathology	Antero-posterior (erect) Lateral (erect)
	Intertuberous sulcus (bicipital groove)	Antero-posterior (basic) Axial
Neck of humerus	Fracture	Antero-posterior Lateral oblique Lateral – supero-superior Lateral – infero-superior

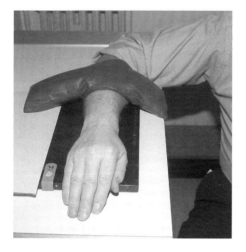

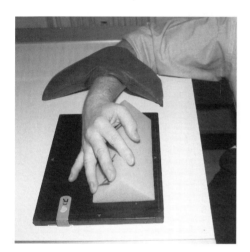

Although radiographic examinations of the upper limb are routine, a high standard of radiography must be maintained. The best possible radiographs are essential, because decisions about injuries, especially of the elbow and the wrist, affect future dexterity, employment and earnings of the patient.

The importance of registering the correct right or left marker at the time of the exposure cannot be overemphasized; neither can the importance of recording the correct patient identification and date of the examination.

To ensure maximum radiation protection, the patient should be seated at the side or end of the table with the lower limbs and gonads away from the primary beam, i.e. with the legs to the side of the table rather than under it; the beam should be collimated within the margins of the cassette. More than one projection can be recorded on the cassette provided that lead-rubber is used to mask off the parts of the cassette not being used.

The limb should be immobilized by the use of non-opaque pads within the radiation field and sandbags outside the field. It is important to remember that the patient will be able to keep the limb still only if it is in a comfortable and relaxed position. When the hand or wrist is being examined, the patient's forearm and hand can rest on the table. For examination of the forearm, elbow and humerus, the shoulder, elbow and wrist should be in a plane parallel to the cassette. With the cassette on the table, this means that the shoulder, elbow and wrist will be at the same horizontal level, i.e. the upper arm, elbow and forearm should be in contact with the table.

2 Hand

Basic projections

It is common practice to obtain two projections, a postero-anterior and an anterior oblique, on one 24 × 30-cm cassette. If possible use a cassette with high-resolution screens. A lead-rubber mask may be used to mask off the half of the film not in use.

Postero-anterior – dorsi-palmar

Position of patient and cassette

- The patient is seated alongside the table with the affected arm nearest to the table.
- The forearm is pronated and placed on the table with the palmer surface of the hand in contact with the cassette.
- The fingers are separated and extended but relaxed to ensure that they remain in contact with the cassette.
- The wrist is adjusted so that the radial and ulna styloid processes are equidistant from the cassette.
- A sandbag is placed over the lower forearm for immobilization.

Direction and centring of the X-ray beam

- The vertical central ray is centred over the head of the third metacarpal.

Essential image characteristics

- The image should demonstrate all the phalanges, including the soft-tissue fingertips, the carpal and metacarpal bones, and the distal end of the radius and ulna.
- The inter-phalangeal and metacarpo-phalangeal and carpo-metacarpal joints should be demonstrated clearly.
- No rotation.

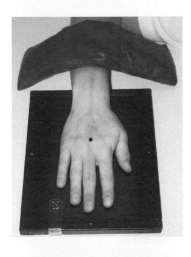

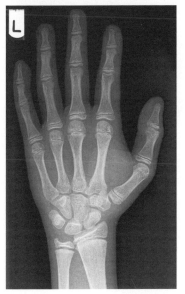

Normal postero-anterior radiograph of left hand

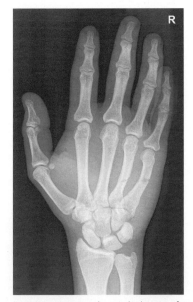

Postero-anterior radiograph showing fractures of fourth and fifth metacarpals

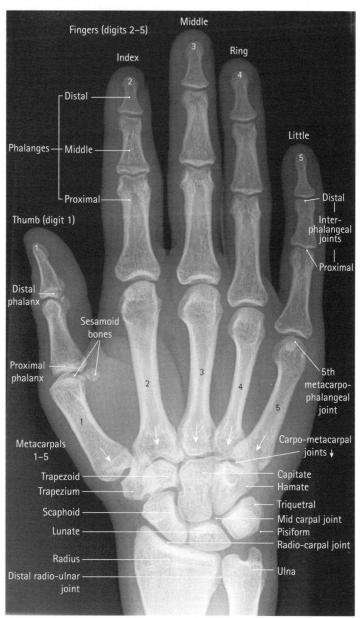

Fingers (digits 2–5)
Middle
Index
Ring
Little
Distal
Phalanges — Middle
Proximal
Thumb (digit 1)
Distal phalanx
Sesamoid bones
Proximal phalanx
Metacarpals 1–5
Trapezoid
Trapezium
Scaphoid
Lunate
Radius
Distal radio-ulnar joint
Distal
Inter-phalangeal joints
Proximal
5th metacarpo-phalangeal joint
Carpo-metacarpal joints ↓
Capitate
Hamate
Triquetral
Mid carpal joint
Pisiform
Radio-carpal joint
Ulna

Right hand postero-anterior

Anterior oblique – dorsi-palmar oblique

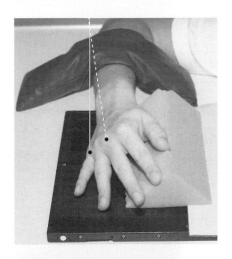

Position of patient and cassette

- From the basic postero-anterior position, the hand is externally rotated 45 degrees with the fingers extended.
- The fingers should be separated slightly and the hand supported on a 45-degree non-opaque pad.
- A sandbag is placed over the lower end of the forearm for immobilization.

Direction and centring of the X-ray beam

- The vertical central ray is centred over the head of the fifth metacarpal.
- The tube is then angled so that the central ray passes through the head of the third metacarpal, enabling a reduction in the size of the field.

Essential image characteristics

- The image should demonstrate all the phalanges, including the soft-tissue of the fingertips, the carpal and metacarpal bones, and the distal end of the radius and ulna.
- The correct degree of rotation has been achieved when the heads of the first and second metacarpals are seen separated whilst those of the fourth and fifth are just superimposed.

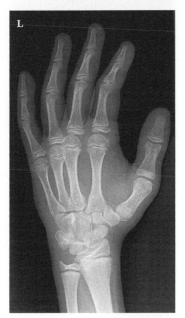

Normal anterior oblique radiograph of left hand

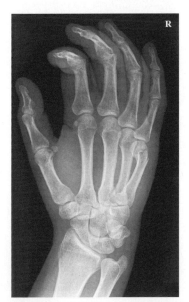

Anterior oblique radiograph of right hand showing fracture neck of fifth metacarpal (Boxer's fracture)

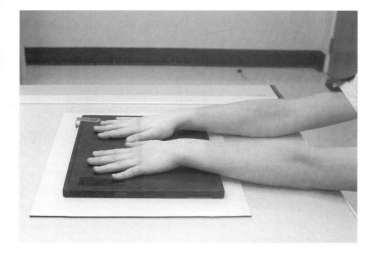

Postero-anterior – both hands

This projection is often used to demonstrate subtle radiographic changes associated with early rheumatoid arthritis and to monitor the progress of the disease.

Position of patient and cassette

- Ideally, the patient is seated alongside the table. However, if this is not possible due to the patient's condition, the patient may be seated facing the table (see Radiation protection, p. 35).
- Both forearms are pronated and placed on the table with the palmer surface of the hands in contact with the cassette.
- The fingers are separated and extended but relaxed to ensure that they remain in contact with the cassette.
- The wrists are adjusted so that the radial and ulna styloid processes are equidistant from the cassette.
- A sandbag is placed over the lower forearms for immobilization.

Direction and centring of the X-ray beam

- The vertical central is centred over a point midway between the inter-phalangeal joints of both thumbs.

Essential image characteristics

- The image should demonstrate all the phalanges, including the soft-tissue fingertips, the carpal and metacarpal bones, and the distal end of the radius and ulna.
- The exposure factors selected must produce a density and contrast that optimally demonstrate joint detail.

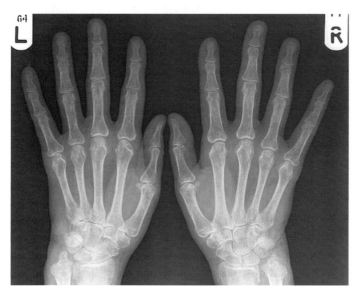

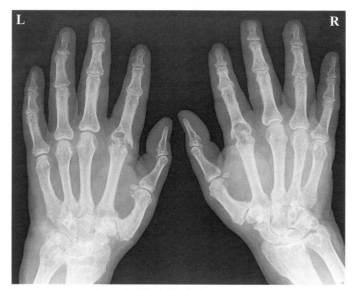

Normal postero-anterior radiograph, both hands

Postero-anterior radiograph of both hands showing severe erosive disease

Posterior oblique – both hands (ball catcher's or Nørgaard projection)

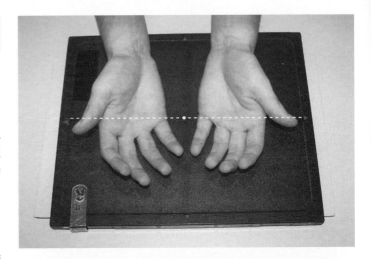

This projection may be used in the diagnosis of rheumatoid arthritis. It can also be used to demonstrate a fracture of the base of the fifth metacarpal.

Position of patient and cassette

- Ideally, the patient is seated alongside the table. However, if this is not possible due to the patient's condition, the patient may be seated facing the table (see Radiation protection, p. 35).
- Both forearms are supinated and placed on the table with the dorsal surface of the hands in contact with the cassette.
- From this position, both hands are rotated internally (medially) 45 degrees into a 'ball-catching' position.
- The fingers and thumbs are separated and extended but relaxed to ensure that they remain in contact with the cassette.
- The hands may be supported using 45-degree non-opaque pads.
- A sandbag is placed over the lower forearms for immobilization.

Direction and centring of the X-ray beam

- The vertical central ray is centred to a point midway between the hands at the level of the fifth metacarpo-phalangeal joints.

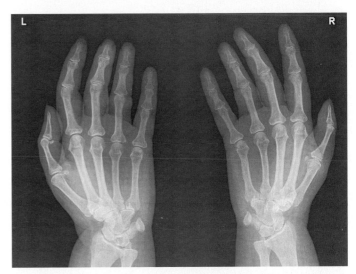

Normal radiograph of hands in ball catcher's position

Essential image characteristics

- The image should demonstrate all the phalanges, including the soft-tissue of the fingertips, the carpal and metacarpal bones, and the distal end of the radius and ulna.
- The exposure factors selected must produce a density and contrast that optimally demonstrate joint detail.
- The heads of the metacarpals should not be superimposed.

Radiation protection

If it has been necessary to position the patient facing the table, it is essential to provide radiation protection for the lower limbs and gonads. This may be achieved by placing a lead-rubber sheet on the table underneath the cassette to attenuate the primary beam.

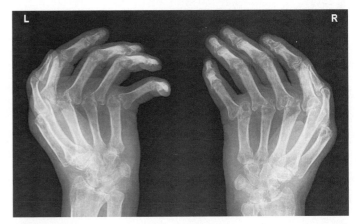

Radiograph of hands in ball catcher's position showing severe erosive disease

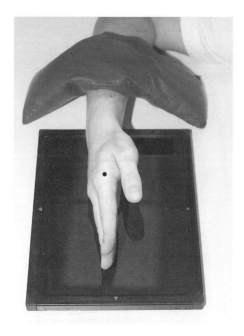

Lateral

This is used in addition to the routine postero-anterior projection to locate a foreign body. It may also be used to demonstrate a fracture or dislocation of the carpal bones.

Position of patient and cassette

- From the postero-anterior position, the hand is externally rotated 90 degrees.
- The palm of the hand is perpendicular to the cassette, with the fingers extended and the thumb abducted and supported parallel to the film on a non-opaque pad.
- The radial and ulnar styloid processes are superimposed.

Direction and centring of the X-ray beam

- The vertical central ray is centred over the head of the second metacarpal.

Essential image characteristics

- The image should include the fingertips, including soft tissue, and the radial and ulnar styloid processes.
- The heads of the metacarpals should be superimposed.
- The thumb should be demonstrated clearly without superimposition of other structures.

Notes

- If the projection has been undertaken to identify the position of a foreign body, the kVp should be lowered to demonstrate or exclude its presence in the soft tissues.
- A metal marker placed adjacent to the puncture site is commonly used to aid localization of the foreign body.

Radiological considerations

- The hand and wrist (like the ankle and foot) have many accessory ossicles, which may trap the unwary into a false diagnosis of pathology.
- 'Boxer's fracture' of the neck of the fifth metacarpal is seen easily, but conspicuity of fractures of the bases of the metacarpals is reduced by over rotation and underexposure.

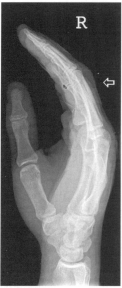

Lateral radiograph of hand with foreign body marker. There is an old fracture of the fifth metacarpal

2 | Fingers

Basic projections

It is common practice to obtain two projections, a postero-anterior and a lateral, on one 18 × 24-cm high-resolution cassette.

It is often necessary to image adjacent fingers, e.g. the second and third or the fourth and fifth. If this is the case, then care should be taken to avoid superimposition, particularly in the lateral projection, by fully extending one finger and partly flexing the other. A non-opaque foam pad is used to support the finger not in contact with the cassette.

A lead-rubber mask may be used to mask off the half of the film not in use.

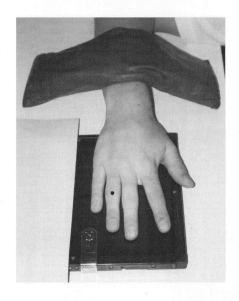

Postero-anterior

Position of patient and cassette

- The patient is positioned seated alongside the table as for a postero-anterior projection of the hand.
- The forearm is pronated with the anterior (palmer) aspect of the finger(s) in contact with the cassette.
- The finger(s) are extended and separated.
- A sandbag is placed across the dorsal surface of the wrist for immobilization.

Direction and centring of the X-ray beam

- The vertical central ray is centred over the proximal interphalangeal joint of the affected finger.

Essential image characteristics

- The image should include the fingertip and the distal third of the metacarpal bone.

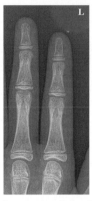 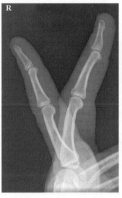

Postero-anterior radiograph of the index and middle fingers

Lateral radiograph of index and middle fingers

Lateral – index and middle fingers

Position of patient and cassette

- The patient is seated alongside the table with the arm abducted and medially rotated to bring the lateral aspect of the index finger into contact with the cassette.
- The raised forearm is supported.
- The index finger is fully extended and the middle finger slightly flexed to avoid superimposition.
- The middle finger is supported on a non-opaque pad.
- The remaining fingers are fully flexed into the palm of the hand and held there by the thumb.

Direction and centring of the X-ray beam

- The vertical central ray is centred over the proximal interphalangeal joint of the affected finger.

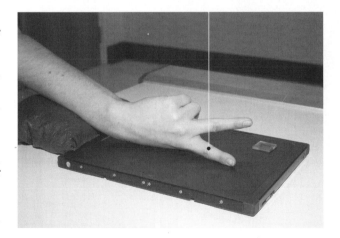

Essential image characteristics

- The image should include the fingertip and the distal third of the metacarpal bone.
- The condyles should be superimposed to avoid obscuring a volar plate fracture.

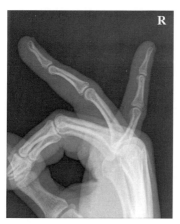

Lateral – ring and little fingers

Position of patient and cassette

- The patient is seated alongside the table with the palm of the hand at right-angles to the table and the medial aspect of the little finger in contact with the film.
- The affected finger is extended and the remaining fingers are fully flexed into the palm of the hand and held there by the thumb in order to prevent superimposition.
- It may be necessary to support the ring finger on a non-opaque pad to ensure that it is parallel to the film.

Direction and centring of the X-ray beam

- The vertical central ray is centred over the proximal inter-phalangeal joint of the affected finger.

Essential image characteristics

- The image should include the tip of the finger and the distal third of the metacarpal bone.

Note

In cases of severe trauma, when the fingers cannot be flexed, it may be necessary to take a lateral projection of all the fingers superimposed, as for the lateral projection of the hand, but centring over the proximal inter-phalangeal joint of the index finger.

Radiological considerations

- Scleroderma (one cause of Raynaud's disease) causes wasting and calcification of the soft tissue of the finger pulp.
- Chip fracture of the base of the dorsal aspect of the distal phalanx is associated with avulsion of the insertion of the extensor digitorum tendon, leading to the mallet finger deformity.

Normal lateral radiograph of ring and little fingers

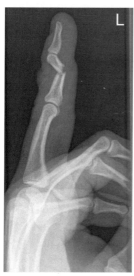

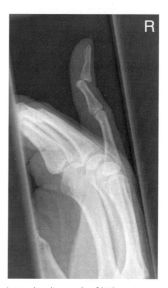

Lateral radiograph of middle finger showing a fracture of the middle phalanx

Lateral radiograph of little finger showing dislocation of the distal interphalangeal joint

2 Thumb

It is common practice to obtain two projections, an antero-posterior and a lateral, on one 18 × 24-cm high-resolution cassette.

In the case of a suspected foreign body in the thenar eminence, a postero-anterior projection is used to maintain the relationship with adjacent structures.

A lead-rubber mask may be used to mask off the half of the cassette not in use.

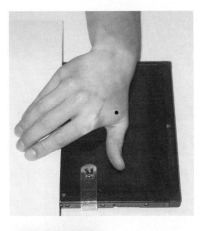

Lateral

Position of patient and cassette

- The patient is seated alongside the table with the arm abducted, the elbow flexed and the anterior aspect of the forearm resting on the table.
- The thumb is flexed slightly and the palm of the hand is placed on the cassette.
- The palm of the hand is raised slightly with the fingers partially flexed and supported on a non-opaque pad, such that the lateral aspect of the thumb is in contact with the cassette.

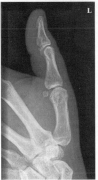

Normal lateral radiograph of thumb

Direction and centring of the X-ray beam

- The vertical central ray is centred over the first metacarpo-phalangeal joint.

Essential image characteristics

- Where there is a possibility of injury to the base of the first metacarpal, the carpo-metacarpal joint must be included on the image.

Antero-posterior

Position of patient and cassette

- The patient is seated facing away from the table with the arm extended backwards and medially rotated at the shoulder. The hand may be slightly rotated to ensure that the second, third and fourth metacarpals are not superimposed on the base of the first metacarpal.
- The patient leans forward, lowering the shoulder so that the first metacarpal is parallel to the tabletop.
- The cassette is placed under the wrist and thumb and oriented to the long axis of the metacarpal.

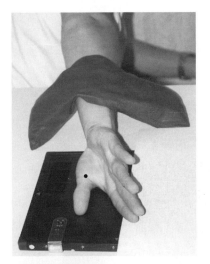

Direction and centring of the X-ray beam

- The vertical central ray is centred over the base of the first metacarpal.

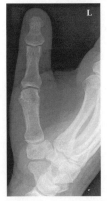

Normal antero-posterior radiograph of thumb

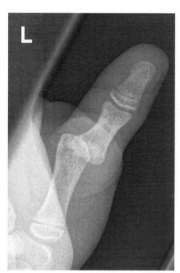

Postero-anterior – foreign body

Position of patient and cassette

- With the hand in the postero-anterior position, the palm of the hand is rotated through 90 degrees to bring the medial aspect of the hand in contact with the table and the palm vertical.
- The cassette is placed under the hand and wrist, with its long axis along the line of the thumb.
- The fingers are extended and the hand is rotated slightly forwards until the anterior aspect of the thumb is parallel to the cassette.
- The thumb is supported in position on a non-opaque pad.

Direction and centring of the X-ray beam

- The vertical central ray is centred to the first metacarpophalangeal joint.

Essential image characteristics

- Where there is a possibility of injury to the base of the first metacarpal, the carpo-metacarpal joint must be included on the image.
- The second, third, fourth and fifth metacarpals should not be superimposed on the first.

Notes

- The postero-anterior projection increases object-to-film distance and hence, potentially, unsharpness, but it is sometimes easier and less painful for the patient.
- The use of the postero-anterior projection maintains the relationship of the adjacent bones, i.e. the radius and ulna, which is essential in cases of suspected foreign body in the thenar eminence.

Radiological considerations

Fracture of the base of the first metacarpal through the joint surface may be associated with dislocation due to the pull of the abductor and extensor tendons of the thumb. This is known as Bennett's fracture and may cause functional impairment and early degenerative disease if not corrected. In contrast, a fracture that does not transgress the articular surface does not dislocate and does not have the same significance (Rolando fracture).

Postero-anterior thumb – showing dislocation at the first metacarpophalangeal joint

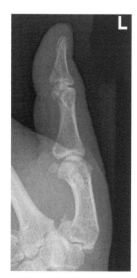

Radiograph of thumb showing Bennett's fracture

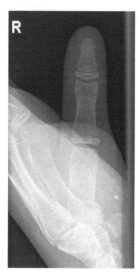

Antero-posterior radiograph of thumb – incorrectly positioned

2 | Scaphoid

Postero-anterior – ulnar deviation

Imaging of the carpal bones is most commonly undertaken to demonstrate the scaphoid. The projections may also be used to demonstrate other carpal bones, as indicated below.

Four projections may be taken to demonstrate all the carpal bones using a 24 × 30-cm cassette, each quarter being used in turn, with the other three-quarters masked off using lead rubber.

For scaphoid fractures, three projections are normally taken: postero-anterior, anterior oblique and lateral.

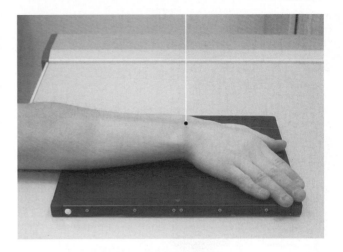

Position of patient and cassette

- The patient is seated alongside the table with the affected side nearest the table.
- The arm is extended across the table with the elbow flexed and the forearm pronated.
- If possible, the shoulder, elbow and wrist should be at the level of the tabletop.
- The wrist is positioned over one-quarter of the cassette and the hand is adducted (ulnar deviation).
- Ensure that the radial and ulnar styloid processes are equidistant from the cassette.
- The hand and lower forearm are immobilized using sandbags.

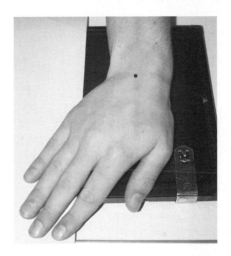

Direction and centring of the X-ray beam

- The vertical central ray is centred midway between the radial and ulnar styloid processes.

Essential image characteristics

- The image should include the distal end of the radius and ulna and the proximal end of the metacarpals.
- The joint space around the scaphoid should be demonstrated clearly.

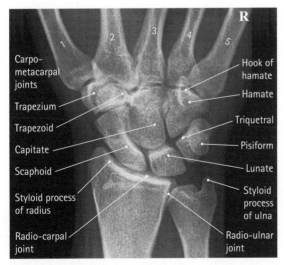

Antero-posterior radiograph of wrist

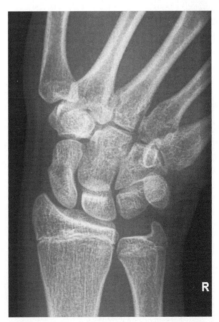

Normal postero-anterior radiograph of scaphoid in ulnar deviation

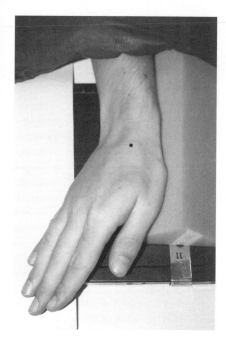

Anterior oblique – ulnar deviation

Position of patient and cassette

- From the postero-anterior position, the hand and wrist are rotated 45 degrees externally and placed over an unexposed quarter of the cassette. The hand should remain adducted in ulnar deviation.
- The hand is supported in position, with a non-opaque pad placed under the thumb.
- The forearm is immobilized using a sandbag.

Direction and centring of the X-ray beam

- The vertical central ray is centred midway between the radial and ulnar styloid processes (see p. 58).

Essential image characteristics

- The image should include the distal end of the radius and ulna and the proximal end of the metacarpals.
- The scaphoid should be seen clearly, with its long axis parallel to the cassette.

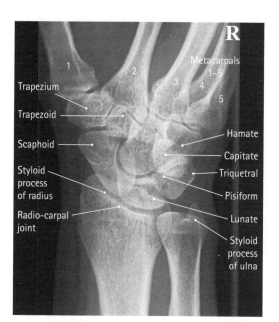

Anterior oblique radiograph of scaphoid

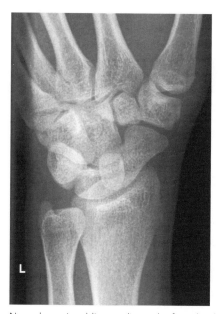

Normal anterior oblique radiograph of scaphoid

51

Posterior oblique

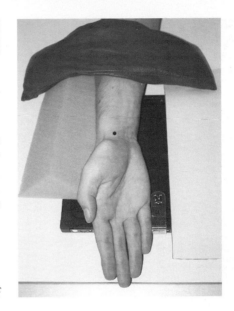

Position of patient and cassette

- From the anterior oblique position, the hand and wrist are rotated externally through 90 degrees, such that the posterior aspect of the hand and wrist are at 45 degrees to the cassette.
- The wrist is placed over an unexposed quarter of the cassette, with the wrist and hand supported on a 45-degree non-opaque foam pad.
- The forearm is immobilized using a sandbag.

Direction and centring of the X-ray beam

- The vertical central ray is centred over the styloid process of the ulna.

Essential image characteristics

- The image should include the distal end of the radius and ulna and the proximal end of the metacarpals.
- The pisiform should be seen clearly in profile situated anterior to the triquetral.
- The long axis of the scaphoid should be seen perpendicular to the cassette.

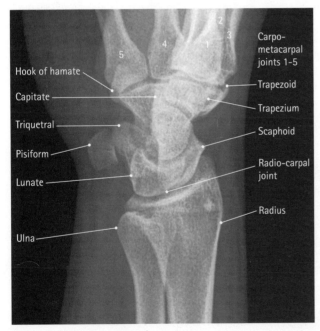

Posterior oblique radiograph of wrist

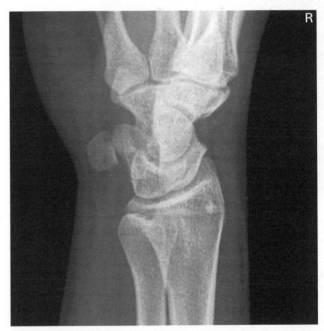

Normal posterior oblique radiograph of wrist

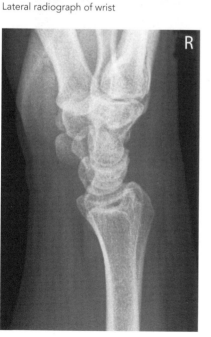

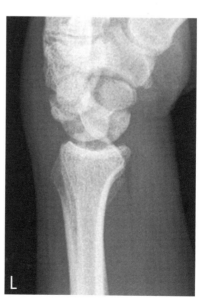

1st metacarpal

Trapezoid

Trapezium

Tubercle of scaphoid

Pisiform

Lunate

Radio-carpal joint

Shaft of radius

Metacarpals 2–5

Hamate

Capitate

Triquetral

Styloid of radius

Styloid process of ulna

Shaft of ulna

Lateral radiograph of wrist

Normal lateral radiograph of wrist

Position of patient and cassette

- From the posterior oblique position, the hand and wrist are rotated internally through 45 degrees, such that the medial aspect of the wrist is in contact with the cassette.
- The hand is adjusted to ensure that the radial and ulnar styloid processes are superimposed.
- The hand and wrist are immobilized using non-opaque pads and sandbags.

Direction and centring of the X-ray beam

- The vertical central ray is centred over the radial styloid process.

Essential image characteristics

- The image should include the distal end of the radius and ulna and the proximal end of the metacarpals.
- The image should demonstrate clearly any subluxation or dislocation of the carpal bones.

Radiological considerations

- Fracture of the waist of the scaphoid may be very poorly visible, if at all, at presentation. It carries a high risk of delayed avascular necrosis of the distal pole, which can cause severe disability. If suspected clinically, the patient may be re-examined after 10 days of immobilization, otherwise a technetium bone scan or magnetic resonance imaging (MRI) may offer immediate diagnosis.

Lateral radiograph of wrist showing dislocation of the lunate. The lunate bone is rotated and anteriorly displaced

2 Carpal tunnel

The carpal bones form a shallow concavity, which, with the bridging flexor retinaculum, forms the carpal tunnel. The flexor retinaculum is attached to the two medial prominences (the pisiform and the hook of the hamate) and to the two lateral prominences (the tubercle of the scaphoid and the tubercle of the trapezium). The median nerve along with the flexor tendons pass through the tunnel, and any swelling here can cause compression of the median nerve, giving rise to the carpal tunnel syndrome. Radiographic examination of the bony part of the tunnel is by an axial projection to demonstrate the medial and lateral prominences and the concavity.

This examination is requested less often nowadays due to improved electrophysiological techniques and the advent of MRI, which gives far better anatomical information.

Two alternative positions using an 18 × 24-cm cassette are described, depending on the condition of the patient.

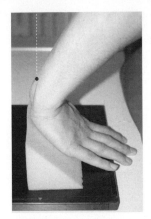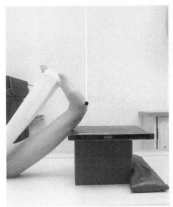

Axial – method 1

Position of patient and cassette

- The patient stand with their back towards the table.
- The cassette is placed level with the edge of the tabletop.
- The palm of the hand is pressed on to the cassette, with the wrist joint dorsiflexed to approximately 135 degrees.
- The fingers are curled around under the table to assist in immobilization.

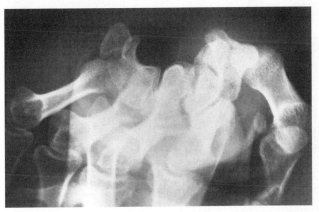

Normal carpal tunnel radiograph

Direction and centring of the X-ray beam

- The vertical central ray is centred between the pisiform and the hook of the hamate medially and the tubercle of the scaphoid and the ridge of the trapezium laterally.

Axial – method 2

Position of patient and cassette

- The patient is seated alongside the table.
- The cassette is placed on top of a plastic block approximately 8 cm high.
- The lower end of the forearm rests against the edge of the block, with the wrist adducted and dorsiflexed to 135 degrees.
- This position is assisted using a traction bandage held by the patient's other hand.

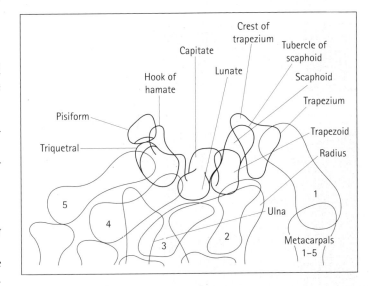

Direction and centring of the X-ray beam

- The vertical central ray is centred between the pisiform and the hook of the hamate medially and the tubercle of the scaphoid and the ridge of the trapezium laterally.

Essential image characteristics

- The image should demonstrate clearly the pisiform and the hook of the hamate medially and the tubercle of the scaphoid and the tubercle of the trapezium laterally.

Basic projection

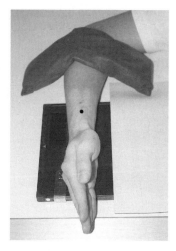

Method 1

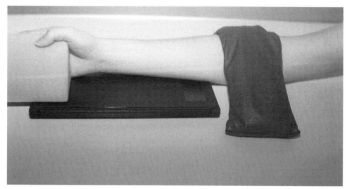

Method 2

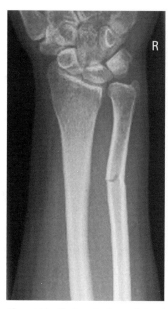
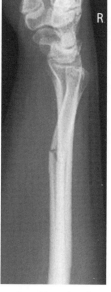

Almost identical projections of the ulna produced by using the postero-anterior projection, and method 1 for the lateral projection. Note the orientation of the fracture of the distal ulna remains the same

Two projections are routinely taken, a postero-anterior and a lateral, using an 18 × 24-cm high-resolution cassette. A lead-rubber sheet can be used to mask the half of the cassette not in use. An additional oblique projection may also be undertaken to provide further information.

When carrying out radiographic examinations of the radius and ulna, it is important to bear in mind the movements that occur at the joints of the upper limb. The hand can be rotated from the palm facing the table to the palm at right-angles to the table with little or no rotation of the ulna. In this movement, the upper end of the radius rotates about its long axis while the lower end rotates around the lower end of the ulna, carrying the hand with it.

The hinge formed by the trochlear surface of the humerus and the trochlear notch of the ulna prevents rotation of the ulna unless the humerus rotates. If, therefore, the wrist is positioned for a postero-anterior projection and then moved into the position for the lateral simply by rotating the hand, we will obtain two projections of the radius but the same projection of the ulna. To achieve two projections at right-angles of both the radius and the ulna, the two positions must be obtained by rotating the humerus (not simply the hand) through 90 degrees, i.e. there should be no rotation at the radio-ulnar joints.

Thus, there are basically two methods of positioning the wrist for a radiographic examination of the lower end of radius and ulna, but only one of these will give two projections of both the radius and the ulna.

Method 1

The forearm remains pronated and the change in position from that for the postero-anterior projection to that for the lateral is achieved by rotation of the hand. In this movement, only the radius, and not the ulna, rotates, giving two projections at right-angles to each other of the radius but the same projection each time for the ulna.

Of the two bones, the radius is the more frequently injured, so this positioning method can be used to demonstrate the injury, provided that the patient can rotate the hand. Very often, the patient cannot rotate the hand, so the second method must be used.

Method 2

The change in position is achieved by rotation of the humerus. Because the humerus rotates, so does the ulna. This method therefore gives us two projections at right-angles to each other of the radius and the ulna.

2 Wrist

Postero-anterior

Position of patient and cassette

- The patient is seated alongside the table, with the affected side nearest to the table.
- The elbow joint is flexed to 90 degrees and the arm is abducted, such that the anterior aspect of the forearm and the palm of the hand rest on the cassette.
- If the mobility of the patient permits, the shoulder joint should be at the same height as the forearm.
- The wrist joint is placed on one half of the cassette and adjusted to include the lower part of the radius and ulna and the proximal two-thirds of the metacarpals.
- The fingers are flexed slightly to bring the anterior aspect of the wrist into contact with the cassette.
- The wrist joint is adjusted to ensure that the radial and ulnar styloid processes are equidistant from the cassette.
- The forearm is immobilized using a sandbag.

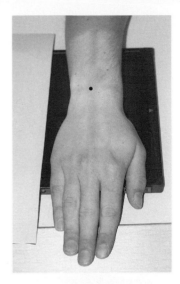

Direction and centring of the X-ray beam

- The vertical central ray is centred to a point midway between the radial and ulnar styloid processes.

Essential image characteristics

- The image should demonstrate the proximal two-thirds of the metacarpals, the carpal bones, and the distal third of the radius and ulna.
- There should be no rotation of the wrist joint.

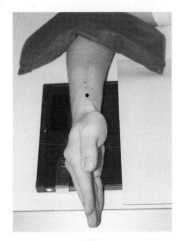

Lateral – method 1

Position of patient and cassette

- From the postero-anterior position, the wrist is externally rotated through 90 degrees, to bring the palm of the hand vertical.
- The wrist joint is positioned over the unexposed half of the cassette to include the lower part of the radius and ulna and the proximal two-thirds of the metacarpals.
- The hand is rotated externally slightly further to ensure that the radial and styloid processes are superimposed.
- The forearm is immobilized using a sandbag.

Direction and centring of the X-ray beam

- The vertical central ray is centred over the styloid process of the radius.

Essential image characteristics

- The exposure should provide adequate penetration to visualize the carpal bones.
- The radial and ulnar styloid processes should be superimposed.

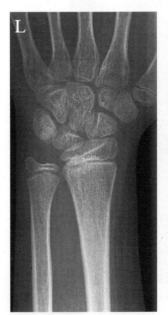

Normal postero-anterior radiograph of wrist

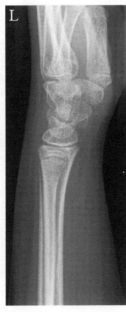

Normal lateral radiograph of wrist, method 1

- The image should demonstrate the proximal two-thirds of the metacarpals, the carpal bones, and the distal third of the radius and ulna.

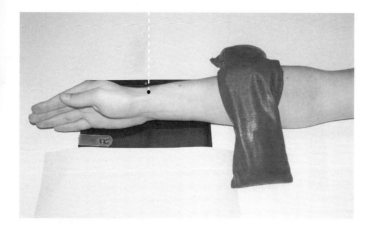

Lateral – method 2

This projection will ensure that both the radius and the ulna will be at right-angles, compared with the postero-anterior projection.

Position of patient and cassette

- From the postero-anterior position, the humerus is externally rotated through 90 degrees.
- The elbow joint is extended to bring the medial aspect of the forearm, wrist and hand into contact with the table.
- The wrist joint is positioned over the unexposed half of the cassette to include the lower part of the radius and ulna and the proximal two-thirds of the metacarpals.
- The hand is rotated externally slightly further to ensure that the radial and styloid processes are superimposed.
- The forearm is immobilized using a sandbag.

Direction and centring of the X-ray beam

- The vertical central ray is centred over the styloid process of the radius.

Essential image characteristics

- The exposure should provide adequate penetration to visualize the carpal bones.
- The radial and ulnar styloid processes should be superimposed.
- The image should demonstrate the proximal two-thirds of the metacarpals, the carpal bones and the distal third of the radius and ulna.

Notes

- If the patient's limb is immobilized in plaster of Paris, then it may be necessary to modify the positioning of the patient to obtain accurate postero-anterior and lateral projections. Increased exposure factors will be necessary to penetrate the plaster, and the resultant image will be of reduced contrast.
- Light-weight plasters constructed from a polyester knit fabric are radio-lucent and require exposure factors similar to uncasted areas.

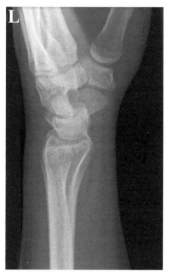

Normal lateral radiograph of wrist, method 2

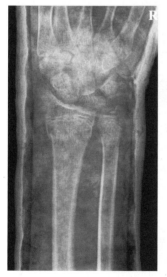

Postero-anterior radiograph of wrist through conventional plaster

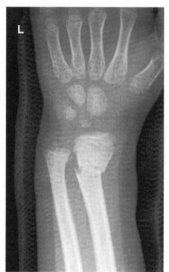

Postero-anterior radiograph of wrist through light-weight plaster

Oblique (anterior oblique)

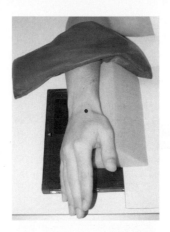

Position of patient and cassette

- The patient is seated alongside the table, with the affected side nearest to the table.
- The elbow joint is flexed to 90 degrees and the arm is abducted, such that the anterior aspect of the forearm and the palm of the hand rest on the tabletop.
- If the mobility of the patient permits, then the shoulder joint should be at the same height as the forearm.
- The wrist joint is placed on the cassette and adjusted to include the lower part of the radius and ulna and the proximal two-thirds of the metacarpals.
- The hand is externally rotated through 45 degrees and supported in this position using a non-opaque pad.
- The forearm is immobilized using a sandbag.

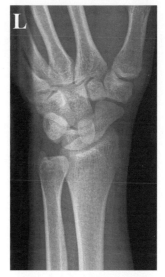

Direction and centring of the X-ray beam

- The vertical central ray is centred midway between the radial and ulnar styloid processes.

Essential image characteristics

- The exposure should provide adequate penetration to visualize the carpal bones.
- The image should demonstrate the proximal two-thirds of the metacarpals, the carpal bones, and the distal third of the radius and ulna.

Normal anterior oblique radiograph of wrist

Notes

- This projection results in an additional oblique projection of the metacarpals, the carpal bones and lower end of the radius. To obtain an additional projection of the lower end of the ulna, it is necessary to rotate the humerus (see Wrist, lateral – method 2, p. 57).
- The three projections, postero-anterior, lateral and oblique, may all be taken on the same cassette using lead rubber to mask off all but the one-third of the cassette being used.

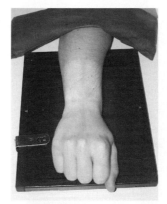
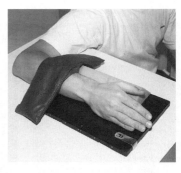

Radiological considerations

- Fracture of the distal radius can be undisplaced, dorsally angulated (Colles' fracture) or ventrally angulated (Smith's fracture). The importance of Smith's fracture lies in the fact that it is less stable than Colles' fracture.
- Dislocations of the carpus are uncommon, but again they carry potential for serious disability. One manifestation of lunate dislocation is an increased gap between it and the scaphoid, which will be missed if the wrist is rotated on the postero-anterior projection.

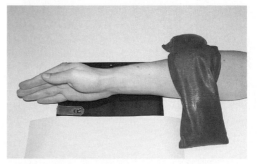

To change the projection of the ulna, the arm must be rotated as shown in the three photographs above

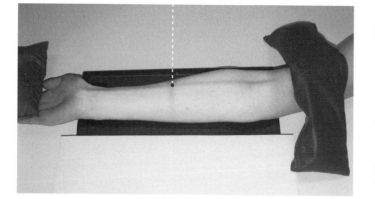

Two projections (antero-posterior and lateral) are required at right-angles to each other to demonstrate the full length of the radius and ulna to include both the elbow and the wrist joint.

The antero-posterior projection with the forearm supinated demonstrates the radius and ulna lying side by side.

A 24 × 30-cm cassette with high-resolution screens may be used and positioned to include both joints on one image. Both projections are normally acquired on one film, with the half of the film not in use being shielded with by lead rubber.

Antero-posterior – basic

Position of patient and cassette

- The patient is seated alongside the table, with the affected side nearest to the table.
- The arm is abducted and the elbow joint is fully extended, with the supinated forearm resting on the table.
- The shoulder is lowered to the same level as the elbow joint.
- The cassette is placed under the forearm to include the wrist joint and the elbow joint.
- The arm is adjusted such that the radial and ulnar styloid processes and the medial and lateral epicondyles are equidistant from the cassette.
- The lower end of the humerus and the hand are immobilized using sandbags.

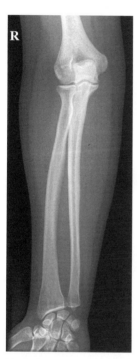

Normal antero-posterior radiograph of forearm

Direction and centring of the X-ray beam

- The vertical central ray is centred in the midline of the forearm to a point midway between the wrist and elbow joints.

Essential image characteristics

- Both the elbow and the wrist joint must be demonstrated on the cassette.
- Both joints should be seen in the true antero-posterior position, with the radial and ulnar styloid processes and the epicondyles of the humerus equidistant from the cassette.

Note

The postero-anterior projection of the forearm with the wrist pronated is not satisfactory because, in this projection, the radius is superimposed over the ulna for part of its length.

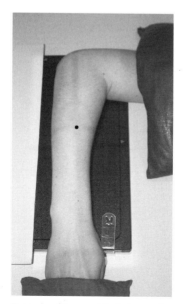

Example of incorrect technique – the radius is superimposed in the postero-anterior projection

Forearm

Lateral – basic

Position of patient and cassette

- From the antero-posterior position, the elbow is flexed to 90 degrees.
- The humerus is internally rotated to 90 degrees to bring the medial aspect of the upper arm, elbow, forearm, wrist and hand into contact with the table.
- The cassette is placed under the forearm to include the wrist joint and the elbow joint.
- The arm is adjusted such that the radial and ulnar styloid processes and the medial and lateral epicondyles are superimposed.
- The lower end of the humerus and the hand are immobilized using sandbags.

Direction and centring of the X-ray beam

- The vertical central ray is centred in the midline of the forearm to a point midway between the wrist and elbow joints.

Essential image characteristics

- Both the elbow and the wrist joint must be demonstrated on the image.
- Both joints should be seen in the true lateral position, with the radial and ulnar styloid processes and the epicondyles of the humerus superimposed.

Notes

- In trauma cases, it may be impossible to move the arm into the positions described, and a modified technique may need to be employed to ensure that two projections at right-angles to each other are obtained.
- If the limb cannot be moved through 90 degrees, then a horizontal beam should be used.
- Both joints should be included on each image.
- No attempt should be made to rotate the patient's hand.

Radiological considerations

- When two or more bones such as the radius and ulna form a ring, fracture of one of the bones is often associated with fracture or dislocation elsewhere in the ring, especially if the fracture is displaced or the bone ends overlap. In Galeazzi fracture there is a fracture of the radius with dislocation of the distal ulna, while in Monteggia fracture there is fracture of the ulna with dislocation of the head of the radius. In forearm fracture, therefore, both ends of both bones, as well as the proximal and distal radio-ulnar joints, must be demonstrated.
- General forearm projections do not give adequate views of the elbow and should not be relied upon for diagnosis of radial head injury.
- If an elbow joint effusion is shown, formal projections of the elbow joint will be required.

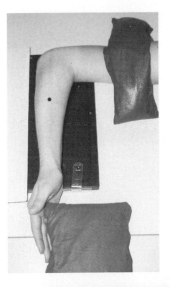

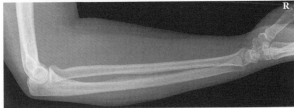

Normal basic lateral radiograph of forearm

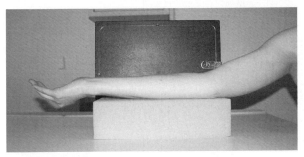

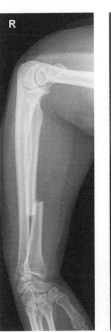 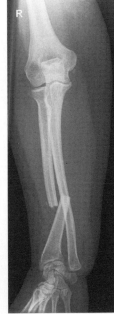

Lateral projection   Antero-posterior projection
Radiographs of the forearm showing Galeazzi fracture

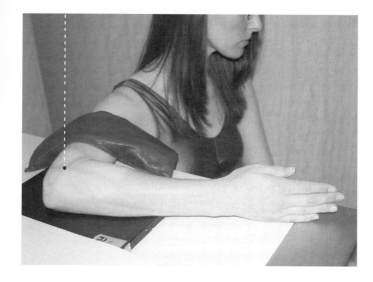

The most satisfactory projections of the elbow joint are obtained when the upper arm is in the same plane as the forearm. For many examinations, the patient will be seated at the table with the shoulder lowered, so that the upper arm, elbow and forearm are on the same horizontal level. To gain the patient's confidence, the lateral projection is taken first, because the patient will find it easier to adopt this position. In changing the position from that for the lateral projection to that for the antero-posterior projection, the humerus must be rotated through 90 degrees to make sure that two projections at right-angles are obtained of the humerus as well as the ulna and radius. Alternatively, if the limb cannot be moved, two projections at right-angles to each other can be taken by keeping the limb in the same position and moving the tube through 90 degrees between projections.

For the lateral projection, the central ray should pass parallel to a line joining the epicondyles of the humerus. For the antero-posterior projection, the central ray should pass at right-angles to this line. In some instances, tube angulation will be necessary.

If the patient cannot extend the elbow fully, modified positioning is necessary for the antero-posterior projection.

Special care should be taken with the child suffering from a supracondylar fracture of the humerus, when basic projections should not be attempted.

Basic lateral and antero-posterior projections can be taken on the same cassette using lead rubber to mask off each half of the cassette in turn. For each projection, care should be taken to place the elbow in the centre of the half of the film being used, so that the two projections of the joint are at the same eye level when viewed.

Lateral

Position of patient and cassette

- The patient is seated alongside the table, with the affected side nearest to the table.
- The elbow is flexed to 90 degrees and the palm of the hand is rotated so that it is at 90 degrees to the tabletop.
- The shoulder is lowered so that it is at the same height as the elbow and wrist, such that the medial aspect of the entire arm is in contact with the tabletop.
- The half of the cassette being used is placed under the patient's elbow, with its centre to the elbow joint and its short axis parallel to the forearm.
- The limb is immobilized using sandbags.

Direction and centring of the X-ray beam

- The vertical central ray is centred over the lateral epicondyle of the humerus.

Essential image characteristics

- The central ray must pass through the joint space at 90 degrees to the humerus, i.e. the epicondyles should be superimposed.
- The image should demonstrate the distal third of humerus and the proximal third of the radius and ulna.

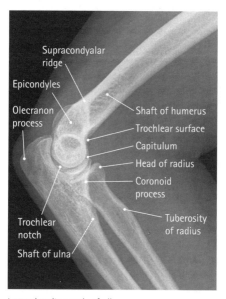

Lateral radiograph of elbow

Supracondyalar ridge
Epicondyles
Olecranon process
Shaft of humerus
Trochlear surface
Capitulum
Head of radius
Coronoid process
Trochlear notch
Tuberosity of radius
Shaft of ulna

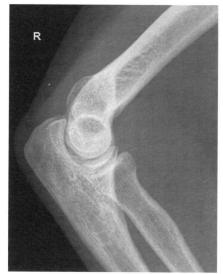

Normal lateral radiograph of elbow

2 | Elbow

Antero-posterior

Position of patient and cassette

- From the lateral position, the patient's arm is externally rotated.
- The arm is then extended fully, such that the posterior aspect of the entire limb is in contact with the tabletop and the palm of the hand is facing upwards.
- The unexposed half of the cassette is positioned under the elbow joint, with its short axis parallel to the forearm.
- The arm is adjusted such that the medial and lateral epicondyles are equidistant from the cassette.
- The limb is immobilized using sandbags.

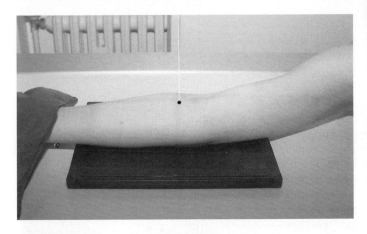

Direction and centring of the X-ray beam

- The vertical central ray is centred through the joint space 2.5 cm distal to the point midway between the medial and lateral epicondyles of the humerus.

Essential image characteristics

- The central ray must pass through the joint space at 90 degrees to the humerus to provide a satisfactory view of the joint space.
- The image should demonstrate the distal third of humerus and the proximal third of the radius and ulna.

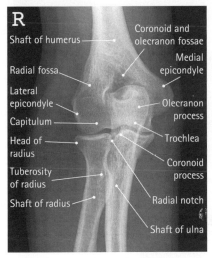

Antero-posterior radiograph of elbow

Notes

- Care should be taken when a supracondylar fracture of the humerus is suspected. In such cases, no attempt should be made to extend the elbow joint, and a modified technique must be employed.
- When the patient is unable to extend the elbow to 90 degrees, a modified technique is used for the antero-posterior projection.
- If the limb cannot be moved, two projections at right-angles to each other can be taken by keeping the limb in the same position and rotating the X-ray tube through 90 degrees.

Antero-posterior – partial flexion

If the patient is unable to extend the elbow fully, the positioning for the antero-posterior projection may be modified. For a general survey of the elbow, or if the main area of interest is the proximal end of the radius and ulna, then the posterior aspect of the forearm should be in contact with the cassette. If the main area of interest is the distal end of the humerus, however, then the posterior aspect of the humerus should be in contact with the cassette.

If the elbow is immobilized in the fully flexed position, then an axial projection must be used instead of the antero-posterior projection.

In both of the above cases, some superimposition of the bones will occur. However, gross injury and general alignment can be demonstrated.

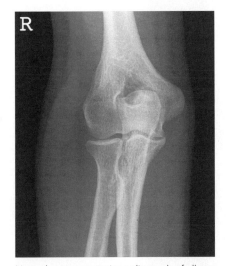

Normal antero-posterior radiograph of elbow

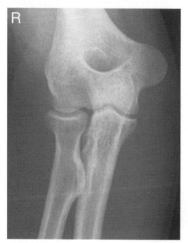

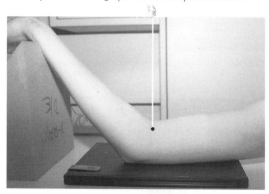

Antero-posterior radiograph of elbow in partial flexion

Antero-posterior – forearm in contact

Position of patient and cassette

- The patient is seated alongside the table, with the affected side nearest to the table.
- The posterior aspect of the forearm is placed on the table, with the palm of the hand facing upwards.
- The cassette is placed under the forearm, with its centre under the elbow joint.
- The arm is adjusted such that the medial and lateral epicondyles of the humerus are equidistant from the cassette.
- The limb is supported and immobilized in this position.

Direction and centring of the X-ray beam

- The vertical central ray is centred in the midline of the forearm 2.5 cm distal to the crease of the elbow.

Essential image characteristics

- The image should demonstrate the distal third of humerus and the proximal third of the radius and ulna.

Antero-posterior – upper arm in contact

Position of patient and cassette

- The patient is seated alongside the table, with the affected side nearest to the table.
- The posterior aspect of the humerus is placed on the table, with the palm of the hand facing upwards.
- The cassette is placed under the forearm, with its centre under the elbow joint.
- The arm is adjusted such that the medial and lateral epicondyles of the humerus are equidistant from the film.
- The limb is supported and immobilized in this position.

Direction and centring of the X-ray beam

- The vertical central ray is centred midway between the epicondyles of the humerus.

Essential image characteristics

- The image should demonstrate the distal third of humerus and the proximal third of the radius and ulna.

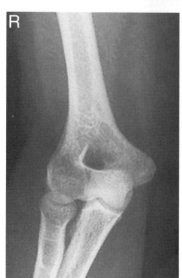

Antero-posterior radiograph of elbow – upper arm in contact with the cassette

Full flexion

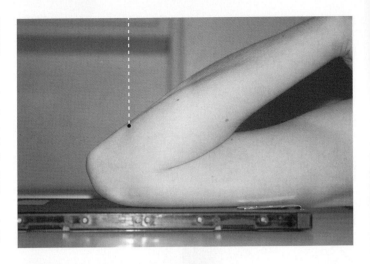

When the patient's elbow is immobilized in full flexion, an axial projection may be substituted for the antero-posterior projection.

It is preferable for the patient's upper arm to be in contact with the cassette for examination of the distal end of the humerus and olecranon process of the ulna, and for the forearm to be in contact with the cassette if the proximal ends of the radius and ulna are to be examined.

In either of these cases, the bones of the forearm will be superimposed on the humerus. However, gross injury and general alignment can be demonstrated.

Axial – upper arm in contact

Position of patient and cassette

- The patient is seated alongside the table, with the affected side nearest to the table.
- The elbow is fully flexed, and the palm of the hand is facing the shoulder.
- The posterior aspect of the upper arm is placed on the cassette, with the arm parallel to the long axis of the cassette.
- The patient's trunk is adjusted in order to bring the medial and lateral epicondyles of the humerus equidistant to the cassette.

Direction and centring of the X-ray beam

- For the lower end of the humerus and the olecranon process of ulna, the vertical central ray is centred 5 cm distal to the olecranon process.
- For the proximal ends of the radius and ulna, including the radio-humeral joint, the central ray is directed at right-angles to the forearm and centred 5 cm distal to the olecranon process.

Essential image characteristics

- The image will include the olecranon process and the lower third of the radius and ulna superimposed on the lower third of the humerus.
- The exposure should be adequate to visualize all three bones.

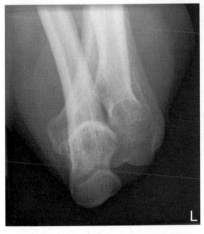

Axial radiograph of elbow – upper arm in contact with the cassette

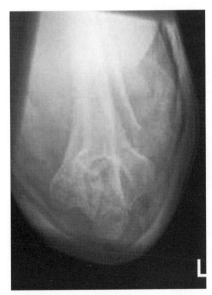

Axial radiograph of elbow – arm in plaster cast with upper arm in contact with the cassette

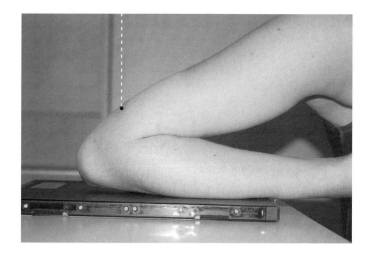

Axial – forearm in contact

Position of patient and cassette

- The patient is seated alongside the table, with the affected side nearest to the table.
- The elbow is fully flexed and the palm of the hand is facing upwards.
- The forearm is fully supinated, with the posterior aspect of the forearm resting on the cassette and the arm parallel to the long axis of the cassette.
- The patient's trunk is adjusted in order to bring the medial and lateral epicondyles of the humerus equidistant to the cassette.

Direction and centring of the X-ray beam

- For the proximal ends of the radius and ulna and the radio-humeral joint, the vertical central ray is directed to a point on the posterior aspect of the upper arm 5 cm proximal to the olecranon process.
- For the lower end of the humerus and the olecranon process of the ulna, the central ray is directed at right-angles to the upper arm centred to a point 5 cm proximal to the olecranon process.

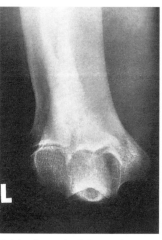

Axial radiograph of elbow – forearm in contact with the cassette

Lateral head of radius

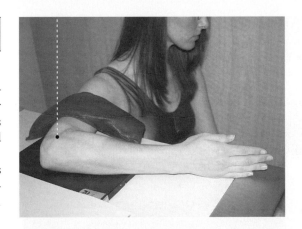

An 18 × 24-cm cassette with high-resolution screens is used for a single projection. Alternatively, an 18 × 43-cm cassette is chosen for multiple projections. A lead-rubber sheet may be used to mask off the area of the cassette not currently in use.

The elbow is positioned as for the lateral elbow. The hand is then moved through different degrees of rotation, enabling visualization of small fissure fractures through the head of the radius.

Position of patient and cassette

- For the first projection, the patient is positioned as for a lateral elbow projection, with the palm of the hand vertical. The forearm is immobilized using a sandbag.
- For the second exposure, the upper arm and elbow are maintained in the same position, whilst the hand is rotated medially until the palm of the hand rests on the table. The forearm is immobilized using a sandbag.
- For the third exposure, the upper arm and elbow are maintained in the same position, whilst the hand is rotated further medially, until the palm of the hand is vertical, facing away from the body. The forearm is immobilized using a sandbag.

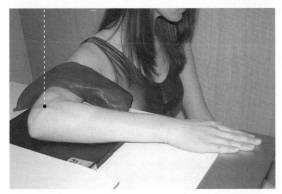

Direction and centring of the X-ray beam

- In each case, the vertical central ray is centred to the lateral epicondyle of the humerus.

Essential image characteristics

- The elbow joint should be seen in the true lateral position in each projection.
- Sufficient detail of bony trabeculae should be demonstrated to enable fine fractures to be detected.

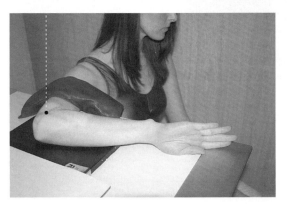

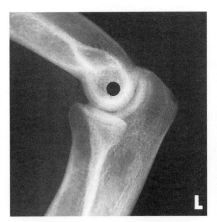

Lateral radiograph of elbow for head of radius – palm at right angles to the table

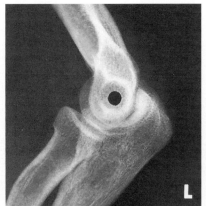

Lateral radiograph of elbow for head of radius – palm in contact with the table

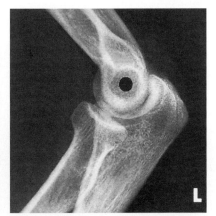

Lateral radiograph of elbow for head of radius – palm facing away from the trunk

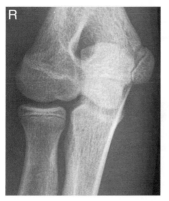

Proximal radio-ulnar joint – oblique

An 18 × 24-cm cassette with high-resolution screens is used.

Position of patient and cassette

- The patient is positioned for an anterior projection of the elbow joint.
- The cassette is positioned under the elbow joint, with the long axis of the cassette parallel to the forearm.
- The humerus is then rotated laterally (or the patient leans towards the side under examination) until the line between the epicondyles is approximately 20 degrees to the cassette.
- The forearm is immobilized using a sandbag.

Direction and centring of the X-ray beam

- The vertical central ray is centred 2.5 cm distal to the mid-point between the epicondyles.

Essential image characteristics

- The image should demonstrate clearly the joint space between the radius and the ulna.

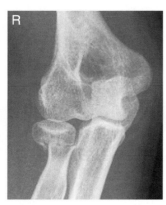

Normal   Fracture radial head
Oblique radiographs of elbow to show proximal radio-ulnar joint

Ulnar groove – axial

The ulnar groove through which the ulnar nerve passes lies between the medial epicondyle and the medial lip of the trochlear of the humerus and is a possible site for ulnar nerve compression.

A modified axial projection with the elbow joint fully flexed demonstrates the groove and any lateral shift of the ulna, which would lead to tightening of the ligaments overlying the ulnar nerve. An 18 × 24-cm cassette with high-resolution screens is used.

Position of patient and cassette

- The patient is seated alongside the X-ray table, with the affected side nearest the table.
- The elbow is fully flexed, and the posterior aspect of the upper arm is placed in contact with the tabletop.
- The cassette is positioned under the lower end of the humerus, with its centre midway between the epicondyles of the humerus.
- With the elbow still fully flexed, the arm is externally rotated through 45 degrees and supported in this position.

Direction and centring of the X-ray beam

- The vertical central ray is centred over the medial epicondyle of the humerus.

Essential image characteristics

- The exposure is chosen to demonstrate the ulnar groove in profile.

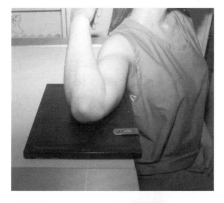

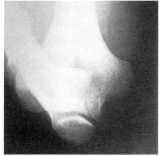

Radiograph of elbow showing ulnar groove

Note

A well-collimated beam is used to reduce degradation of the image by scattered radiation.

Radiological considerations

- An effusion is a useful marker of disease and may be demonstrated in trauma, infection and inflammatory conditions. It is seen as an elevation of the fat pads anteriorly and posteriorly (see below) and requires a good lateral projection with no rotation. It may be an important clue to otherwise occult fracture of the radial head or a supracondylar fracture of the humerus.
- Radial head fracture may be nearly or completely occult, showing as the slightest cortical infraction or trabecular irregularity at the neck or just a joint effusion.
- Avulsion of one of the epicondyles of the humerus may be missed if the avulsed bone is hidden over other bone or in the olecranon or coronoid fossae. Recognition of their absence requires knowledge of when and where they should be seen.

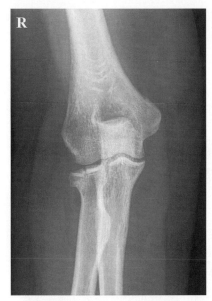

Antero-posterior radiograph of elbow showing vertical fracture of the head of the radius

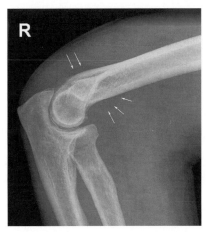

Lateral radiograph of elbow showing elevation of anterior and posterior fat pads

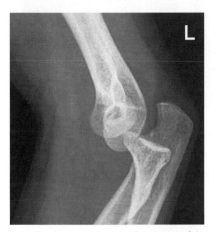

Lateral radiograph showing dislocation of the elbow

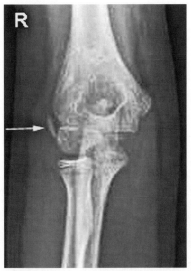

Antero-posterior radiograph of elbow showing avulsion injury of the lateral epicondyle

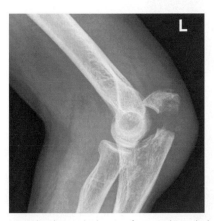

Lateral radiograph showing fracture through the olecranon process, with displacement due to triceps muscle pull

A type of injury commonly found in children is a fracture of the lower end of the humerus just proximal to the condyles. The injury is very painful and even small movements of the limb can

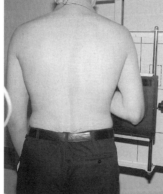

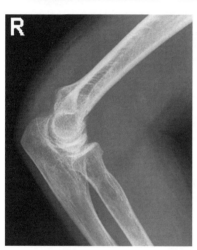

Lateral radiograph of elbow showing undisplaced supracondylar fracture

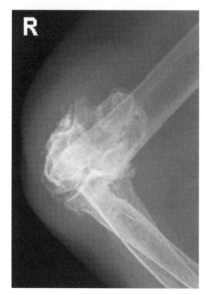

Lateral radiograph of elbow showing supracondylar fracture with displacement and bone disruption

exacerbate the injury, causing further damage to adjacent nerves and blood vessels.

Any supporting sling should not be removed, and the patient should not be asked to extend the elbow joint or to rotate the arm or forearm.

A 24 × 30-cm cassette is used.

Lateral

Position of patient and cassette

Method 1

- The patient sits or stands facing the X-ray tube.
- A cassette is supported between the patient's trunk and elbow, with the medial aspect of the elbow in contact with the cassette.
- A lead-rubber sheet or other radiation protection device is positioned to protect the patient's trunk from the primary beam.

Method 2

- A cassette is supported vertically in a cassette holder.
- The patient stands sideways, with the elbow flexed and the lateral aspect of the injured elbow in contact with the cassette. The arm is gently extended backwards from the shoulder. The patient is rotated forwards until the elbow is clear of the rib cage but still in contact with the cassette, with the line joining the epicondyles of the humerus at right-angles to the cassette.

Direction and centring of the X-ray beam

Method 1

- The X-ray tube is angled so that the central ray is directed perpendicular to the shaft of the humerus and centred to the lateral epicondyle.

Method 2

- The horizontal central ray is directed to the medial epicondyle and the beam collimated to the elbow.

Essential image characteristics

- The image should include the lower end of the humerus and the upper third of the radius and ulna.

Notes

- The patient should be made as comfortable as possible to assist immobilization.
- An erect cassette holder, or similar device, may be used to assist the patient in supporting the cassette.
- The X-ray beam should be collimated carefully to ensure that the primary beam does not extend beyond the area of the cassette.

Humerus – supracondylar fracture

Antero-posterior

As in the lateral projection, the cassette is held in a vertical cassette holder with the patient either standing or sitting during the procedure.

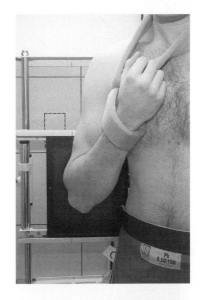

Position of patient and cassette

- From the lateral position, the patient's upper body is rotated towards the affected side.
- The cassette is placed in an erect cassette holder, and the patient's position is adjusted so that the posterior aspect of the upper arm is in contact with the cassette.

Direction and centring of the X-ray beam

- If the elbow joint is fully flexed, the central ray is directed at right-angles to the humerus to pass through the forearm to a point midway between the epicondyles of the humerus.
- If the elbow joint is only partially flexed, the central ray is directed at right-angles to the humerus to a point midway between the epicondyles of the humerus without first passing through the forearm.

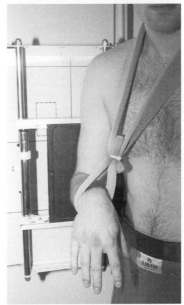

Essential image characteristics

- If the elbow joint is fully flexed, sufficient exposure must be selected to provide adequate penetration of the forearm.

Notes

- It is essential that no movement of the elbow joint occurs during positioning of the patient.
- Particular attention should be paid to radiation protection measures.

Radiological considerations

- Signs of supracondylar fracture can be very subtle. Demonstration of the position of the condyles in relation to the anterior cortical line of the humeral shaft may be crucial and demands a true lateral image.

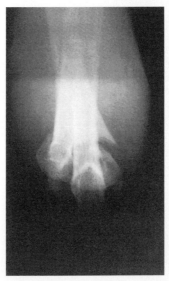

Antero-posterior radiograph in full flexion showing supracondylar fracture

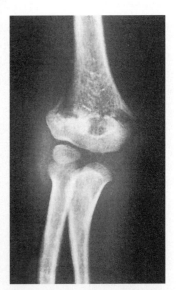

Antero-posterior radiograph in partial flexion showing supracondylar fracture

Antero-posterior – supine

A 35 × 43-cm cassette fitted with regular-speed screens can be used, providing it is large enough to demonstrate the elbow and shoulder joint on one film. To reduce the risk of patient movement, exposures are made on arrested respiration.

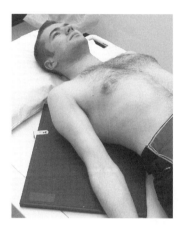
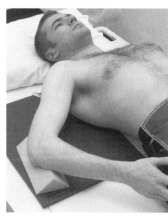

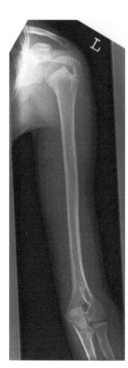
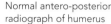
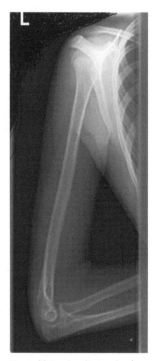

Normal antero-posterior radiograph of humerus

Normal lateral radiograph of humerus

When movement of the patient's arm is restricted, a modified technique may be required.

Position of patient and cassette

- The patient lies supine on the X-ray table, with the unaffected side raised and supported on pads.
- The cassette is positioned under the affected limb and adjusted to include the shoulder and elbow joints.
- The arm is slightly abducted and the elbow joint is fully extended, so that the posterior aspect of the upper arm is in contact with the cassette.
- The arm is adjusted to ensure that the medial and lateral epicondyles are equidistant from the cassette.
- The forearm is immobilized using a sandbag.

Direction and centring of the X-ray beam

- The vertical central ray is centred to a point midway between the shoulder and elbow joints.

Lateral – supine

Position of patient and cassette

- From the antero-posterior position, the elbow joint is flexed to 90 degrees.
- The arm is abducted and then medially rotated through 90 degrees to bring the medial aspect of the arm, elbow and forearm in contact with the table.
- The cassette is placed under the arm and adjusted to include both the shoulder and the elbow joints.
- The humerus is adjusted to ensure that the medial and lateral epicondyles of the humerus are superimposed.
- The forearm is immobilized using a sandbag.

Direction and centring of the X-ray beam

- The vertical central ray is centred to a point midway between the shoulder and elbow joints.

Notes

- When rotating the humerus, it is essential to ensure that the forearm and hand rest on the tabletop and not the trunk.
- The humerus is normally examined with the patient erect and the cassette placed in an erect cassette holder. The radiographic technique is similar (except that a horizontal central ray is used) but additional care should be taken to ensure that the patient is immobilized adequately, as described below.

Essential image characteristics

- Both joints should be seen on the image.
- The elbow joint should be seen in the true lateral and antero-posterior positions.

Humerus – shaft

Antero-posterior – erect

Position of patient and cassette

- The cassette is placed in an erect cassette holder.
- The patient sits or stands with their back in contact with the cassette.
- The patient is rotated towards the affected side to bring the posterior aspect of the shoulder, upper arm and elbow into contact with the cassette.
- The position of the patient is adjusted to ensure that the medial and lateral epicondyles of the humerus are equidistant from the cassette.

Direction and centring of the X-ray beam

- The central ray is directed at right-angles to the shaft of the humerus and centred midway between the shoulder and elbow joints.

Lateral – erect

If the arm is immobilized in order to obtain a true lateral projection, i.e. one that is at right-angles to the antero-posterior, then it will be necessary to have the patient's median sagittal plane parallel to the cassette and the lateral aspect of the injured arm in contact with the cassette, and to direct the horizontal central ray through the thorax to the injured arm. This has the disadvantage that the ribs and lungs will be superimposed on the humerus, obscuring details of the injury and signs of healing and adding to the radiation dose to the patient. The position described, although not fully at right-angles to the antero-posterior projection, avoids this superimposition.

Position of patient and cassette

- The cassette is placed in an erect cassette holder.
- From the anterior position, the patient is rotated through 90 degrees until the lateral aspect of the injured arm is in contact with the cassette.
- The patient is now rotated further until the arm is just clear of the rib cage but still in contact with the cassette.

Direction and centring of the X-ray beam

- The horizontal central ray is directed at right-angles to the shaft of the humerus and centred midway between the shoulder and elbow joint.

Essential image characteristics

- The exposure should be adjusted to ensure that the area of interest is clearly visualized.

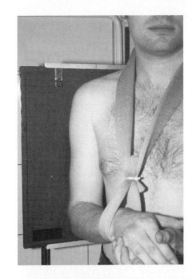

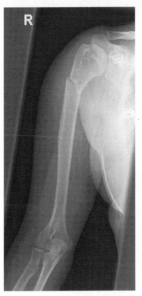

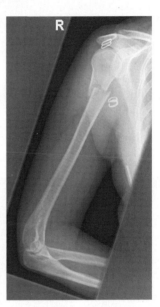

Antero-posterior radiograph of humerus showing a fracture of the proximal shaft of the humerus

Lateral radiograph of the humerus in the same patient

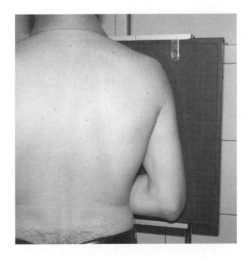

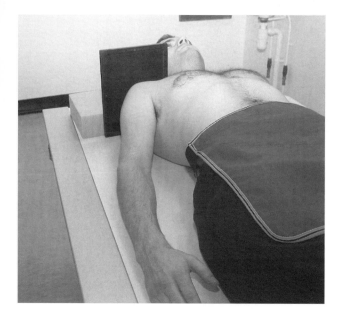

The intertuberous sulcus or bicipital groove is situated between the greater and lesser tuberosities of the humerus. It transmits the tendon of the long head of the biceps.

An 18 × 24-cm cassette with high-resolution screens is used.

Axial

Position of patient and cassette

- The patient lies supine on the X-ray table.
- The cassette is supported vertically above the shoulder.
- The arm is rested on the tabletop with the palm of the hand facing the patient's side and the line joining the epicondyles of the humerus at 45 degrees to the table.

Direction and centring of the X-ray beam

- The central ray is directed almost horizontally and centred to the anterior part of the head of the humerus.

Essential image characteristics

- The sulcus should be seen in profile, and the exposure is such as to demonstrate lesions within or impingements on the sulcus.

Notes

- To reduce the risk of patient movement, the exposure is made on arrested respiration.
- The exposure is adjusted to demonstrate soft-tissue structures within the sulcus.

Alternative axial projection

Direction and centring of the X-ray beam

- The patient sits with their shoulder joint against a vertical cassette holder.
- Ideally, this holder should be angled 15 degrees forwards, but if this facility is not available the cassette can be supported above the shoulder.
- The arm is abducted anteriorly and supported to bring the long axis of the shaft of the humerus perpendicular to the cassette.
- The hand is rotated 45 degrees laterally from the prone position to bring the bicipital groove in profile with the central beam.

Direction and centring of the X-ray beam

- The central ray is directed cranially along the long axis of the humerus and centred to the anterior part of the head of the humerus. The beam is collimated to the humeral head.

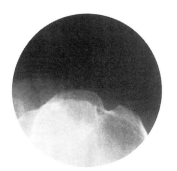

Radiograph of bicipital groove taken with standard technique

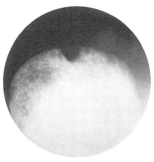

Radiograph of bicipital groove taken with alternative technique

2 Humerus – neck

The most common reason for radiography of the neck of the humerus is suspected fracture, either pathological or traumatic.

Two projections at right-angles are necessary: an antero-posterior and an axial or a lateral projection. Movement of the arm may be limited, and the technique may need to be modified accordingly. Where possible, the supporting sling should be removed.

Depending on the condition of the patient, the examination may be undertaken with the patient erect, providing adequate immobilization is used, supine on the X-ray table, or, in cases of multiple trauma, on a trolley.

The exposure is made on arrested respiration.

A 24 × 30-cm cassette fitted with a regular-speed screen is used.

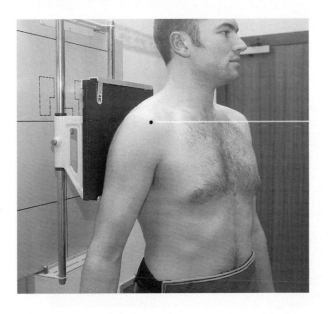

Antero-posterior

Position of patient and cassette

- The patient stands or lies supine facing the X-ray tube.
- The patient is rotated towards the affected side to bring the posterior aspect of the injured shoulder into contact with the midline of the cassette.
- The cassette is positioned to include the acromion process and the proximal half of the humerus.

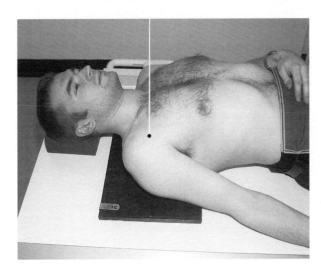

Direction and centring of the X-ray beam

- The central ray is directed at right-angles to the humerus and centred to the head of the humerus.

Essential image characteristics

- The image should include the acromion process and proximal half of the shaft of the humerus.
- The exposure should demonstrate adequately the neck of the humerus clear of the thorax.

Notes

- Exposure should be made on arrested respiration.
- The patient should immobilize the affected forearm by supporting its weight with the other arm. If the patient is supine, a sandbag should be placed over the forearm.

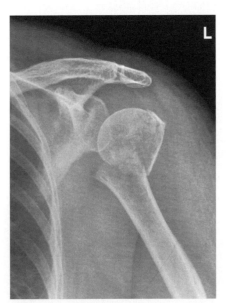

Antero-posterior radiograph of neck of humerus taken erect to show fracture of the neck of the humerus

Axial projection

Positioning for the lateral projection will depend on how much movement of the arm is possible.

If the patient is able to abduct the arm, then a supero-inferior projection is recommended with the patient sitting at the end of the X-ray table. Alternatively, if the patient is lying on a trolley, then an infero-superior projection is acquired. If, however, the arm is fully immobilized, then an alternative lateral oblique (as for the lateral scapula) may be taken.

Lateral – supero-inferior

This projection can be taken even when only a small degree of abduction is possible. It is important that no attempt should be made to increase the amount of movement that the patient is able or willing to make.

An 18 × 24-cm cassette is selected.

Position of patient and cassette

- The patient is seated at one end of the table, with the trunk leaning towards the table, the arm of the side being examined in its maximum abduction, and the elbow resting on the table.
- The height of the table is adjusted to enable the patient to adopt a comfortable position and to maximize full coverage of the neck of the humerus and the shoulder joint.
- The cassette rests on the table between the elbow and the trunk.

Direction and centring of the X-ray beam

- The vertical central ray is directed from above to the acromion process of the scapula.
- Owing to increased object-to-cassette distance, a small focal spot together with an increased FFD should be selected.

Essential image characteristics

- The image should include the acromion and coracoid processes, the glenoid cavity and the proximal head and neck of the humerus.
- The exposure should demonstrate adequately the neck of the humerus.

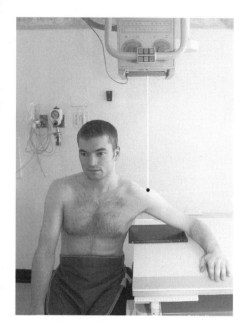

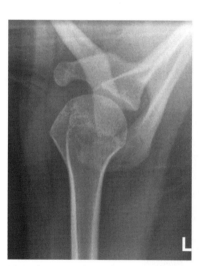

Normal supero-inferior projection to show neck of humerus

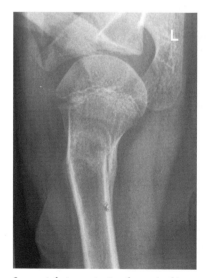

Supero-inferior projection for neck of humerus, showing healing angulated fracture of proximal shaft of humerus

Humerus – neck

Lateral – infero-superior

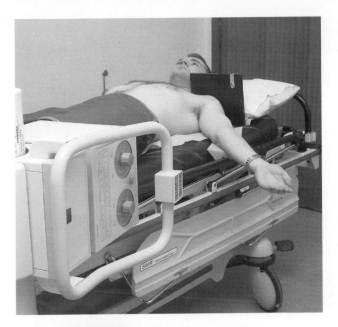

This projection is usually undertaken with the patient supine on a trolley or the X-ray table.

Position of patient and cassette

- The patient lies supine on the trolley, with the arm of the affected side abducted as much as possible (ideally at right-angles to the trunk), the palm of the hand facing upwards, and the medial and lateral epicondyles of the humerus equidistant from the tabletop.
- The shoulder and arm are raised slightly on non-opaque pads, and a cassette supported vertically against the shoulder is pressed against the neck to include as much of the scapula as possible in the image.

Direction and centring of the X-ray beam

The horizontal central ray is directed upwards and centred to the patient's axilla with minimum angulation towards the trunk.

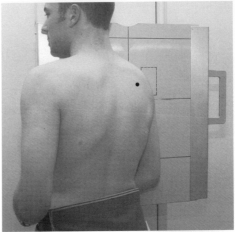

Essential image characteristics

- The image should include the acromion and coracoid processes, the glenoid cavity and the proximal head and neck of the humerus.
- The exposure should demonstrate adequately the neck of the humerus.

Notes

- Exposure should be made on arrested respiration.
- It is important that no attempt is made to increase the amount of movement that the patient is able or willing to make.

Lateral oblique

This projection is used when the arm is immobilized and no abduction of the arm is possible. A vertical Bucky technique may be necessary to improve image quality.

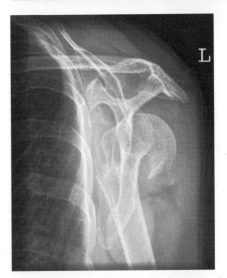

Position of patient and cassette

- The patient stands or sits with the lateral aspect of the injured arm against the cassette or vertical Bucky.
- The patient is rotated forwards until the line joining the medial and lateral borders of the scapula is at right-angles to the cassette.
- The cassette is positioned to include the head of the humerus and the whole scapula.

Lateral oblique projection of neck of humerus, showing fracture

Direction and centring of the X-ray beam

- The horizontal X-ray beam is directed to the medial border of the scapula and centred to the head of the humerus.

Essential image characteristics

- The scapula and the upper end of the humerus should be demonstrated clear of the thoracic cage.

CONTENTS

INTRODUCTION	78
Radiological considerations	78
RECOMMENDED PROJECTIONS	79
BASIC PROJECTIONS	80
Antero-posterior (15 degrees) erect – survey image	81
Supero-inferior (axial)	81
Infero-superior (alternate)	82
OUTLET PROJECTIONS	83
Antero-posterior (outlet projection)	83
Lateral (outlet projection)	84
GLENOHUMERAL JOINT	85
Antero-posterior – erect	85
Antero-posterior – supine (trauma)	86
Lateral oblique 'Y' projection (alternate) dislocation/fracture proximal humerus	86
MODIFICATIONS IN TECHNIQUE (POST-MANIPULATION)	87
Antero-posterior – 25 degrees caudad	87
RECURRENT DISLOCATION	88
Antero-posterior (lateral humerus)	88
Antero-posterior (oblique humerus)	89
Antero-posterior (modified) – Stryker's	90
Infero-superior	90

CALCIFIED TENDONS	91
Antero-posterior	92
Antero-posterior – 25 degrees caudad	93
Infero-superior	93
ACROMIOCLAVICULAR JOINTS	94
Antero-posterior	94
CLAVICLE	95
Postero-anterior – erect (basic)	95
Antero-posterior – supine (alternate)	96
Infero-superior	97
Infero-superior – supine	98
STERNOCLAVICULAR JOINTS	99
Postero-anterior oblique (basic)	99
Semi-prone (alternate)	99
Postero-anterior	100
Lateral	100
SCAPULA	101
Antero-posterior (basic) – erect	101
Lateral (basic)	102
Lateral (alternate)	102
CORACOID PROCESS	103
Antero-posterior (arm abducted)	103

3 Introduction

Radiographic examinations of the shoulder joint and shoulder girdle can be carried out with the patient supine on the X-ray table or trolley, but in most cases it will be more comfortable for the patient to sit or stand with the back of the shoulder in contact with the cassette. The erect position affords ease of positioning, allows the head of humerus to be assessed more accurately for potential impingement syndrome, and can sometimes demonstrate a lipohaemarthrosis where there is a subtle intra-articular fracture.

For radiation protection, particularly of the eyes, the patient's head should be rotated away from the side being examined.

The central ray can be directed caudally after centring to the coracoid process so that the primary beam can be collimated to the area under examination.

For a general survey of the shoulder, e.g. for injury, the field size must be large enough to cover the whole of the shoulder girdle on the injured side. When localized areas are being examined, however, e.g. tendon calcifications or joint spaces, the X-ray beam should be well collimated.

To improve radiographic contrast, a secondary radiation grid can be used for large patients; however, the increased contrast resolution of a computed radiography (CR) imaging system reduces the need for this.

When examining the shoulder joint, it is important to check on the position of the head of the humerus by palpating and positioning the epicondyles at the distal end of the humerus. When the line joining the epicondyles is parallel to the tabletop (or vertical cassette), the humerus is in position for an antero-posterior projection of the head of the humerus. To judge the degree of rotation of the humerus by the position of the hand can be very misleading.

The image appearance is affected significantly by the posture of the patient. If the patient leans back into the cassette, adopting a lordotic stance, then the head of humerus will overlie the acromion process. Conversely, if the patient leans forward, the head of humerus becomes projected inferiorly, appearing to be subluxated.

As in all other skeletal examinations, radiographs showing good bone detail are required to demonstrate minor fractures and bone changes associated with pathology, including injuries to tendon insertions.

Radiological considerations

The rounded humeral head articulates with a rather flat glenoid to maximize the possible range of movement at the joint. The stability of the joint is maintained by the cartilage of the glenoid labrum, ligaments, and the tendons of the rotator cuff. The rotator cuff is four broad tendons encircling the glenohumeral joint. The most superior of these is the supraspinatus, which traverses the subacromial tunnel between the undersurface of the acromion and the upper surface of the humerus to reach its insertion.

Impingement is a common orthopaedic problem occurring when the subacromial space is compromised by degenerative disease, often exacerbated by congenital anomalies of the acromion. The tendon of supraspinatus then becomes compressed between the humerus and the acromion, causing mechanical pain, tendinitis and tendon tears. Radiological signs are non-specific, but radiographs help to assess the width of the subacromial space and the shape of the acromion. It is important that projections of the shoulder in patients with suspected impingement show the subacromial space adequately. Rotation of the patient or incorrect angulation of the beam can obscure the signs.

Tendinitis (inflammation) may cause visible calcification and is seen most frequently in the supraspinatus tendon on a good antero-posterior (AP) projection, although an outlet projection may be a useful addition. The calcification can be obscured by poor technique.

In the various forms of arthritis, the glenohumeral articulation is primarily affected. The width of this joint space is a marker of the severity and progression of disease, and obtaining a projection along the joint line is therefore crucial.

Posterior dislocation is uncommon. Signs on the AP image may be no more than subtle loss of the normal congruity between the glenoid and humeral articular surfaces; therefore, if this is suspected, an axial projection is particularly important.

Detailed examination of the entire shoulder mechanism would require multiple projections. The practitioner must therefore be familiar with the reasons for examination to ensure selection of the appropriate projections to address the clinical problem.

Ultrasound in experienced hands is a valuable tool for assessment of the shoulder, especially for rotator cuff tears. It may be more sensitive than plain radiography for some calcifications. It is often easier to obtain than magnetic resonance imaging (MRI), although it cannot image the glenohumeral joint.

MRI can show all the joint structures, including the rotator cuff, and will be required if there is concern regarding areas not seen well on ultrasound, if ultrasound is equivocal, or if ultrasound expertise is not available.

Unenhanced computed tomography (CT) has a role in assessing the severity of complex fractures around the shoulder.

For recurrent dislocations, accurate imaging of the bony glenoid and labrum, the capsule and glenohumeral ligaments, as well as the rotator cuff is needed. Cross-sectional imaging (MRI or CT) with arthrography is often required.

Shoulder – survey	Antero-posterior (15 degrees) – erect/supine
	Supero-inferior (axial)
	Infero-superior (axial) – alternate
	Antero-posterior – outlet projection
	Lateral oblique – outlet projection
Glenohumeral joint trauma	Antero-posterior – erect
	Antero-posterior – supine
	Lateral oblique 'Y' projection
Post-manipulation	Antero-superior (30 degrees) – 25 degrees caudad
Recurrent dislocation	Antero-posterior (lateral humerus)
	Antero-posterior (oblique humerus)
	Antero-posterior (modified) – Stryker's
	Infero-superior
Calcified tendons	Antero-posterior
	Antero-posterior with medical rotation of the humerus
	Antero-posterior with lateral rotation of the humerus
	Antero-posterior 25 degrees caudad
	Infero-superior
Acromioclavicular joints	Antero-posterior – erect
Clavicle	Postero-anterior – erect
	Antero-posterior – supine (alternate)
	Infero-superior
	Infero-superior – supine (alternate)
Sternoclavicular joints	Postero-anterior oblique – erect
	Postero-anterior oblique – semi-prone (alternate)
Scapula	Antero-posterior – erect
	Lateral – erect
	Lateral – prone (alternate)
Coracoid process	Antero-posterior (arm abducted)
	Supero-inferior (axial)
	Infero-superior (axial) (alternate)

3 Basic projections

It is common practice to obtain two views of the shoulder joint, particularly in cases of suspected dislocation: an antero-posterior (supine) view using a 24 × 30-cm cassette and a supero-inferior (axial) view using an 18 × 24-cm cassette. An avulsion fracture of the greater tuberosity is often seen only on the axial projection.

Modified projections may be undertaken to demonstrate the anterior portion of the acromion process in cases of suspected shoulder impingement syndrome.

These projections may be undertaken with the patient seated or standing, provided that adequate immobilization is used.

If the patient is obese, then the use of a grid cassette or Bucky may improve the contrast of the image but will result in an increased radiation dose.

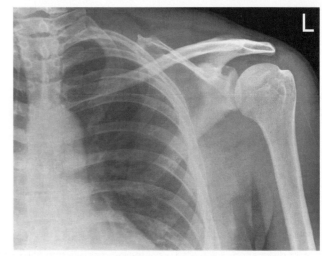

Normal antero-posterior radiograph of shoulder

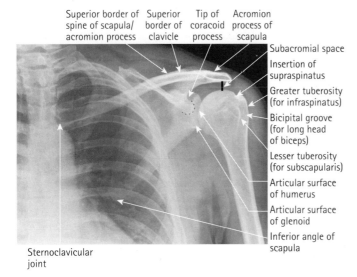

Superior border of spine of scapula/ acromion process — Superior border of clavicle — Tip of coracoid process — Acromion process of scapula — Subacromial space — Insertion of supraspinatus — Greater tuberosity (for infraspinatus) — Bicipital groove (for long head of biceps) — Lesser tuberosity (for subscapularis) — Articular surface of humerus — Articular surface of glenoid — Inferior angle of scapula — Sternoclavicular joint

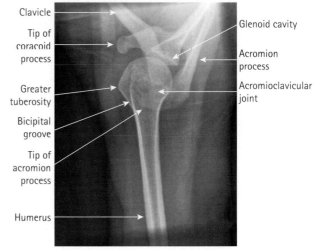

Clavicle — Tip of coracoid process — Greater tuberosity — Bicipital groove — Tip of acromion process — Humerus — Glenoid cavity — Acromion process — Acromioclavicular joint

Antero-posterior (15 degrees) erect – survey image

Position of patient and cassette

- The patient stands with the affected shoulder against the cassette and is rotated 15 degrees to bring the shoulder closer to the cassette and the plane of the acromioclavicular joint parallel to the central beam.

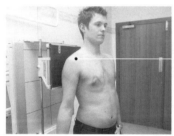

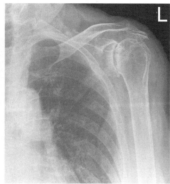

Antero-posterior radiograph of shoulder showing severe arthritic disease

- The arm is supinated and slightly abducted away from the body. The medial and lateral epicondyles of the distal humerus should be parallel to the cassette.
- The cassette is positioned so that its upper border is at least 5 cm above the shoulder to ensure that the oblique rays do not project the shoulder off the cassette.

Direction and centring of the X-ray beam

- The horizontal central ray is directed to the palpable coracoid process of the scapula. The beam can then be directed caudally and collimated.
- The central ray passes through the upper glenoid space to separate the articular surface of the humerus from the acromion process.

Essential image characteristics

- The image should demonstrate the head and proximal end of the humerus, the inferior angle of the scapula and the whole of the clavicle.
- The head of the humerus should be seen slightly overlapping the glenoid cavity but separate from the acromion process.
- Arrested respiration aids good rib detail in acute trauma.

Supero-inferior (axial)

Position of patient and cassette

- The patient is seated at the side of the table, which is lowered to waist level.
- The cassette is placed on the tabletop, and the arm under examination is abducted over the cassette.
- The patient leans towards the table to reduce the object-to-film distance (OFD) and to ensure that the glenoid cavity is included in the image. A curved cassette, if available, can be used to reduce the OFD.
- The elbow can remain flexed, but the arm should be abducted to a minimum of 45 degrees, injury permitting. If only limited abduction is possible, the cassette may be supported on pads to reduce the OFD.

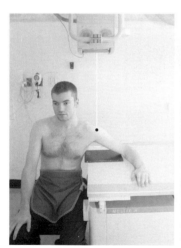

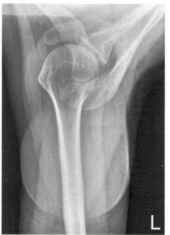

Normal supero-inferior image of the shoulder

Direction and centring of the X-ray beam

- The vertical central ray is directed through the proximal aspect head of the humeral head. Some tube angulation, towards the palm of the hand, may be necessary to coincide with the plane of the glenoid cavity.
- If there is a large OFD, it may be necessary to increase the overall focus-to-film distance (FFD) to reduce magnification.

Basic projections

Infero-superior (alternate)

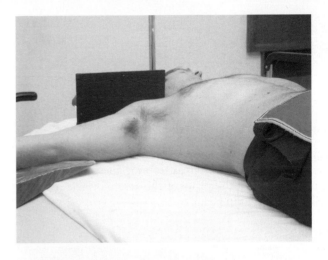

This projection may be used as an alternative to the supero-inferior projection in cases of dislocation or when the patient is supine, since it can be taken even when the patient is able to abduct the arm only slightly. No attempt should be made to increase the amount of abduction that the patient is able and willing to make. An 18 × 24-cm cassette is used.

Position of patient and cassette

- The patient lies supine, with the arm of the affected side slightly abducted and supinated without causing discomfort to the patient.
- The affected shoulder and arm are raised on non-opaque pads.
- A cassette is supported vertically against the shoulder and is pressed against the neck to include as much as possible of the scapula on the film.

Direction and centring of the X-ray beam

- The horizontal central ray is directed towards the axilla with minimum angulation towards the trunk.
- The FFD will probably need to be increased, since the tube head will have to be positioned below the end of the trolley.

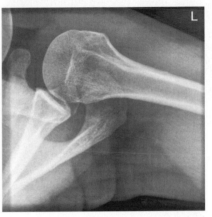

Normal infero-superior radiograph of the shoulder

Essential image characteristics

- The image should demonstrate the head of the humerus, the acromion process, the coracoid process and the glenoid cavity of the scapula.
- The lesser tuberosity will be in profile, and the acromion process and the superior aspect of the glenoid will be seen superimposed on the head of humerus.

Note

The most common type of dislocation of the shoulder is an anterior dislocation, where the head of the humerus displaces below the coracoid process, anterior to the glenoid cavity. Much rarer is a posterior dislocation. In some instances, although the antero-posterior projection shows little or no evidence of a posterior dislocation, it can always be demonstrated in an infero-superior or supero-inferior projection of the shoulder.

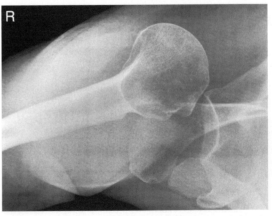

Axial radiograph of the shoulder showing posterior dislocation

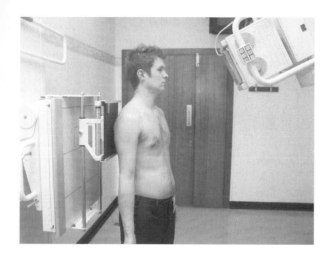

In cases of suspected shoulder impingement syndrome, it is important to visualize the anterior portion of the acromion process. Routine projections described above are frequently unsatisfactory because the anterior portion of the acromion is superimposed on the body of the acromion. If the antero-posterior projection is undertaken with the X-ray beam angled 30 degrees caudally, the anterior part of the acromion is projected inferiorly to the body of the acromion and is visualized more clearly.

A modified lateral projection (outlet view) with 10-degree caudal angulation may also be undertaken.

Antero-posterior (outlet projection)

Position of patient and cassette (as for the antero-posterior survey image)

- The patient stands with the affected shoulder against a cassette and is rotated 15 degrees to bring the plane of the scapula parallel with the cassette.
- The arm is supinated and slightly abducted away from the body. The medial and lateral epicondyles of the distal humerus should be parallel to the cassette.
- The cassette is positioned so that its upper border is at least 5 cm above the shoulder to ensure that the oblique rays do not project the shoulder off the cassette.

Direction and centring of the X-ray beam

- The horizontal central ray is directed 30 degrees caudally and centred to the palpable coracoid process of the scapula.
- An 18 × 24-cm cassette is used with the beam collimated to the glenohumeral joint.

Essential image characteristics

- The image should demonstrate the anterior part of the acromion projected inferiorly to the body to visualize the presence of bony spurs or abnormally long acromion process.
- The subacromial joint space should be shown above the humeral head.

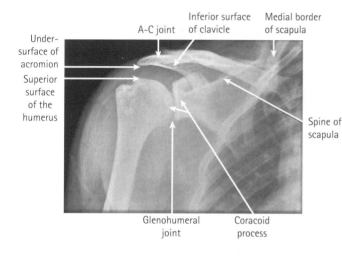

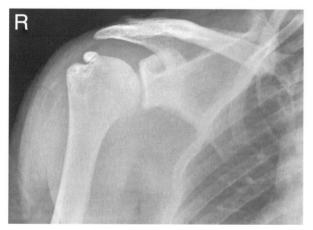

Antero-posterior radiograph of shoulder outlet showing normal undersurface of acromion (incidental calcification of the supraspinatus tendon)

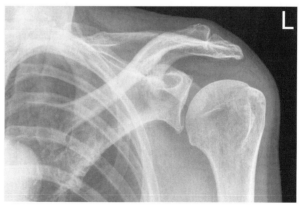

Antero-posterior projection of the shoulder showing bony spur on the lateral undersurface of the acromion process

3 | Outlet projections

Lateral (outlet projection)

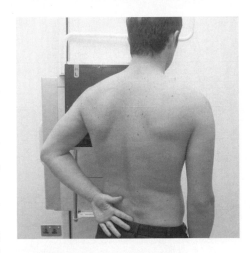

Position of patient and cassette

- The patient stands or sits facing the cassette, with the lateral aspect of the affected arm in contact.
- The affected arm is extended backwards, with the dorsum of the hand resting on the patient's waist.
- The patient is adjusted so that the head of the humerus (coracoid process) is in the centre of the cassette.
- The patient is now rotated forward until a line joining the medial and lateral borders of the affected scapula is at right-angles to the cassette. The body of the scapula is now at right-angles to the cassette, and the scapula and the proximal end of the humerus are clear of the rib cage.

Direction and centring of the X-ray beam

- The horizontal central ray is angled 10 degrees caudally and centred to the head of the humerus.
- The beam is collimated to an 18 × 24-cm cassette.

Essential image characteristics

- The image should demonstrate the extent of the anterior projection of the acromion and the subacromial space.

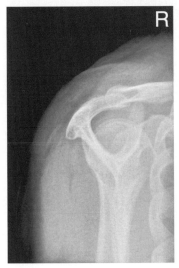

Normal radiograph of lateral shoulder outlet

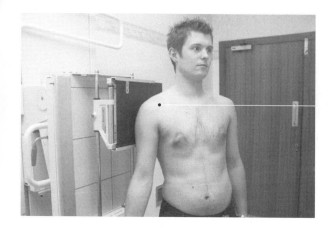

Antero-posterior – erect

To demonstrate the glenoid cavity and glenohumeral joint space, the body of the scapula should be parallel to the cassette so that the glenoid cavity is at right-angles to the cassette. The horizontal central ray can now pass through the joint space parallel to the glenoid cavity of the scapula.

Position of patient and cassette

- The patient stands with the affected shoulder against the cassette and is rotated approximately 30 degrees to bring the plane of the glenoid fossa perpendicular to the cassette.
- The arm is supinated and slightly abducted away from the body.
- The cassette is positioned so that its upper border is at least 5 cm above the shoulder to ensure that the oblique rays do not project the shoulder off the cassette.

Direction and centring of the X-ray beam

- The horizontal central ray is centred to the palpable coracoid process of the scapula.
- The primary beam is collimated to an 18 × 24-cm cassette.

Essential image characteristics

- The image should demonstrate clearly the joint space between the head of the humerus and the glenoid cavity.
- The image should demonstrate the head, the greater and lesser tuberosities of the humerus, together with the lateral aspect of the scapula and the distal end of the clavicle.

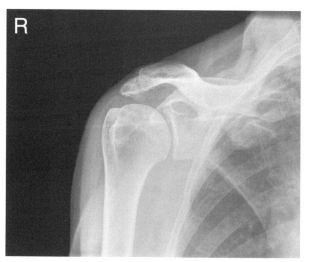

Normal antero-posterior radiograph of the shoulder to show glenohumeral joint

3 Glenohumeral joint

Antero-posterior – supine (trauma)

There are occasions when the patient cannot be examined in the erect position, e.g. due to multiple trauma or immobility. Often, such patients present on a trolley in the emergency situation.

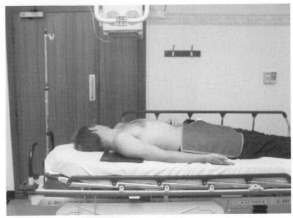

Position of patient and cassette

- The patient lies supine on the trolley, and the unaffected shoulder is raised slightly to bring the scapula on the affected side parallel to the cassette.
- The arm is partially abducted and supinated clear of the trunk.
- The cassette is positioned under the patient so that its upper border is at least 5 cm above the shoulder to ensure that the oblique rays do not project the shoulder off the film. If the patient cannot be moved, then the cassette tray under the trolley can be used.

Direction and centring of the X-ray beam

- The vertical central ray is centred to the palpable coracoid process of the scapula.
- It may be necessary to direct the primary beam caudally in order to project the head of the humerus below the acromion process.

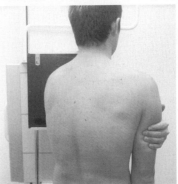

Essential image characteristics

- The subacromial space should be visible.
- The proximal end of the humerus, the lateral aspect of the scapula and the whole of the clavicle need to be included.
- The greater tuberosity will be in profile when the arm is supinated.
- If the arm cannot be supinated, then the head of humerus has the appearance of a 'lightbulb' shape.

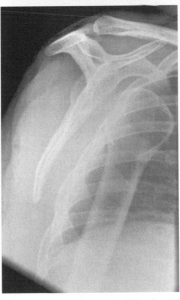

Lateral oblique 'Y' projection (alternate) dislocation/fracture proximal humerus

If the arm is immobilized and no abduction of the arm is possible, then a lateral oblique 'Y' projection is taken using a 24 × 30-cm cassette in an erect cassette holder or vertical Bucky if the patient is particularly large.

Position of patient and cassette

- The patient stands or sits with the lateral aspect of the injured arm against an erect cassette and is adjusted so that the axilla is in the centre of the film.
- The unaffected shoulder is raised to make the angle between the trunk and cassette approximately 60 degrees. A line joining the medial and lateral borders of the scapula is now at right-angles to the cassette.
- The cassette is positioned to include the superior border of the scapula.

Lateral oblique radiograph of the shoulder showing anterior dislocation

Direction and centring of the X-ray beam

- The horizontal central ray is directed towards the medial border of the scapula and centred to the head of the humerus.

Essential image characteristics

- The body of the scapula should be at right-angles to the cassette, and the scapula and the proximal end of the humerus are clear of the rib cage.
- The exposure should demonstrate the position of the head of the humerus in relation to the glenoid cavity between the coracoid and acromion processes.

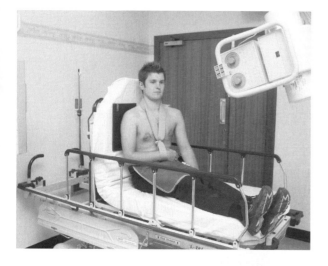

A revised shoulder technique may be necessary immediately following manipulation to check that a shoulder dislocation has been reduced successfully. The affected arm will be immobilized, usually in a collar and cuff support. An image of the joint space is taken in the antero-posterior position on an 18 × 24-cm cassette; this is achieved by raising the unaffected side approximately 30 degrees.

It is important that accurate assessment of the glenohumeral joint is possible from the resultant image in order that an avulsion fracture from around the glenoid rim is demonstrated clearly.

Poor positioning technique may be the result of the following:

- The patient not being X-rayed erect and not enough compensatory caudal angulation being applied.
- The immobilized arm will be nursed with the humerus internally rotated. This has the effect that the coronal plane is often tilted towards the unaffected side.

Such a poor technique results in no joint space being seen, the humeral head overlying the acromion process, and the humeral head appearing as a 'lightbulb' with the greater tuberosity not being demonstrated.

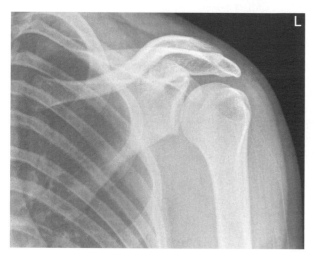

Antero-posterior radiograph of the shoulder, post manipulation, showing good technique

Antero-posterior – 25 degrees caudad

Position of patient and cassette

- The patient sits fully erect, if possible, on the accident and emergency (A&E) trolley, with the head section of the trolley raised to a vertical position to support the patient.
- With the arm immobilized in a collar and cuff, the patient is turned 30 degrees towards the affected side.
- The unaffected shoulder is supported on pads to bring the posterior aspect of the affected shoulder into closer contact with the cassette, which is positioned under the affected arm and held in position with the patient's body weight.
- The cassette is positioned so that its upper border is at least 5 cm above the shoulder to ensure that the oblique rays do not project the shoulder off the film.

Direction and centring of the X-ray beam

- The horizontal central ray is angled 25 degrees caudally and directed to the palpable coracoid process of the scapula.
- The beam is collimated to the 18 × 24-cm cassette.

Essential image characteristics

- The glenoid rim should be clear of the humeral head and the articular surface of the head of the humerus should be clear of the acromion process.
- Any avulsion fragments should be seen clearly in the joint space.

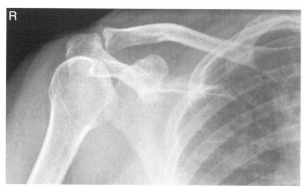

Antero-posterior radiograph of the shoulder, post manipulation, showing poor technique – joint space not adequately demonstrated

3 Recurrent dislocation

Compression defects, sometimes referred to as hatchet-shaped defects, on the head of the humerus are associated with recurrent dislocation of the shoulder. In the case of recurrent anterior dislocation, the defect will occur on the postero-lateral aspect of the head of the humerus (Hill–Sach's lesion). In the case of recurrent posterior dislocation, the defect will be on the anterior part of the head. In each case, this is where the dislocated head of the humerus impacts on the glenoid rim.

The radiographic examination for recurrent dislocation of the shoulder requires a projection of the glenoid cavity for signs of fracture affecting the inferior rim (Bankart lesion) as well as different projections of the head of the humerus to demonstrate the defect. It is important to remember that the angle formed between the epicondyles of the humerus and the cassette indicates the degree of rotation of the humerus. To judge the rotation of the humerus by the position of the hand can be very misleading.

Projections may be selected from the following:

- antero-posterior with the humerus lateral;
- antero-posterior with the humerus oblique;
- antero-posterior (modified) – Stryker's;
- infero-superior.

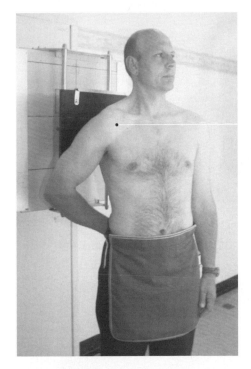

Antero-posterior (lateral humerus)

If the patient is able to cooperate fully, these projections may be taken erect. If not, the patient is positioned supine to reduce the risk of movement. An 18 × 24-cm cassette is selected.

Position of patient and cassette

- The patient is positioned erect, with the unaffected shoulder raised approximately 30 degrees to bring the glenoid cavity at right-angles to the centre of the cassette.
- The arm is partially abducted, the elbow flexed and the arm medially rotated. The palm of the hand rests on the patient's waist.
- The cassette is placed with its upper border 5 cm above the shoulder and centred to the joint.

Direction and centring of the X-ray beam

- The horizontal central ray is directed to the head of the humerus and the centre of the cassette.
- Exposure is made on arrested respiration.

Essential image characteristics

- The image should demonstrate the head and neck of the humerus and the glenoid cavity with the glenohumeral joint shown well.

Note

To improve image quality and reduce radiation dose, careful collimation of the beam is employed.

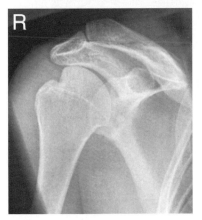

Antero-posterior shoulder (lateral humerus projection) showing Hill-Sachs deformity due to recurrent dislocation

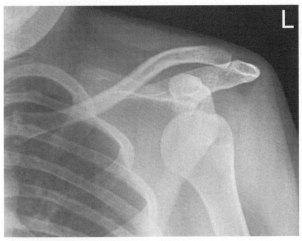

Antero-posterior shoulder showing anterior dislocation

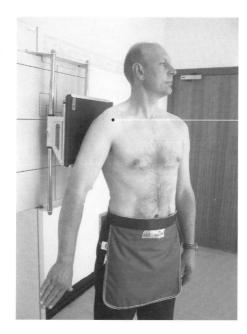

Antero-posterior (oblique humerus)

Position of patient and cassette

- The patient is positioned erect, with the unaffected shoulder raised approximately 30 degrees to bring the glenoid cavity at right-angles to the centre of the cassette.
- The elbow is extended, allowing the arm to rest in partial abduction by the patient's side.
- The humerus is now in an oblique position midway between that for the antero-posterior projection and that for a lateral projection.
- The cassette is placed with its upper border 5 cm above the shoulder and centred to the joint.

Direction and centring of the X-ray beam

- The horizontal central ray is directed to the head of the humerus and the centre of the cassette.
- Exposure is made on arrested respiration.

Essential image characteristics

- The image should demonstrate the head and neck of the humerus and the glenoid cavity, with the glenohumeral joint shown clearly.

Note

To improve image quality and reduce radiation dose, careful collimation of the beam is employed.

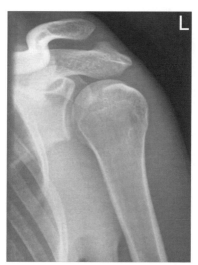

Normal antero-posterior oblique radiograph of humerus for recurrent dislocation

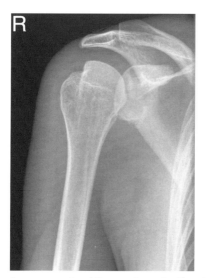

Antero-posterior oblique radiograph of head of humerus showing Hill-Sach's deformity of recurrent dislocation

Antero-posterior (modified) – Stryker's

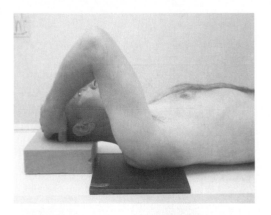

This position will demonstrate a Hills–Sachs deformity of the humeral head.

Position of patient and cassette

- The patient lies supine on the X-ray table.
- The arm of the affected side is extended fully and the elbow then flexed to allow the hand to rest on the patient's head.
- The line joining the epicondyles of the humerus remains parallel to the tabletop.
- The centre of the cassette is positioned 2.5 cm superior to the head of the humerus.

Direction and centring of the X-ray beam

- The central ray is angled 10 degrees cranially and directed through the centre of the axilla to the head of the humerus and the centre of the cassette.

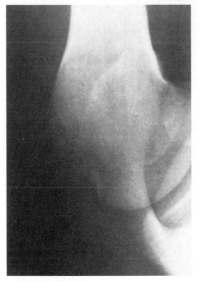

Infero-superior

This will give a second projection of the glenoid cavity as well as a further projection of the head of the humerus.

Stryker's projection

Position of patient and cassette

- The patient lies supine on the X-ray table, with the arm of the affected side abducted without causing discomfort to the patient.
- The palm of the hand is turned to face upwards, with the medical and lateral epicondyles of the humerus equidistant from the tabletop.
- A cassette is supported vertically against the shoulder and is pressed against the neck to include as much as possible of the scapula on the film.
- The shoulder and arm are raised slightly on non-opaque pads.

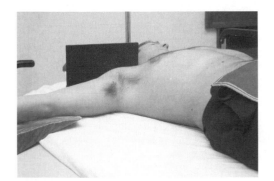

Direction and centring of the X-ray beam

- The horizontal central ray is directed towards the axilla with minimum angulation towards the trunk.

Essential image characteristics

- The image should demonstrate the head of the humerus, the acromion process, the coracoid process and the glenoid cavity of the scapula.
- The lesser tuberosity will be in profile, and the acromion process and the superior aspect of the glenoid will be seen superimposed on the head of the humerus.

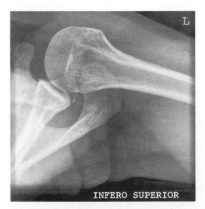

Normal infero-superior radiograph of shoulder

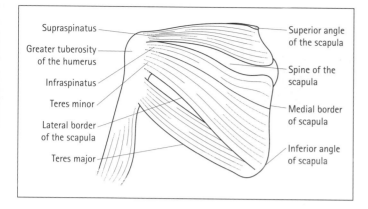

Supraspinatus
Greater tuberosity of the humerus
Infraspinatus
Teres minor
Lateral border of the scapula
Teres major
Superior angle of the scapula
Spine of the scapula
Medial border of scapula
Inferior angle of scapula

Most tendon pathology is best demonstrated by MRI or ultrasound. Calcification does not show well on MRI and calcific tendonitis is thus best depicted by plain radiographs or ultrasound. The radiographic technique is described below.

To demonstrate calcifications in the tendons around the shoulder joint by radiography, the course of each tendon, unobstructed by overlaying bone, should be demonstrated, including a profile of each region of the proximal end of the humerus into which a tendon is inserted. The tendons affected are those of the supraspinatus, subscapularis, infraspinatus, and rarely teres minor muscles. The illustration shows the origins, courses and insertions of most of these muscles.

The supraspinatus muscle has its origin in the supraspinatus fossa on the posterior aspect of the scapula superior to the spine of the scapula. Its tendon passes beneath the acromion process then over the upper posterior part of the shoulder joint, to be inserted into the highest of the three impressions of the greater tuberosity.

The infraspinatus muscle has its origin in the infraspinatus fossa on the posterior surface of the scapula inferior to the spine of the scapula. Its tendon glides over the posterior border of the acromion and then passes behind the capsule of the shoulder joint, to be inserted into the middle impression of the greater tuberosity of the humerus.

The teres minor muscle has its origin on the lateral border of the scapula and its tendon passes behind the lower part of the capsule of the shoulder joint, to be inserted into the lowest of the three impressions of the greater tuberosity of the humerus and to the shaft just distal to this lowest impression.

The subscapularis muscle has its origin in the subscapularis fossa on the deep (anterior) surface of the scapula and its tendon crosses the shoulder joint anteriorly, to be inserted into the lesser tuberosity of the humerus.

The recommended projections for each of the tendons are given in the table below (remember ultrasound is very effective in localizing calcification and may also give information about the soft tissue of the tendon).

Tendon	Projection	Variation
Supraspinatus	Antero-posterior	No rotation of humerus
	Lateral outlet view	
Subscapularis	Infero-superior	
	Antero-posterior	Lateral rotation of humerus
Infraspinatus	Antero-posterior	25° caudad angulation
	Infero-superior	
Teres minor	Antero-superior	Medial rotation of humerus

3 Calcified tendons

Antero-posterior

An 18 × 24-cm cassette is used in a vertical cassette holder.

Position of patient and cassette

- The patient stands with the affected shoulder against the vertical cassette holder and rotated 15 degrees to bring the plane of the scapula parallel with the cassette.
- The cassette is positioned so that its upper border is at least 5 cm above the shoulder to ensure that the oblique rays do not project the shoulder off the film.

Position of the arm

- The arm is supinated at the patient's side, palm facing forwards, with the line joining the medial and lateral epicondyles of the humerus parallel to the vertical cassette holder.
- With the elbow flexed, the arm is partially abducted and **medially rotated**, with the dorsum of the hand resting on the rear waistline. The line joining the medial and lateral epicondyles of the humerus is now perpendicular to the vertical cassette holder.
- With the elbow flexed, the arm is abducted and **laterally rotated**, with the hand raised above the shoulder. The palm of the hand faces forward, with the lateral epicondyle facing backwards. The line joining the medial and lateral epicondyles of the humerus should be perpendicular to the vertical cassette holder.

Direction and centring of the X-ray beam

- In each case, the horizontal central ray is directed to the head of the humerus and to the centre of the film.

Essential image characteristics

- In each case, the image should demonstrate the proximal end of the humerus in profile to the tendon under examination.
- Different degrees of rotation will demonstrate whether the calcification moves in relation to the humerus.
- The exposure should be adjusted to show the soft-tissue details – usually 5 kVp less than for general images.

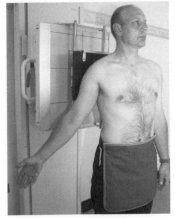
No rotation (arm in position 1)

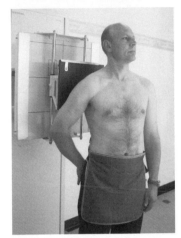
Medial rotation (arm in position 2)

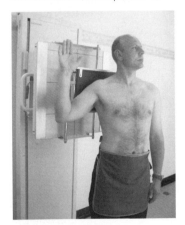
Lateral rotation (arm in position 3)

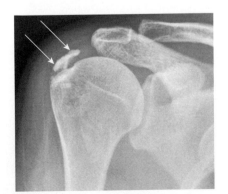
No rotation (arm in position 1)

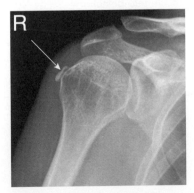
Medial rotation (arm in position 2)

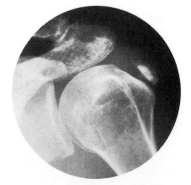
Lateral rotation (arm in position 3)

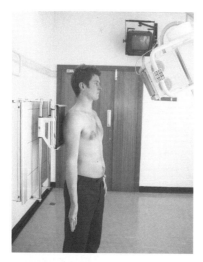

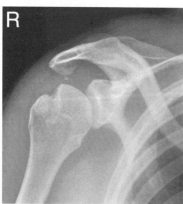

Antero-posterior radiograph of shoulder with 25 degrees caudad angulation to show calcifications

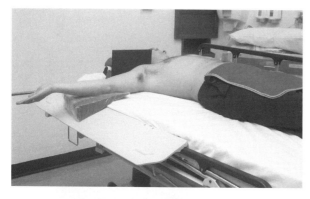

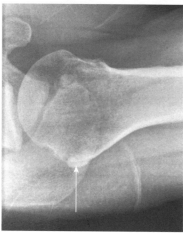

Infero-superior radiograph of shoulder showing calcification

Antero-posterior – 25 degrees caudad

Position of patient and cassette

- The patient stands with the affected shoulder against a vertical cassette holder and rotated 15 degrees to bring the plane of the scapula parallel with the cassette.
- The arm is supinated at the patient's side, palm facing forwards, with the line joining the medial and lateral epicondyles of the humerus parallel to the vertical cassette holder.
- To allow for caudal angulation of the X-ray beam, the cassette is adjusted vertically, so that the centre of the cassette is approximately 5 cm distal to the head of the humerus.

Direction and centring of the X-ray beam

- The collimated central ray is angled 25 degrees caudally and centred to the head of the humerus and to the centre of the film.

Demonstrates: insertion of infraspinatus and the subacromial part of the supraspinatus tendon.

Infero-superior

Position of patient and cassette

- The patient lies supine on the table, with the arm of the side being examined abducted to a right-angle.
- The palm of the hand faces upwards and the line joining the medial and lateral epicondyles is in a plane parallel to the tabletop.
- The cassette is supported vertically against the upper border of the shoulder and pressed into the neck.

Direction and centring of the X-ray beam

- The horizontal central ray is directed to the centre of the axilla, with the minimum angulation towards the trunk.

Demonstrates: the insertion of the subscapularis and teres minor and the course of tendons anterior and posterior to the capsule of the shoulder joint.

Essential image characteristics

- In each case, the image should demonstrate the proximal end of the humerus in profile to the tendon under examination.

3 Acromioclavicular joints

Antero-posterior

An antero-posterior projection of the joint in question is all that is normally required. In certain circumstances, subluxation of the joint may be confirmed with the patient holding a heavy weight.

An 18 × 24-cm cassette is placed in a vertical cassette holder.

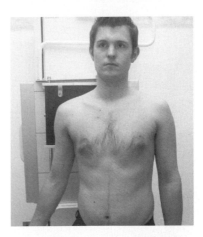

Position of patient and cassette

- The patient stands facing the X-ray tube, with the arms relaxed to the side. The posterior aspect of the shoulder being examined is placed in contact with the cassette, and the patient is then rotated approximately 15 degrees towards the side being examined to bring the acromioclavicular joint space at right-angles to the film.
- The cassette is positioned so that the acromion process is in the centre of the film.

Direction and centring of the X-ray beam

- The horizontal central ray is centred to the palpable lateral end of the clavicle at the acromioclavicular joint.
- To avoid superimposition of the joint on the spine of the scapula, the central ray can be angled 25 degrees cranially before centring to the joint.

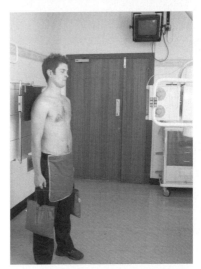

Essential image characteristics

- The image should demonstrate the acromioclavicular joint and the clavicle projected above the acromion process.
- The exposure should demonstrate soft tissue around the articulation.

Notes

- The normal joint is variable (3–8 mm) in width. The normal difference between the sides should be less than 2–3 mm (Manaster 1997).
- The inferior surfaces of the acromion and clavicle should normally be in a straight line.

Weight-bearing antero-posterior projection

- The acromioclavicular joint has a weak joint capsule and is vulnerable to trauma. Subluxation may be difficult to diagnose in the standard antero-posterior image, because the width of the joint can be variable and may look widened in a normal joint.
- To prove subluxation, it may be necessary to do weight-bearing comparison projections of both acromioclavicular joints (separate joint images).
- The positions of the patient and cassette are as described above.
- It is advisable to 'strap' the weights used for the procedure around the lower arms rather than getting the patient to hold on to them, as the biomechanics involved may lead to a false negative appearance.

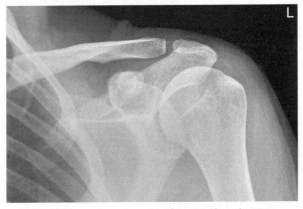

Normal antero-posterior radiograph of acromioclavicular joint

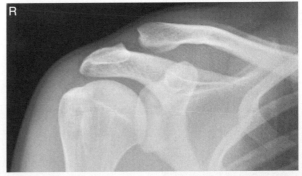

Antero-posterior radiograph of acromioclavicular joint showing subluxation

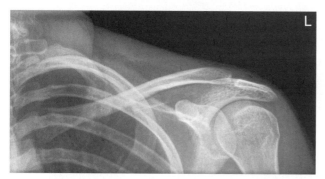

Postero-anterior – erect (basic)

Although the clavicle is demonstrated on the antero-posterior 'survey' image, it is desirable to have the clavicle as close to the cassette as possible to give optimum bony detail. The postero-anterior position also reduces the radiation dose to the thyroid and eyes, an important consideration in follow-up fracture images. Alternatively, the patient may be supine on the table or trolley for the antero-posterior projection in which immobility and movement are considerations.

A 24 × 30-cm cassette is placed transversely in an erect cassette holder (or a vertical Bucky if the patient is particularly large).

Position of patient and cassette

- The patient sits or stands facing an erect cassette holder.
- The patient's position is adjusted so that the middle of the clavicle is in the centre of the cassette.
- The patient's head is turned away from the side being examined and the affected shoulder rotated slightly forward to allow the affected clavicle to be brought into close contact with the Bucky.

Direction and centring of the X-ray beam

- The horizontal central ray is directed to the centre of the clavicle and the centre of the image, with the beam collimated to the clavicle.

Essential image characteristics

- The entire length of the clavicle should be included on the image.
- The lateral end of the clavicle will be demonstrated clear of the thoracic cage.
- There should be no foreshortening of the clavicle.
- The exposure should demonstrate both the medial and the lateral ends of the clavicle.

Note

Exposure is made on arrested respiration to reduce patient movement.

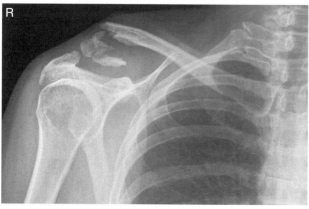

Normal postero-anterior radiograph of clavicle

Postero-anterior radiograph of clavicle showing comminuted fracture

3 | Clavicle

Antero-posterior – supine (alternate)

Position of patient and cassette

- The patient is supine on the X-ray table.
- A small sandbag is placed under the opposite shoulder to rotate the patient slightly towards the affected side to make sure that the medial end of the clavicle is not superimposed on the vertebral column.
- The arm of the side being examined is in a relaxed position by the side of the trunk.
- A 24 × 30-cm cassette is placed transversely behind the patient's shoulder and adjusted so that the clavicle is in the middle.

Direction and centring of the X-ray beam

- The vertical central ray is directed to the middle of the clavicle.

Essential image characteristics

- The entire length of the clavicle should be included on the image.
- The lateral end of the clavicle will be demonstrated clear of the thoracic cage.
- There should be no foreshortening of the clavicle.
- The exposure should demonstrate both the medial and the lateral ends of the clavicle.

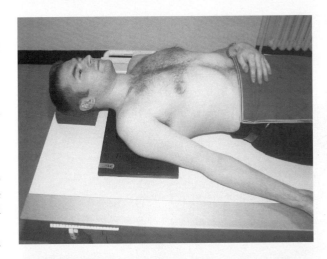

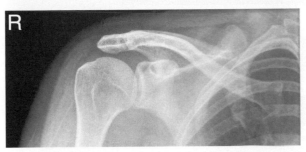

Normal antero-posterior supine radiograph of clavicle

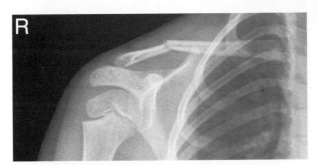

Antero-posterior supine radiograph of clavicle showing fracture

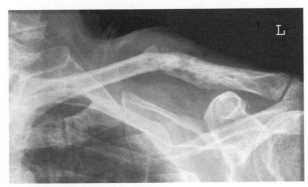

Antero-posterior supine radiograph of clavicle showing a pathological fracture through a sclerotic metastasis

Infero-superior

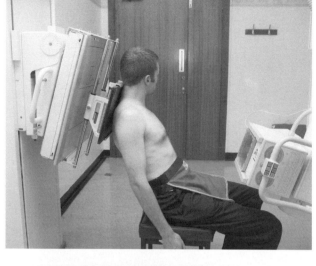

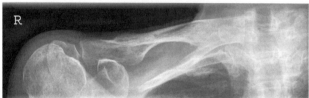

Erect infero-superior radiograph of clavicle

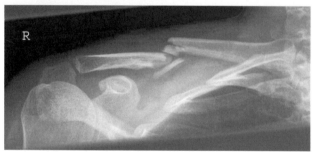

Infero-superior radiograph of clavicle showing fracture

This projection can be very useful to confirm a possible fracture seen on the postero-anterior/antero-posterior projection, to assess the degree of any fracture displacement and to show the medial end of clavicle clear of underlying ribs.

In cases of acute injury, it is more comfortable for the patient to be examined in the erect position.

Position of patient and cassette

- The patient sits facing the X-ray tube with a 24 × 30-cm cassette placed in the cassette holder. Some holders allow forward-angulation of the cassette of 15 degrees towards the shoulder. This reduces the distortion caused by the cranially projected central beam.
- The unaffected shoulder is raised slightly to bring the scapula in contact with the cassette.
- The patient's head is turned away from the affected side.
- The cassette is displaced above the shoulder to allow the clavicle to be projected into the middle of the image.

Direction and centring of the X-ray beam

- The central ray is angled 30 degrees cranially and centred to the centre of the clavicle.
- The 30 degrees needed to separate the clavicle from the underlying ribs can be achieved by a combination of patient positioning and central ray angulation.
- The medial end of the clavicle can be shown in greater detail by adding a 15-degree lateral angulation to the beam.

Essential image characteristics

- The image should demonstrate the entire length of the clavicle, including the sternoclavicular and acromioclavicular joints.
- The entire length of the clavicle, with the exception of the medial end, should be projected clear of the thoracic cage.
- The clavicle should be horizontal.

Radiological considerations

- If a fracture occurs together with fracture of the upper ribs, then this implies a severe injury and may be associated with subclavian vessel damage or pneumothorax.

Clavicle

Infero-superior – supine

Position of patient and cassette

- The patient lies supine on the table, with the shoulder of the side being examined raised on a non-opaque pad and with the arm relaxed by the side.
- The patient's head is turned away from the affected side.
- The cassette is tilted back about 20 degrees from the vertical and is supported by sandbags against the upper border of the shoulder and pressed into the side of the neck.

Direction and centring of the X-ray beam

- The central ray is angled 45 degrees cranially and centred to the centre of the clavicle.

Essential image characteristics

- The image should demonstrate the entire length of the clavicle, including the sternoclavicular and acromioclavicular joints.
- The entire length of the clavicle, with the exception of the proximal end, should be projected clear of the thoracic cage.
- The clavicle should be horizontal.

Note

If the cassette cannot be pressed well into the side of the neck, then the medial end of the clavicle might not be included on the cassette. In this case, with the central ray again angled 45 degrees cranially, the central ray is first centred to the sternoclavicular joint of the affected side and then the tube is rotated until the central ray is directed to the centre of the clavicle.

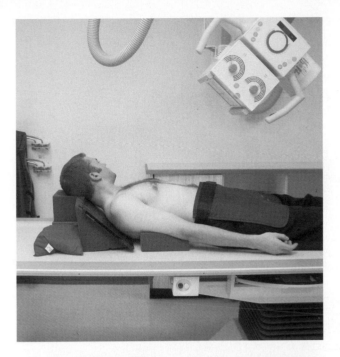

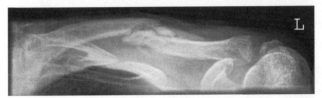

Supine infero-superior radiograph of clavicle showing early healing of a fracture

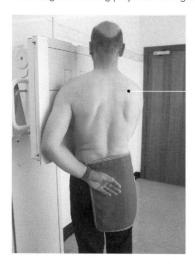

Axial diagram showing projection for right sternoclavicular joint

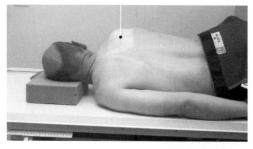

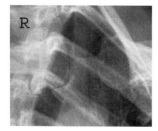

Radiograph of normal right sternoclavicular join

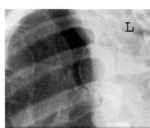

Radiograph of normal left sternoclavicular joint

In an antero-posterior or postero-anterior projection, the vertebral column will be superimposed on, and obscure, the sternoclavicular joints, hence an oblique projection is required to show the joint space clear of the vertebral column. An oblique projection is chosen that will bring the joint space as near as possible at right-angles to the film. Both sides may be imaged for comparison.

Postero-anterior oblique (basic)

Position of patient and cassette

- The patient stands facing the Bucky.
- The patient is then rotated through 45 degrees so that the median sagittal plane of the body is at 45 degrees to the cassette with the sternoclavicular joint being examined nearer the cassette and centred to it.
- The patient holds the vertical stand to help immobilization and continues to breathe during the exposure.

Direction and centring of the X-ray beam

- The horizontal central ray is centred at the level of the fourth thoracic vertebra to a point 10 cm away from the midline on the side away from the cassette.

Essential image characteristics

- The sternoclavicular joint should be demonstrated clearly in profile away from the vertebral column.

Note

Superimposed lung detail may be reduced by asking the patient to breathe gently during the exposure.

Semi-prone (alternate)

Alternatively, the patient may be examined in the semi-prone position. Starting with the patient prone, the side not being examined is raised from the table until the median sagittal plane is at 45 degrees to the table, with the joint being examined in the midline of the table. The centring point is to the raised side, 10 cm from the midline at the level of the fourth thoracic vertebra.

Radiological considerations

- These joints are difficult to demonstrate, even with good technique. Alternatives include ultrasound, CT (especially with three-dimensional or multiplanar reconstructions) and MRI.

3 Sternoclavicular joints

Postero-anterior

Using a single-exposure technique, both joints are imaged for comparison in a case of suspected subluxation.

A 24 × 30-cm cassette is used, placed transversely in an erect cassette holder.

Position of patient and cassette

- The patient sits or stands facing an erect cassette holder with their chin resting on the top of the cassette holder.
- The patient's position is adjusted so that the median sagittal plane is at right angles to the vertical central line of the cassette.
- The cassette is adjusted vertically to the level of the middle of the manubrium.
- The arms are extended by the sides of the body or alternatively the patient can hold onto the cassette holder.

Direction and centring of the X-ray beam

- The horizontal central ray is centred in the midline of the thorax at the level of the head of the humerus.

Notes

- The radiographic exposure is similar to that given for an antero-posterior shoulder projection on the patient.
- The beam is collimated to the sternoclavicular joints.

Lateral

An 18 × 24-cm cassette is used, placed vertically in an erect cassette holder.

Position of patient and cassette

- The patient sits or stands sideways with the affected side adjacent to the cassette.
- The median sagittal plane is adjusted parallel to the cassette with the upper arm in contact with it.
- the patient clasps the hands behind and pulls the shoulders well back to avoid any obscuring of the joints.
- The centre of the cassette is adjusted to coincide with the level of the sternoclavicular joints.

Direction and centring of the X-ray beam

- The horizontal central ray is centred to the palpable sternoclavicular joints just below the sternal notch.

Note

- Ideally anterior subluxation is diagnosed clinically. Posterior subluxation compromises the airway.

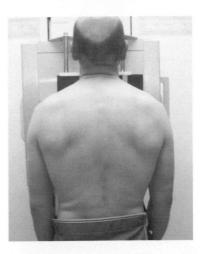

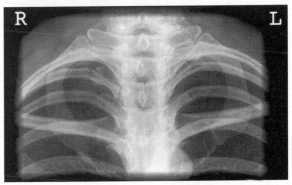

Radiograph of normal sternoclavicular joints in postero-anterior projection

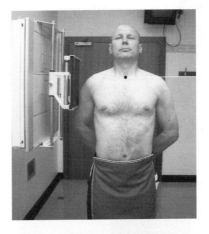

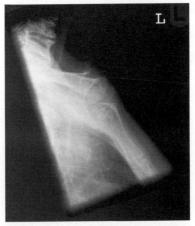

Radiograph of normal sternoclavicular joints in lateral projection

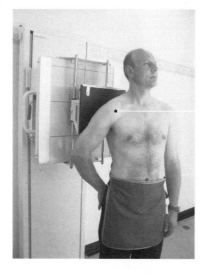

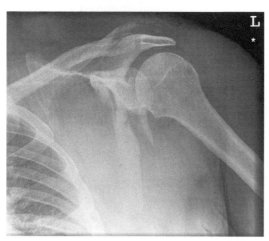

Antero-posterior radiograph of scapula showing a fracture through the neck of the glenoid

The position of the scapula relative to the thorax changes as the arm moves through abduction, adduction, flexion, extension and rotation. When the shoulders are pressed back, the medial borders for the scapulae are parallel to and near the vertebral column, so that most of the scapula would be superimposed on the thoracic cage in the antero-posterior projection of the scapula. With the arm in full medial rotation, the scapula glides laterally over the ribs, allowing more of the body of the scapula to be shown clearly against the rib cage.

A 24 × 30-cm cassette is used, placed vertically in an erect cassette holder or a Bucky if the patient is large.

Antero-posterior (basic) – erect

The scapula can be shown on the antero-posterior basic survey projection of the shoulder but with the arm in medial rotation. It is preferable for the patient to be examined in the erect position when there is suspected injury as it is more comfortable. There may also be underlying rib fractures.

Position of patient and cassette

- The patient stands with the affected shoulder against a cassette and rotated slightly to bring the plane of the scapula parallel with the cassette.
- The arm is slightly abducted away from the body and medially rotated.
- The cassette is positioned so that its upper border is at least 5 cm above the shoulder to ensure that the oblique rays do not project the shoulder off the cassette.

Direction and centring of the X-ray beam

- The horizontal ray is directed to the head of the humerus.

Note

A long exposure time may be chosen and the patient allowed to continue quiet breathing during the exposure, so that images of overlying lung and rib are blurred in cases of non-trauma.

Essential image characteristics

- The entire scapula should be demonstrated on the image.
- The medial border of the scapula should be projected clear of the mediastinum.
- The medial border of the scapula should be projected clear of the ribs.

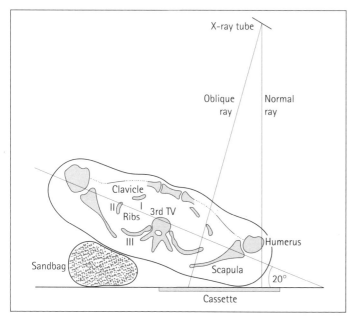

Axial diagram showing the relationship of cassette and X-ray beam to the scapula

3 | Scapula

Lateral (basic)

Position of patient and cassette

- The patient stands with the side being examined against a vertical Bucky.
- The patient's position is adjusted so that the centre of the scapula is at the level of the centre of the cassette.
- The arm is either adducted across the body or abducted with the elbow flexed to allow the back of the hand to rest on the hip.
- Keeping the affected shoulder in contact with the Bucky, the patient's trunk is rotated forward until the body of the scapula is at right-angles to the cassette. This can be checked by palpating the medial and lateral borders of the scapula near the inferior angle.

Direction and centring of the X-ray beam

- The horizontal central ray is directed to the midpoint of the medial border of the scapula and to the middle of the cassette.

Essential image characteristics

- The scapula should be demonstrated clear of the ribs.
- The medial and lateral borders should be superimposed.
- The humerus should be projected clear of the area under examination.
- The exposure should demonstrate adequately the whole of the scapula.

Lateral (alternate)

Position of patient and cassette

- The patient lies prone on the X-ray table.
- The arm on the side being examined is slightly abducted and the elbow flexed.
- The unaffected side is raised until the palpable body of the scapula is at right-angles to the table and in the midline of the table.

Direction and centring of the X-ray beam

- The vertical central ray is directed just medial to the midpoint of the palpable medial border of the scapula and to the middle of the Bucky table.

Radiological considerations

- This is a very thin sheet of bone with several dense appendages overlying the upper ribs, making fractures, and their full extent, hard to assess. CT may be very useful for complete evaluation, in particular the multiplanar reconstruction facility, once a fracture has been detected.

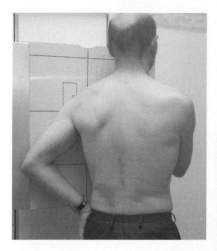
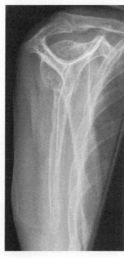

Normal lateral radiograph of scapula

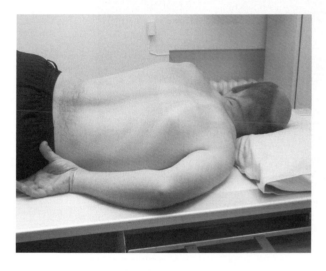

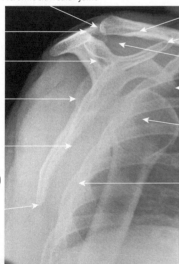

Acromioclavicular joint

Body of the acromion

Spine of scapula

Posterior border of glenoid

Anterior surface of scapula (fossa for subscapularis)

Inferior tip of scapula

Clavicle

Superior border of scapula

Supraspinatus fossa

Tip of the coracoid process

Head of the humerus (dislocated anteriorly)

Posterolateral ribs

Shaft of the humerus

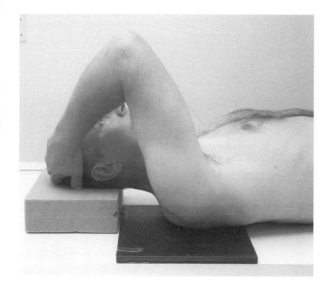

The coracoid process is demonstrated more clearly in an antero-posterior projection, with the arm abducted to above-shoulder level. Additionally, the process is demonstrated in the axial (supero-inferior and infero-inferior) projections of the shoulder (see pp. 81 and 82).

Antero-posterior (arm abducted)

A 24 × 30-cm cassette is placed in an erect cassette holder or a vertical Bucky if the patient is large.

Position of patient and cassette

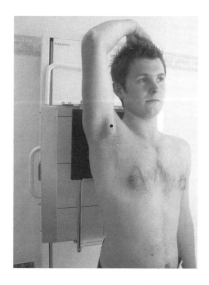

- The patient is supine or erect, with the posterior aspect of the affected shoulder against the cassette.
- The arm of the affected side is abducted to above-shoulder level and the elbow flexed, allowing the hand to rest on the patient's head.
- The patient is now rotated slightly to bring the affected side away from the cassette.
- The position of the cassette is adjusted so that it is centred to the axilla.

Direction and centring of the X-ray beam

- The central ray is directed at right-angles to the cassette and centred to the axilla of the affected side.

Note

This projection will also demonstrate the acromioclavicular joint of the same side free from overlaying structures.

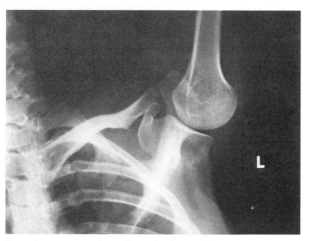

Normal antero-posterior radiograph of coracoid process

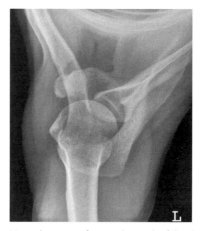

Normal supero-inferior radiograph of the shoulder demonstrating the coracoid process

Reference

Manaster BJ (1997). *Handbook of Skeletal Radiology*, 2nd edn. St Louis: Mosby.

Section 4

The Lower Limb

CONTENTS

RECOMMENDED PROJECTIONS 106

POSITIONING TERMINOLOGY 107

FOOT 108
Basic projections 108
Dorsi-plantar (basic) 108
Dorsi-plantar oblique 109
Lateral 110
Lateral – erect 111
Dorsi-plantar – erect 111

TOES 112
Basic projections 112
Dorsi-plantar – basic 112
Dorsi-plantar oblique – basic 112
Lateral (basic) – hallux 113
First metatarsal-phalangeal sesamoid
　bones 113
Lateral 113
Axial 113

ANKLE JOINT 114
Basic projections 114
Antero-posterior – basic
　(Mortice projection) 114
Lateral (basic) – medio-lateral 115
Alternative projection methods 116
Antero-posterior 116
Lateral (alternate) – latero-medial
　(horizontal beam) 116
Stress projections for subluxation 117
Antero-posterior – stress 117
Lateral – stress 117

CALCANEUM 118
Basic projections 118
Lateral – basic 118
Axial – basic 119

SUBTALAR JOINTS 120
Recommended projections 120
Oblique medial 121

Oblique lateral 122
Lateral oblique 123

TIBIA AND FIBULA 124
Basic projections 124
Antero-posterior – basic 124
Lateral – basic 124

PROXIMAL TIBIO-FIBULAR JOINT 125
Basic projections 125
Lateral oblique – basic 125
Antero-posterior oblique 125

KNEE JOINT 126
Basic projections 126
Antero-posterior 126
Lateral – basic 127
Additional projections 128
Lateral – horizontal beam 128
Antero-posterior – standing projections 129
Stress projections for subluxation 129
Antero-posterior – stress 129
Patella 130
Postero-anterior 130
Skyline projections 131
Conventional infero-superior projection 131
Supero-inferior 132
Infero-superior – patient prone 133
Postero-anterior oblique 134
Antero-posterior oblique 134
Intercondylar notch (tunnel) 135

SHAFT OF FEMUR 136
Basic projections 136
Antero-posterior 136
Lateral – basic 137
Additional projection – lateral horizontal
　beam 137

LEG ALIGNMENT 138
Conventional film/screen method 138
Digital computed radiography method 139

Foot	Fracture/dislocation of the metatarsal	Dorsi-plantar (basic)	Dorsi-plantar oblique (basic)	Lateral (on request)
	Fracture/dislocation of the tarsal bone	Dorsi-plantar (basic)	Dorsi-plantar oblique (basic)	Lateral (on request)
	Foreign body	Dorsi-plantar (basic)	Lateral (basic)	
	Pathology	Dorsi-plantar (basic)	Dorsi-plantar oblique (basic)	
	Pes planus	Lateral – erect (both sides for comparison)		
	Hallux valgus	Dorsi-plantar – erect (both sides for comparison)		
Toe	Trauma or pathology – hallux	Dorsi-plantar (basic)	Lateral (basic)	
	Trauma or pathology – other toe	Dorsi-plantar (basic)	Dorsi-plantar oblique (basic)	
First metatarso-phalangeal sesamoid bone	Trauma or pathology	Lateral	Axial	
Ankle joint	Trauma or pathology	Antero-posterior (basic)	Lateral (basic or alternate)	Antero-posterior oblique (on request)
	Subluxation (torn lateral ligament)	Antero-posterior (basic)	Lateral (basic or alternate)	
	Provided that no fracture is seen, these are followed by:		Antero-posterior (stress)	Lateral (stress)
Calcaneum (heel)	Trauma	Axial (basic)	Lateral (basic)	
	Pathology	Lateral (basic)	Axial on request (basic or alternate)	
Subtalar joint	Trauma or pathology	Projections on request		
Tibia/fibula	Trauma or pathology	Antero-posterior (basic)	Lateral (basic or alternate)	
Proximal tibio-fibular joint	Trauma or pathology	Lateral oblique (basic) or antero-posterior oblique (alternate)		
Knee joint	Trauma	Antero-posterior (basic)	Lateral horizontal beam	
	Additional trauma projections	Obliques	Skyline – infero-superior or supero-inferior	Intercondylar notch
	Loose bodies	Antero-posterior (basic)	Lateral (basic)	Intercondylar notch
	Pathology	Antero-posterior (basic)	Lateral (basic)	Antero-posterior (erect)
	Subluxation	Antero-posterior (stress)		
Femur/shaft	Trauma or pathology	Antero-posterior (basic)	Lateral – basic or horizontal beam	
Lower limb	Leg alignment and measurement	Conventional method	Digital method	

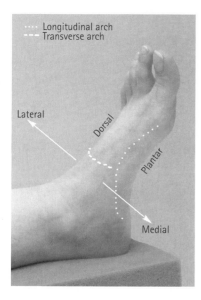

Longitudinal arch
Transverse arch

Lateral

Dorsal

Plantar

Medial

Rotation of the lower limb occurs at the hip joint. The position of the foot relates to the direction of rotation.

- **Dorsal surface:** the superior surface of the foot is known as the dorsal surface and slopes downwards, at a variable angle, from the ankle to the toes and from medial to lateral.
- **Plantar aspect:** the inferior surface of the foot is known as the plantar aspect.
- **Medial aspect:** the surface nearer the midline of the body is the medial aspect.
- **Lateral aspect:** the surface further from the midline of the body is the lateral aspect.
- **Medial rotation:** the lower limb is rotated inwards, so that the anterior surface faces medially. This will produce internal rotation of the hip joint.
- **Lateral rotation:** the lower limb is rotated outwards, so that the anterior surface faces laterally. This will produce external rotation of the hip joint.
- **Dorsiflexion:** dorsiflexion of the ankle joint occurs when the dorsal surface of the foot is moved in a superior direction.
- **Plantarflexion:** plantarflexion of the ankle joint occurs when the plantar surface of the foot is moved in an inferior direction.
- **Inversion:** inversion of the foot occurs when the plantar surface of the foot is turned to face medially, with the limb extended.
- **Eversion:** eversion of the foot occurs when the plantar surface of the foot is turned to face laterally, with the limb extended.
- **Flexion of the knee joint:** the degree of flexion of the knee joint relates to the angle between the axis of the tibia when the knee is extended and the angle of the axis of the tibia when the knee is flexed.

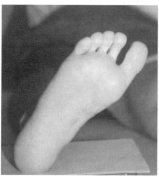

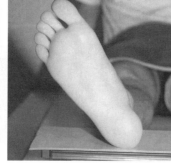

Medial rotation

Lateral rotation

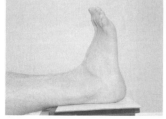

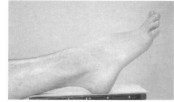

Dorsiflexion

Plantarflexion

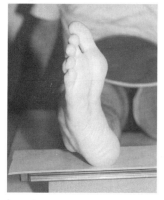

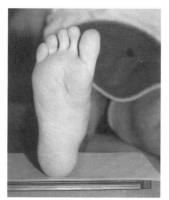

Inversion

Eversion

4 Foot

Basic projections

It is common practice to obtain two projections, a dorsi-plantar and a dorsi-plantar oblique, using a 24 × 30-cm high-resolution cassette. A lead-rubber mask is used to mask off each half of the cassette not in use.

Dorsi-plantar (basic)

To ensure the tarsal and tarso-metatarsal joints are demonstrated, the foot is X-rayed with the foot flat on the cassette and with the X-ray tube angled 15 degrees cranially. Alternatively, the foot is raised on a 15-degree non-opaque pad using a vertical central beam. The angulation compensates for the inclination of the longitudinal arch and reduces overshadowing of the tarsal bones.

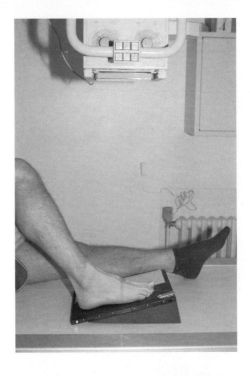

Position of patient and cassette

- The patient is seated on the X-ray table, supported if necessary, with the affected hip and knee flexed.
- The plantar aspect of the affected foot is placed on the cassette and the lower leg is supported in the vertical position by the other knee.
- Alternatively, the cassette can be raised on a 15-degrees foam pad for ease of positioning.

Direction and centring of the X-ray beam

- The central ray is directed over the cuboid-navicular joint, midway between the palpable navicular tuberosity and the tuberosity of the fifth metatarsal.
- The X-ray tube is angled 15 degrees cranially when the cassette is flat on the table.
- The X-ray tube is vertical when the cassette is raised on a 15-degree pad.

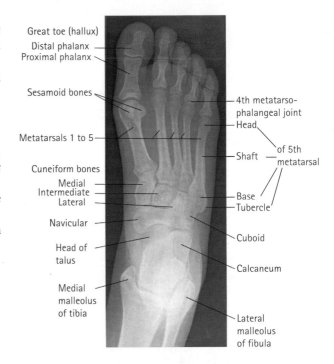

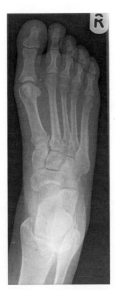

Normal dorsi-plantar radiograph of foot

Essential image characteristics

- The tarsal and tarso-metatarsal joints should be demonstrated when the whole foot is examined.
- The kVp selected should reduce the difference in subject contrast between the thickness of the toes and the tarsus to give a uniform radiographic contrast over the range of foot densities.

Note

A wedge filter can be used to compensate for the difference in tissue thickness.

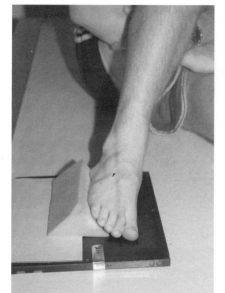

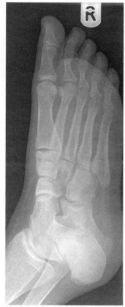

Normal dorsi-plantar oblique radiograph of foot

Dorsi-plantar oblique

This projection allows the alignment of the metatarsals with the distal row of the tarsus to be assessed.

Position of patient and cassette

- From the basic dorsi-plantar position, the affected limb is allowed to lean medially to bring the plantar surface of the foot approximately 30–45 degrees to the cassette.
- A non-opaque angled pad is placed under the foot to maintain the position, with the opposite limb acting as a support.

Direction and centring of the X-ray beam

- The vertical central ray is directed over the cuboid-navicular joint.

Essential image characteristics

- The kVp selected should reduce the difference in subject contrast between the thickness of the toes and the tarsus to give a uniform radiographic contrast over the range of foot densities.
- A wedge filter may also be used to give a uniform range of densities.
- The dorsi-plantar oblique should demonstrate the inter-tarsal and tarso-metatarsal joints.

Note

For non-ambulant/wheelchair-bound patients, the cassette may be placed on a pad or stool directly in contact with the plantar aspect of the foot.

Radiological considerations

- There are numerous possible accessory ossicles in the foot and around the ankle, as at the wrist. These may give rise to confusion with small avulsion injuries.
- The base of the fifth metatarsal ossifies from the accessory ossification centre, which is oriented parallel to the long axis of the bone. This should not be confused with a fracture, which usually runs transversely.
- If the accessory ossification centre is not parallel to the metatarsal, then this may be due to an avulsion injury.
- Lisfranc fracture dislocations at the bases of the metatarsals are difficult to see, except on oblique projections, and will be masked by underexposure.

Great toe (hallux)
- Distal phalanx
- Proximal phalanx
- Sesamoid bones

Metatarsals 1 to 5
Cuneiform bones
- Medial
- Intermediate
- Lateral
- Navicular
- Talonavicular joint
- Head of talus

- Ankle joint

- Tibia
- Fibula

Phalanges of 4th toe
- Distal
- Middle
- Proximal

- 5th metatarso-phalangeal joint

5th metatarsal
- Head
- Shaft
- Base

- 3rd tarso-metatarsal joint
- Cuboid
- Calcaneo-cuboid joint

- Calcaneum

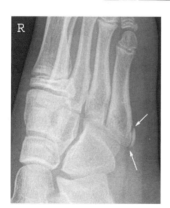

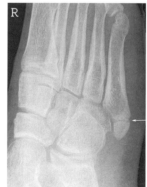

Radiographs showing normal fifth metatarsal ossification centre on the left, and fracture base fifth metatarsal on right (arrow)

Lateral

This is used in addition to the routine dorsi-planter projection to locate a foreign body. It may also be used to demonstrate a fracture or dislocation of the tarsal bones, or base of metatarsal fractures or dislocation.

Position of patient and cassette

- From the dorsi-plantar position, the leg is rotated outwards to bring the lateral aspect of the foot in contact with the cassette.
- A pad is placed under the knee for support.
- The position of the foot is adjusted slightly to bring the plantar aspect perpendicular to the cassette.

Direction and centring of the X-ray beam

- The vertical central ray is centred over the navicular cuneiform joint.

Essential image characteristics

- If examining for a suspected foreign body, the kVp selected should be adequate to show the foreign body against the soft-tissue structures.

Note

A metal marker placed over the puncture site is commonly used to aid localization of the foreign body.

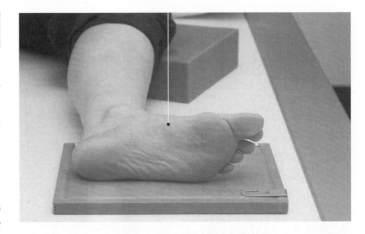

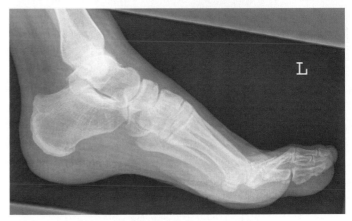

Normal lateral radiograph of foot

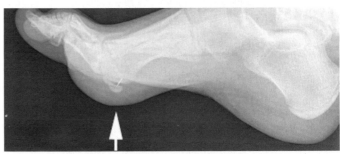

Lateral radiograph of foot showing metallic foreign body

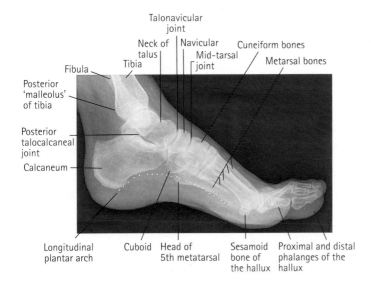

Talonavicular joint
Neck of talus | Navicular
Tibia | Mid-tarsal joint
Cuneiform bones
Metatarsal bones
Fibula
Posterior 'malleolus' of tibia
Posterior talocalcaneal joint
Calcaneum
Longitudinal plantar arch
Cuboid
Head of 5th metatarsal
Sesamoid bone of the hallux
Proximal and distal phalanges of the hallux

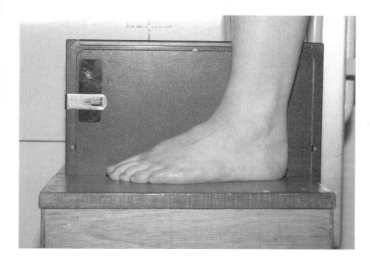

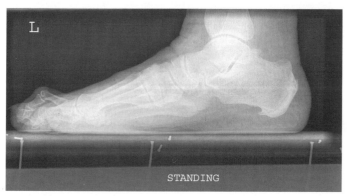

Lateral – erect

This projection is used to demonstrate the condition of the longitudinal arches of the foot, usually in pes planus (flat feet). Both feet are examined for comparison.

Position of patient and cassette

- The patient stands on a low platform with a cassette placed vertically between the feet.
- The feet are brought close together The weight of the patient's body is distributed equally.
- To help maintain the position, the patient should rest their forearms on a convenient vertical support, e.g. the vertical Bucky.

Direction and centring of the X-ray beam

- The horizontal central ray is directed towards the tubercle of the fifth metatarsal.

Dorsi-plantar – erect

This projection can be used to show the alignment of the metatarsals and phalanges in cases of hallux valgus. Both forefeet are taken for comparison.

Position of patient and cassette

- The patient stands with both feet on the cassette.
- The cassette is positioned to include all the metatarsals and phalanges.
- The weight of the patient's body is distributed equally.
- To help maintain the position, the patient should rest the forearms on a convenient vertical support, e.g. the vertical Bucky.

Direction and centring of the X-ray beam

- The vertical ray is centred midway between the feet at the level of the first metatarso-phalangeal joint.

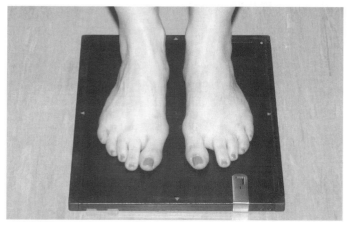

Normal erect lateral projection of foot

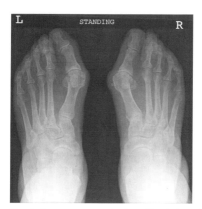

Dorsi-plantar erect projection of both feet showing hallux valgus

4 Toes

Basic projections

It is common practice to obtain two projections, a dorsi-plantar and a dorsi-plantar oblique, using a 18 × 24-cm high-resolution cassette. A lateral projection is taken for fractures of the hallux phalanx. A lead-rubber mask can be used to mask off each half of the cassette not in use.

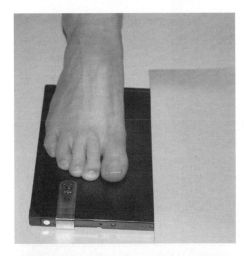

Dorsi-plantar – basic

Position of patient and cassette

- The patient is seated on the X-ray table, supported if necessary, with hips and knees flexed.
- The plantar aspect of the affected foot is placed on the cassette. This cassette may be supported on a 15-degree pad.
- The leg may be supported in the vertical position by the other knee.

Direction and centring of the X-ray beam

- The vertical central ray is directed over the third metatarso-phalangeal joint, perpendicular to the cassette if all the toes are to be imaged.
- For single toes, the vertical ray is centred over the metatarso-phalangeal joint of the individual toe and collimated to include the toe either side.

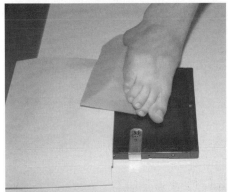

Dorsi-plantar oblique – basic

Position of patient and cassette

- From the basic dorsi-plantar position, the affected limb is allowed to lean medially to bring the plantar surface of the foot approximately 45 degrees to the cassette.
- A 45-degree non-opaque pad is placed under the side of the foot for support, with the opposite leg acting as a support.

Direction and centring of the X-ray beam

- The vertical ray is centred over the first metatarso-phalangeal joint if all the toes are to be imaged and angled sufficiently to allow the central ray to pass through the third metatarso-phalangeal joint.
- For single toes, the vertical ray is centred over the metatarso-phalangeal joint of the individual toe, perpendicular to the cassette.

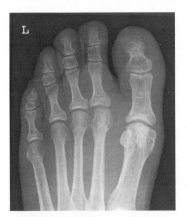

Normal dorsi-plantar projection of all toes

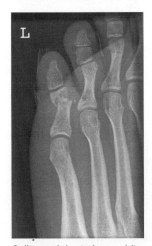

Collimated dorsi-plantar oblique projection of fifth toe, showing fracture of the proximal phalanx

Position of patient and cassette

- From the dorsi-plantar position, the foot is rotated medially until the medial aspect of the hallux is in contact with the cassette. A bandage is placed around the remaining toes (provided that no injury is suspected) and they are gently pulled forwards by the patient to clear the hallux. Alternatively, they may be pulled backwards; this shows the metatarso-phalangeal joint more clearly.

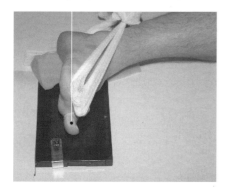 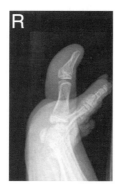

Normal lateral basic projection of hallux

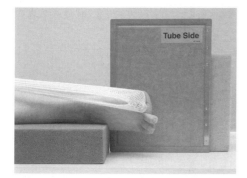

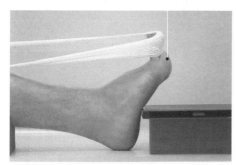

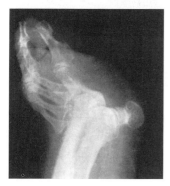 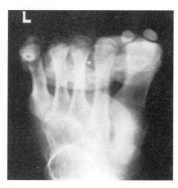

Lateral projection of first metatarsal sesamoids, note exostosis on medial sesamoid

Normal axial projection of first metatarsal sesamoids

Lateral (basic) – hallux

Direction and centring of the X-ray beam

- The vertical ray is centred over the first metatarso-phalangeal joint.

First metatarsal-phalangeal sesamoid bones

The sesamoid bones are demonstrated on the lateral foot projection. However, when requested specifically, a modified lateral and an axial projection may be necessary for further demonstration.

Lateral

Position of patient and cassette

- The patient lies on the unaffected side, and the medial aspect of the affected leg and foot is placed in contact with the table.
- The cassette is placed under the foot to include the phalanges of the hallux and the distal part of the first metatarsal.
- The hallux is then dorsiflexed with the aid of a bandage and held by the patient.

Direction and centring of the X-ray beam

- Centre with the vertical ray perpendicular to the cassette, over the first metatarso-phalangeal joint.

Axial

Position of patient and cassette

There is a choice of two positions for this projection:

1. The patient is positioned as for the lateral projection of the foot. The foot is raised on a support and the cassette is supported vertically and well into the instep. A horizontal beam is used in this case.
2. The patient sits on the X-ray table, with legs extended. The hallux is then dorsiflexed with the aid of a bandage and held by the patient. The cassette is raised on a support and positioned firmly against the instep.

Direction and centring of the X-ray beam

- Centre to the sesamoid bones with the central ray projected tangentially to the first metatarso-phalangeal joint.

4 | Ankle joint

Basic projections

Two projections are routinely taken, an antero-posterior and a lateral, using an 18 × 24-cm high-resolution cassette. A lead-rubber mask can be used to mask off the half of the film not in use.

Antero-posterior – basic (Mortice projection)

Position of patient and cassette

- The patient is either supine or seated on the X-ray table with both legs extended.
- A pad may be placed under the knee for comfort.
- The affected ankle is supported in dorsiflexion by a firm 90-degree pad placed against the plantar aspect of the foot. The limb is rotated medially (approximately 20 degrees) until the medial and lateral malleoli are equidistant from the cassette.
- The lower edge of the cassette is positioned just below the plantar aspect of the heel.

Direction and centring of the X-ray beam

- Centre midway between the malleoli with the vertical central ray at 90 degrees to an imaginary line joining the malleoli.

Essential image characteristics

- The lower third of the tibia and fibula should be included.
- A clear joint space between the tibia, fibula and talus should be demonstrated (commonly called the Mortice view).

Common faults and remedies

- Insufficient dorsiflexion results in the calcaneum being superimposed on the lateral malleolus.
- Insufficient medial rotation causes overshadowing of the tibiofibular joint with the result that the joint space between the fibula and talus is not demonstrated clearly.

- If internal rotation of the limb is difficult, then the central ray is angled to compensate, making sure that it is still at 90 degrees to the imaginary line joining the malleoli.

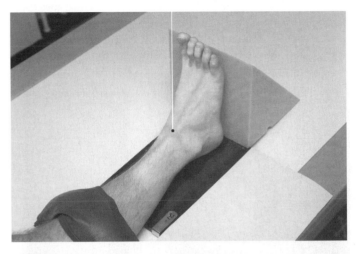

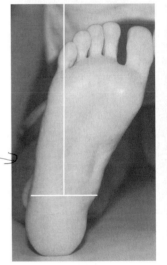

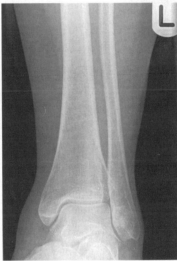

Normal antero-posterior radiograph of ankle

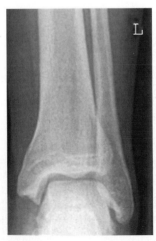

Insufficient medial rotation

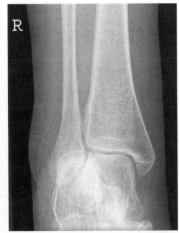

Insufficient dorsiflexion

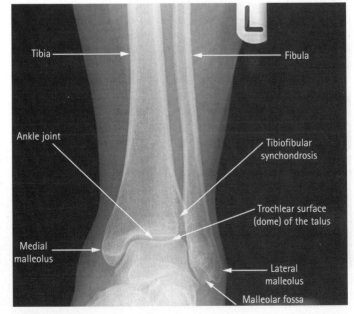

Annotated antero-posterior radiograph

Position of patient and cassette

- With the ankle dorsiflexed, the patient turns on to the affected side until the malleoli are superimposed vertically and the tibia is parallel to the cassette.

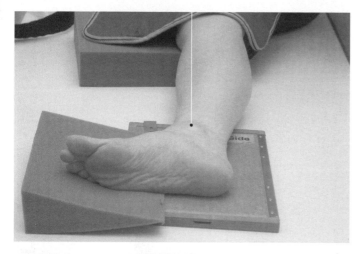

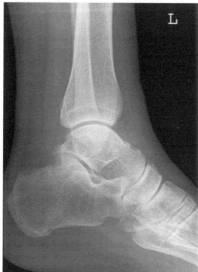

Normal lateral radiograph of ankle

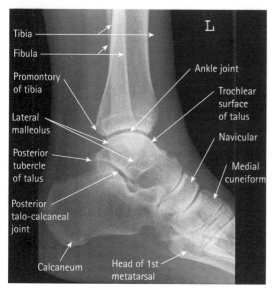

Annotated radiograph of lateral ankle

Lateral (basic) – medio-lateral

- A 15-degree pad is placed under the lateral border of the forefoot and a pad is placed under the knee for support. The lower edge of the cassette is positioned just below the plantar aspect of the heel.

Direction and centring of the X-ray beam

- Centre over the medial malleolus, with the central ray at right-angles to the axis of the tibia.

Essential image characteristics

- The lower third of the tibia and fibula should be included.
- The medial and lateral borders of the trochlear articular surface of the talus should be superimposed on the image.

Common faults and remedies

- Over-rotation causes the fibula to be projected posterior to the tibia and the medial and lateral borders of the trochlear articulations are not superimposed.
- Under-rotation causes the shaft of the fibula to be superimposed on the tibia and the medial and lateral borders of the trochlear articulations are not superimposed.
- The base of the fifth metatarsal and the navicular bone should be included on the image to exclude fracture.

Radiological considerations

- Inversion injury of the ankle is common and may result in fracture of the lateral malleolus or the base of the fifth metatarsal. Investigation of the injury should therefore cover both areas.
- Tear of the collateral ligaments without bone fracture may make the ankle unstable, despite a normal radiograph. Stress projections may clarify this problem and ultrasound or MRI may be useful. Complex injuries may occur with fracture of both malleoli, rendering the ankle mortise very unstable, especially if associated with fracture of the posterior tibia – the so-called trimalleolar fracture – and/or disruption of the distal tibio-fibular synchondrosis. These injuries frequently require surgical fixation.

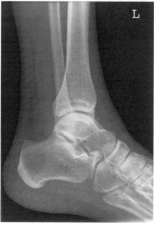

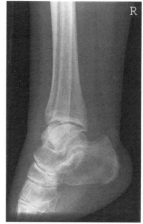

Over rotation

Under rotation

Alternative projection methods

In cases of trauma, the techniques may be modified to obtain the basic radiographs without moving the patient from a wheelchair or turning the leg of a patient lying on a trolley. This also applies to those patients from the fracture clinic with below-knee plaster casts. In the latter case, for conventional film processing, radiography cassettes with standard-speed screens are used because of the increase in radiation dose necessary to penetrate the cast.

The horizontal techniques described can be undertaken only in X-ray rooms that have the capability of lowering the ceiling tube suspension sufficiently to centre the X-ray beam on the ankle joint.

Antero-posterior

Position of patient and cassette

- From the sitting position, whilst the patient is in a wheelchair, the whole limb is raised and supported on a stool and a pad is placed under the raised knee for support.
- The lower limb is rotated medially, approximately 20 degrees, until the medial and lateral malleoli are equidistant from the cassette. A non-opaque angled pad is placed against the medial border of the foot and sandbags are placed at each side of the leg for support.
- The lower edge of the cassette is placed just below the plantar aspect of the heel.

Direction and centring of the X-ray beam

- Centre midway between the malleoli, with the vertical central ray at 90 degrees to the imaginary line joining the malleoli or compensatory angulation of the beam if the foot is straight.

Note

If the foot remains straight, there will be overshadowing of the tibio-fibular joint combined with a vertical central ray.

Lateral (alternate) – latero-medial (horizontal beam)

Position of patient and cassette

- With the patient maintaining the sitting position or lying on the trauma trolley, the limb is raised and supported on a firm non-opaque pad.
- A cassette is placed against the medial aspect of the limb. The lower edge of the cassette is placed just below the plantar aspect of the heel.

Direction and centring of the X-ray beam

- The horizontal central ray is directed to the lateral malleolus.

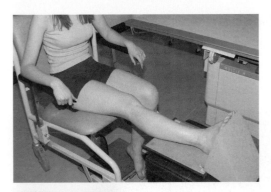

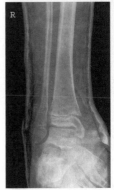

Antero-posterior radiograph through plaster showing fracture of the distal fibula

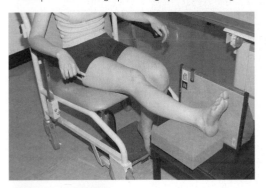

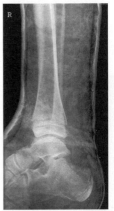

Horizontal beam lateral radiograph of ankle through plaster

Note

If there is no internal rotation of the foot, then the distal fibula will be projected behind the distal tibia and a 'true lateral' image is not produced. If the foot cannot be rotated to superimpose the malleoli, then compensatory superior angulation (approximately 20 degrees) can be applied to the beam.

Stress projections of the ankle joint are taken to demonstrate subluxation due to rupture of the lateral ligaments. Although these projections may be done in the department, they are now commonly done in theatre using a mobile image intensifier.

Stress projections for subluxation

Stress is applied to the joint by medical personnel, usually an orthopaedic surgeon.

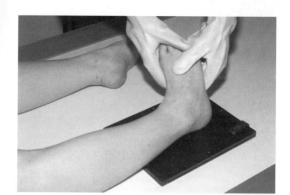

Antero-posterior – stress

Position of patient and cassette

- The patient and cassette are positioned for the routine antero-posterior projection.
- The doctor in charge forcibly inverts the foot without internally rotating the leg.

Direction and centring of the X-ray beam

- Centre midway between the malleolus, with the central ray at right-angles to the imaginary line joining the malleoli.

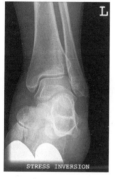
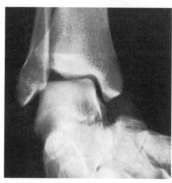

Normal   Subluxation

Antero-posterior projection with inversion stress

Lateral – stress

Position of patient and cassette

- The patient lies supine on the table, with the limb extended.
- The foot is elevated and supported on a firm pad.
- The ankle is dorsiflexed and the limb rotated medially until the malleoli are equidistant from the tabletop.
- The film is supported vertically against the medial aspect of the foot.
- The doctor applies firm downward pressure on the lower leg.

Direction and centring of the X-ray beam

- Centre to the lateral malleoli with a horizontal beam.

Notes

- The antero-posterior stress projection demonstrates widening of the joint space if the calcaneo-fibular joint space is torn.
- The lateral stress views demonstrate anterior subluxation if the anterior talo-fibular ligament is torn.
- Similar techniques are used in theatre, with the image intensifier positioned above the ankle. The degree of stress applied is viewed and recorded.

Radiation protection

- The doctor applying the stress must wear a suitable lead protective apron and gloves.
- If the technique is done using a mobile image intensifier, then local rules must be implemented and all staff must be provided with protective clothing.

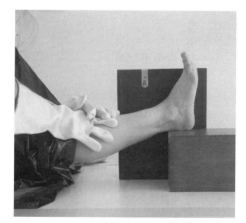

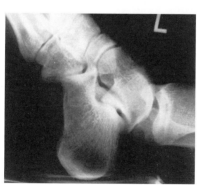

Lateral projection with stress showing subluxation

4 Calcaneum

Basic projections

It is common practice to take two projections, a lateral and an axial, using an 18 × 24-cm cassette fitted with high-resolution intensifying screens. A lead-rubber mask may be used to mask off each half of the film not in use.

Lateral – basic

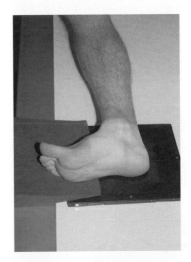

Position of patient and cassette

- From the supine position, the patient rotates on to the affected side.
- The leg is rotated until the medial and lateral malleoli are superimposed vertically.
- A 15-degree pad is placed under the anterior aspect of the knee and the lateral border of the forefoot for support.
- The cassette is placed with the lower edge just below the plantar aspect of the heel.

Direction and centring of the X-ray beam

- Centre 2.5 cm distal to the medial malleolus, with the vertical central ray perpendicular to the cassette.

Essential image characteristics

- The adjacent tarsal bones should be included in the lateral projection, together with the ankle joint.

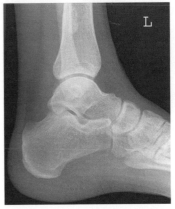

Normal lateral radiograph of calcaneum

Note

This projection is used to demonstrate calcaneal spurs. For comparison, a radiograph of both heels in the lateral position may be necessary.

Radiological considerations

- The normal juvenile calcaneal apophysis is dense and often appears fragmented. The appearance rarely obscures a fracture and should rarely, if ever, require projections of the contralateral side for assessment.
- The primary trabeculae of bones follow lines of maximum load. In the calcaneum, this results in an apparent lucency in the central area. This should not be mistaken for pathology.
- Fracture of the calcaneum due to heavy landing on the heel causes a compression injury with depression of the central area by the talus. This is seen as flattening of the Bohler's angle to less than 40 degrees, as shown in the diagram.
- Small spurs or 'tug' lesions at attachments of the Achilles tendon and plantar ligament are common. If significant, they are usually ill-defined and clinically tender. Ultrasound may help in their assessment. Computed tomography (CT) is very useful for the complete evaluation of complex calcaneal fractures, especially utilizing the direct coronal plane, multiplanar and three-dimensional reconstructions.

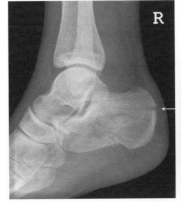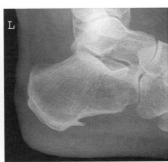

Fracture of the calcaneum   Calcaneal spur
Lateral radiographs of the calcaneum

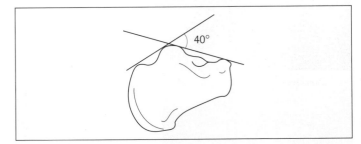

Line diagram showing Bohler's angle

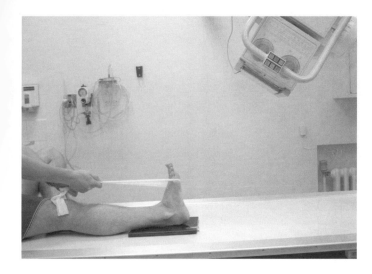

Axial – basic

Position of patient and cassette

- The patient sits or lies supine on the X-ray, table with both limbs extended.
- The affected leg is rotated medially until both malleoli are equidistant from the film.
- The ankle is dorsiflexed The position is maintained by using a bandage strapped around the forefoot and held in position by the patient.
- The cassette is positioned with its lower edge just distal to the plantar aspect of the heel.

Direction and centring of the X-ray beam

- Centre to the plantar aspect of the heel at the level of the tubercle of the fifth metatarsal.
- The central ray is directed cranially at an angle of 40 degrees to the plantar aspect of the heel.

Essential image characteristics

- The subtalar joint should be visible on the axial projection.

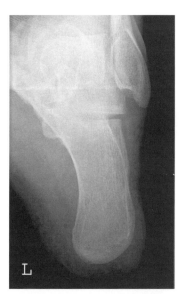

Normal axial projection of calcaneum

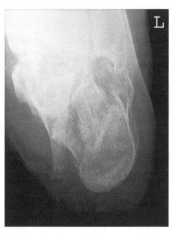

Axial projection of calcaneum showing comminuted fracture

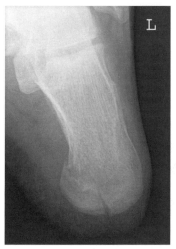

Axial projection of calcaneum showing fracture

4 Subtalar joints

Recommended projections

There are three articular surfaces of the subtalar joint: anterior, middle and posterior. The projections undertaken with the articulations demonstrated are shown in the table below, with matching images also given.

Projection	Articulation
Lateral oblique – 20-degree caudal tilt	Middle and posterior articulations
Dorsi-plantar oblique	Anterior articulation
45-degree oblique – medial with 10-degree cranial tilt	Posterior articulation from an anterior direction
45-degree oblique – lateral with 15-degree cranial tilt	Posterior articulation from a lateral direction

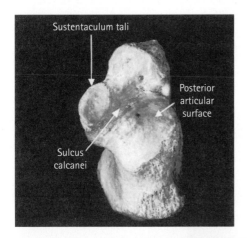

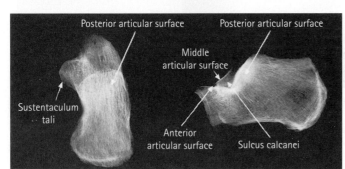

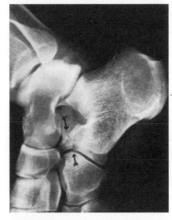

Dorsi-plantar oblique

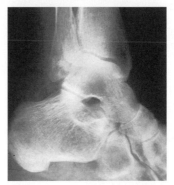

Lateral oblique 20-degree caudal tilt

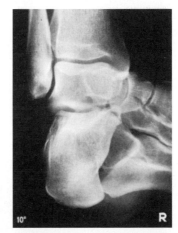

45-degree oblique lateral with 10-degree cranial tilt

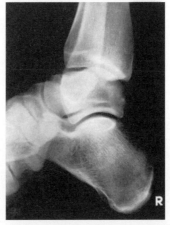

45-degree oblique lateral with 15-degree cranial tilt

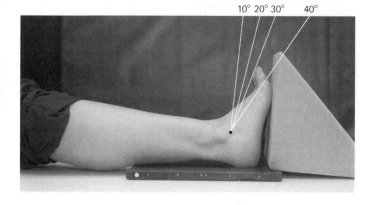

10° 20° 30°   40°

Oblique medial

Position of patient and cassette

- The patient lies supine on the X-ray table, with the affected limb extended.
- The ankle joint is dorsiflexed and the malleoli are equidistant from the film.
- The leg is internally rotated through 45 degrees.
- A pad is placed under the knee for support.
- A non-opaque square pad and sandbag may be placed against the plantar aspect of the foot to keep the ankle joint in dorsiflexion.
- The lower edge of the cassette is placed at the level of the plantar aspect of the heel.

Direction and centring of the X-ray beam

- Centre 2.5 cm distal to the lateral malleolus with the following cranial angulations:

10 degrees	Posterior part of the posterior articulation
20–30 degrees	Middle part of the posterior articulation and the middle articulation
40 degrees	Anterior part of the posterior articulation

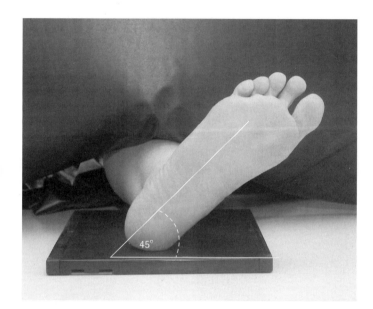

45°

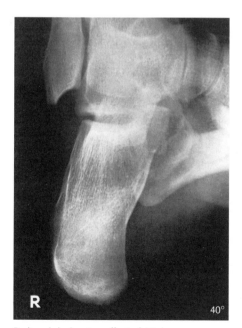

R   40°

Radiograph showing effect of 40-degree angulation

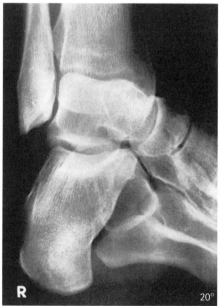

R   20°

Radiograph showing effect of 20-degree angulation

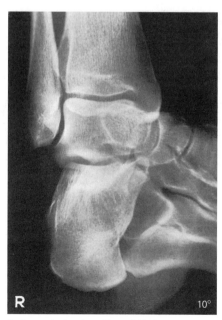

R   10°

Radiograph showing effect of 10-degree angulation

4 | Subtalar joints

Oblique lateral

Position of patient and cassette

- The patient lies supine on the X-ray table, with the affected limb extended.
- The ankle joint is dorsiflexed and the malleoli are equidistant from the cassette.
- The leg is externally rotated through 45 degrees.
- A pad is placed under the knee for support.
- A non-opaque square pad and sandbag may be placed against the plantar aspect of the foot to keep the ankle joint in dorsiflexion.
- The lower edge of the cassette is placed at the level of the plantar aspect of the heel.

Direction and centring of the X-ray beam

- Centre 2.5 cm distal to the medial malleolus, with the central ray angled 15 degrees cranially.

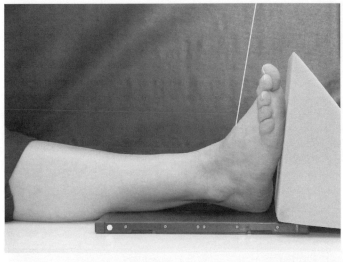

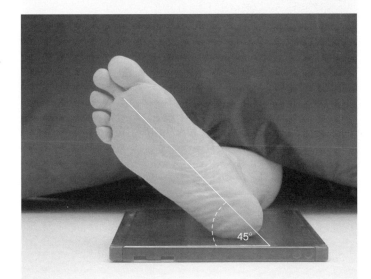

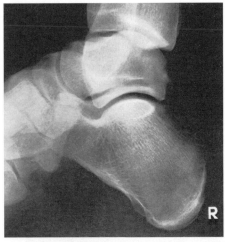

Oblique lateral with 15 degrees cranial tube angulation

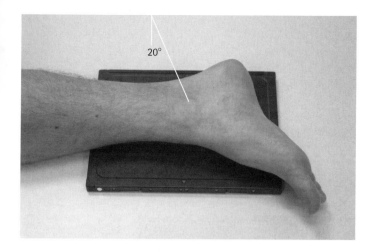

Lateral oblique

Position of patient and cassette

- The patient lies on the affected side.
- The opposite limb is flexed and brought in front of the affected limb.
- The affected foot and leg are now further rotated laterally until the plantar aspect of the foot is approximately 45 degrees to the cassette.
- The lower edge of the cassette is positioned just below the plantar aspect of the heel.

Direction and centring of the X-ray beam

- Centre to the medial malleolus, with the central ray angled 20 degrees caudally.

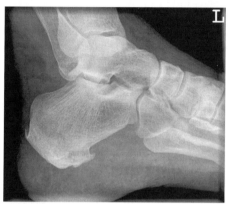

Radiograph of subtalar joints – lateral oblique projection

Tibia and fibula

Basic projections

Two projections are taken of the full length of the lower leg. A cassette fitted with standard intensifying screens is chosen that is large enough to accommodate the entire length of the tibia and fibula.

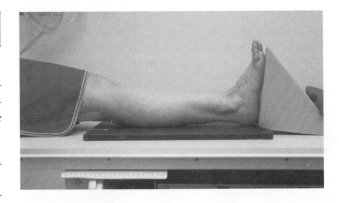

Antero-posterior – basic

Position of patient and cassette

- The patient is either supine or seated on the X-ray table, with both legs extended.
- The ankle is supported in dorsiflexion by a firm 90-degree pad placed against the plantar aspect of the foot. The limb is rotated medially until the medial and lateral malleoli are equidistant from the cassette.
- The lower edge of the cassette is positioned just below the plantar aspect of the heel.

Direction and centring of the X-ray beam

- Centre to the middle of the cassette, with the central ray at right-angles to both the long axis of the tibia and an imaginary line joining the malleoli.

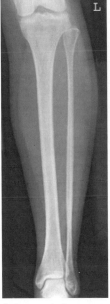 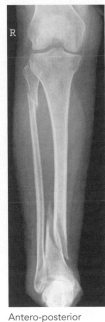

Antero-posterior   Lateral   Antero-posterior radiograph showing fracture of proximal fibula and distal tibia

Lateral – basic

Position of patient and cassette

- From the supine/seated position, the patient rotates on to the affected side.
- The leg is rotated further until the malleoli are superimposed vertically.
- The tibia should be parallel to the cassette.
- A pad is placed under the knee for support.
- The lower edge of the cassette is positioned just below the plantar aspect of the heel.

Direction and centring of the X-ray beam

- Centre to the middle of the cassette, with the central ray at right-angles to the long axis of the tibia and parallel to an imaginary line joining the malleoli.

Essential image characteristics

- The knee and ankle joints must be included, since the proximal end of the fibula may also be fractured when there is a fracture of the distal fibula.

Notes

- If it is impossible to include both joints on one image, then two films should be exposed separately, one to include the ankle and the other to include the knee. Both images should

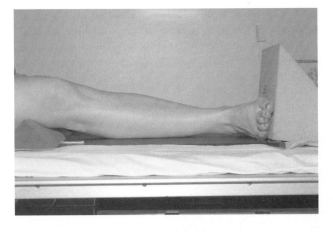

include the middle third of the lower leg, so the general alignment of the bones may be seen.
- If it is impossible for the patient to rotate on to the affected side, then the cassette should be supported vertically against the medial side of the leg and the beam directed horizontally to the middle of the cassette.

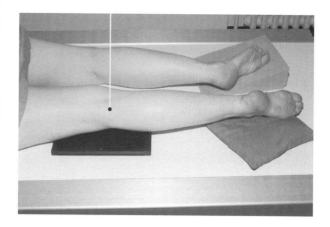

Basic projections

Either a lateral oblique or an anterior oblique projection is taken to demonstrate the tibio-fibular articulation.

Lateral oblique – basic

Position of patient and cassette

- The patient lies on the affected side, with the knee slightly flexed.
- The other limb is brought forward in front of the one being examined and supported on a sandbag.
- The head of the fibula and the lateral tibial condyle of the affected side are palpated and the limb rotated laterally to project the joint clear of the tibial condyle.
- The centre of the cassette is positioned at the level of the head of the fibula.

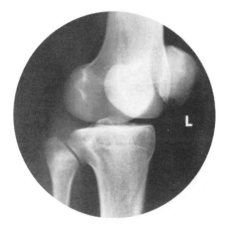

Direction and centring of the X-ray beam

- The vertical central ray is directed to the head of the fibula.

Antero-posterior oblique

Position of patient and cassette

- The patient is either supine or seated on the X-ray table, with both legs extended.
- Palpate the head of fibula and the lateral tibial condyle.
- Rotate the limb medially to project the tibial condyle clear of the joint.
- The limb is supported by pads and sandbags.
- The centre of the cassette is positioned at the level of the head of the fibula.

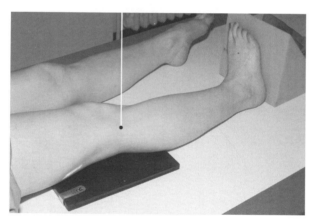

Direction and centring of the X-ray beam

- The vertical central ray is directed to the head of the fibula.

Radiological considerations

This pair of bones constitutes a ring. As for other bony rings, a fracture at one site may be associated with a fracture elsewhere. An example is the Maissonneuve's fracture, which is a fracture of the distal tibia and proximal fibula. If a fracture of one of the pair is seen, with overlap or shortening, then the entire length of both bones must be demonstrated.

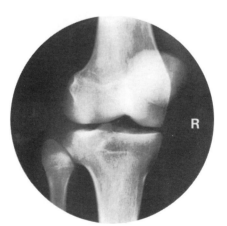

4 Knee joint

Basic projections

Two projections are taken routinely: an antero-posterior and a lateral. Each image is normally acquired using a 18 × 24-cm cassette with standard-speed intensifying screens.

Antero-posterior

Position of patient and cassette

- The patient is either supine or seated on the X-ray table, with both legs extended. The affected limb is rotated to centralize the patella between the femoral condyles, and sandbags are placed against the ankle to help maintain this position.
- The cassette should be in close contact with the posterior aspect of the knee joint, with its centre level with the upper borders of the tibial condyles.

Direction and centring of the X-ray beam

- Centre 2.5 cm below the apex of the patella through the joint space, with the central ray at 90 degrees to the long axis of the tibia.

Essential image characteristics

- The patella must be centralized over the femur.

Notes

- To enable correct assessment of the joint space, the central ray must be at 90 degrees to the long axis of the tibia and, if necessary, angled slightly cranially. If the central ray is not perpendicular to the long axis of the tibia, then the anterior and posterior margins of the tibial plateau will be separated widely and assessment of the true width of the joint space will be difficult.
- If the central ray is too high, then the patella is thrown down over the joint space and the joint space appears narrower.
- If the knee joint is flexed and the patient is unable to extend the limb, then the cassette may be raised on pads to bring it as close as possible to the posterior aspect of the knee.
- In the antero-posterior projection, the patella is remote from the cassette. Although the relationship of the patella to the surrounding structures can be assessed the trabecular pattern of the femur is superimposed. Therefore, this projection is not ideal for demonstrating discrete patella bony abnormalities.

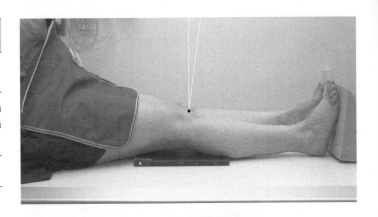

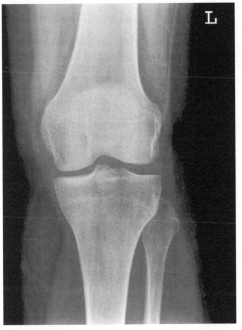

Normal antero-posterior radiograph

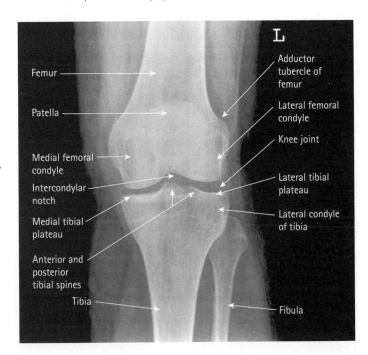

Femur —
Patella —
Medial femoral condyle
Intercondylar notch
Medial tibial plateau
Anterior and posterior tibial spines
Tibia

Adductor tubercle of femur
Lateral femoral condyle
Knee joint
Lateral tibial plateau
Lateral condyle of tibia
Fibula

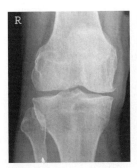

Effect of internal rotation

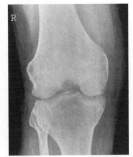

Effect of flexion of the knee

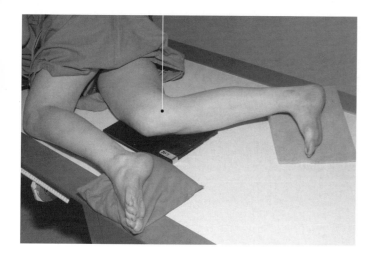

Lateral – basic

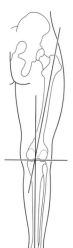

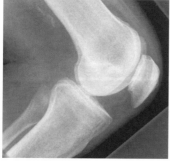

Lateral radiograph of the knee with 90 degrees of flexion

Position of patient and cassette

- The patient lies on the side to be examined, with the knee flexed at 45 or 90 degrees (see below).
- The other limb is brought forward in front of the one being examined and supported on a sandbag.
- A sandbag is placed under the ankle of the affected side to bring the long axis of the tibia parallel to the cassette.
- The position of the limb is now adjusted to ensure that the femoral condyles are superimposed vertically.
- The centre of the cassette is placed level with the medial tibial condyle.

Direction and centring of the X-ray beam

- Centre to the middle of the superior border of the medial tibial condyle, with the central ray at 90 degrees to the long axis of the tibia.

Essential image characteristics

- The patella should be projected clear of the femur.
- The femoral condyles should be superimposed.
- The proximal tibio-fibular joint is not clearly visible.

Notes

- If over-rotated, the medial femoral condyle is projected in front of the lateral condyle and the proximal tibio-fibular joint will be well demonstrated.
- If under-rotated, the medial femoral condyle is projected behind the lateral condyle and the head of the fibula is superimposed on the tibia.
- If the central ray is not at 90 degrees to the long axis of the tibia, the femoral condyles will not be superimposed.
- Flexion of the knee at 90 degrees is the most easily reproducible angle and allows assessment of any degree of patella alta or patella baja (patella riding too high or too low). With the knee flexed at 90 degrees, a patella in normal position will lie between two parallel lines drawn along the anterior and posterior surfaces of the femur.
- In patients who are unable to flex to 90 degrees, the examination should be performed at 45-degree flexion. This may permit a clearer view of the patello-femoral articulation.

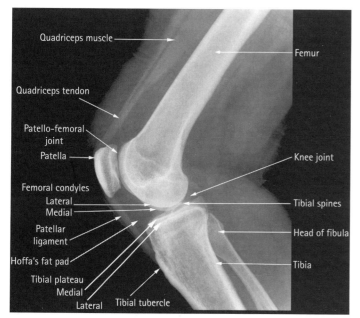

Quadriceps muscle
Femur
Quadriceps tendon
Patello-femoral joint
Patella
Knee joint
Femoral condyles
Lateral
Medial
Tibial spines
Patellar ligament
Head of fibula
Hoffa's fat pad
Tibia
Tibial plateau
Medial
Lateral
Tibial tubercle

Lateral radiograph of the knee with 45 degrees of flexion

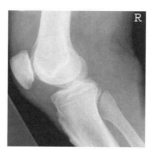

Effect of over rotation

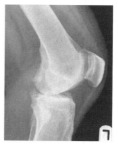

Effect of under rotation

Knee joint

Additional projections

Further projections are used to demonstrate fracture of the patella and the intercondylar notch. Stress views may also be taken in suspected ligamental tears.

A lateral projection of the knee and tibial tubercle may be useful in Osgood Schlatter's disease, although this is primarily a clinical diagnosis and radiography is reserved for exclusion of other pathology in cases of doubt. Ultrasound may also be useful in this clinical situation.

Lateral – horizontal beam

This projection replaces the conventional lateral in all cases of gross injury and suspected fracture of the patella.

Position of patient and cassette

- The patient remains on the trolley/bed, with the limb gently raised and supported on pads.
- If possible, the leg may be rotated slightly to centralize the patella between the femoral condyles.
- The film is supported vertically against the medial aspect of the knee.
- The centre of the cassette is level with the upper border of the tibial condyle.

Direction and centring of the X-ray beam

- The horizontal central ray is directed to the upper border of the lateral tibial condyle, at 90 degrees to the long axis of the tibia.

Notes

- No attempt must be made to either flex or extend the knee joint.
- Additional flexion may result in fragments of a transverse patellar fracture being separated by the opposing muscle pull.
- Any rotation of the limb must be from the hip, with support given to the whole leg.
- By using a horizontal beam, fluid levels may be demonstrated, indicating lipohaemarthrosis.

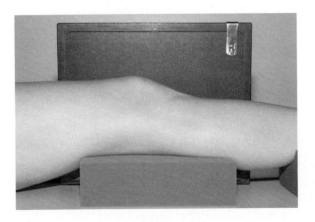

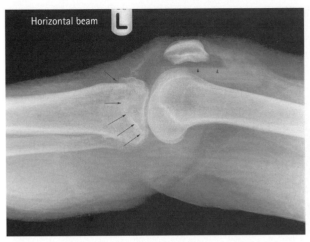

Horizontal beam lateral showing depressed fracture of tibial plateau (arrows) and lipohaemarthrosis (arrowheads)

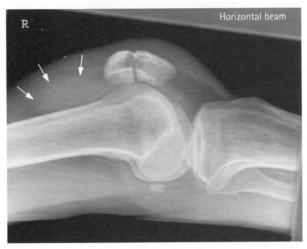

Horizontal beam lateral showing transverse fracture of the patella and joint effusion in suprapatellar bursa (arrows)

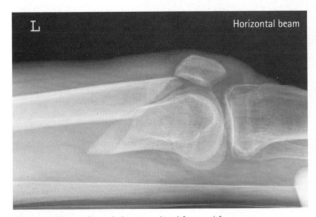

Horizontal beam lateral showing distal femoral fracture

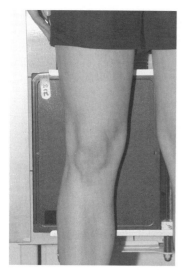

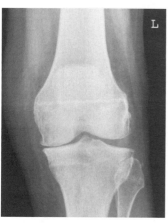

Standing antero-posterior knee radiograph showing loss of height of the medial compartment due to osteoarthritis

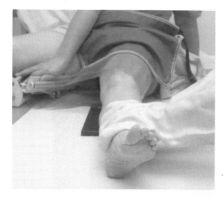

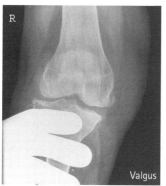

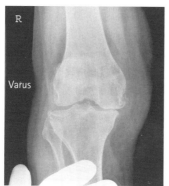

Antero-posterior knee with valgus stress

Antero-posterior knee with varus stress

Antero-posterior – standing projections

This projection is useful to demonstrate alignment of the femur and tibia in the investigation of valgus (bow leg) or varus (knock knee) deformity. Any such deformity will be accentuated when weight bearing, which more closely resembles the real-life situation. It is commonly requested to assess alignment prior to joint replacement, as narrowing of one side to the joint space more than the other will produce varus or valgus tilt. Both knees may be included for comparison.

Position of patient and cassette

- The cassette is supported in the chest stand.
- The patient stands with their back against the vertical Bucky, using it for support if necessary.
- The patient's weight is distributed equally.
- The knee is rotated so that the patella lies equally between the femoral condyles.
- The limb is rotated slightly medially to compensate for the obliquity of the beam when the central ray is centred midway between the knees.
- The centre of the cassette is level with the palpable upper borders of the tibial condyles.

Direction and centring of the X-ray beam

- The horizontal beam is centred midway between the palpable upper borders of the tibial condyles.

Stress projections for subluxation

Stress projections of the knee joint are taken to show subluxation due to rupture of the collateral ligaments. Although these projections may be done in the department, they are now commonly done in theatre using a mobile image intensifier. Stress is applied to the joint by medical personnel, usually an orthopaedic surgeon.

Antero-posterior – stress

Position of patient and cassette

- The patient and cassette are positioned for the routine antero-posterior projection.
- The doctor forcibly abducts or adducts the knee, without rotating the leg.

Direction and centring of the X-ray beam

- Centre midway between the upper borders of the tibial condyles, with the central ray at 90 degrees to the long axis of the tibia.

4 | Knee joint

Patella

Additional projections may be necessary to demonstrate the patella adequately.

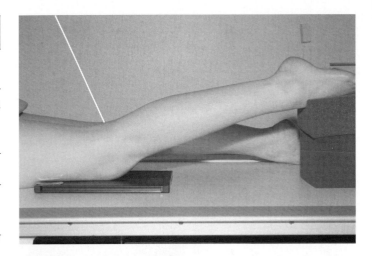

Postero-anterior

Position of patient and cassette

- The patient lies prone on the table, with the knee slightly flexed.
- Foam pads are placed under the ankle and thigh for support.
- The limb is rotated to centralize the patella.
- The centre of the cassette is level with the crease of the knee.

Direction and centring of the X-ray beam

- Centre midway between the upper borders of the tibial condyles at the level of the crease of the knee, with the central ray at 90 degrees to the long axis of the tibia.

Notes

- The beam may have to be angled caudally to be at right-angles to the long axis of the tibia.
- The patella may be demonstrated more clearly as it is now adjacent to the image receptor and not distant from it, as in the conventional antero-posterior projection.
- Subtle abnormalities may not be detected, as the trabecular pattern of the femur will still predominate.
- This projection depends on the fitness of the patient and must not be attempted if it results in undue discomfort or if it may exacerbate the patient's condition.

Radiological considerations

- A joint effusion is well demonstrated on the lateral projection as an ovoid density rising above the postero-superior aspect of the patella. Its significance varies according to the clinical setting. Causes include infection, haemorrhage and arthritis, but it may also be a marker of occult fracture, e.g. tibial spine or tibial plateau fracture. Lipohaemarthrosis occurs when a fracture passes into the marrow-containing medullary space. Fat (bone marrow) leaks into the joint, producing a fluid level between fat and fluid (blood) that can be seen when a horizontal beam is used.
- Fracture of the anterior tibial spine may be subtle, with demonstration requiring attention to exposure and rotation. It is important as the attachment of the anterior cruciate ligament, avulsion of which may cause debilitating instability of the knee.
- Vertical fracture of the patella is not visible on the lateral projection and will be seen on the antero-posterior projection only if exposed properly (i.e. not underexposed). If clinically suspected, then a skyline view maybe requested.

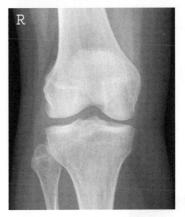

Postero-anterior radiograph of normal patella

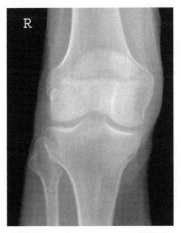

Radiograph of patella showing transverse fracture

- Tibial plateau fractures can be subtle and hard to detect, but again they are functionally very important. Good technique is the key. Full evaluation may be aided by three-dimensional CT in some cases.
- The fabella is a sesamoid bone in the tendon of medial head of gastrocnemius, behind the medial femoral condyle, and should not be confused with loose body.
- Osgood–Schlatters disease is a clinical diagnosis and does not usually require radiography for diagnosis. Ultrasound may be useful if confirmation is required. Projections of the contralateral knee should not normally be needed.

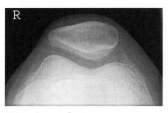
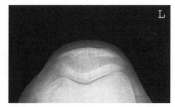

Thirty-degree flexion
Infero-superior (conventional) projection

Sixty-degree flexion

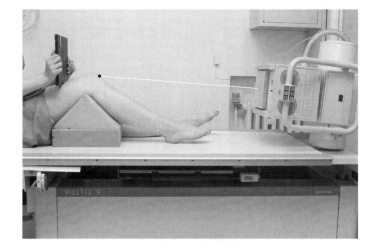

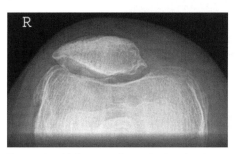

Conventional infero-superior projection showing osteophytosis affecting the retro-patellar joint

Skyline projections

The skyline projection can be used to:

- assess the retro-patellar joint space for degenerative disease;
- determine the degree of any lateral subluxation of the patella with ligament laxity;
- diagnose chondromalacia patellae;
- confirm the presence of a vertical patella fracture in acute trauma.

The optimum retro-patellar joint spacing occurs when the knee is flexed approximately 30–45 degrees. Further flexion pulls the patella into the intercondylar notch, reducing the joint spacing; as flexion increases, the patella tracks over the lateral femoral condyle. The patella moves a distance of 2 cm from full extension to full flexion.

There are three methods of achieving the skyline projection:

- conventional infero-superior;
- supero-inferior – beam directed downwards;
- infero-superior – patient prone.

Conventional infero-superior projection

The procedure is undertaken using an 18 × 24-cm cassette.

Position of patient and cassette

- The patient sits on the X-ray table, with the knee flexed 30–45 degrees and supported on a pad placed below the knee.
- A cassette is held by the patient against the anterior distal femur and supported using a non-opaque pad, which rests on the anterior aspect of the thigh.

Direction and centring of the X-ray beam

- The tube is lowered. Avoiding the feet, the central ray is directed cranially to pass through the apex of the patella parallel to the long axis.
- The beam should be closely collimated to the patella and femoral condyles to limit scattered radiation to the trunk and head.

Radiation protection

- Examination of the individual single knee is recommended, rather than including both knees in one exposure when both knees are requested.
- The total radiation field can be reduced, thus limiting the scattered radiation.
- A lead-rubber apron is worn for protection, with additional lead-rubber protection placed over the gonads.

4 Knee joint

Supero-inferior

This projection has the advantage that the radiation beam is not directed towards the gonads.

Position of patient and cassette

- The patient sits on the X-ray table, with the affected knee flexed over the side.
- Ideally, the leg should be flexed to 45 degrees to reflect a similar knee position to the conventional skyline projection. Too much flexion reduces the retro-patellar spacing. Sitting the patient on a cushion helps to achieve the optimum position.
- The cassette is supported horizontally on a stool at the level of the inferior tibial tuberosity border.

Direction and centring of the X-ray beam

- The vertical beam is directed to the posterior aspect of the proximal border of the patella. The central ray should be parallel to the long axis of the patella.
- The beam is collimated to the patella and femoral condyles.

Notes

- Not enough flexion will cause the tibial tuberosity to overshadow the retro-patellar joint.
- Too much flexion will cause the patella to track over the lateral femoral condyle.

Radiation protection

Radiation protection should be provided to the gonads, and the patient should lean backwards, away from the primary beam.

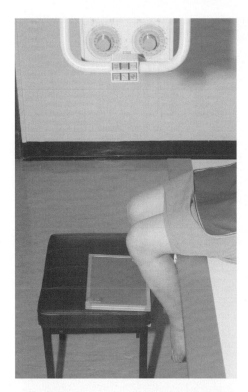

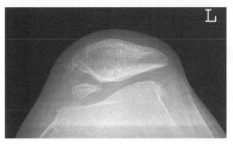

Supero-inferior image showing some degenerative changes and a loose bone fragment

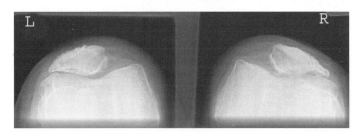

Supero-inferior projections showing advanced degenerative changes but the knees have been flexed too much, giving the appearance of lateral subluxation of the patella

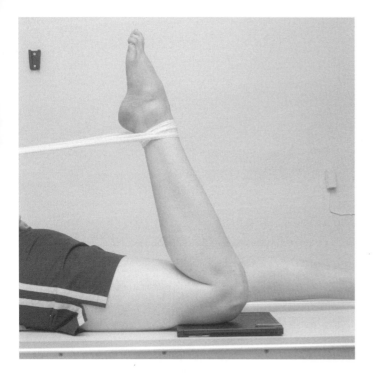

Infero-superior – patient prone

This projection has the advantage in that the primary beam is not directed towards the gonads, as is the case with the conventional infero-superior projection. However, the patient has to be able to adopt the prone position, which may not be suitable for all patients.

Position of patient and cassette

- The patient lies prone on the X-ray table, with the cassette placed under the knee joint and the knee flexed through 90 degrees.
- A bandage placed around the ankle and either tethered to a vertical support or held by the patient may prevent unnecessary movement.

Direction and centring of the X-ray beam

- Centre behind the patella, with the vertical central ray angled approximately 15 degrees towards the knee, avoiding the toes.

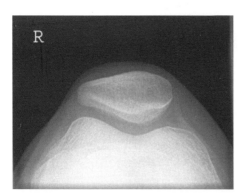

Normal infero-superior radiograph of patella, patient prone

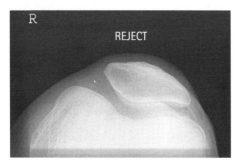

Infero-superior radiograph with insufficient flexion causing the tibia to be projected over the patella

Knee joint

Postero-anterior oblique

Position of patient and cassette

- The patient lies prone on the X-ray table.
- The trunk is then rotated on to each side in turn to bring either the medial or the lateral aspect of the knee at an angle of approximately 45 degrees to the cassette.
- The knee is then flexed slightly.
- A sandbag is placed under the ankle for support.
- The centre of the cassette is level with the uppermost tibial condyle.

Direction and centring of the X-ray beam

- The vertical central ray is directed to the uppermost tibial condyle.

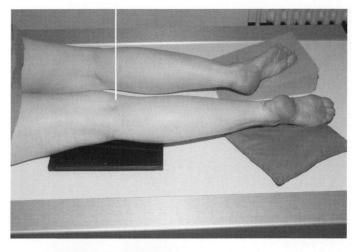

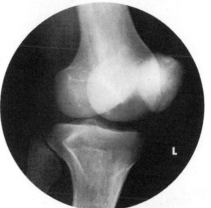

Antero-posterior oblique

Position of patient and cassette

- The patient lies supine on the X-ray table.
- The trunk is then rotated to allow rotation of the affected limb either medially or laterally through 45 degrees.
- The knee is flexed slightly.
- A sandbag is placed under the ankle for support.
- The centre of the cassette is level with the upper border of the uppermost tibial condyle.

Direction and centring of the X-ray beam

- The vertical central ray is directed to the middle of the uppermost tibial condyle.

Notes

- These projections may be taken in addition to the basic images to show each half of the patella clear of the femur.
- The choice of either postero-anterior oblique or antero-posterior oblique is dependent upon the condition of the patient. The postero-anterior projection will give a better quality image by placing the patella in closer proximity to the cassette.

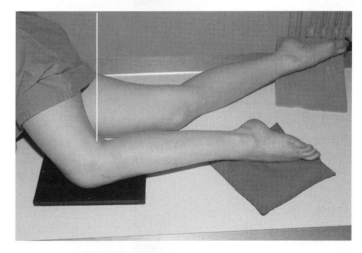

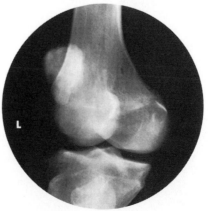

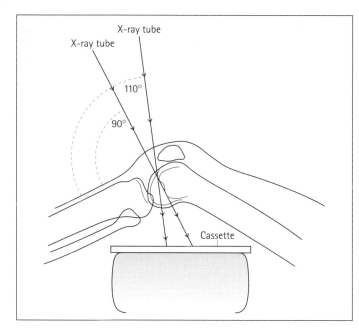

Intercondylar notch (tunnel)

This projection is taken to demonstrate loose bodies within the knee joint. A curved cassette with standard-speed intensifying screens, if available, is used to acquire the image. Curved cassettes are not available with digital imaging systems, in which case an 18 × 24 cm cassette will be used.

Position of patient and cassette

- The patient is either supine or seated on the X-ray table, with the affected knee flexed to approximately 60 degrees.
- A suitable pad is placed under the knee to help maintain the position.
- The limb is rotated to centralize the patella over the femur.
- The cassette is placed on top of the pad as close as possible to the posterior aspect of the knee and displaced towards the femur.

Direction and centring of the X-ray beam

- Centre immediately below the apex of the patella, with the following angulations to demonstrate either the anterior or posterior aspects of the notch:

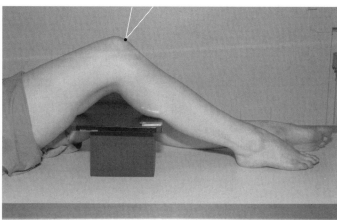

Angulation to the long axis of the tibia	Anatomy demonstrated
110 degrees	Anterior aspect of the notch
90 degrees	Posterior aspect of the notch

Notes

- Commonly only the 90 degree angulation is used.
- This projection may be requested occasionally to demonstrate a fracture of the tibial spines, where cruciate ligaments are attached. Care must be taken when flexing the knee.

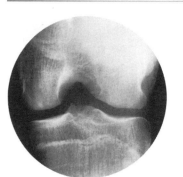

110 degrees

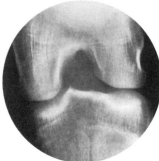

90 degrees

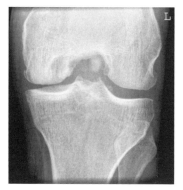

Radiograph of intercondylar notch showing loose body

135

4 Shaft of femur

Basic projections

Two projections are taken routinely, preferably with both the knee and hip joints included on the image. If this is impossible to achieve, then the joint nearest the site of injury should be included.

A large cassette is placed in the table Bucky so that the effects of scatter are reduced. However, should only an image of the distal aspect of the femur be required, then the use of the Bucky can be eliminated in order to reduce patient dose.

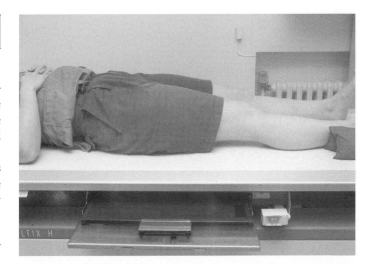

Antero-posterior

Position of patient and cassette

- The patient lies supine on the X-ray table, with both legs extended.
- The affected limb is rotated to centralize the patella over the femur.
- Sandbags are placed below the knee to help maintain the position.
- The cassette is positioned in the Bucky tray immediately under the limb, adjacent to the posterior aspect of the thigh to include both the hip and the knee joints.
- Alternatively, the cassette is positioned directly under the limb, against the posterior aspect of the thigh to include the knee joint.

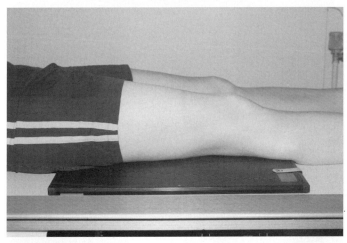

Direction and centring of the X-ray beam

- Centre to the middle of the cassette, with the vertical central ray at 90 degrees to an imaginary line joining both femoral condyles.

Notes

- In cases of suspected fracture, the limb must not be rotated.
- If both joints are not included on one film, then a single antero-posterior projection of the joint distal to the fracture site must be taken. This ensures that no fracture is missed and allows assessment of any rotation at the fracture site.
- Remember that the divergent beam will project the hip cranially and the knee caudally, and therefore care must be taken when positioning the cassette to ensure that the joint will be on the top/bottom of the film.

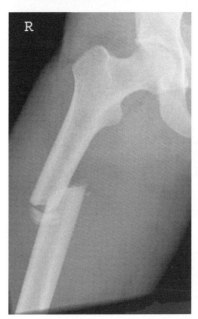
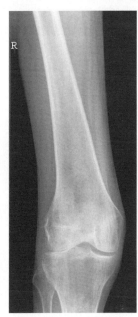

Antero-posterior radiograph of femur, hip down, showing fracture of upper femoral shaft

Antero-posterior radiograph of normal femur, knee up

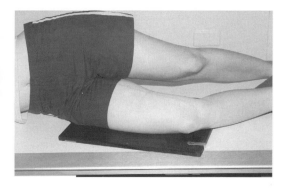

Position of patient and cassette

- From the antero-posterior position, the patient rotates on to the affected side, and the knee is slightly flexed.
- The pelvis is rotated backwards to separate the thighs.
- The position of the limb is then adjusted to vertically super-impose the femoral condyles.
- Pads are used to support the opposite limb behind the one being examined.
- The cassette is positioned in the Bucky tray under the lateral aspect of the thigh to include the knee joint and as much of the femur as possible.
- Alternatively, the cassette is positioned directly under the limb, against the lateral aspect of the thigh, to include the knee joint.

Direction and centring of the X-ray beam

- Centre to the middle of the cassette, with the vertical central ray parallel to the imaginary line joining the femoral condyles.

Additional projection – lateral horizontal beam

This projection replaces the conventional lateral in all cases of gross injury and suspected fracture.

Position of patient and cassette

- The patient remains on the trolley/bed. If possible, the leg may be slightly rotated to centralize the patella between the femoral condyles.
- The cassette is supported vertically against the lateral aspect of the thigh, with the lower border of the cassette level with the upper border of the tibial condyle.
- The unaffected limb is raised above the injured limb, with the knee flexed and the lower leg supported on a stool or specialized support.

Direction and centring of the X-ray beam

- Centre to the middle of the cassette, with the beam horizontal.

Note

If the injury involves only the lower two-thirds of femur, then place the cassette vertically against the medial aspect of the thigh, directing the beam from the lateral aspect of the limb to the middle of the cassette.

Radiation protection

- In all cases, the beam must be well collimated.
- Gonad protection must be applied in all non-trauma cases, as extra-focal radiation and scattered radiation will irradiate the gonads if not protected.
- In trauma cases, gonad protection is not used in the first instance as it may obscure injury. In subsequent follow-up radiographs, gonad protection must be used.

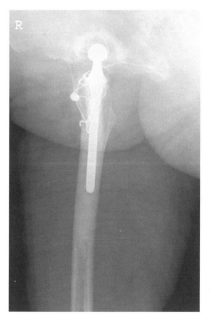

Lateral radiograph of femur, hip down, showing prosthetic hip

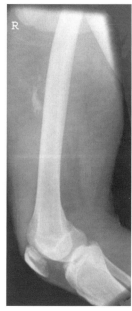

Lateral radiograph of femur, knee up, showing an area of myositis ossificans

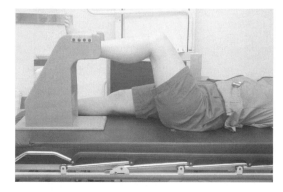

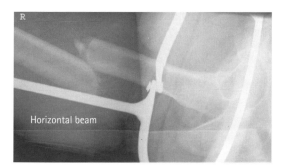

Horizontal beam

4 Leg alignment

Images of both lower limbs are required to demonstrate leg alignment. This is undertaken for a variety of reasons, but predominately in adults before and after artificial joint replacement and in children for bow legs and knocked knees. The technique for children is similar to that described for leg-length measurement in the paediatric chapter (see p. 417).

In adults, this technique is undertaken with the patient erect and therefore weight bearing, and is described below for both conventional film/screen and digital computed radiography (CR).

Conventional film/screen method

Assessment by conventional film/screen radiography is undertaken using a single-exposure technique using a long cassette (35 × 105 cm) fitted with graduated screens and preferably loaded with a single film (triple-fold film) and a large FFD (typically 180–200 cm). The fastest end of the screens is placed behind the hips and the slowest at the ankle joints. The cassette is mounted vertically in a special holder to facilitate radiography in the erect position. With this technique, the divergent beam will magnify the limbs; however, the degree of inaccuracy is considered surgically insignificant and is not a factor when assessing the limbs for alignment (see Section 14, pp. 417–418, for further information).

Position of patient and cassette

- The patient stands on a low step, with the posterior aspect of the legs against the long cassette. The arms are folded across the chest. The anterior superior iliac spines should be equidistant from the cassette. The medial sagittal plane should be vertical and coincident with the central longitudinal axis of the cassette.
- The legs should be, as far as possible, in a similar relationship to the pelvis, with the feet separated so that the distance between the ankle joints is similar to the distance between the hip joints and with the patella of each knee facing forward.
- Ideally, the knees and ankle joints should be in the anteroposterior position. However, if this impossible to achieve, it is more important that the knees rather than the ankle joints are placed in the antero-posterior position.
- Foam pads and sandbags are used to stabilize the legs and maintain the position. If necessary, a block may be positioned below a shortened leg to ensure that there is no pelvic tilt and that the limbs are aligned adequately.

Direction and centring of the X-ray beam

- The horizontal central ray is directed towards a point midway between the knee joints.
- The X-ray beam is collimated to include both lower limbs from hip joints to ankle joints.

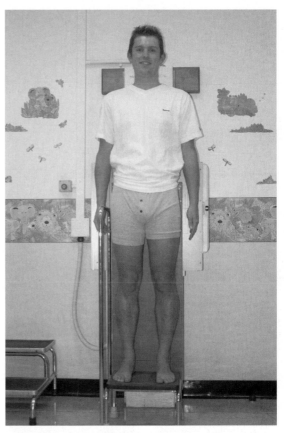

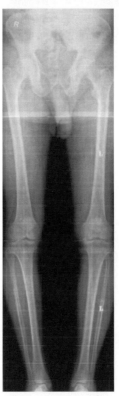

Preoperative CR image to show limb alignment

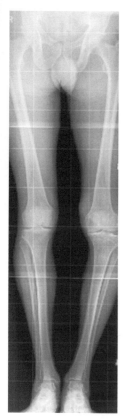

Limb alignment on CR showing genu varus secondary to osteoarthritis of the knee. This can cause difficulty fitting the whole of the limbs onto one image

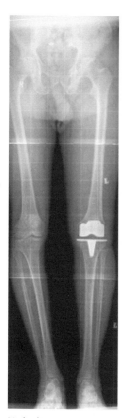

Limb alignment on CR image following total knee replacement (same patient as radiograph on p. 138)

Digital computed radiography method

A special three-cassette-holding device is secured in a vertical position to allow horizontal beam radiography using a large FFD, as described for the conventional film/screen method. Using this method, three individual images of the lower limbs are acquired using one exposure. These are then 'stitched together' electronically using a special imaging software package.

Positioning of the patient and the direction and centring of the X-ray beam are similar to that described for the conventional film/screen method.

Image acquisition

Three 35 × 43-cm cassettes are inserted lengthways into the vertical cassette-holding device. This is designed to accommodate the cassettes in three separate slots, allowing for a slight overlap in the images. The holding device itself can be adjusted vertically to accommodate patients of different heights. If a patient is small in stature, then only two cassettes may be necessary.

It is important that anatomical markers are secured on to the front of the vertical cassette-holding device and placed in such a way that they are visible on each individual image. A minimum of three is recommended to distinguish between right and left limbs.

The X-ray beam is collimated to the whole area of interest from hips to ankles. The central ray is angled two to three degrees caudally to assist the stitching software.

Image analysis

Following the exposure, the cassettes are carefully identified and presented for image reading, after which post-processing of the images is undertaken to correct for differences in anatomical thicknesses. The three images are then 'stitched' together following the manufacturer's protocol to produce one full-length image. This final image is correctly windowed and annotated.

An assessment of leg alignment can then be undertaken using various post-processing tools. One technique involves drawing a line along the femur from mid-femoral head to mid-femoral condyles and a line along the length of the tibia from mid-ankle joint to mid-knee joint, which is then extended. The angle intersecting the femoral line to a continuation of the tibial line is then measured. This angle should normally be less than three degrees. Alternatively, a line (the mechanical axis) can be drawn from the mid-femoral head to midpoint of the ankle; this should pass through the centre of the knee. Deflexion of the mechanical axis can be measured and the angle derived from $(m/3 + 1)$ degrees, where m is the deflection measured in millimetres.

Radiological considerations

The image must demonstrate the endpoints of the mechanical axis clearly, i.e. all three joints (hip, knee and ankle) must be exposed correctly and both legs must be in correct neutral anatomical position, with the patella facing forward and symmetrical.

Section 5

The Hip, Pelvis and Sacro-iliac Joints

CONTENTS

RECOMMENDED PROJECTIONS   142

ANATOMY AND IMAGE APPEARANCES   143
Introduction   145

EFFECT OF ROTATION AND
ABDUCTION OF THE LOWER LIMB   147

HIP JOINT, UPPER THIRD OF FEMUR
AND PELVIS   148
Antero-posterior – pelvis (basic projection)
  and both hips (basic projection)   148

HIP JOINT AND UPPER THIRD
OF FEMUR   150
Antero-posterior – single hip (basic)   150
Posterior oblique (commonly known as
  Lauenstein's projection)   151
True lateral – neck of femur (basic)   152
Lateral – single hip (alternative
  projections) modification of technique   153

Lateral oblique modified – alternative 1   153
Lateral modified – alternative 2   153
Lateral – both hips ('frog's legs position')   154

ACETABULUM AND HIP JOINT   155
Anterior oblique (Judet's projection)   155
Posterior oblique (reverse Judet's
  projection)   155

PELVIS   156
Ilium   156
Posterior oblique – basic projection   156
Posterior oblique (alternate)   156
Lateral   157
Symphysis pubis   158
Antero-posterior – erect   158

SACRO-ILIAC JOINTS   159
Postero-anterior   159
Antero-posterior   160
Antero-posterior oblique   161

5 Recommended projections

Hip joint	Fractured proximal end of femur	Antero-posterior – both hips (basic) Lateral neck of femur (basic) Lateral – single hip (alternative 1 projection) Lateral – modified (alternative 2 projection)
	Dislocation	Antero-posterior – both hips (basic) Antero-posterior – single hip (post-reduction) Lateral neck of femur (basic)
	Fractured acetabulum	Antero-posterior – both hips (basic) Lateral neck of femur (basic) Posterior oblique Anterior oblique (Judet's projection)
	Other pathology	Antero-posterior – both hips (basic) Other projections on request
	Paediatric disorders: – Development dysplasia (DDH/CDH) – Irritable hips – Postoperative for slipped epiphysis – Trauma	See Section 14
Pelvis	Fractures and pathology	Antero-posterior – both hips (basic) Posterior oblique (basic) Posterior oblique (alternate) Lateral
	Subluxation of the symphysis pubis	Antero-posterior – erect
Sacro-iliac joints	Pathology	Postero-anterior (basic) Antero-posterior Posterior obliques on request

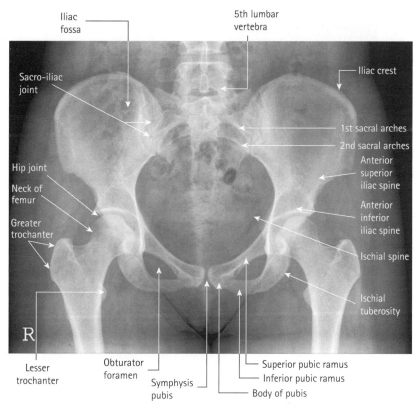

Iliac fossa

5th lumbar vertebra

Sacro-iliac joint

Iliac crest

1st sacral arches

2nd sacral arches

Anterior superior iliac spine

Hip joint

Neck of femur

Anterior inferior iliac spine

Greater trochanter

Ischial spine

Ischial tuberosity

R

Lesser trochanter

Obturator foramen

Symphysis pubis

Body of pubis

Superior pubic ramus

Inferior pubic ramus

Antero-posterior projection of pelvis

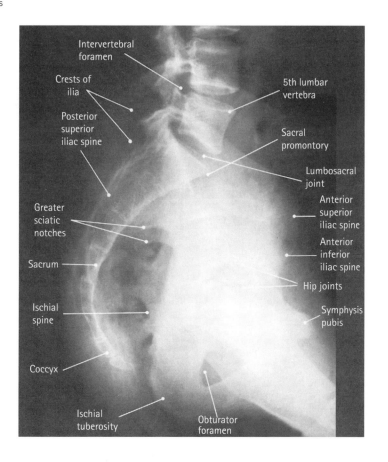

Intervertebral foramen

Crests of ilia

5th lumbar vertebra

Posterior superior iliac spine

Sacral promontory

Lumbosacral joint

Anterior superior iliac spine

Greater sciatic notches

Anterior inferior iliac spine

Sacrum

Hip joints

Ischial spine

Symphysis pubis

Coccyx

Ischial tuberosity

Obturator foramen

Lateral projection of pelvis

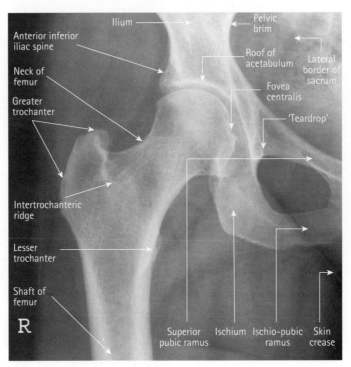

Antero-posterior projection of hip

Labels: Ilium; Pelvic brim; Anterior inferior iliac spine; Roof of acetabulum; Lateral border of sacrum; Neck of femur; Fovea centralis; Greater trochanter; 'Teardrop'; Intertrochanteric ridge; Lesser trochanter; Shaft of femur; R; Superior pubic ramus; Ischium; Ischio-pubic ramus; Skin crease

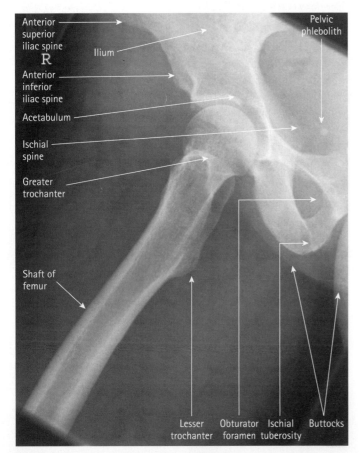

Posterior oblique (Lauenstein's) projection of hip

Labels: Anterior superior iliac spine; Ilium; Pelvic phlebolith; R; Anterior inferior iliac spine; Acetabulum; Ischial spine; Greater trochanter; Shaft of femur; Lesser trochanter; Obturator foramen; Ischial tuberosity; Buttocks

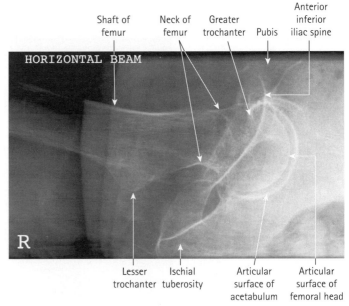

True lateral projection of hip (neck of femur)

Labels: Shaft of femur; Neck of femur; Greater trochanter; Pubis; Anterior inferior iliac spine; HORIZONTAL BEAM; R; Lesser trochanter; Ischial tuberosity; Articular surface of acetabulum; Articular surface of femoral head

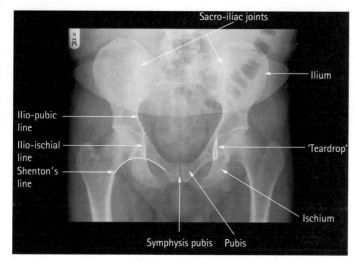

Antero-posterior projection of pelvis

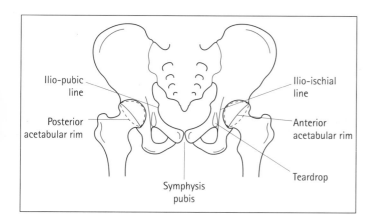

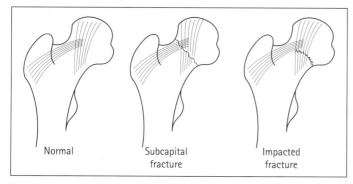

Trabecular patterns in the femoral neck.

Introduction

The hip joint is a ball-and-socket joint in which the smooth, almost spherical head of the femur articulates with the acetabulum, which is formed by the three parts of the innominate bone.

The proximal aspect of the femur consists of the head, neck and greater and lesser trochanters. The neck lies at an angle of approximately 130 degrees with the shaft and is angulated anteriorly approximately 130 degrees when articulated normally with the acetabulum (Rogers, 2002).

The annotated images on p. 144 illustrate the anatomical references used in the text.

Two principal groups of trabeculae exist within the femoral head and neck. The trabecular pattern is more obvious in the elderly, and subtle fractures can cause these pattern lines to become distorted.

The pelvis is formed by the two innominate bones and the sacrum (the innominate bones are themselves formed from the ilium, ischium and pubis). It provides a protective girdle for the pelvic organs and supports the lower limbs. The innominate bones articulate anteriorly at the symphysis pubis and posteriorly with the sacrum at the sacro-iliac joints. As the pelvis is a ring of bone with only slightly moveable joints, bony trauma to one side can result in a corresponding injury to the opposite side.

There are several bony prominences in the pelvic region, which serve as important surface landmarks in radiography. These are:

- the symphysis pubis, upper border: anterior to the bladder, and aligned to the coccyx;
- the anterior superior iliac spine (ASIS): second sacral segment;
- the iliac crests: L4/5; bifurcation of the aorta;
- the posterior superior iliac spines: L5/S1; sacro-iliac joints.

There are also several anatomical radiographic lines that can be used to assess the integrity of the pelvis and hips in trauma:

- 'Shenton's line': a line following the curve of the lower border of the superior pubic ramus and the inferior border of the femoral neck. The shape of the curves on both sides of the pelvis should be the same in the absence of an acute bony injury.
- 'Teardrop' sign: medial wall of the acetabulum.
- Ilio-pubic line: anterior column of the acetabulum.
- Ilio-ischial line: posterior column of the acetabulum.

Introduction (*contd*)

Posture

When the patient is supine, the pelvic brim is tilted according to the degree of angulation at the L5/S1 junction. This results in considerable variation in image appearance. A pronounced lordosis in the lower back can cause the obturator foramen to appear very elliptical and the symphysis pubis to be foreshortened. A small pad placed under the knees can reduce this lordosis and improve the image appearance.

This increased L5/S1 angulation in females when compared with the male pelvis contributes to the differing image appearance.

Subject type

There is a variable difference in the breadth and depth of the pelvis, according to subject type and sex, as seen in the images. The male pelvis is narrower but has greater depth. Careful positioning is often required to include the full width of a female pelvis in the image.

Radiation protection

Protection of the gonads from unnecessary X-radiation is an important factor when examining the hip joints, upper femora, pelvis and lower lumbar vertebrae. Exposure of the patient to X-radiation should be made in accordance with the as low as reasonably practicable (ALARP) principle and, in the UK, Ionising Radiations (Medical Exposure) Regulations (IRMER) 2000.

Primary lead protection should be applied to the gonads of patients from infancy to middle-age, as appropriate. It is not recommended for initial examinations, however, when its use may obscure anatomical information.

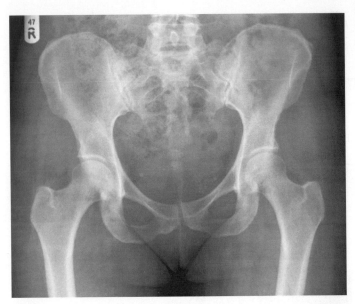

Female pelvis

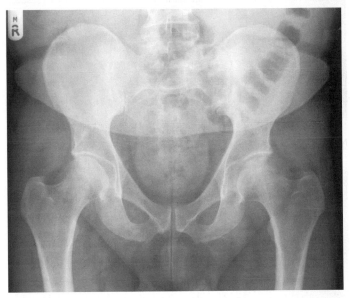

Male pelvis

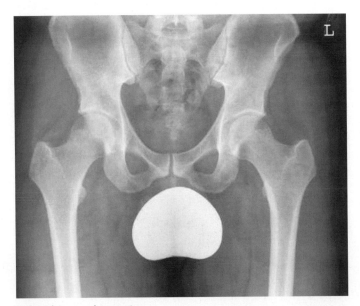

Male pelvis gonad protection

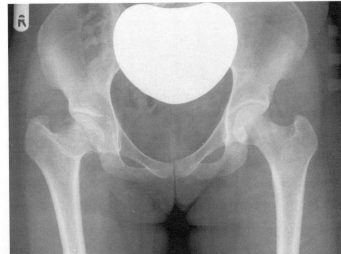

Female pelvis with gonad protection positioned wrongly

Position of limb	Anatomical appearance
Neutral – long axis of foot vertical	Femoral neck oblique Lesser trochanter just visible
Internal rotation	Femoral neck elongated and lying parallel to the cassette Lesser trochanter obscured by shaft of femur
External rotation	Femoral neck foreshortened Lesser trochanter clearly visible

Different positions of the lower limb result in different anatomical projections of the hip joint. The head of the femur lies anterior to the trochanteric bone of the femur when articulating normally with the acetabulum. There is an approximate angulation anteriorly of 125–130 degrees, which is best appreciated on the true lateral projection of the hip (Rogers, 2002).

Internal rotation of the hip joint by approximately 50 degrees will bring the neck of the femur parallel to the cassette and the head and trochanteric bone on the same level.

In abnormal conditions of the hip joint, the position of the foot is a significant clue to the type of injury sustained. Displaced fractures involving the neck and trochanteric region will cause external rotation and usually foreshortening of the affected leg.

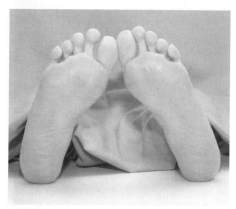

Neutral

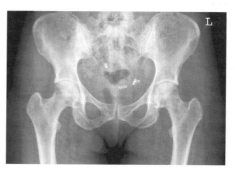

Lesser trochanters visible

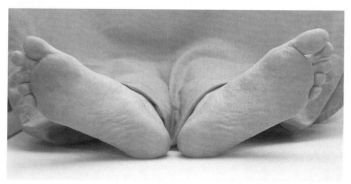

Internal rotation

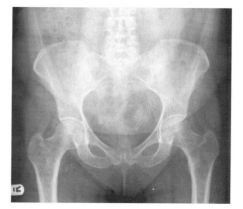

Femoral neck parallel to cassette, lesser trochanters not visible

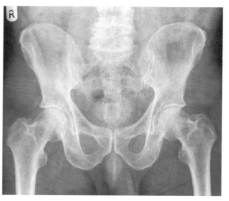

Lesser trochanter clearly visible

External rotation

5 Hip joint, upper third of femur and pelvis

Antero-posterior – pelvis (basic projection) and both hips (basic projection)

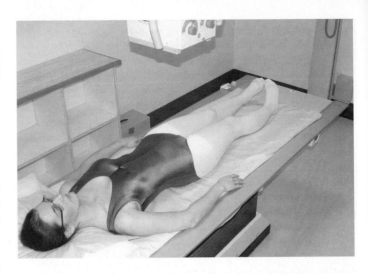

The antero-posterior projection is a general image used as a first assessment of the pelvic bones and hip joints. The position of the patient is identical for imaging both the hips and the pelvis, but the centring of the beam may differ. For the hip joints and upper femora, the centring may be more inferior, e.g. in trauma cases.

The antero-posterior image allows a comparison of both hips to be made; in trauma cases, it ensures that a fracture to the distal pelvis is not missed, e.g. a fractured pubic ramus.

In cases of suspected fracture of the hip, the injured limb is commonly externally rotated and must not be moved. If possible, the opposite limb should be externally rotated to the same degree of rotation so that a more accurate comparison can be made.

Position of patient and cassette

- The patient lies supine and symmetrical on the X-ray table, with the median sagittal plane perpendicular to the tabletop.
- The midline of the patient must coincide with the centred primary beam and table Bucky mechanism.
- If the patient remains on a trolley, ideally they should be positioned down the midline and adjusted to achieve an optimum projection dependent on their degree of mobility.
- To avoid pelvic rotation, the anterior superior iliac spines must be equidistant from the tabletop. A non-opaque pad placed under a buttock can be used to make the pelvis level. The coronal plane should now be parallel to the tabletop.
- The limbs are slightly abducted and internally rotated to bring the femoral necks parallel to the cassette.
- Sandbags and pads are placed against the ankle region to help maintain this position.

Direction and centring of the X-ray beam

- Centre in the midline, with a vertical central beam.
- The centre of the cassette is placed midway between the upper border of the symphysis pubis and anterior superior iliac spine for the whole of the pelvis and proximal femora. The upper edge of the cassette should be 5 cm above the upper border of the iliac crest to compensate for the divergent beam and to ensure that the whole of the bony pelvis is included.
- The centre of the cassette is placed level with the upper border of the symphysis pubis for the hips and upper femora.

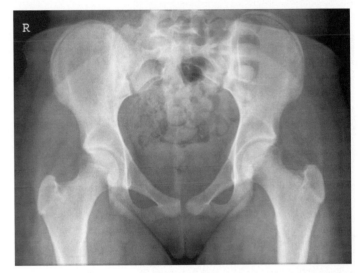

Antero-posterior projection of the whole pelvis, with internal rotation of the femora

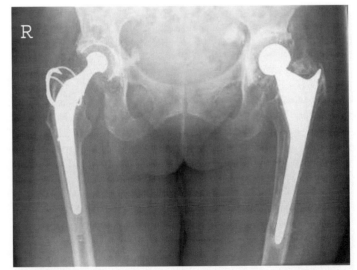

Antero-posterior radiograph of both hips and upper femora showing bilateral prostheses

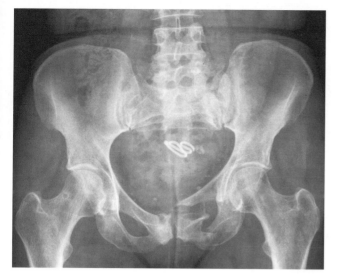

Antero-posterior pelvis showing fracture of ischium and pubis with disruption of Shenton's line. Associated fracture of the left side of the sacrum

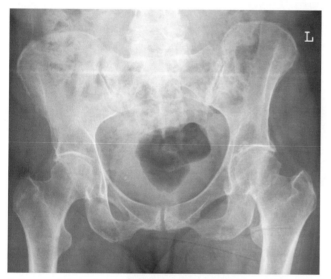

Antero-posterior radiograph showing a subcapital fracture of the neck of the left femur

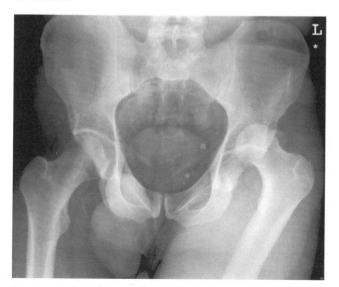

Antero-posterior radiograph of pelvis showing posterior dislocation of the left hip

Antero-posterior – pelvis (basic projection) and both hips (basic projection)

Essential image characteristics

- For the basic projection of both hips, both trochanters and the upper third of the femora must be visible on the image.
- For the basic pelvis projection, both iliac crests and proximal femora, including the lesser trochanters, should be visible on the image.
- No rotation. The iliac bones should be of equal size and the obturator foramina the same size and shape.
- It should be possible to identify Shenton's line, which forms a continuous curve between the lesser trochanter, femoral neck and lower border of the symphysis pubis.
- The optical density, ideally, should be similar throughout the bones of the pelvis and the proximal femora. If the kVp is too low and the mAs is too high, then the supero-lateral part of the ilia and the greater trochanters may not be visualized, particularly in slender patients.
- The image contrast must also allow visualization of the trabecular patterns in the femoral necks. Using compression on appropriate patients, who have excess soft tissue overlying their pelvic bones, can improve image contrast.
- No artefacts from clothing should be visible.

Notes

- Internal rotation of the limb compensates for the X-ray beam divergence when centring in the midline. The resultant image will show both greater and lesser trochanters.
- Patient breathing to blur out overlying structures can be used to diminish obvious bowel shadows over the sacrum and iliac bones.

Radiation protection

- At the first clinic visit and in trauma cases, it is normal practice to not apply gonad protection, which may obscure the pelvic bones and result in missed information. In follow-up visits, gonad protection must be used and must be positioned carefully to avoid obscuring the region of interest resulting in an unnecessary repeat radiograph.
- The primary beam should be optimally collimated to the size of the cassette. Ideally, evidence of collimation should be visible on the image.
- The correct use of automatic exposure control (AEC) reduces the number of repeats due to poor choice of exposure factors.
- Exposure factors or dose–area product (DAP) readings should be recorded.

5 Hip joint and upper third of femur

Antero-posterior – single hip (basic)

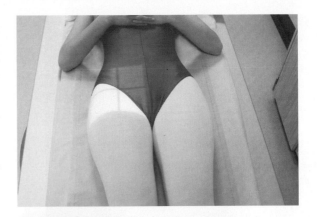

Position of patient and cassette

The patient is positioned as described for the basic pelvis and basic bilateral hip projections.

- The patient lies supine and symmetrical on the X-ray table, with the median sagittal plane perpendicular to the tabletop.
- To avoid pelvic rotation, the anterior superior iliac spines must be equidistant from the tabletop.
- The affected limb is internally rotated to bring the neck of the femur parallel to the tabletop, and is then supported by sandbags.

Direction and centring of the X-ray beam

- The vertical central ray is directed 2.5 cm distally along the perpendicular bisector of a line joining the anterior superior iliac spine and the symphysis pubis over the femoral pulse.
- The primary beam should be collimated to the area under examination and gonad protection applied where appropriate.

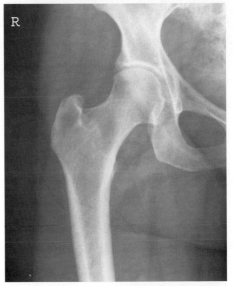

Antero-posterior radiograph of single hip

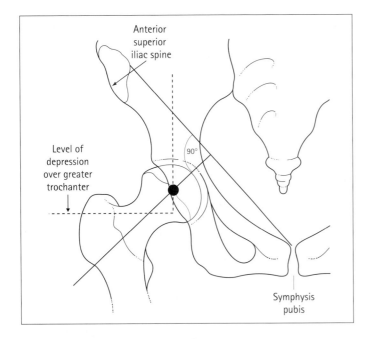

Notes

- The image must include the upper third of the femur. When taken to show the positioning and integrity of an arthroplasty, the whole length of the prosthesis, including the cement, must be visualized.
- Together with the oblique lateral projection, this is used for checking internal fixations following a fracture.
- If too high an mAs is used, the optical density around the greater trochanter may be too great for adequate visualization, particularly in very slender patients.

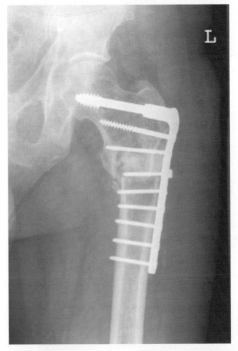

Antero-posterior radiograph of single hip showing pin and plate *in situ*

- Over-rotating the limb internally will bring the greater trochanter into profile. This may be a useful supplementary projection for a suspected avulsion fracture to this bone.

Posterior oblique (commonly known as Lauenstein's projection)

This projection demonstrates the upper third of the femur in the lateral position and the relationship between the head of the femur and the acetabulum. The posterior rim of the acetabulum is shown.

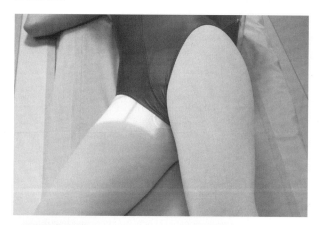

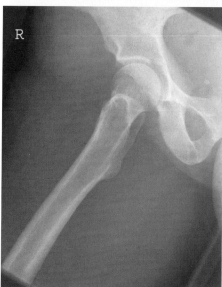

Normal posterior oblique projection of hip

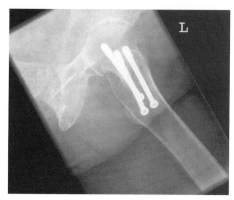

Posterior oblique projection showing position of Garden screws

Position of patient and cassette

- The patient lies supine on the X-ray table, with the legs extended. The median sagittal plane coincides with the long axis of the table Bucky.
- The patient rotates through 45 degrees on to the affected side, with the hip abducted 45 degrees and flexed 45 degrees, and is supported in this position by non-opaque pads.
- The knee is flexed to bring the lateral aspect of the thigh into contact with the tabletop. The knee falls into a lateral position.
- The opposite limb is raised and supported behind the limb being examined.
- A 24 × 30-cm cassette is used and placed longitudinally and possibly obliquely in the Bucky tray.
- The cassette is centred at the level of the femoral pulse in the groin and should include the upper third of the femur. The upper border of the cassette should be level with the anterior superior iliac spine.

Direction and centring of the X-ray beam

- Centre to the femoral pulse in the groin of the affected side, with the central ray perpendicular to the cassette.
- The long axis of the primary beam is adjusted by turning the light beam diaphragm (LBD) to coincide with the long axis of the femur.
- The primary beam needs to be collimated to the area under examination.

Notes

- If the unaffected side is raised greater than 45 degrees, then the superior pubic ramus may be superimposed on the acetabulum.
- The shaft of the femur will be positioned at 45 degrees to the long axis of the body.

Radiological considerations

- This projection should not be used for the primary investigation of suspected fracture. A full antero-posterior projection of the pelvis is required for that purpose to assess other bony pelvic injuries.
- The patient requires a degree of mobility to be positioned satisfactorily and should not experience any great discomfort in maintaining the position.
- Used with the antero-posterior projection, it shows the satisfactory position of internal fixation pins and plates.
- The whole of the acetabular rim can be assessed when this image is used in conjunction with the anterior oblique projection (Judet's projection).

Hip joint and upper third of femur

True lateral – neck of femur (basic)

This projection is used routinely in all cases of suspected fracture of the neck of femur. It is commonly carried out with the patient remaining on a stretcher, as it is not advisable to move patients with a clinical suspicion of a fracture (affected foot in external rotation, foreshortening of the limb and pain when moving). Patients who sustain a fracture of the hip are often elderly and can be quite frail. It is common practice for these patients to be 'fast-tracked' through Casualty and for them to have received some pain relief. Care and consideration for their dignity is necessary during the examination.

Either a 24 × 30-cm grid cassette, a cassette and stationary grid, or an erect Bucky and AEC can be used. An air-gap technique, with or without a filter, can also be used.

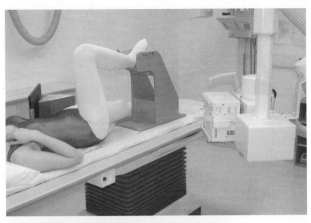

Position of patient and cassette

- The patient lies supine on the stretcher or X-ray table.
- The legs are extended and the pelvis adjusted to make the median sagittal plane perpendicular to the tabletop. This may not always be possible if the patient is in great pain.
- If the patient is very slender, it may be necessary to place a non-opaque pad under the buttocks so that the whole of the affected hip can be included in the image.
- The grid cassette is positioned vertically, with the shorter edge pressed firmly against the waist, just above the iliac crest.
- The longitudinal axis of the cassette should be parallel to the neck of femur. This can be approximated by placing a 45-degree foam pad between the front of the cassette and the lateral aspect of the pelvis.
- The cassette is supported in this position by sandbags or a special cassette holder attached to the table.
- The unaffected limb is then raised until the thigh is vertical, with the knee flexed. This position is maintained by supporting the lower leg on a stool or specialized equipment.

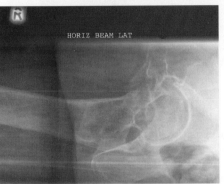

Lateral projection of hip showing subcapital fracture of neck and femur

Direction and centring of the X-ray beam

- Centre through the affected groin, midway between the femoral pulse and the palpable prominence of the greater trochanter, with the central ray directed horizontally and at right-angles to the cassette. The central beam should be adjusted vertically to pass in line with the femoral neck and should be collimated closely to the area to improve the image contrast.

Notes

- If the erect Bucky is used, then the stretcher is turned so that its long axis makes an angle of 45 degrees with the Bucky. The neck of the femur is now parallel with the cassette placed in the Bucky. The middle AEC chamber is positioned in line with the femoral neck, which will mean an air gap exists between the patient and the erect Bucky. The resultant magnification can be compensated for by increasing the

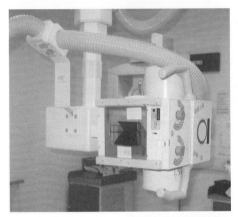

Example of filter in place on light beam diaphragm

focus-to-film distance (FFD). The air gap improves the image contrast.

- In trauma cases, when a fracture is suspected, the limb is often externally rotated. On no account should the limb be rotated from this position. The antero-posterior and lateral projections are taken with the limb in that position.
- A relatively high kVp (e.g. 100 kVp) is necessary to penetrate the thigh without blackening the trochanteric region. Using a filter improves the overall optical density.
- Loss of bony resolution can occur when using a grid cassette or stationary grid and cassette due to the X-ray beam not being aligned correctly to the grid lines.

Radiological considerations

This projection is routinely used for suspected neck of femur fracture. It is similarly invaluable for assessment of suspected slipped upper femoral epiphysis, and fracture of the acetabulum.

Lateral – single hip (alternative projections) modification of technique

These projections may be used when it is impossible either to rotate the patient on to the affected side or to elevate the unaffected limb.

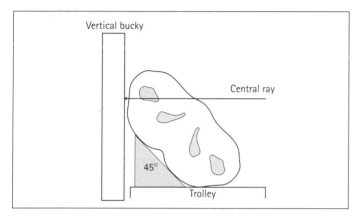

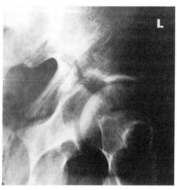

Modified technique lateral projection showing fracture of the acetabulum

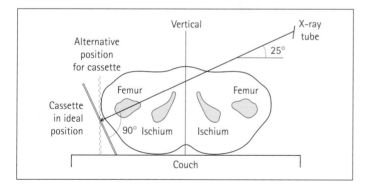

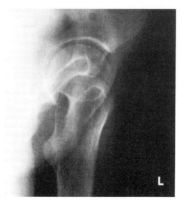

Modified technique lateral projection of hip joint

Lateral oblique modified – alternative 1

Position of patient and cassette

- From the supine position, the patient is rotated through approximately 45 degrees on to the unaffected side, depending on the degree of mobility and pain.
- The trunk and limb are supported on non-opaque pads.
- If the patient is being examined on a trolley, the trolley is positioned against the vertical Bucky. If not, a grid cassette is supported vertically against the side being examined.

The cross-sectional diagram shows the position of the two hips when the pelvis is tilted, the cassette in position and the direction of the X-ray beam.

Direction and centring of the X-ray beam

- Centre to the femoral pulse on the side being examined, with the central ray directed horizontally and at right-angles to the cassette or vertical Bucky.
- It may be necessary to use a combination of patient rotation and inferior angulation of the central beam to achieve a diagnostic image.
- Collimate the beam to the area under examination.

Lateral modified – alternative 2

This projection is used if both limbs are injured or abducted and in a plaster cast, and the patient cannot be moved from the supine position.

Position of patient and cassette

- The patient remains supine.
- The cassette is positioned vertically against the lateral aspect of the affected hip and centred at the level of the femoral pulse.
- The cassette is tilted backwards through 25 degrees and placed a little under the affected buttock. It is supported using pads and sandbags.

The cross-sectional diagram shows the relationship between the tube and cassette about the affected hip, enabling the two sides to be separated.

Direction and centring of the X-ray beam

- Centre to the femoral pulse, with the central ray tilted 25 degrees vertically downwards from the horizontal and at right-angles to the cassette.
- Collimate the beam to the area under examination.

5 Hip joint and upper third of femur

Lateral – both hips ('frog's legs position')

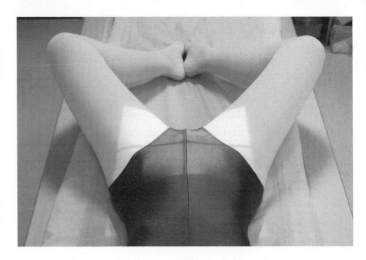

Radiography of the hip in children is discussed in detail in Chapter 14.

When there is freedom of movement, both hips can be exposed simultaneously for a general lateral projection of the femoral necks and heads. The resultant lateral hip image is similar to that obtained through the oblique lateral projection (Lauenstein's) described previously (p. 151).

This projection may be used in addition to the basic antero-posterior of both hips when comparison of both hips is required. This may apply in children, e.g. when diagnosing osteochondritis of the capital epiphysis (Perthes' disease). The position of the patient is often referred to as the 'frog' position.

Gonad-protection devices must be positioned correctly and secured firmly.

Depending on the age and size of the patient, either a 43 × 35-cm or a 30 × 40-cm cassette is placed horizontally in the Bucky tray.

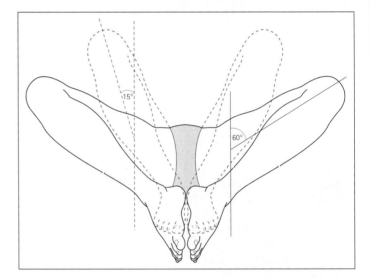

Position of patient and cassette

- The patient lies supine on the X-ray table, with the anterior superior iliac spines equidistant from the tabletop to avoid rotation of the pelvis.
- The median sagittal plane is perpendicular to the table and coincident with the centre of the table Bucky mechanism.
- The hips and knees are flexed and the limbs rotated laterally through approximately 60 degrees. This movement separates the knees and brings the plantar aspect of the feet in contact with each other.
- The limbs are supported in this position by pads and sandbags.
- The cassette is centred at the level of the femoral pulse to include both hip joints.

Direction and centring of the X-ray beam

- Centre in the midline at the level of the femoral pulse, with the central ray perpendicular to the cassette. Collimate to the area under examination.

Notes

- A lateral rotation of 60 degrees demonstrates the hip joints.
- A modified technique with the limbs rotated laterally through 15 degrees and the plantar aspect of the feet in contact with the tabletop demonstrates the neck of femur.
- If the patient is unable to achieve 60-degree rotation, it is important to apply the same degree of rotation to both limbs without losing symmetry.
- In very young children, a Bucky grid is not required. The child may be placed directly on to the X-ray cassette.

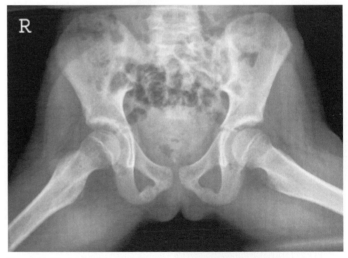

Normal radiograph showing both hips in lateral projection (frog legs)

Radiation protection

Gonad protection must be applied correctly and secured firmly in position.

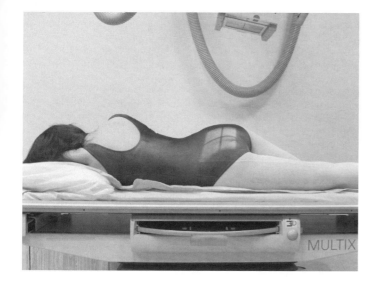

Anterior oblique (Judet's projection)

This projection may be used to assess the acetabulum when a fracture is suspected. Although the acetabulum is seen on the antero-posterior pelvis, the anterior and posterior rims are superimposed over the head of the femur and the ischium. If the patient is immobile or in pain, then a reverse Judet's projection is taken.

Judet's projection demonstrates the anterior rim of the acetabulum, with the patient prone.

A posterior oblique projection (Lauenstein's projection) shows the posterior rim of the acetabulum, with the patient supine.

Position of patient and cassette

- The patient lies prone on the X-ray table.
- The trunk is then rotated approximately 45 degrees on to the **unaffected side** and the **affected side** is raised and supported on non-opaque pads.
- In this position, the rim of the acetabulum nearest the table-top is approximately parallel to the cassette.
- A 24 × 30-cm cassette is placed longitudinally in the Bucky tray.

Direction and centring of the X-ray beam

- Centre just distal to the coccyx, with the central beam directed 12 degrees towards the head. Collimate to the affected area.

Posterior oblique (reverse Judet's projection)

Position of patient and cassette

- The patient lies supine on the X-ray table.
- The **affected side** is raised approximately 45 degrees and supported on non-opaque pads.

Direction and centring of the X-ray beam

- Centre to the femoral pulse on the raised side, with the central ray directed 12 degrees towards the feet.
- The cassette is centred at the level of the femoral pulse and collimated to the area under examination.

Notes

- It is necessary in trauma cases to adequately demonstrate fractures of the pelvis and acetabulum, as there is a high incident of damage to the surrounding anatomy (lower urinary tract, blood vessels, nerves). These fractures can be classified as stable/unstable depending on the stability of the bony fragments.
- Computed tomography (CT) scanning is used to assess the position of intra-articular bony fragments and soft-tissue injuries.

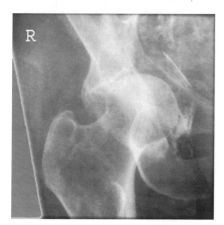

Judet's projection of hip showing a central fracture of the acetabulum

5 Pelvis

Ilium

Although the ilium is seen on the basic pelvic projection, an oblique projection may be necessary to show the entire bone. The procedure is undertaken with the patient supine for bony trauma; however, it may not be possible to turn a badly injured patient into this position.

The posterior oblique shows the iliac wing, fossa, ischium ischial spine, sciatic notches and acetabulum. It is a similar projection to that already described for the hip and upper femora (p. 151), but with less patient rotation and centred more superiorly.

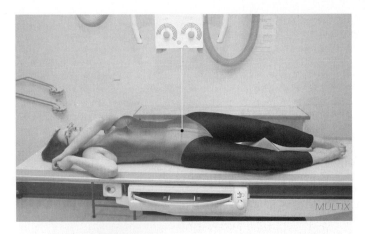

Posterior oblique – basic projection

Position of patient and cassette

- The patient lies supine on the X-ray table and is positioned for a basic antero-posterior pelvic projection.
- From this position, the patient is rotated approximately 40 degrees on to the **affected** side; the **unaffected** side is raised and supported.
- Both hips and knees are flexed and the raised limb is supported on a pad.
- The iliac fossa is now parallel to the cassette.
- A 24 × 30-cm cassette is placed crossways in the Bucky tray, with the top margin 5 cm above the iliac crest.

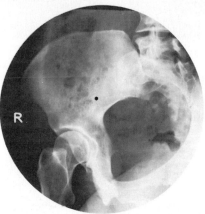

Normal posterior oblique projection of ilium

Direction and centring of the X-ray beam

- Centre midway between the anterior superior iliac spine of the affected side and the midline of the pelvis, with the vertical central ray perpendicular to the film.

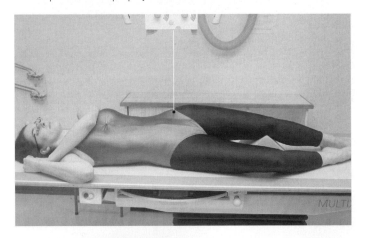

Posterior oblique (alternate)

This is an uncommon projection that can be used when additional information is required regarding the posterior aspect of the iliac bone.

Position of patient and cassette

- The patient lies supine on the X-ray table.
- From this position, the patient is rotated approximately 45 degrees on to the **unaffected** side, with the **affected side** raised and supported.
- A 24 × 30-cm cassette is placed longitudinally in the Bucky tray 5 cm above the iliac crest.

Direction and centring of the X-ray beam

- The vertical central ray is directed to the anterior superior iliac spine on the side being examined.

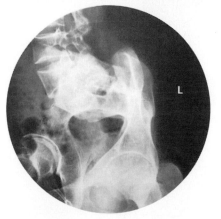

Normal posterior oblique (alternate) projection of ilium

Lateral

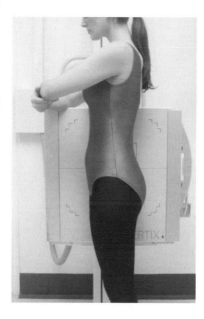

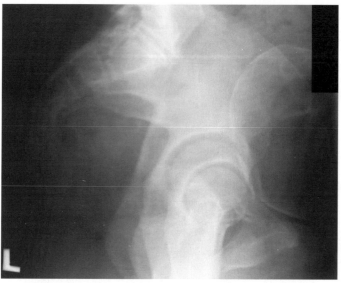

Lateral erect radiograph of pelvis at full term of pregnancy (pelvimetry)

The patient may be examined in the erect, lateral decubitus or supine position.

The projection is uncommon for general imaging, as it will deliver a high radiation dose for limited diagnostic value. It may be used as part of a specific pelvimetry series for assessing the pelvic inlet and outlet during pregnancy, but this is now rarely practiced. For assessment of major pelvic trauma, CT is usually the preferred option.

The erect projection only is described.

Position of patient and cassette (erect position)

- The patient stands with either side in contact with the vertical Bucky, which is adjusted vertically to the pelvic level.
- To ensure that the patient's stance is firm, the feet are separated.
- The median sagittal plane is parallel and the coronal plane is perpendicular to the image receptor.
- A careful check should be made to ensure that the vertebral column is parallel to the image receptor and that the coronal plane is at right angles to the image receptor. The latter may be assessed by palpating either the anterior or posterior superior iliac spines and rotating the patient as necessary so that an imaginary line joining the two sides is at right angles to the image receptor.
- The arms are folded across the chest and the arm nearest the Bucky can rest on top of the Bucky for support.

Direction and centring of the X-ray beam

- A cassette of suitable size is placed horizontally in the vertical Bucky.
- The central ray is directed horizontally to a depression immediately superior to the greater trochanter and collimated to include the symphysis pubis, ischium and the iliac crests.

5 Pelvis

Symphysis pubis

This projection may be done to demonstrate postpartum widening of the symphysis pubis, although this is rarely clinically relevant. Non-weight-bearing views may show subluxation of the symphisis pubis. Alternatively, two antero-posterior radiographs may be obtained in the erect position, with the patient weight-bearing on alternate feet. The dose implications of this study must be assessed against the likely benefit.

Antero-posterior – erect

Position of patient and cassette

- The patient stands with the posterior aspect of the trunk against the vertical Bucky.
- The arms are folded across the chest with the feet separated, so that the patient can comfortably adopt a standing position on one foot, and then the other.
- The anterior superior iliac spines should be equidistant from the image receptor, with the median sagittal plane perpendicular to the vertical central line of Bucky.
- The vertical Bucky is adjusted so that the horizontal central line is at the same level as the symphysis pubis.
- For the single projection a 24 × 30-cm cassette is exposed with the weight equally distributed on both feet.
- For the weight bearing projection, a 24 × 30-cm cassette is exposed, with the full weight of the body on one limb. A second cassette is then exposed with the weight on the opposite limb.

Direction and centring of the X-ray beam

- Centre to the midline at the level of the symphysis pubis, with the horizontal central ray perpendicular to the image receptor.

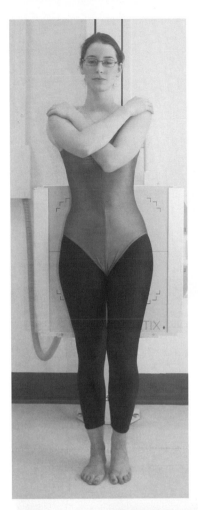

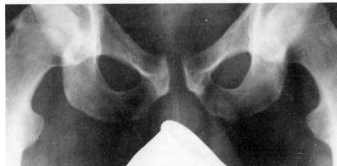

Antero-posterior projection of symphysis pubis showing widening of the symphysis

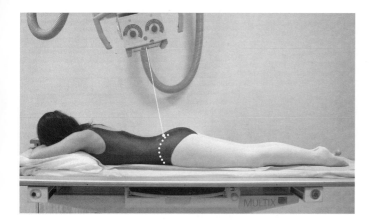

Postero-anterior

The sacrum is situated posteriorly between the two iliac bones, the adjacent surfaces forming the sacro-iliac joints. These joint surfaces are oblique in direction, sloping backward, inward and downward.

In the prone position, the oblique rays coincide with the direction of the joints.

The postero-anterior projection demonstrates the joints more effectively than the antero-posterior projection. It also reduces the radiation dose to the gonads in comparison with the antero-posterior projection.

Position of patient and cassette

- The patient lies prone, with the median sagittal plane perpendicular to the tabletop.
- The posterior superior iliac spines should be equidistant from the tabletop to avoid rotation.
- The midline of the patient should coincide with the centred primary beam and the table Bucky mechanism.
- The forearms are raised and placed on the pillow.
- A 24 × 30-cm cassette is placed transversely in the Bucky tray and positioned so that the central ray passes through the centre of the cassette.

Direction and centring of the X-ray beam

- Centre in the midline at the level of the posterior superior iliac spines.
- The central ray is angled 5–15 degrees caudally from the vertical, depending on the sex of the patient. The female requires greater caudal angulation of the beam.
- The primary beam is collimated to the area of interest.

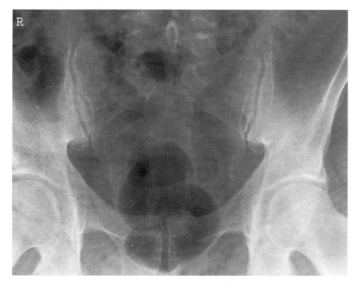

Normal postero-anterior projection of sacro-iliac joints

5 Sacro-iliac joints

Antero-posterior

The antero-posterior projection shows both sacro-iliac joints on one image and can be done when the patient is unable to turn prone.

The positions of the patient and the film and the direction of the beam are the same as those described for the antero-posterior projection of the sacrum.

The sacro-iliac joints are included routinely on the antero-posterior projection of the lumbar spine in some protocols, as some pathologies can give rise to lower back pain.

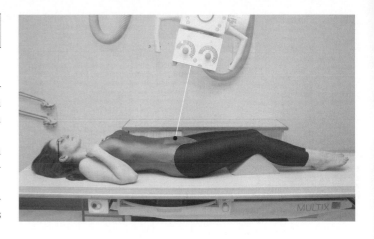

Position of patient and cassette

- The patient lies supine and symmetrical on the X-ray table, with the median sagittal plane perpendicular.
- The midline of the patient must coincide with the centred primary beam and the table Bucky mechanism.
- To avoid rotation, the anterior superior iliac spines must be equidistant from the tabletop.
- A 24 × 30-cm cassette, placed transversely in the Bucky tray, is centred at a level to coincide with the central ray.
- The shoulders are raised over a pillow to eliminate the lumbar arch.
- The knees should be flexed over foam pads for comfort.

Direction and centring of the X-ray beam

- Centre in the midline at a level midway between the anterior superior iliac spines and the superior border of the symphysis pubis.
- The central ray is directed between 5 and 15 degrees cranially, depending on the sex of the patient. The female requires greater caudal angulation of the beam.
- The primary beam is collimated to the area of interest.

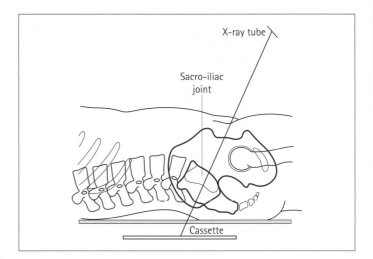

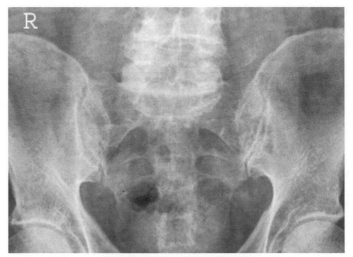

Normal antero-posterior projection of sacro-iliac joints

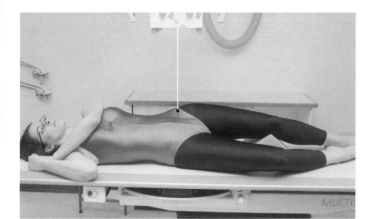

Antero-posterior oblique

Both sides are examined for comparison.

Position of patient and cassette

- The patient lies supine on the table.
- From this position, the patient is rotated 15–25 degrees on to the side **not** being examined.
- The anterior superior iliac spine on the raised side should lie just lateral to the posterior superior iliac spine.
- The raised side is supported with non-opaque pads placed under the trunk and the raised thigh.
- Pads may be placed between the knees for comfort.

Direction and centring of the X-ray beam

- Centre 2.5 cm medial to the anterior superior iliac spine on the raised side (the side under examination), with the central ray perpendicular to the cassette.

Note

If it is necessary to demonstrate the inferior part of the joint more clearly, the central ray is angled 15 degrees cranially and centred 2.5 cm medial to and 5 cm inferior to the anterior superior iliac spine on the side under examination (raised side).

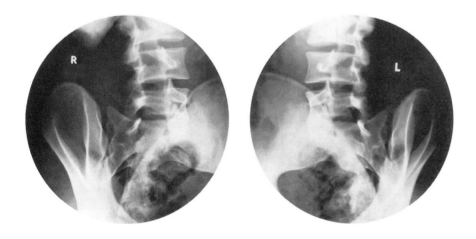

Reference

Rogers LF (2002). *Radiology of Skeletal Trauma*, 3rd edn. London: Churchill Livingstone.

Section 6

The Vertebral Column

CONTENTS

RECOMMENDED PROJECTIONS 164

VERTEBRAL CURVES 165
VERTEBRAL LEVELS 166

CERVICAL VERTEBRAE 168
Basic projections 168
Lateral erect 168
Lateral supine 169
Antero-posterior – first and second
  cervical vertebrae (open mouth) 170
Antero-posterior third to seventh
  vertebrae 172
Axial – upper cervical vertebra 174
Lateral – flexion and extension 175
Right and left posterior oblique – erect 176
Right and left posterior oblique – supine 177

CERVICO-THORACIC VERTEBRAE 178
Lateral swimmers' 178

THORACIC VERTEBRAE 179
Antero-posterior – basic 179
Lateral – basic 180
Localized projections 181

LUMBAR VERTEBRAE 182
Antero-posterior – basic 182
Lateral – basic 183
Lateral horizontal beam 185
Lateral flexion and extension 186
Right or left posterior oblique 187

LUMBO-SACRAL JUNCTION 188
Lateral 188
Antero-posterior 189
Right or left posterior oblique 189

SACRUM 190
Antero-posterior/postero-anterior 190
Lateral 191

COCCYX 192
Antero-posterior 192
Lateral 192

6 Recommended projections

The projections recommended below are only a guide,
as practice may vary according to local departmental protocols.

Cervical vertebrae	Severe trauma (patient on trolley with neck brace)	Lateral supine with horizontal beam (basic) Antero-posterior supine (basic) Antero-posterior C1/2, 'open mouth', supine (basic) Swimmers' lateral supine or oblique supine if C7/T1 not demonstrated (additional) Flexion and extension (additional), consultant request after initial images cleared
	Minor trauma (patient walking)	Lateral erect (basic) Antero-posterior, erect or supine (basic) Antero-posterior C1/2, 'open mouth', erect or supine (basic) Swimmers' lateral or oblique if C7/T1 not demonstrated (additional) Flexion and extension (additional), consultant request after initial images cleared
	Non-traumatic pathology	Lateral erect (basic) Antero-posterior, erect or supine (basic) Flexion and extension (additional) Oblique erect (additional) Flexion and extension (additional) Swimmers' lateral if cervico-thoracic region is of particular interest (additional)
Thoracic vertebrae	Trauma (patient on trolley)	Lateral supine with horizontal beam (basic) Antero-posterior supine (basic)
	Non-traumatic pathology	Lateral (basic) Antero-posterior supine (basic)
Lumbar vertebrae	Trauma (patient on trolley)	Lateral supine with horizontal beam (basic) Antero-posterior supine (basic)
	Non-traumatic pathology	Lateral (basic) Antero-posterior supine or postero-anterior (basic) Oblique (additional) Flexion and extension (additional)
Lumbo-sacral junction	Trauma (patient on trolley)	Lateral supine with horizontal beam (basic) Antero-posterior supine (basic)
	Non-traumatic pathology	Lateral (basic) Antero-posterior supine (basic) Oblique (additional)
Sacrum	Trauma	Lateral (basic), horizontal beam if patient cannot turn Antero-posterior supine (basic)
	Non-traumatic pathology	Lateral (basic) Antero-posterior (basic) See Chapter 5
Coccyx	Trauma/pathology	Projections not normally performed unless patient considered for coccyxectomy Lateral (basic), antero-posterior (basic)
Scoliosis and kyphosis	See Section 14	

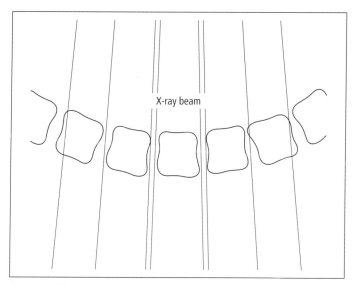

Concavity of vertebral curve towards X-ray tube

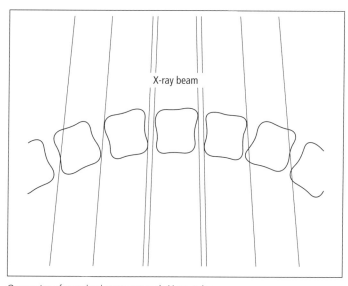

Convexity of vertebral curve towards X-ray tube

At birth, the majority of the vertebral column is curved, with its concavity facing forward. As development occurs, and the child starts to lift its head and begins to walk, additional curvatures develop with the spine in response to these activities. The anterior concavity is maintained in the thoracic and sacro-coccygeal regions, hence they are given the name **primary curves**. The cervical and lumbar regions become convex anteriorly. These are the **secondary curves**.

A knowledge of vertebral curves is important in radiography as their position with respect to the direction of the X-ray beam will determine the quality of the final image in terms of ability to make an accurate diagnosis.

Important considerations in spinal radiography

- Remember that the X-ray beam diverges from the focal spot on the anode. The X-rays are not parallel to each other.
- Ideally, the vertebral bodies will not be superimposed over one another and will be separated on the image.
- Disc spaces should be demonstrated clearly, without superimposition of vertebral bodies.
- The vertebral endplates will be parallel with the X-ray beam at a given point. This will ensure that the lateral borders are superimposed and will give the typical quadrangular appearance on the final image.
- In order to achieve the above, the concavity of the part of the spine under examination should always face the X-ray tube (see diagrams).
- The curves are variable along the area of interest, thus making it impossible to achieve separation of individual vertebra. In this instance, it may be worth considering individual exposures, with the beam angled to achieve the required degree of separation.

6 Vertebral levels

The photographs below and the diagram on the next page illustrate the surface markings of the vertebral levels, which are useful in radiographic positioning. The relative positions may vary according to the patient's build and posture.

Useful landmarks

- The easily palpated tip of the mastoid process indicates the level of C1.
- The spinous process of C7 produces a visible protuberance on the posterior aspect of the inferior part of the neck. Below this, the spinous process of the thoracic spine can be palpated. NB: the thoracic spinous processes are directed steeply downwards, so their palpable tips will be adjacent to the vertebral body below.

- The inferior angle of the scapula indicates the level of T7 when the arms are placed by the side.
- The sternal notch lies at the junction between T2 and T3.
- T4 is indicated by the sternal angle with T9 corresponding to the xiphisternal joint, although the size of this structure is variable.
- The lower costal margin indicates L3 and is located easily. This is a very useful aid to positioning in spinal radiography.
- A line joining the most superior parts of the iliac crests indicates the level of L4, whilst the tubercle of the iliac crest discloses the location of L5.
- The anterior and posterior iliac spines lie at the level of the second sacral vertebra.
- The coccyx can be palpated between the buttocks and lies at the level of the symphysis pubis.

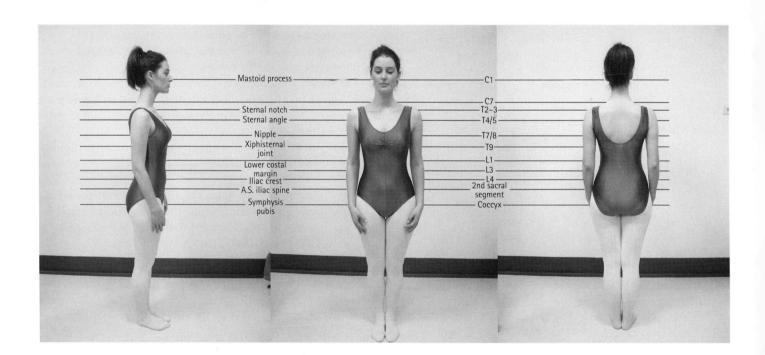

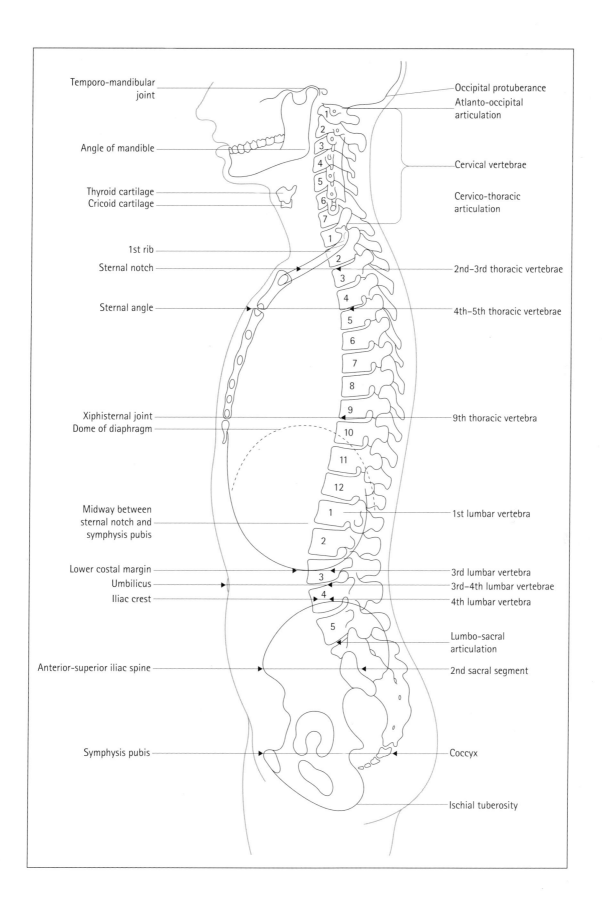

Temporo-mandibular joint

Occipital protuberance

Atlanto-occipital articulation

Angle of mandible

Cervical vertebrae

Cervico-thoracic articulation

Thyroid cartilage
Cricoid cartilage

1st rib

Sternal notch

2nd–3rd thoracic vertebrae

Sternal angle

4th–5th thoracic vertebrae

Xiphisternal joint
Dome of diaphragm

9th thoracic vertebra

Midway between sternal notch and symphysis pubis

1st lumbar vertebra

Lower costal margin

3rd lumbar vertebra

Umbilicus

3rd–4th lumbar vertebrae

Iliac crest

4th lumbar vertebra

Lumbo-sacral articulation

Anterior-superior iliac spine

2nd sacral segment

Symphysis pubis

Coccyx

Ischial tuberosity

Cervical vertebrae

Basic projections

Many centres perform an antero-posterior and a lateral projection, with the addition of a further image to demonstrate the C1/2 region if the patient has a history of trauma.

18 × 24-cm cassettes are employed routinely, but 24 × 30-cm cassettes are often used in difficult cases.

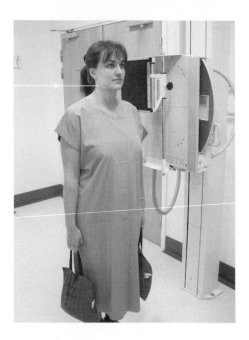

Lateral erect

Position of patient and cassette

- The patient stands or sits with either shoulder against the cassette.
- The median sagittal plane should be adjusted such that it is parallel with the cassette.
- The head should be flexed or extended such that the angle of the mandible is not superimposed over the upper anterior cervical vertebra or the occipital bone does not obscure the posterior arch of the atlas.
- To aid immobilization, the patient should stand with the feet slightly apart and with the shoulder resting against the cassette stand.
- In order to demonstrate the lower cervical vertebra, the shoulders should be depressed, as shown in the photograph. This can be achieved by asking the patient to relax their shoulders downwards. The process can be aided by asking the patient to hold a weight in each hand (if they are capable) and making the exposure on arrested expiration.

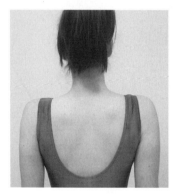
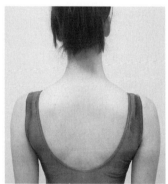

Shoulders depressed

Direction and centring of the X-ray beam

- The horizontal central ray is centred to a point vertically below the mastoid process at the level of the prominence of the thyroid cartilage.

Essential image characteristics

- The whole of the cervical spine should be included, from the atlanto-occipital joints to the top of the first thoracic vertebra.
- The mandible or occipital bone does not obscure any part of the upper vertebra.
- Angles of the mandible and the lateral portions of the floor of the posterior cranial fossa should be superimposed.
- Soft tissues of the neck should be included.
- The contrast should produce densities sufficient to demonstrate soft tissue and bony detail.

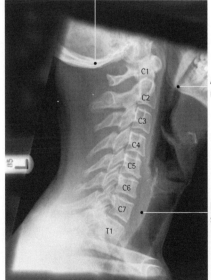

Floor of posterior
cranial fossa
(occipital bone)

Angle of
mandible

Prevertebral
soft tissue

C1
C2
C3
C4
C5
C6
C7
T1

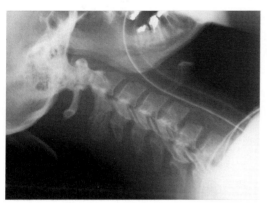

Lateral supine projection showing fracture dislocation of C5/C6

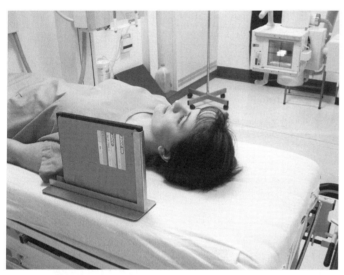

Positioning for lateral supine projection

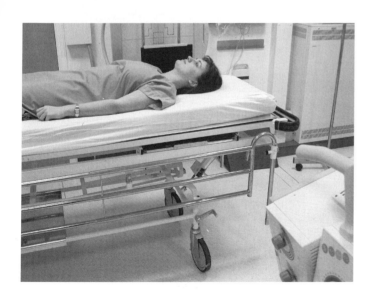

Lateral erect

Radiological considerations

- Atlanto-axial subluxation is seen on the lateral projection, especially in flexion (where appropriate). Care is needed in making this diagnosis in children, in whom the normal space is larger (adults <2 mm, children 3–5 mm).
- Visualization of the margins of the foramen magnum can be difficult but is necessary for diagnosis of various skull-base abnormalities, such as basilar invagination. It will be obscured by incorrect exposure or the presence of earrings.
- A secondary sign of a vertebral injury is swelling of the soft tissues anterior to the vertebral body (normal thickness is less than the depth of a normal vertebral body). This can be mimicked by flexion of the neck – always try to obtain films in the neutral position.

Common faults and remedies

- Failure to demonstrate C7/T1: if the patient cannot depress the shoulders, even when holding weights, then a swimmers' projection should be considered.
- Care should be taken with the position of the lead name blocker. Important anatomy may easily be obscured, especially when using a small cassette.

Notes

- The large object-to-film distance (OFD) will increase geometric unsharpness. This is overcome by increasing the focus-to-film distance (FFD) to 150 cm.
- An air gap between the neck and the film eliminates the need to employ a secondary radiation grid to attenuate scatter.

Radiation protection

- Care should be taken when collimating to avoid including the eyes within the primary beam.

Lateral supine

For trauma cases, the patient's condition usually requires the examination to be performed on a casualty trolley. The lateral cervical spine projection is taken first, without moving the patient. The resulting radiograph must be examined by a medical officer to establish whether the patient's neck can be moved for other projections. See Section 16 for additional information.

Position of patient and cassette

- The patient will normally arrive in the supine position.
- It is vitally important for the patient to depress the shoulders (assuming no other injuries to the arms).
- The cassette can be either supported vertically or placed in the erect cassette holder, with the top of the cassette at the same level as the top of the ear.

(contd)

Lateral supine (*contd*)

- To further depress the shoulders, one or two suitably qualified individuals can apply caudal traction to the arms. NB: refer to departmental local rules for staff working within a controlled area.

Common faults and remedies

- Failure to demonstrate C7/T1: if the patient's shoulders are depressed fully, then the application of traction will normally show half to one extra vertebra inferiorly. Should the cervical thoracic junction still remain undemonstrated, then a swimmers' lateral or oblique projections should be considered.

Radiological considerations

- This projection is part of the Advanced Trauma and Life Support (ATLS) primary screen.
- Clear demonstration of the C7/T1 junction is essential, as this is a common site of injury and is associated with major neurological morbidity. It is often not covered fully on the initial trauma screen and must always be demonstrated in the setting of trauma, by supplementary projections if necessary.

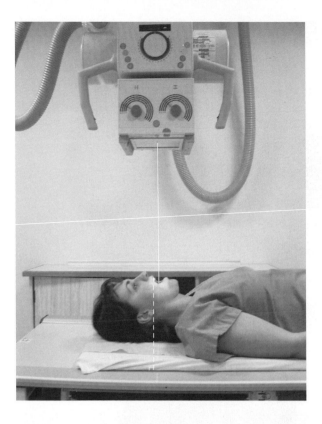

Antero-posterior – first and second cervical vertebrae (open mouth)

Position of patient and cassette

- The patient lies supine on the Bucky table or, if erect positioning is preferred, sits or stands with the posterior aspect of the head and shoulders against the vertical Bucky.
- The medial sagittal plane is adjusted to coincide with the midline of the cassette, such that it is at right-angles to the cassette.
- The neck is extended, if possible, such that a line joining the tip of the mastoid process and the inferior border of the upper incisors is at right-angles to the cassette. This will superimpose the upper incisors and the occipital bone, thus allowing clear visualization of the area of interest.
- The cassette is centred at the level of the mastoid process.

Direction and centring of the X-ray beam

- Direct the perpendicular central ray along the midline to the centre of the open mouth.
- If the patient is unable to flex the neck and attain the position described above, then the beam must be angled, typically five to ten degrees cranially or caudally, to superimpose the upper incisors on the occipital bone.
- The cassette position will have to be altered slightly to allow the image to be centred after beam angulation.

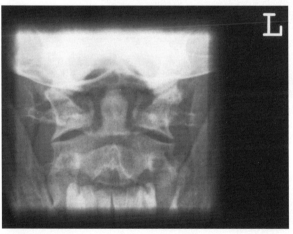

Example of correctly positioned radiograph

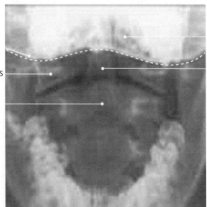

Occipital bone

Lateral mass of C1

Body of C2

Upper incisor

Odontoid process of C2

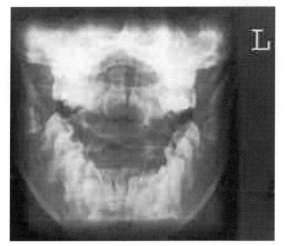
Incorrect positioning – upper teeth superimposed

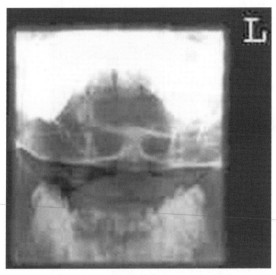
Incorrect positioning – occipital bone superimposed

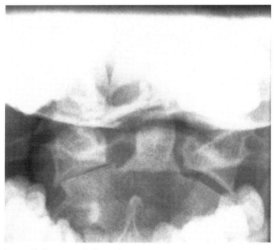
Loss of alignment in lateral masses

Antero-posterior – first and second cervical vertebrae (open mouth)

Essential image characteristics

- The inferior border of the upper central incisors should be superimposed over the occipital bone.
- The whole of the articulation between the atlas and the axis must be demonstrated clearly.
- Ideally, the whole of the dens, the lateral masses of the atlas and as much of the axis as possible should be included within the image.

Radiological considerations

- Fracture of the odontoid peg usually occurs across the base, below the suspensory ligament supporting the atlas. Good initial plain images are therefore essential. The base of the peg must not be obscured by any overlying bone or tooth. Failure to demonstrate the peg will lead to the need for more complex imaging. In a patient who is to have computed tomography (CT) of the head for associated trauma, scans of areas of the spine not already covered adequately are recommended in ATLS. In other patients, failure to show C1/2 either will result in the need for a CT scan for the spine alone or will lead to the patient being fully immobilized for a long period of time, with the morbidity attendant upon that.
- A burst (Jefferson) fracture is seen on the antero-posterior view as a loss of alignment of the margins of the lateral masses. Rotated images make this harder to appreciate (this fracture is seen very well on CT).

Common faults and remedies

- Failure to open the mouth wide enough: the patient can be reminded to open their mouth as wide as possible just before the exposure.
- A small degree of rotation may result in superimposition of the lower molar over the lateral section of the joint space. Check for rotation during positioning.
- If the front teeth are superimposed over the area of interest (top left photograph), then the image should be repeated with the chin raised or with an increased cranial angulation of the tube.
- If the occipital bone is superimposed, then the chin should be lowered or a caudal angulation should be employed.
- It is worth noting that some individuals have a very prominent maxilla. It will be very difficult to produce an image without some degree of superimposition in these cases, so an alternative projection or modality should be considered.

Antero-posterior – first and second cervical vertebrae (open mouth) (*contd*)

Note

A decrease in patient dose can be obtained by not using a grid. This will produce an image of lower contrast due to the increased scatter incident on the film, but it should still be of diagnostic quality. The choice of whether to use a grid will vary according to local needs and preferences.

Radiation protection

- Local protocols may state that this projection is not routinely used for degenerative disease.

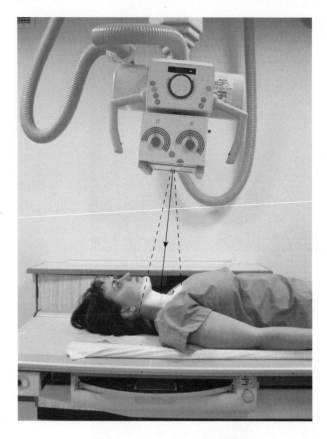

Antero-posterior third to seventh vertebrae

Position of patient and cassette

- The patient lies supine on the Bucky table or, if erect positioning is preferred, sits or stands with the posterior aspect of the head and shoulders against the vertical Bucky.
- The median sagittal plane is adjusted to be at right-angles to the cassette and to coincide with the midline of the table or Bucky.
- The neck is extended (if the patient's condition will allow) so that the lower part of the jaw is cleared from the upper cervical vertebra.
- The cassette is positioned in the Bucky to coincide with the central ray. The Bucky tray will require some cranial displacement if the tube is angled.

Direction and centring of the X-ray beam

- A 5–15-degree cranial angulation is employed, such that the inferior border of the symphysis menti is superimposed over the occipital bone.
- The beam is centred in the midline towards a point just below the prominence of the thyroid cartilage through the fifth cervical vertebra.

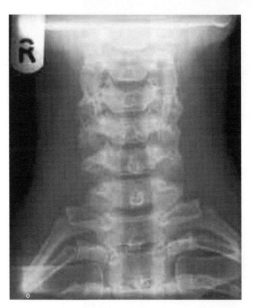

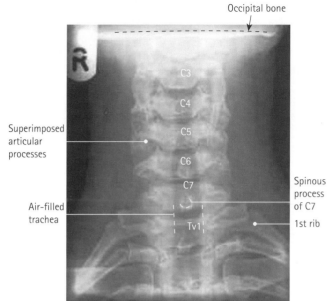

Occipital bone

C3
C4
C5
C6
C7
Tv1

Superimposed
articular
processes

Air-filled
trachea

Spinous
process
of C7

1st rib

Radiological considerations

- A unifacet dislocation can be diagnosed by loss of continuity of the line of spinous processes (or a line bisecting the bifid processes). This is made more difficult if the patient is rotated or the image is underexposed.

Common faults and remedies

- Failure to demonstrate the upper vertebra: an increase in the tube angle or raising the chin should provide a solution.

Notes

- Work is currently being undertaken to investigate the advantages of performing this projection postero-anteriorly. The positioning is similar to the antero-posterior projection, except that the patient faces the cassette and a 15-degree caudal angulation is applied to the tube. Indications suggest that this projection has the advantage of showing the disc spaces more clearly and substantially reducing the dose to the thyroid.
- The moving jaw technique uses auto-tomography to diffuse the image of the mandible, thus demonstrating the upper vertebra more clearly. The patient's head must be immobilized well, and an exposure time that is long enough to allow the jaw to open and close several times must be used.
- Linear tomography has also been used to demonstrate the cervical vertebra obscured by the mandible and facial bones.

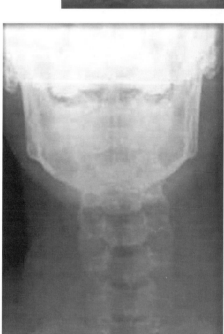

Poor quality image with mandible obscuring upper cervical spine

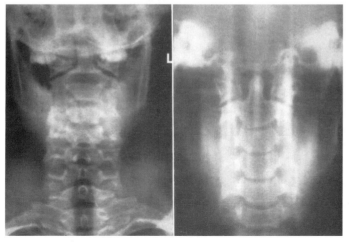

Moving jaw technique   Tomogram

Cervical vertebrae

Axial – upper cervical vertebra

This is a useful projection if the odontoid peg cannot be demonstrated using the open mouth projection. Remember that the neck must not be flexed in acute injuries.

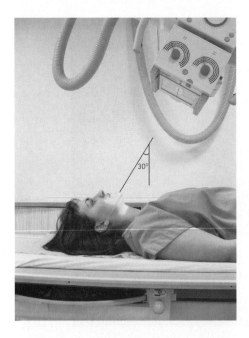

Position of patient and cassette

- The patient lies supine on the Bucky table, with the median sagittal plane coincident with the midline of the table and at right-angles to the cassette.
- The neck is extended so that that the orbito-meatal baseline is at 45 degrees to the tabletop. The head is then immobilized.
- The cassette is displaced cranially so that its centre coincides with the central ray.

Direction and centring of the X-ray beam

- The beam is angled 30 degrees cranially from the vertical and the central ray directed towards a point in the midline between the external auditory meatuses.

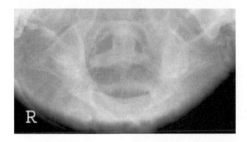

Essential image characteristics

- The odontoid peg will be projected over the occipital bone but clear of other confusing surrounding structures.

Notes

- Additional beam angulation may be used if the patient is wearing a rigid collar.
- Linear tomography has also been used to demonstrate this region.

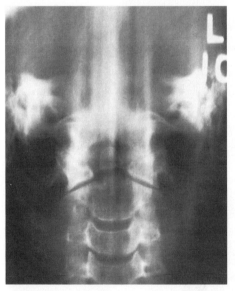

Example of linear tomogram

Lateral – flexion and extension

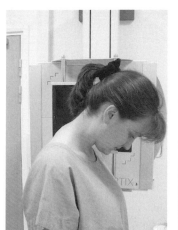
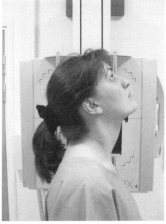

These projections may be required, but only at the request of a medical officer, to supplement the basic projections in cases of trauma, e.g. subluxation, or pathology, e.g. rheumatoid arthritis (and often before surgery to assess movement in the neck for insertion of an endotracheal tube). The degree of movement and any change in the relationship of the cervical vertebrae can also be assessed. If an injury is suspected or is being followed up, then an experienced trauma doctor must be present to supervise flexion and extension of the neck.

Position of patient and cassette

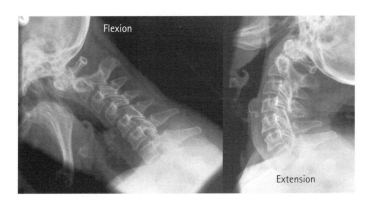

Flexion

Extension

- The patient is positioned as for the lateral basic or lateral supine projections; however, erect positioning is more convenient. The patient is asked to flex the neck and to tuck the chin in towards the chest as far as is possible.
- For the second projection, the patient is asked to extend the neck by raising the chin as far as possible.
- Immobilization can be facilitated by asking the patient to hold on to a solid object, such as the back of a chair.
- The cassette is centred to the mid-cervical region and may have to be placed transversely for the lateral in flexion, depending on the degree of movement and the cassette size used.
- If imaged supine, the neck can be flexed by placing pads under the neck. Extension of the neck can be achieved by placing pillows under the patient's shoulders.

Direction and centring of the X-ray beam

- Direct the central ray horizontally towards the mid-cervical region (C4).

Essential image characteristics

- The final image should include all the cervical vertebra, including the atlanto-occipital joints, the spinous processes and the soft tissues of the neck.

Notes

- The large OFD will increase geometric unsharpness. This is overcome by increasing the focal film distance to 150 cm.
- An air gap between the neck and the film eliminates the need to employ a secondary radiation grid to attenuate scatter.
- Refer to local protocols for the removal of immobilization collars when undertaking these examinations.

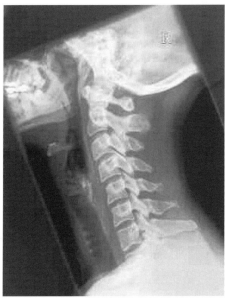

Whiplash injury (spine in neutral position)

Right and left posterior oblique – erect

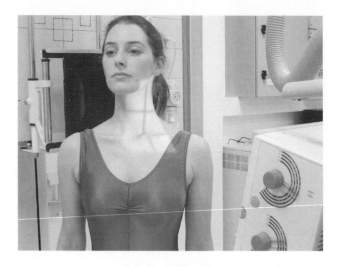

Oblique projections are requested mainly to supplement the basic projections in cases of trauma. The images demonstrate the intervertebral foramina, the relationship of the facet joints in suspected dislocation or subluxation as well as the vertebral arches. Oblique projections have also been used with certain pathologies, such as degenerative disease.

Position of patient and cassette

- The patient stands or sits with the posterior aspect of their head and shoulders against the vertical Bucky (or cassette if no grid is preferred).
- The median sagittal plane of the trunk is rotated through 45 degrees for right and left sides in turn.
- The head can be rotated so that the median sagittal plane of the head is parallel to the cassette, thus avoiding superimposition of the mandible on the vertebra.
- The cassette is centred at the prominence of the thyroid cartilage.

Direction and centring of the X-ray beam

- The beam is angled 15 degrees cranially from the horizontal and the central ray is directed to the middle of the neck on the side nearest the tube.

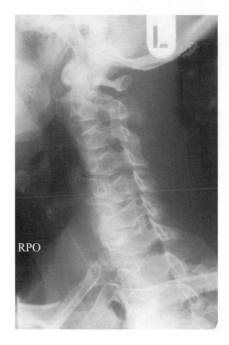

Essential image characteristics

- The intervertebral foramina should be demonstrated clearly.
- C1 to T1 should be included within the image.
- The mandible and the occipital bone should be clear of the vertebrae.

Radiological considerations

If this and the swimmers' projections are not successful, the patient may require more complex imaging (e.g. CT).

Notes

- Anterior oblique projections are usually undertaken on mobile patients. The position used is exactly the opposite to the posterior oblique projection, i.e. the patient faces the cassette and a 15-degree caudal angulation is used. Use of this projection will reduce the radiation dose to the thyroid.
- The foraminae demonstrated on the posterior oblique are those nearest the X-ray tube.

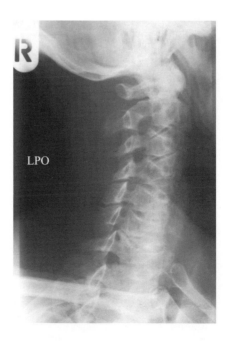

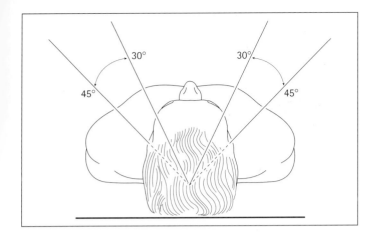

Right and left posterior oblique – supine

This positioning is often necessary in cases of severe injury, particularly if other basic projections have failed to demonstrate the lower cervical vertebrae.

Position of patient and cassette

- The patient remains in the supine position on the casualty trolley.
- To avoid moving the neck, the cassette should ideally be placed in the cassette tray underneath the trolley.
- If no cassette tray is available, then the cassette can be slid carefully into position without moving the patient's neck.

Direction and centring of the X-ray beam

- The beam is angled 30–45 degrees to the median sagittal plane (the degree of angulation will depend on local protocols).
- The central ray is directed towards the middle of the neck on the side nearest the tube at the level of the thyroid cartilage.

Radiological considerations

- If this and the swimmers' projections are not successful, the patient may require more complex imaging (e.g. CT).

Common faults and remedies

- Unless the equipment used allows alignment of the grid slats with the tube angle, then a grid cut-off will result.
- Grid cut-off can be prevented by not using a grid. Alternatively, the gridlines can be positioned to run transversely. This will result in suboptimal demonstration of the intervertebral foramina, but the image will be of diagnostic quality.

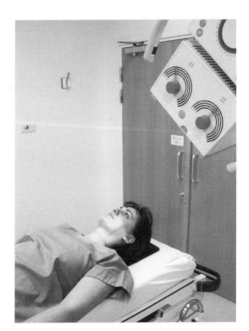

6 Cervico-thoracic vertebrae

Lateral swimmers'

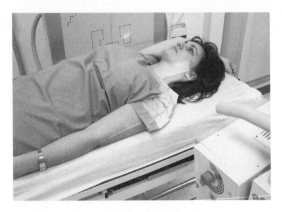

In all trauma radiography, it is imperative that all of the cervical vertebrae and the cervico-thoracic junction are demonstrated. This is particularly important, as this area of the spine is particularly susceptible to injury. The superimposition of the shoulders over these vertebra and subsequent failure to produce an acceptable image is a familiar problem to all radiographers. In the majority of cases, the use of the swimmers' lateral will produce an image that reveals the alignment of these vertebrae and provides an image suitable for diagnosis.

Position of patient and cassette

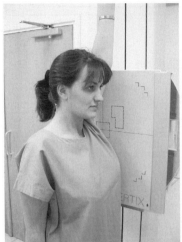

- This projection is usually carried out with the patient supine on a trauma trolley. The trolley is positioned adjacent to the vertical Bucky, with the patient's median sagittal plane parallel with the cassette.
- The arm nearest the cassette is folded over the head, with the humerus as close to the trolley top as the patient can manage. The arm and shoulder nearest the X-ray tube are depressed as far as possible.
- The shoulders are now separated vertically.
- The Bucky should be raised or lowered, such that the line of the vertebrae should coincide with the middle of the cassette.
- This projection can also be undertaken with the patient erect, either standing or sitting or supine.

Direction and centring of the X-ray beam

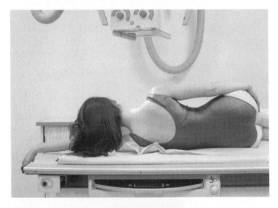

- The horizontal central ray is directed to the midline of the Bucky at a level just above the shoulder remote from the cassette.

Essential image characteristics

- It is imperative to ensure that the C7/T1 junction has been included on the image. It is therefore useful to include an anatomical landmark within the image, e.g. atypical CV2. This will make it possible to count down the vertebrae and ensure that the junction has been imaged.

Radiological considerations

- See Right and left posterior oblique – supine (previous page).

Common faults and remedies

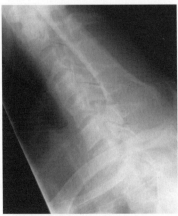

- Failure to ensure that the raised arm is as flat as possible against the stretcher may result in the head of the humerus obscuring the region of interest.

Notes

- For some patients, it may be useful to rotate the side further from the cassette sufficiently forward to separate the shoulders transversely. This positioning will produce a lateral oblique projection of the vertebrae.

- Image quality will be increased if the erect Bucky is used in preference to a stationary grid. This is due to the better scatter attenuation properties of the grid within the Bucky.

Antero-posterior – basic

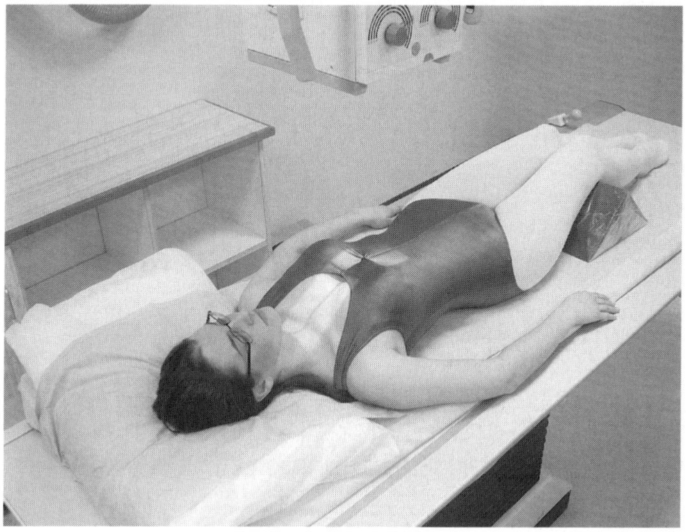

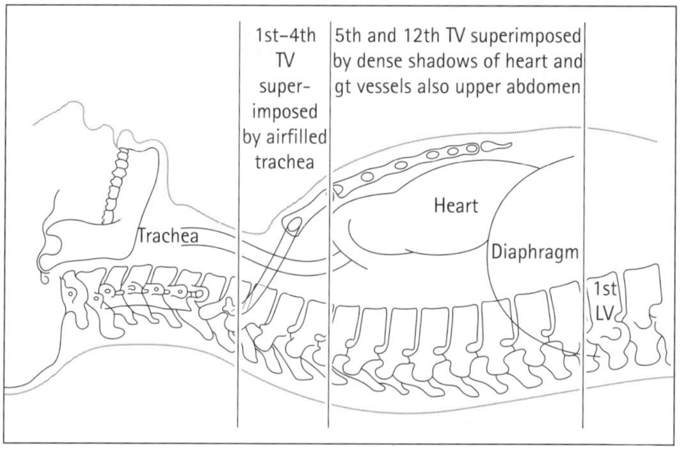

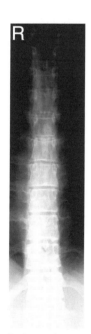

Position of patient and cassette

- The patient is positioned supine on the X-ray table, with the median sagittal plane perpendicular to the tabletop and coincident with the midline of the Bucky.
- The upper edge of a cassette, which should be at least 40 cm long for an adult, should be at a level just below the prominence of the thyroid cartilage to ensure that the upper thoracic vertebrae are included.
- Make exposure on arrested inspiration. This will cause the diaphragm to move down over the upper lumbar vertebra, thus reducing the chance of a large density difference appearing on the image from superimposition of the lungs.

Direction and centring of the X-ray beam

- Direct the central ray at right-angles to the cassette and towards a point 2.5 cm below the sternal angle.
- Collimate tightly to the spine.

Essential image characteristics

- The image should include the vertebrae from C7 to L1.
- The image density should be sufficient to demonstrate bony detail for the upper as well as the thoracic lower vertebrae.

Radiological considerations

- The presence of intact pedicles is an important sign in excluding metastatic disease. Pedicles are more difficult to see on an underexposed or rotated film.

Common faults and remedies

- The cassette and beam are often centred too low, thereby excluding the upper thoracic vertebrae from the image.
- The lower vertebrae are also often not included. L1 can be identified easily by the fact that it usually will not have a rib attached to it.
- High radiographic contrast (see below) causes high density over the upper vertebrae and low density over the lower vertebra.

Notes

- This region has an extremely high subject contrast. This is due to the superimposition of the air-filled trachea over the upper thoracic vertebrae. This produces a relatively lucent area and a high density on the radiograph. The heart and liver superimposed over the lower thoracic vertebrae will attenuate more X-rays and yield a much lower film density.

(contd)

Diagram labels:

1st–4th TV superimposed by airfilled trachea

5th and 12th TV superimposed by dense shadows of heart and gt vessels also upper abdomen

Trachea

Heart

Diaphragm

1st LV

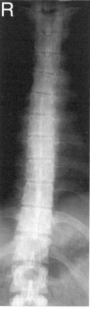

Radiographic contrast too high

Lower contrast producing acceptable density for upper and lower vertebra

6 | Thoracic vertebrae

Antero-posterior – basic (*contd*)

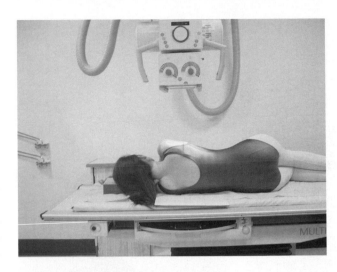

- The radiographer can employ a number of strategies to reduce the high radiographic contrast associated with this region. The use of a relatively high kVp (80 kVp or more) will usually lower the radiographic contrast, thus demonstrating all the vertebrae within the useful density range.
- The anode heel effect can also be exploited by positioning the anode cranially and the cathode caudally.
- The use of graduated screens, wedge filters placed on the light beam diaphragm or attenuators positioned over the upper thoracic vertebrae have also proved effective in reducing the contrast.

Lateral – basic

Position of patient and cassette

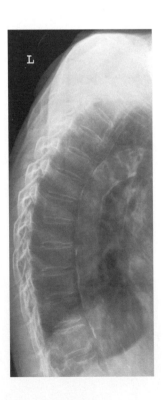

- Usually undertaken with the patient in the lateral decubitus position on the X-ray table, although this projection can also be performed erect.
- The median sagittal plane should be parallel to the cassette and the midline of the axilla coincident with the midline of the table or Bucky.
- The arms should be raised well above the head.
- The head can be supported with a pillow, and pads may be placed between the knees for the patient's comfort.
- The upper edge of the cassette should be at least 40 cm in length and should be positioned 3–4 cm above the spinous process of C7.

Direction and centring of the X-ray beam

- The central ray should be at right-angles to the long axis of the thoracic vertebrae. This may require a caudal angulation.
- Centre 5 cm anterior to the spinous process of T6/7. This is usually found just below the inferior angle of the scapula (assuming the arms are raised), which is easily palpable.

Essential image characteristics

- The upper two or three vertebrae may not be demonstrated due to the superimposition of the shoulders.
- Look for the absence of a rib on L1 at the lower border of the image. This will ensure that T12 has been included within the field.
- The posterior ribs should be superimposed, thus indicating that the patient was not rotated too far forwards or backwards.
- The trabeculae of the vertebrae should be clearly visible, demonstrating an absence of movement unsharpness.
- The image density should be adequate for diagnosis for both the upper and lower thoracic vertebrae. The use of a wide-latitude imaging system/technique is therefore desirable.

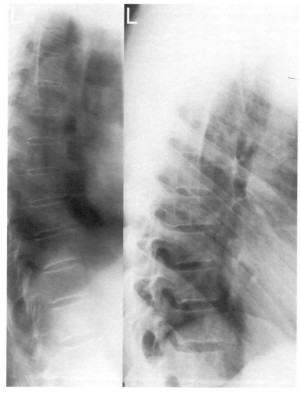

The use of autotomography (left) will prevent lung and rib shadows from obscuring the spine

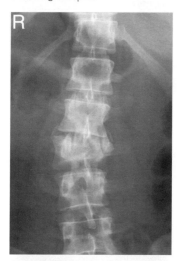

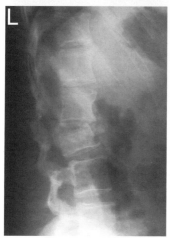

Examples of localized spine projections

Radiological considerations

- Mild endplate changes (e.g. early osteoporotic collapse or partial wedge fractures) are more difficult to see if the X-ray beam does not pass cleanly through all the disc spaces.
- 7–10 per cent of cervical spine fractures are associated with fractures of the thoracic or lumbar vertebrae, and current ATLS and Royal College of Radiologists (RCR) advice is that radiographs of the whole spine are recommended in patients with cervical spine fractures.

Common faults and remedies

- If the exposure is made on arrested inspiration, then the rib shadows will be superimposed over the vertebrae and detract from the image quality. The use of auto-tomography (see below) should resolve this problem.

Note

The vertebrae will be demonstrated optimally if auto-tomography is used to diffuse the lung and rib shadows. This involves setting a low mA (10–20 mA) and a long exposure time (3–5 s). The patient is allowed to breathe normally during the exposure.

Localized projections

Localized projections or tomography are requested occasionally, e.g. when following up a fracture. The centring point must be adjusted to the appropriate vertebrae. The following anterior surface markings can be used as a guide to the appropriate centring point:

- Cricoid cartilage: sixth cervical vertebra.
- Sternal notch: second to third thoracic vertebra.
- Sternal angle: lower border of fourth thoracic vertebra.
- Xiphisternal joint: ninth thoracic vertebra.

Posterior surface markings are more convenient for lateral projections. The level of the upper and middle thoracic vertebrae may be found by first palpating the prominent spinous process of the seventh cervical vertebrae and then counting the spinous processes downwards. The lower vertebrae can be identified by palpating the spinous process of the third lumbar vertebrae at the level of the lower costal margin and then counting the spinous processes upwards.

It is important to remember that the tips of the spinous processes of T5 to T10 are opposite to the bodies of the vertebrae below.

6 Lumbar vertebrae

Antero-posterior – basic

Position of patient and cassette

- The patient lies supine on the Bucky table, with the median sagittal plane coincident with, and at right-angles to, the midline of the table and Bucky.
- The anterior superior iliac spines should be equidistant from the tabletop.
- The hips and knees are flexed and the feet are placed with their plantar aspect on the tabletop to reduce the lumbar arch and bring the lumbar region of the vertebral column parallel with the cassette.
- The cassette should be large enough to include the lower thoracic vertebrae and the sacro-iliac joints and is centred at the level of the lower costal margin.
- The exposure should be made on arrested expiration, as the diaphragm will cause the diaphragm to move superiorly. The air within the lungs would otherwise cause a large difference in density and poor contrast between the upper and lower lumbar vertebrae.

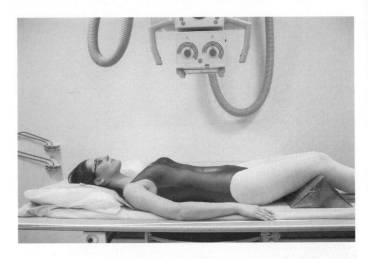

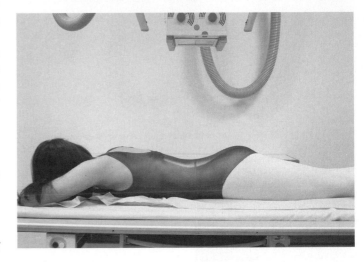

Direction and centring of the X-ray beam

- Direct the central ray towards the midline at the level of the lower costal margin (L3).

Essential image characteristics

- The image should include from T12 down, to include all of the sacro-iliac joints.
- Rotation can be assessed by ensuring that the sacro-iliac joints are equidistant from the spine.
- The exposure used should produce a density such that bony detail can be discerned throughout the region of interest.

Radiological considerations

- The same considerations apply as to the thoracic spine.
- See p. 184.

See p. 184.

Common faults and remedies

- The most common fault is to miss some or all of the sacro-iliac joint. An additional projection of the sacro-iliac joints should be performed.

Note

For relatively fit patients, this projection can be performed with the patient in the postero-anterior position. This allows better visualization of the disc spaces and sacro-iliac joints, as the concavity of the lumbar lordosis faces the tube so the diverging beam passes directly through these structures. Although the magnification is increased, this does not seriously affect image quality.

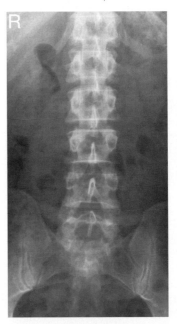

Antero-posterior projection

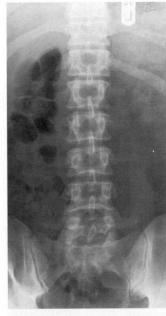

Postero-anterior projection: better visualization of disc spaces and SI joints

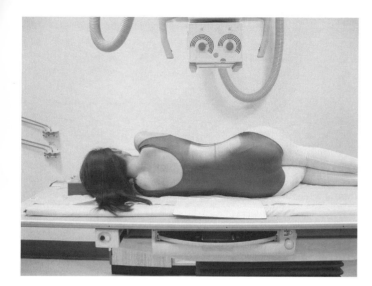

Position of patient and cassette

- The patient lies on either side on the Bucky table. If there is any degree of scoliosis, then the most appropriate lateral position will be such that the concavity of the curve is towards the X-ray tube.
- The arms should be raised and resting on the pillow in front of the patient's head. The knees and hips are flexed for stability.
- The coronal plane running through the centre of the spine should coincide with, and be perpendicular to, the midline of the Bucky.
- Non-opaque pads may be placed under the waist and knees, as necessary, to bring the vertebral column parallel to the film.
- The cassette is centred at the level of the lower costal margin.
- The exposure should be made on arrested expiration.
- This projection can also be undertaken erect with the patient standing or sitting.

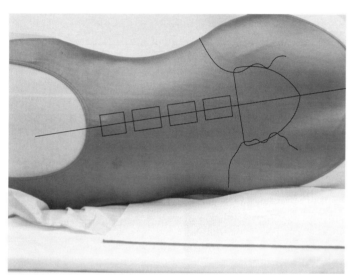

Incorrect – vertebral column not parallel with table

Direction and centring of the X-ray beam

- Direct the central ray at right-angles to the line of spinous processes and towards a point 7.5 cm anterior to the third lumbar spinous process at the level of the lower costal margin.

Essential image characteristics

- The image should include T12 downwards, to include the lumbar sacral junction.
- Ideally, the projection will produce a clear view through the centre of the intervertebral disc space, with individual vertebral endplates superimposed.
- The cortices at the posterior and anterior margins of the vertebral body should also be superimposed.
- The imaging factors selected must produce an image density sufficient for diagnosis from T12 to L5/S1, including the spinous processes.

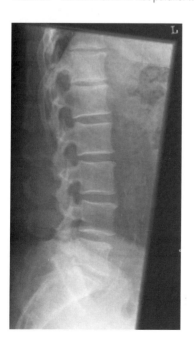

Lateral – basic (*contd*)

Radiological considerations

- The same conditions apply as to the thoracic spine.
- Transitional vertebrae (see diagram opposite) are common at the lumbosacral junction and can make counting the level of an abnormality difficult. A sacralized L5 has a shape similar to S1, with large transverse processes, and is partially incorporated into the upper sacrum. The converse is lumbarization of S1, in which the body and appendages of S1 resemble L5 and the sacro-iliac joints are often reduced in height. These anomalies may cause errors in counting the level of an abnormality, in which case the twelfth rib and thoracic vertebra must be seen clearly to enable counting down from above. This is of particular importance when plain images are used to confirm the level of an abnormality detected on other imaging modalities, e.g. MRI.

Common faults and remedies

- High-contrast images will result in an insufficient or high image density over areas of high or low patient density, i.e. the spinous processes and L5/S1. A high kVp or the use of other wide-latitude techniques is recommended.
- The spinous processes can easily be excluded from the image as a result of overzealous collimation.
- Poor superimposition of the anterior and posterior margins of the vertebral bodies is an indication that the patient was rolled too far forward or backward during the initial positioning (i.e. mean sagittal plane not parallel to cassette).
- Failure to demonstrate a clear intervertebral disc space usually results as a consequence of the spine not being perfectly parallel with the cassette or is due to scoliosis or other patient pathology.

Note

A piece of lead rubber or other attenuator placed behind the patient will reduce scatter incident on the film. This will improve overall image quality as well as reduce the chance of automatic exposure control error.

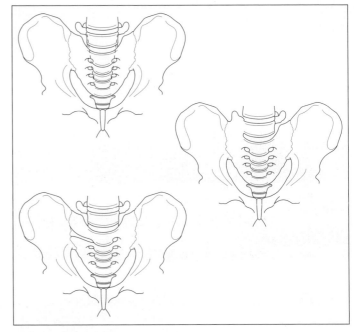

Lumbar transitional vertebra

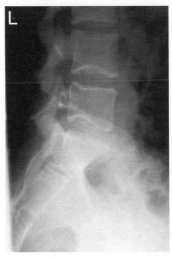

Rudimentary disc at S1/S2

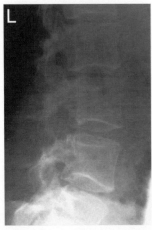

Poor superimposition of anterior and posterior vertebral body margins due to poor positioning

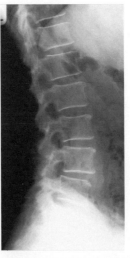

Inappropriately high-contrast image

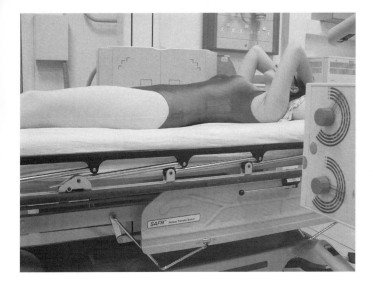

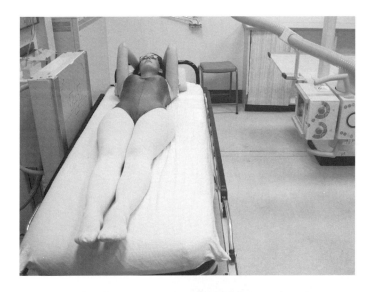

Lateral horizontal beam

A patient with a suspected fracture to the lumbar vertebrae should not be moved from the casualty trolley without medical supervision. Similarly, the patient should not be moved into the lateral decubitus position in these circumstances. This will necessitate the use of a horizontal beam technique in order to obtain the second projection required for a complete examination.

Horizontal beam techniques are discussed further in Section 16.

Position of patient and cassette

- The trauma trolley is placed adjacent to the vertical Bucky.
- Adjust the position of the trolley so that the lower costal margin of the patient coincides with the vertical central line of the Bucky and the median sagittal plane is parallel to the cassette.
- The Bucky should be raised or lowered such that the patient's mid-coronal plane is coincident with the midline of the cassette within the Bucky, along its long axis.
- If possible, the arms should be raised above the head.

Direction and centring of the X-ray beam

- Direct the horizontal central ray parallel to a line joining the anterior superior iliac spines and towards a point 7.5 cm anterior to the third lumbar spinous process at the level of the lower costal margin.

Essential image characteristics

- Refer to lateral lumbar spine (p. 183).
- Extreme care must be taken if using the automatic exposure control. The chamber selected must be directly in line with the vertebrae, otherwise an incorrect exposure will result.
- If a manual exposure is selected, them a higher exposure will be required than with a supine lateral. This is due to the effect of gravity on the internal organs, causing them to lie either side of the spine.

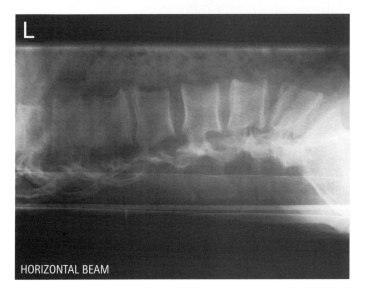

HORIZONTAL BEAM

Lateral flexion and extension

Lateral projections in flexion and extension may be requested to demonstrate mobility and stability of the lumbar vertebrae.

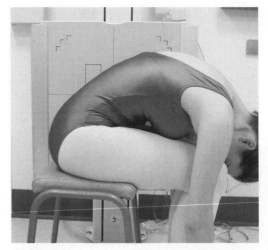

Flexion

Position of patient and cassette

- This projection may be performed supine, but it is most commonly performed erect with the patient seated on a stool with either side against the vertical Bucky.
- A seated position is preferred, since apparent flexion and extension of the lumbar region is less likely to be due to movement of the hip joints when using the erect position.
- The dorsal surface of the trunk should be at right-angles to the cassette and the vertebral column parallel to the cassette.
- For the first exposure the patient leans forward, flexing the lumbar region as far as possible, and grips the front of the seat to assist in maintaining the position.
- For the second exposure the patient then leans backward, extending the lumbar region as far as possible, and grips the back of the seat or another support placed behind the patient.
- The cassette is centred at the level of the lower costal margin, and the exposure is made on arrested expiration.

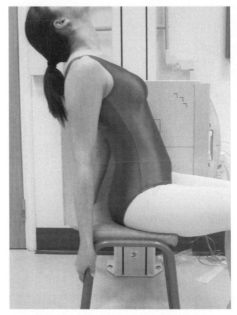

Extension

Direction and centring of the X-ray beam

- Direct the central ray at right-angles to the film and towards a point 7.5 cm anterior to the third lumbar spinous process at the level of the lower costal margin.

Essential image characteristics

Refer to lateral lumbar spine (p. 183). All of the area of interest must be included on both projections.

Common faults and remedies

- Extreme care must be taken if using the automatic exposure control. The chamber selected must be directly in line with the vertebrae, otherwise an incorrect exposure will result.
- If a manual exposure is selected, a higher exposure will be required than with a supine lateral. This is due to the effect of gravity on the internal organs, causing them to lie either side of the spine.
- A short exposure time is desirable, as it is difficult for the patient to remain stable.

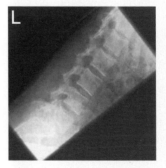

Flexion

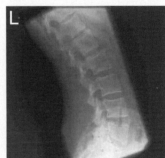

Extension

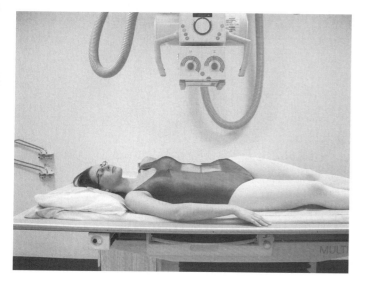

Right or left posterior oblique

These projections demonstrate the pars interarticularis and the apophyseal joints on the side nearest the cassette. Both sides are taken for comparison.

Position of patient and cassette

- The patient is positioned supine on the Bucky table and is then rotated 45 degrees to the right and left sides in turn. The patient's arms are raised, with the hands resting on the pillow.
- The hips and knees are flexed and the patient is supported with a 45-degree foam pad placed under the trunk on the raised side.
- The cassette is centred at the lower costal margin.

Direction and centring of the X-ray beam

- Direct the vertical central ray towards the midclavicular line on the raised side at the level of the lower costal margin.

Essential image characteristics

- The degree of obliquity should be such that the posterior elements of the vertebra are aligned in such as way as to show the classic 'Scottie dog' appearance (see diagram).

Radiological considerations

A defect in the pars interarticularis can be congenital or due to trauma. It is a weakness in the mechanism that prevents one vertebra slipping forward on the one below (spondylolisthesis) and can be a cause of back pain. If bilateral, a spondylolisthesis is more likely. The defect appears as a 'collar' on the 'Scottie dog', hence the importance of demonstrating the 'dog'.

Common faults and remedies

- A common error is to centre too medially, thus excluding the posterior elements of the vertebrae from the image.

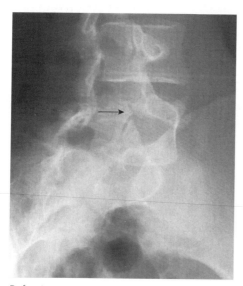

Normal left posterior oblique

Defect in pars interarticularis at L5

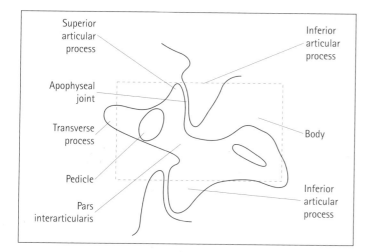

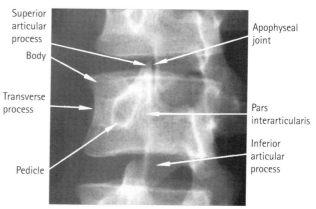

6 Lumbo-sacral junction

Lateral

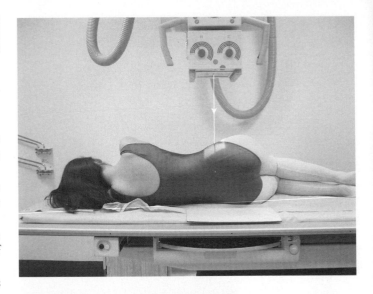

Position of patient and cassette

- The patient lies on either side on the Bucky table, with the arms raised and the hands resting on the pillow. The knees and hips are flexed slightly for stability.
- The dorsal aspect of the trunk should be at right-angles to the cassette. This can be assessed by palpating the iliac crests or the posterior superior iliac spines.
- The coronal plane running through the centre of the spine should coincide with, and be perpendicular to, the midline of the Bucky.
- The cassette is centred at the level of the fifth lumbar spinous process.
- Non-opaque pads may be placed under the waist and knees, as necessary, to bring the vertebral column parallel to the cassette.

Direction and centring of the X-ray beam

- Direct the central ray at right-angles to the lumbo-sacral region and towards a point 7.5 cm anterior to the fifth lumbar spinous process. This is found at the level of the tubercle of the iliac crest or midway between the level of the upper border of the iliac crest and the anterior superior iliac spine.
- If the patient has particularly large hips and the spine is not parallel with the tabletop, then a five-degree caudal angulation may be required to clear the joint space.

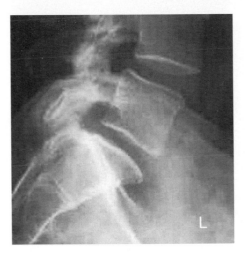

Essential image characteristics

- The area of interest should include the fifth lumbar vertebra and the first sacral segment.
- A clear joint space should be demonstrated.

Radiation protection

- This projection requires a relatively large exposure so should not be undertaken as a routine projection. The lateral lumbar spine should be evaluated and a further projection for the L5/S1 junction considered if this region is not demonstrated to a diagnostic standard.

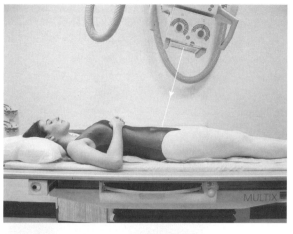

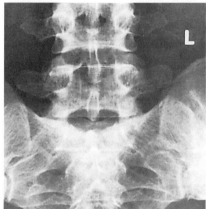

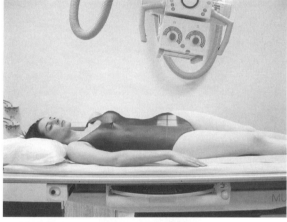

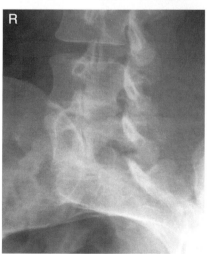

Antero-posterior

The lumbo-sacral articulation is not always demonstrated well on the antero-posterior lumbar spine, due to the oblique direction of the articulation resulting from the lumbar lordosis. This projection may be requested to specifically demonstrate this articulation.

Position of patient and cassette

- The patient lies supine on the Bucky table, with the median sagittal plane coincident with, and perpendicular to, the midline of the Bucky.
- The anterior superior iliac spines should be equidistant from the tabletop.
- The knees can be flexed over a foam pad for comfort and to reduce the lumbar lordosis.
- The cassette is displaced cranially so that its centre coincides with the central ray.

Direction and centring of the X-ray beam

- Direct the central ray 10–20 degrees cranially from the vertical and towards the midline at the level of the anterior superior iliac spines.
- The degree of angulation of the central ray is normally greater for females than for males and will be less for a greater degree of flexion at the hips and knees.

Essential image characteristics

- The image should be collimated to include the fifth lumbar and first sacral segment.

Right or left posterior oblique

These projections demonstrate the pars interarticularis and the apophyseal joints on the side nearer the film.

Position of patient and cassette

- The patient is positioned supine on the Bucky table and is then rotated to the right and left sides in turn so that the median sagittal plane is at an angle of approximately 45 degrees to the tabletop.
- The hips and knees are flexed and the patient is supported with 45-degree foam pads placed under the trunk on the raised side.
- The cassette is displaced cranially at a level to coincide with the central ray.

Essential image characteristics

- The posterior elements of L5 should appear in the 'Scottie dog' configuration (see oblique lumbar spine, p. 187).

Common faults and remedies

- A common error is to centre too medially, thus excluding the posterior elements of the vertebrae from the image.

6 Sacrum

Antero-posterior/postero-anterior

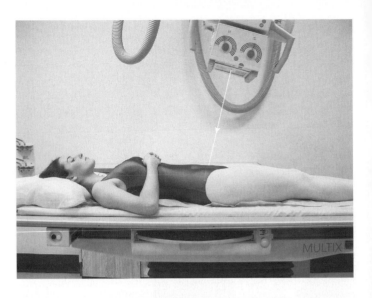

The sacrum may be either imaged antero-posteriorly or postero-anteriorly. If imaged postero-anteriorly, there will be various advantages, including a lower dose to the gonads and better demonstration of the sacro-iliac joints, as the joint spaces will be more parallel with the divergent central ray. The antero-posterior position may be a more realistic option when the patient is infirm or injured and therefore would find it difficult to maintain the prone position.

Position of patient and cassette

- The patient lies supine or prone on the Bucky table, with the median sagittal plane coincident with, and at right-angles to, the midline of the Bucky.
- The anterior superior iliac spines should be equidistant from the tabletop.
- If the patient is examined supine (antero-posteriorly), the knees can be flexed over a foam pad for comfort. This will also reduce the pelvic tilt.
- The cassette is displaced cranially for antero-posterior projection, or caudally for postero-anterior projections, such that its centre coincides with the angled central ray.

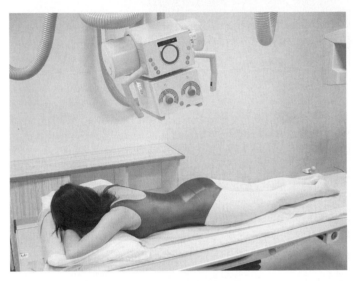

Direction and centring of the X-ray beam

- Antero-posterior: direct the central ray 10–25 degrees cranially from the vertical and towards a point midway between the level of the anterior superior iliac spines and the superior border of the symphysis pubis.
- The degree of angulation of the central ray is normally greater for females than for males and will be less for a greater degree of flexion at the hips and knees.
- Postero-anterior: palpate the position of the sacrum by locating the posterior superior iliac spine and coccyx. Centre to the middle of the sacrum in the midline.
- The degree of beam angulation will depend on the pelvic tilt. Palpate the sacrum and then simply apply a caudal angulation, such that the central ray is perpendicular to the long axis of the sacrum (see photograph opposite).

Radiological considerations

- The sacrum is a thin bone. Problems with exposure can easily lead to important pathologies such as fractures and metastases being missed.

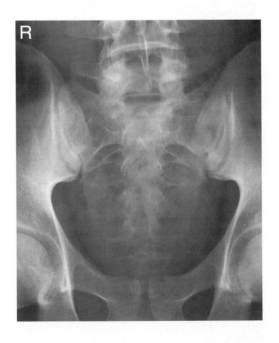

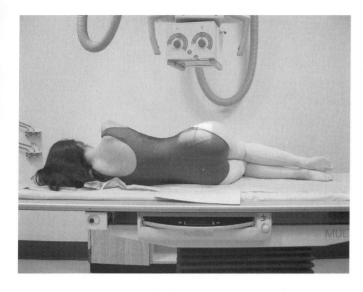

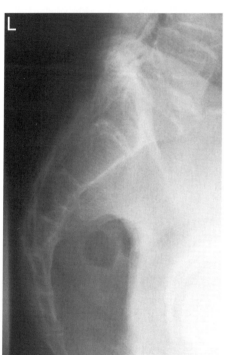

Position of patient and cassette

- The patient lies on either side on the Bucky table, with the arms raised and the hands resting on the pillow. The knees and hips are flexed slightly for stability.
- The dorsal aspect of the trunk should be at right-angles to the cassette. This can be assessed by palpating the iliac crests or the posterior superior iliac spines. The coronal plane running through the centre of the spine should coincide with, and be perpendicular to, the midline of the Bucky.
- The cassette is centred to coincide with the central ray at the level of the midpoint of the sacrum.

Direction and centring of the X-ray beam

- Direct the central ray at right-angles to the long axis of the sacrum and towards a point in the midline of the table at a level midway between the posterior superior iliac spines and the sacro-coccygeal junction.

Radiological considerations

- Fractures are easily missed if the exposure is poor or a degree of rotation is present.

Common faults and remedies

- If using an automatic exposure control, centring too far posteriorly will result in an underexposed image.

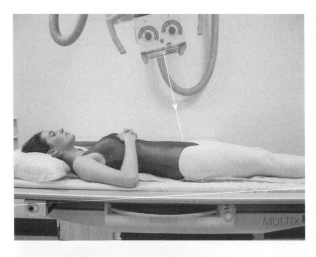

Antero-posterior

Position of patient and cassette

- The patient lies supine on the Bucky table, with the median sagittal plane coincident with, and at right-angles to, the midline of the Bucky.
- The anterior superior iliac spines should be equidistant from the tabletop.
- The knees can be flexed over a foam pad for comfort and to reduce the pelvic tilt.
- The cassette is displaced caudally so that its centre coincides with the central ray.

Direction and centring of the X-ray beam

- Direct the central ray 15 degrees caudally towards a point in the midline 2.5 cm superior to the symphysis pubis.

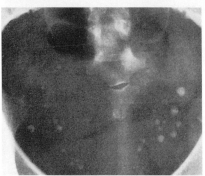

Radiological considerations

- Anatomy of the coccyx is very variable (number of segments, angle of inclination, etc.).
- This is a high dose investigation with little yield unless the patient is to have a coccyxectomy.

Lateral

Position of patient and cassette

- The patient lies on either side on the Bucky table, with the palpable coccyx in the midline of the Bucky. The arms are raised, with the hands resting on the pillow. The knees and hips are flexed slightly for stability.
- The dorsal aspect of the trunk should be at right-angles to the cassette. This can be assessed by palpating the iliac crests or the posterior superior iliac spines. The median sagittal plane should be parallel with the Bucky.
- The cassette is centred to coincide with the central ray at the level of the coccyx.

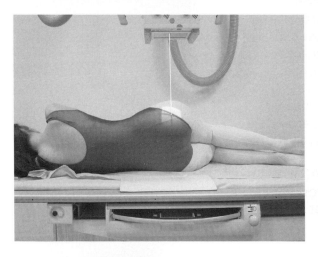

Direction and centring of the X-ray beam

- Direct the central ray at right-angles to the long axis of the sacrum and towards the palpable coccyx.

Radiological considerations

- See above.

Common faults and remedies

Care must be taken when using an automatic exposure control, as underexposure can easily result if the chamber is positioned slightly posterior to the coccyx.

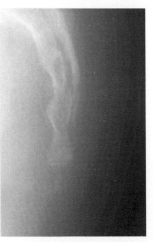

Section 7

The Thorax and Upper Airways

CONTENTS

THORAX: PHARYNX AND LARYNX	194	Postero-anterior	216
Antero-posterior	194	Left lateral	218
Lateral	195	Right anterior oblique	219
THORAX: TRACHEA (INCLUDING		BONES OF THE THORAX	220
THORACIC INLET)	196	Introduction	220
Antero-posterior	196	Recommended projections	221
Lateral	197		
		LOWER RIBS	222
LUNGS	198	Antero-posterior (basic)	222
Introduction	198	Right and left posterior oblique	223
Radiographic anatomy	204		
General radiological considerations	205	UPPER RIBS	224
Postero-anterior – erect	206	Right and left posterior oblique	224
Antero-posterior – erect	208	First and second – antero-posterior	225
Antero-posterior – supine	209	Cervical – antero-posterior	225
Antero-posterior – semi-erect	210		
Lateral	211	STERNUM	226
Apices	212	Anterior oblique – tube angled	226
Upper anterior region – lateral	213	Anterior oblique – trunk rotated	227
Lordotic	213	Lateral	228
HEART AND AORTA	214		
Introduction	214		
Anatomy	215		

7 Thorax: pharynx and larynx

Plain radiography is requested to investigate the presence of soft-tissue swellings and their effects on the air passages, as well as to locate the presence of foreign bodies or assess laryngeal trauma. Tomography, computed tomography (CT) and/or magnetic resonance imaging (MRI) may be needed for full evaluation of other disease processes.

It is common practice to take two projections, an antero-posterior and a lateral, using a 24 × 30-cm cassette.

Antero-posterior

Position of patient and cassette

- The patient lies supine, with the median sagittal plane adjusted to coincide with the central long axis of the couch.
- The chin is raised to show the soft tissues below the mandible and to bring the radiographic baseline to an angle of 20 degrees from the vertical.
- The cassette is centred at the level of the fourth cervical vertebra.

Direction and centring of the X-ray beam

- Direct the central ray 10 degrees cephalad and in the midline at the level of the fourth cervical vertebra.
- Exposure is made on forced expiration.

Essential image characteristics

- The beam should be collimated to include an area from the occipital bone to the seventh cervical vertebra.

Notes

- Image acquisition may be made either with or without a Bucky grid.
- Assessment of possible small foreign bodies may not require the antero-posterior projection, as such foreign bodies are likely to be obscured by virtue of the overlying cervical spine.
- Air in the pharynx and larynx will result in an increase in subject contrast in the neck region. This may be reduced using a high-kilovoltage technique.

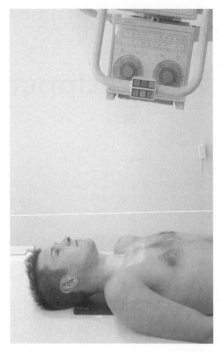

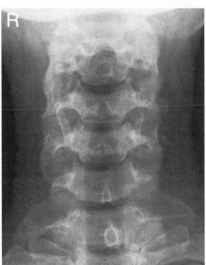

Antero-posterior radiograph showing normal larynx

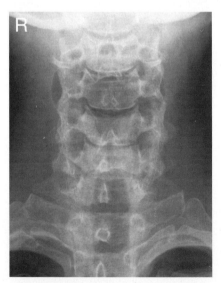

Antero-posterior radiograph of larynx showing a laryngocoele

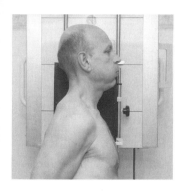

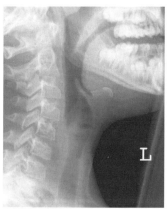

Lateral radiograph showing normal air-filled larynx

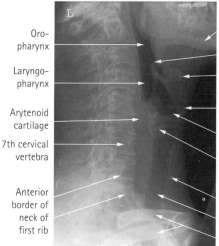

Oro-pharynx

Laryngo-pharynx

Arytenoid cartilage

7th cervical vertebra

Anterior border of neck of first rib

Mandible

Tip of epiglottis

Hyoid bone

Anterior border of thyroid cartilage

Laryngeal ventricle

Cricoid cartilage

Benign thyroid calcification

Tracheal air shadow

Clavicles

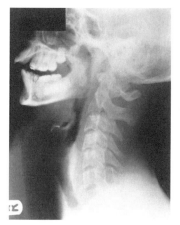

Lateral radiograph showing fracture of the hyoid bone

Position of patient and cassette

- The patient stands or sits with either shoulder against a vertical cassette. Two 45-degree pads may be placed between the patient's head and the cassette to aid immobilization.
- The median sagittal plane of the trunk and head are parallel to the cassette.
- The jaw is raised slightly so that the angles of the mandible are separated from the bodies of the upper cervical vertebrae.
- A point 2.5 cm posterior to the angle of the mandible should be coincident with the vertical central line of the cassette.
- The cassette is centred at the level of the prominence of the thyroid cartilage opposite the fourth cervical vertebra.
- Immediately before exposure, the patient is asked to depress the shoulders forcibly so that their structures are projected below the level of the seventh cervical vertebra.
- When carrying out this manoeuvre, the head and trunk must be maintained in position.
- Exposure is made on forced expiration.

Direction and centring of the X-ray beam

- The horizontal central ray is directed to a point vertically below the mastoid process at the level of the prominence of the thyroid cartilage through the fourth cervical vertebra.

Essential image characteristics

- The soft tissues should be demonstrated from the skull base to the root of the neck (C7).
- Exposure should allow clear visualization of laryngeal cartilages and any possible foreign body.

Radiological considerations

- If the prevertebral soft tissues at the level of C4–C6 are wider than the corresponding vertebral body, then soft-tissue swelling can be diagnosed (this may be the only sign of a lucent foreign body). This sign may be mimicked if the neck is flexed or may be masked if the projection is oblique. A true lateral is therefore essential.
- The cartilages of the larynx typically calcify in a patchy fashion and may mimic foreign bodies.

7 Thorax: trachea (including thoracic inlet)

Plain radiography is requested to investigate the presence of soft-tissue swellings in the neck and the upper thorax and to demonstrate the effects on the air passages, e.g. the presence of retrosternal goitre.

Consideration should also be given to the fact that radiography in the lateral position will involve exposure of the neck and the relatively thicker upper thorax. A high-kilovoltage technique should therefore be employed to demonstrate the full length of the trachea on one image.

Two projections, an antero-posterior and a lateral, are taken using a moving grid technique. A cassette size is selected that will include the full length of the trachea.

CT or tomography of the trachea may be required for more complex problems.

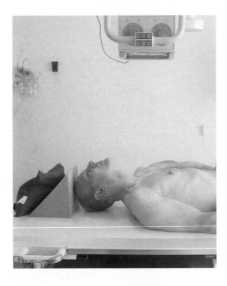

Antero-posterior

Position of patient and cassette

- The patient lies supine, with the median sagittal plane adjusted to coincide with the central long axis of the imaging couch.
- The chin is raised to show the soft tissues below the mandible and to bring the radiographic baseline to an angle of 20 degrees from the vertical.
- The cassette is centred at the level of the sternal notch.

Direction and centring of the X-ray beam

- Direct the vertical ray in the midline at the level of the sternal notch.
- Exposure is made on forced expiration.

Essential image characteristics

The beam should be collimated to include the full length of the trachea.

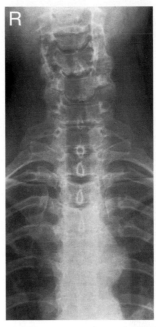

Antero-posterior radiograph showing normal trachea

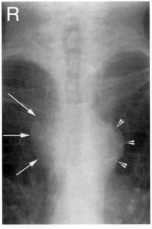

Antero-posterior radiograph of trachea showing paratracheal lymph node mass (arrows). The arrowheads indicate the aortic arch

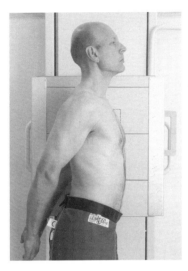

Lateral

Image acquisition is best performed with the patient erect, thus enabling the patient to position the shoulders away from the area of interest.

Position of patient and cassette

- The patient stands or sits with either shoulder against a vertical Bucky.
- The median sagittal plane of the trunk and head are parallel to the cassette.
- The cassette should be large enough to include from the lower pharynx to the lower end of the trachea at the level of the sternal angle.
- The shoulders are pulled well backwards to enable the visualization of the trachea.
- This position is aided by the patient clasping their hands behind the back and pulling their arms backwards.
- The cassette is centred at the level of the sternal notch.

Direction and centring of the X-ray beam

- The horizontal central ray is directed to the cassette at the level of the sternal notch.
- The exposure is made on forced expiration.

Note

The full length of the trachea can be demonstrated on a single image using a high-kilovoltage technique (p. 29), which reduces the contrast between the neck and the denser upper thorax.

Radiological considerations

- This projection is sometimes helpful in confirming retrosternal extension of the thyroid gland. Most assessments of the trachea itself will be by bronchoscopy and/or CT (especially multislice CT with MPR reconstructions and virtual bronchoscopy).
- An anterior mediastinal mass (e.g. retrosternal thyroid) causes increased density of the anterior mediastinal window. This can also be mimicked by superimposed soft tissue if the patient's arms are not pulled backwards sufficiently away from the area of interest.

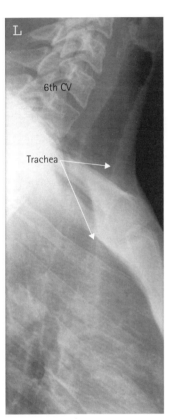

Lateral radiograph showing normal air-filled trachea

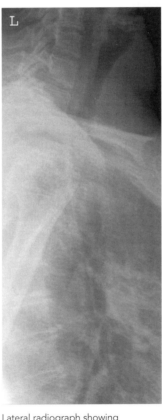

Lateral radiograph showing compression and posterior deviation of the trachea by an enlarged thyroid. Note the shoulders are not pulled back to the ideal position and the humeral heads just overlap the trachea

7 Lungs

Introduction

Radiographic examination of the lungs is performed for a wide variety of medical conditions, including primary lung disease and pulmonary effects of diseases in other organ systems. Such effects produce significant changes in the appearance of the lung parenchyma and may vary over time depending on the nature and extent of the disease.

Imaging may also be performed using a variety of imaging modalities, notably CT and radionuclide imaging.

Recommended projections

Examination is performed by means of the following projections:

Basic	Postero-anterior – erect
Alternative	Antero-posterior – erect
	Antero-posterior – supine
	Antero-posterior – semi-erect
Supplementary	Lateral
	Postero-anterior – expiration
	Apices
	Lateral – upper anterior region
	Decubitus with horizontal beam
	Tomography

Positioning

The choice of erect or decubitus technique is governed primarily by the condition of the patient, with the majority of patients positioned erect. Very ill patients and patients who are immobile are X-rayed in the supine or semi-erect position (see Section 12). With the patient erect, positioning is simplified, control of respiration is more satisfactory, the gravity effect on the abdominal organs allows for the disclosure of the maximum area of lung tissue, and fluid levels are defined more easily with the use of a horizontal central ray.

The postero-anterior projection is generally adopted in preference to the antero-posterior because the arms can be arranged more easily to enable the scapulae to be projected clear of the lung fields. Heart magnification is also reduced significantly compared with the antero-posterior projection.

This projection also facilitates compression of breast tissue with an associated reduction in dose to the breast tissue. Additionally, the dose to the thyroid is reduced.

The mediastinal and heart shadows, however, obscure a considerable part of the lung fields, and a lateral radiograph may be necessary in certain situations.

Supplementary projections may be required for specific indications at the request of a clinician or radiologist (see table above).

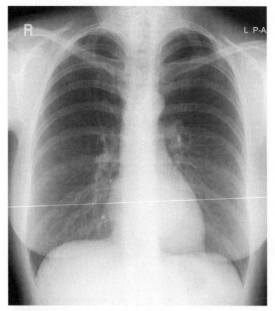

Normal postero-anterior radiograph of chest

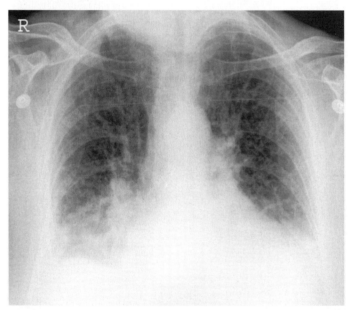

Abnormal postero-anterior radiograph of chest showing lung bases obscured by bilateral basal pulmonary oedema

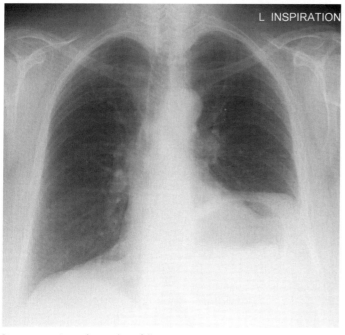

Postero-anterior radiograph on full inspiration

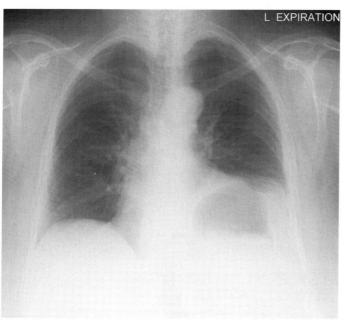

Postero-anterior radiograph on expiration

Introduction

Respiration

Images are normally acquired on arrested deep inspiration, which ensures maximum visualization of the air-filled lungs. The adequacy of inspiration of an exposed radiograph can be assessed by the position of the ribs above the diaphragm. In the correctly exposed image, it should be possible to visualize either six ribs anteriorly or ten ribs posteriorly.

A brief explanation to the patient, along with a rehearsal of the procedure, should ensure a satisfactory result. Respiratory movements should be repeated several times before the performance is considered to be satisfactory. With the patient having taken a deep breath, a few moments should be allowed to elapse to ensure stability before the exposure is made. Risk of movement is minimal by using equipment capable of using exposures in the region of 20 ms. On inspiration, there is a tendency to raise the shoulders, which should be avoided, as the shadows of the clavicles then obscure the lung apices.

A normal nipple may be visible projected over the lower part of one or both lung fields on a frontal radiograph, typically having a well-defined lateral border with an indistinct medial border. In cases of doubt, a simple metallic marker can be taped to the nipple and a repeat radiograph performed. If the opacity corresponds to the metal marker, then it is likely to be nipple. This may be confirmed further by an expiratory radiograph to show that both marker and opacity move together with respiration. Due to the radiation dose involved, these additional exposures should be made under the guidance of a radiologist. Soft-tissue artefacts are discussed on p. 494.

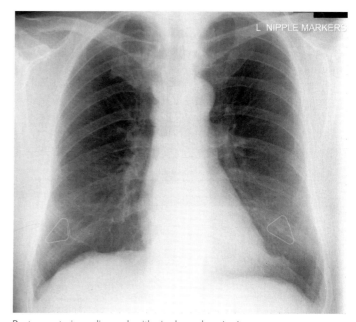

Postero-anterior radiograph with nipple markers *in situ*

Introduction (*contd*)

Image acquisition

Radiography of the lung fields may be performed by a variety of imaging techniques. The following systems are available:

- conventional screen – film with low kVp
- conventional screen – film with high kVp
- conventional screen – film with selective filter device
- asymmetric screen – film system
- digital acquisition using storage phospors
- digital acquisition using semiconductor technology
- digital scanning with selenium detectors.

Selection of the imaging system to be used will be dependent on the operational protocols of the imaging department. However, the overriding objective of the system selected is to acquire an image of the thorax that will demonstrate all of the anatomical structures present, including lung parenchyma behind the mediastinum and in the regions of the costophrenic angles where the lung fields may be obscured by abdominal structures.

The following table illustrates the optimum high- and low-contrast resolution criteria expected of an imaging system where the entrance surface dose for a standard patient is 0.3 mGy using a conventional screen–film system.

	High contrast	*Low contrast*
Small, round details	0.7 mm diameter	2 mm diameter
Linear and reticular details	0.3 mm width	2 mm width

Imaging parameters

For adults, a vertical chest stand with a stationary or moving grid is selected for patients who are able to stand unaided. Imaging without a grid is selected when a low-kVp technique is preferred.

The technique is modified when examining children and babies or examining adults whose medical condition is such that they require to be examined using mobile or portable equipment.

The following table illustrates the parameters necessary to provide optimum and consistent image resolution and contrast.

Item	*Comment*
Focal spot size	≤1.3 mm
Total filtration	≥3.0 mm Al equivalent
Anti-scatter grid	R = 12; 40/cm
Film-screen combination	Speed class 200–400
FFD	180 (range 140–200) cm
Radiographic voltage	100–150 kVp
Automatic exposure control	Chamber selected – lateral
Exposure time	<20 ms

FFD, focus-to-film distance

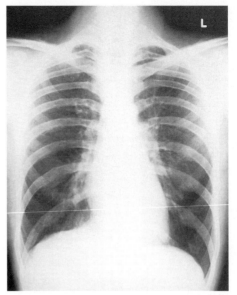

Postero-anterior chest radiograph taken using conventional screen/film combination at low kVp

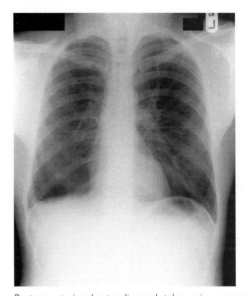

Postero-anterior chest radiograph taken using conventional screen/film combination at high kVp

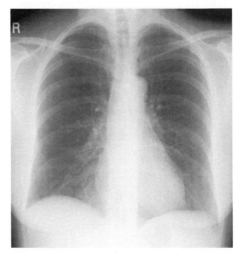

Postero-anterior chest radiograph taken using digital acquisition by storage phosphor technology

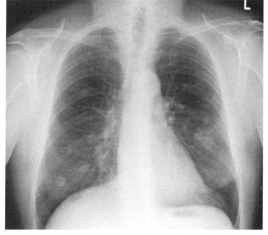

Dual energy digital postero-anterior radiograph without subtraction

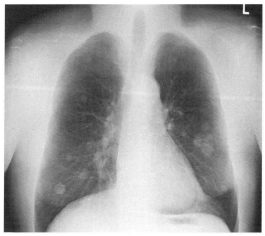

Dual energy digital postero-anterior radiograph with bone subtracted

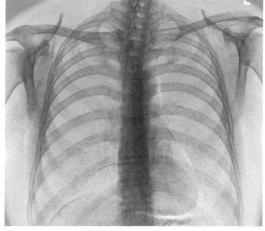

Dual energy digital postero-anterior radiograph showing bone detail. The above example of standard, soft-tissue and bone images acquired using a dual-energy technique, with an exposure of less than 200 ms, illustrates how chest nodules can be best demonstrated on the soft-tissue image by removing overlying ribs

Introduction

Choice of kilovoltage/dual-energy subtraction

Selection of an appropriate kilovoltage should primarily provide adequate penetration from the hila to the periphery of the lung fields and should be in keeping with the patient thickness, habitus and pathology. In general, 60–70 kVp provides adequate penetration for the postero-anterior projection, in which case there will be minor penetration of the mediastinum and heart. An increase in kilovoltage is necessary for penetration of the denser mediastinum and heart to show the lung behind those structures and behind the diaphragm, as well as the lung bases in a very large or heavy-breasted patient.

A high-kilovoltage technique (120–150 kVp), appropriate to the film speed, reduces the dynamic range of information that needs to be recorded, thus enabling visualization of the lung fields and mediastinum with one exposure. This technique also has the advantage of reducing radiation dose. However, with this technique there is a loss of subject contrast and therefore visualization of small lesions of soft-tissue density becomes difficult. Additionally, rib lesions are more difficult to visualize adequately using a high-kilovoltage technique.

A range of kilovoltages (80–100 kVp) midway between non-grid and high kilovoltages is used to compromise between the advantages and disadvantages of the two techniques.

Dual-energy digital subtraction can be used to overcome the problem of pathology obscured by overlying bones. In this technique, high- and low-energy images are acquired less than 200 ms apart during the same breath-hold. The low-energy image is subtracted from the standard high-kVp image to produce bone and soft-tissue images. Three images are presented for viewing, similar to those shown opposite. Typically, there is up to 80 kVp separating the exposures.

Maintaining general contrast/use of grid

Scattered radiation has the effect of reducing subject contrast and adding image noise. To combat these effects, especially when using a high-kVp technique, selection of a grid with a grid ratio of at least 10 : 1 is necessary. For dedicated Bucky work, a grid designed to work at a focus-to-film distance (FFD) of 180 cm with a ratio of 12 : 1 is usually selected.

Grids with a lower grid ratio need less precise grid alignment and may be used for mobile radiography.

Air-gap technique

This technique employs the displacement of the subject from the film by a distance of 15 cm. To reduce any geometric unsharpness, the FFD is increased to 300 cm. A high proportion of oblique scattered radiation from the subject will no longer fall on the film because of the increased distance between subject and the film. A patient support, which is 15 cm in front of the cassette, is used to steady the patient and provide the subject-to-film distance.

Introduction (*contd*)

Magnification factor and focus-to-film distance

To obtain minimal magnification of the intra-thoracic structures, especially the heart, and structural detail at differing distances from the film, FFDs in the range of 150–180 cm are selected. However, the FFD must be kept constant for any one department to allow comparison of successive films. At these distances, geometric unsharpness is greatly reduced. The selection of the focal spot size is governed by the maximum output of the generator, which enables the shortest exposure time to be selected for the examination at the kilovoltage set. Ideally, the focal spot size should be no greater than 1.3 mm for an FFD of 180 cm.

An FFD less than those recommended increases the image magnification. However, such a reduction in distance to 120 cm is a satisfactory means of obtaining a short exposure time when using low-output machines such as conventional mobile units.

Exposure time related to subject movement

Involuntary subject movement is reduced by the selection of the shortest exposure time available, preferably in the millisecond range. Ideally, exposure times should be less than 20 ms. This can be obtained with high-output units at the higher mA settings, balanced to the speed of the film and screen combination and the kilovoltage selected. The use of rare earth screens and fast film combinations is essential to ensure short exposure times.

With high kilovoltage, shorter exposure times are also possible, with the added advantage of selecting a smaller focal spot within the tube rating.

Uniformity

Automatic exposure control and use of automatic processors, which are monitored for constant performance, enable films to be obtained of comparable good quality over a period of time at each repeat examination. However, even without automatic exposure control, comparable good-quality films can be obtained for the same patient by the adoption of a technique that relates kVp to chest thickness. This technique will also improve the possibility of greater uniformity throughout the range of patients.

If, for an average 22.5 cm thickness, for example, 67.5 kVp is judged to give the required penetration and density at a selected mAs factor, then for each 1 cm difference in measured thickness, a 2–3 kVp adjustment is added either as the thickness increases or as the thickness decreases.

A record of exposure factors, used for each projection, should be made on either the X-ray request card or the computer records. Reference to these records will enable films of comparable good quality to be obtained over a period of time and in different sections of the same imaging department or hospital.

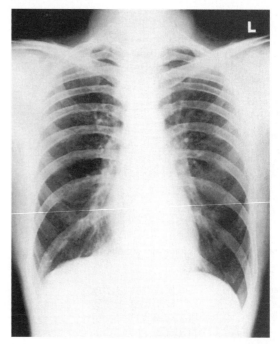

FFD = 180 cm

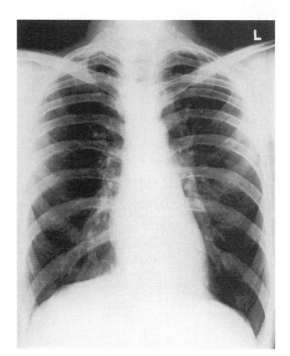

FFD = 75 cm

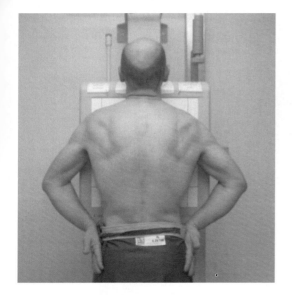

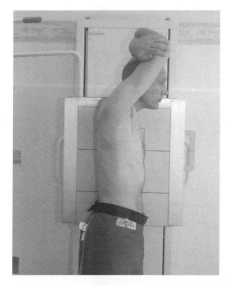

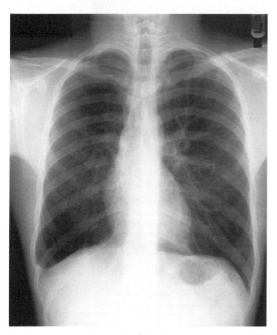

Postero-anterior radiograph of chest using asymmetrical film/screen combination

Introduction

Radiation protection

An adjustable rectangular diaphragm is used to collimate the radiation field to the size of the lung fields. This reduces the radiation dose to the patient. The effects of back-scatter from walls can be reduced by suspending a piece of lead rubber on the rear of the chest stand immediately behind the cassette holder or vertical Bucky.

For all projections of the thorax, an adjustable mobile lead protective screen or waist lead-rubber apron should be placed to shield the trunk below the diaphragm from the tube aspect.

The radiation dose to the sternum and mammary glands is minimized by employing, where possible, the postero-anterior projection of the chest in preference to the antero-posterior projection.

Film/intensifying screen combinations

Intensifying screens are selected that enable the production of good-quality radiographs that are free of movement unsharpness and quantum mottle. The radiation dose to the patient can be reduced considerably by selecting a 200–400-speed film/screen combination. Faster speed systems, although reducing patient dose, have the disadvantage of introducing quantum mottle.

The use of asymmetrical films and screens may also be employed to record large differences in absorption on one film. Such systems are comprised of two screens differing in speed and spatial resolution and an asymmetrical dual-emulsion film with built in anti-crossover technology. The front high-resolution screen and high-contrast emulsion records the lung fields, while the faster rear screen and film emulsion records the mediastinum, retro-cardiac and subdiaphragmatic areas. This combination provides high-exposure latitude and a fast-speed system.

A major necessity in maintaining good-quality radiographs is the assurance of good film/screen contact to eliminate unsharpness. Cassettes should be tested for this as well as inspecting them for damage around the hinges and corners. Intensifying screens should be cleaned regularly in accordance with the manufacturer's instructions.

Identification

Accurate identification of chest radiographs is essential, with information such as right and left sides, patient's name, date, hospital number and radiology identification number being distinguished clearly. Congenital transposition of the organs occurs in a small number of people, and without the correct side marker the condition may be misdiagnosed. Additional information relating to orientation of the patient and tube different from the norm should also be recorded.

7 | Lungs

Radiographic anatomy

The lungs lie within the thoracic cavity on either side of the mediastinum, separated from the abdomen by the diaphragm. The right lung is larger than the left due to the inclination of the heart to the left side. In normal radiographs of the thorax, some lung tissue is obscured by the ribs, clavicles and, to a certain extent, the heart, and also by the diaphragm and upper abdominal organs in the postero-anterior projection.

The right lung is divided into upper, middle and lower lobes, and the left lung is divided into upper and lower lobes. The fissures that separate the lobes can be demonstrated in various projections of the thorax, when the plane of each fissure is parallel to the beam. On a postero-anterior radiograph, however, the main lobes overlap, so that for descriptive purposes the lungs are divided into three zones separated by imaginary horizontal lines. The upper zone is above the anterior end of the second ribs, the midzone is between the second and fourth ribs anteriorly, and the lower zone is below the level of the fourth ribs. On a lateral radiograph, where horizontal and oblique fissures are visible, upper, middle and lower lobes can be defined separately. On a postero-anterior radiograph, a horizontal fissure separating the upper and middle lobes may be seen extending from the right hilum to the level of the right sixth rib laterally. An accessory lobe called the azygos lobe is sometimes seen in the right upper zone as a result of aberrant embryological migration of the azygos vein to the normal medial position. The azygos vein, surrounded by a double layer of visceral and parietal pleura, is seen as opacity at the lower end of the accessory fissure, resembling an inverted comma.

The trachea is seen centrally as a radiolucent air-filled structure in the upper thorax, which divides at the level of the fourth thoracic vertebra into the right and left main bronchi. The right main bronchus is wider, shorter and more vertical than the left, and as a result inhaled foreign bodies are more likely to pass into the right bronchial tree. The main bronchi enter the hila, beyond which they divide into bronchi, bronchioles and, finally, alveolar air spaces, each getting progressively smaller.

As these passages are filled with air, they do not appear on a normal radiograph of the thorax, since the surrounding lung is also air-filled. If the parenchyma is consolidated, however, an air-filled bronchogram is shown.

The hilar regions appear as regions of increased radio-opacity and are formed mainly by the main branches of the pulmonary arteries. The lung markings that spread out from the hilar regions are branches of these pulmonary arteries, and are seen diminishing in size as they pass distally from the hilar regions. The right dome of the diaphragm lies higher than the left, due mainly to the presence of the liver on the right. The costophrenic angles and lateral chest walls should be defined clearly.

Special landmarks that may be seen, although not in every image, are the subclavian vein over the apex of the left lung and

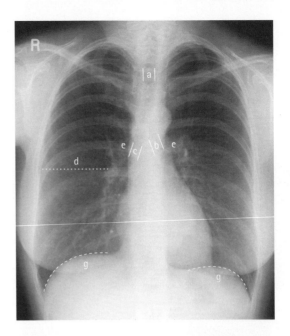

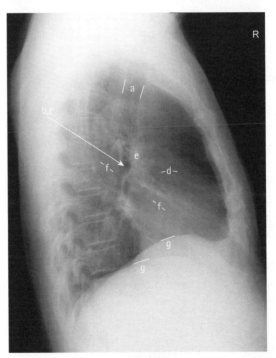

(a) Trachea; (b) left main bronchus; (c) right main bronchus; (d) horizontal fissure; (e) pulmonary arteries; (f) oblique fissure; (g) diaphragm

the inferior vena cava appearing as a triangular shadow within the cardiophrenic angle of the right lung. Both appear as low-density shadows, as does the hair-like line of the fissure between the upper and middle lobes of the right lung.

Viewing radiographs of lung fields

Apart from antero-posterior projections, all other radiographs are viewed as if the observer was looking towards the X-ray tube.

General observations

The chest X-ray (CXR) examination is a vital part of the investigation of many lung and cardiac conditions, often providing a diagnosis or the clue to the next appropriate test. The CXR is complex and not easy to read, but a high-technical quality examination with appropriate exposure on a modern film–screen combination can provide a wealth of initial detail about the heart, mediastinum and thoracic cage, as well as the lung parenchyma and pulmonary vessels.

The amount of information available to the reader, and thereby the diagnostic usefulness of the test, can be reduced by a variety of technical errors and problems. Many radiographs are initially read and acted upon by non-radiologists, who may be less aware of the diagnostic limitations of a poor-quality examination. The aim is, therefore, to demonstrate the intra-thoracic organs as fully as possible, though some areas (e.g. retrocardiac) will always be partially obscured.

Inspiration

Sub-maximal inspiration has several potential effects:

- The heart will swing up to a more horizontal lie and may thus appear enlarged.
- The lung bases will be less well inflated, which may simulate a variety of pathologies or cause abnormal areas to lie hidden.
- Under-inflation of the lower lobes causes diversion of blood to the upper lobe vessels, mimicking the early signs of heart failure.

Supine position

This posture is sometimes the best that can be achieved in a sick patient, but it alters the appearance of some structures; these are detailed in the relevant sections.

Semi-erect projection

The degree to which the patient is leaning from the vertical in such a projection varies according to circumstances, e.g. age, fitness, location of patient, availability of assistance. The patient may also lean to one side or the head may droop over the upper chest. It will be more difficult to ensure that the central ray is at right-angles to the film. The viewer will have difficulty assessing how much allowance to make for posture and technical factors; for these reasons, a supine film (being more standardized) is regarded by some radiologists as preferable to the semi-erect radiograph.

Antero-posterior projection

Magnification makes heart size difficult to assess in this projection.

Rotation

Obliquity causes the side of the chest furthest removed from the film plane to appear enlarged and hypodense, whilst the other side is partially obscured by the spine and more dense. A thoracic scoliosis may produce similar artefacts. The differing densities may simulate either abnormal density (e.g. consolidation or pleural effusion) on one side or abnormal lucency (e.g. emphysema, air-trapping) on the other.

General radiological considerations

Rotation markedly affects the appearance of the mediastinum and hila. The hilum of the raised side appears more prominent and may simulate a mass. The other hilum is hidden by the spine, tending to obscure any mass that may be present. Difficulty in assessing the mediastinum in the emergency setting is especially critical when evaluating a possible thoracic aortic aneurysm.

Lordosis

An apical lordotic projection is a useful image for a clearer depiction of the apices, but lordotic projection on an antero-posterior radiograph obscures more of the posterior basal part of the lung.

Exposure (See pp. 200 and 201.)

- Overexposed films reduce the visibility of lung parenchymal detail, masking vascular and interstitial changes and reducing the conspicuity of consolidation and masses. Pneumothorax becomes harder to detect.
- Underexposure can artificially enhance the visibility of normal lung markings, leading to them being interpreted wrongly as disease (e.g. pulmonary fibrosis or oedema).
- Underexposure also obscures the central areas, causing failure to diagnose abnormalities of the mediastinum, hila and spine.

Collimation

Good collimation is essential to good practice and dose reduction. Excessive collimation will exclude areas such as the costophrenic sulci (which may be the only site to indicate pleural disease). Failure to demonstrate the whole of the rib cage may lead to missed diagnosis of metastases, fractures, etc. (this is especially important in patients with unexplained chest pains). Collimating off the apices can obscure early tuberculosis (TB), apical (Pancoast) tumours, and small pneumothoraces.

Soft-tissue artefacts

Soft-tissue artefacts are a common cause of confusion. One of the commonest of these is the normal nipple, diagnosis of which is discussed on p. 199. Other rounded artefacts may be produced by benign skin lesions such as simple seborrhoeic warts and neurofibromata. Dense normal breast tissue or breast masses may also cause confusion with lung lesions. Breast implants may be obvious as a density with a thin curved line at the edge of the implant. Linear artefacts may be due to clothing or gowns, or in thin (often elderly) patients due to skin folds and creases. These are usually easy to spot, but they may be mistaken for the edge of the lung in a pneumothorax. Absence of soft tissue, as for example with a mastectomy, will produce hypertransradiancy of the ipsilateral thorax, although the lung itself is normal.

Postero-anterior – erect

A 35 × 43-cm or 35 × 35-cm cassette is selected, depending on the size of the patient. Orientation of the larger cassette will depend on the width of the thorax.

Position of patient and cassette

- The patient is positioned facing the cassette, with the chin extended and centred to the middle of the top of the cassette.
- The feet are paced slightly apart so that the patient is able to remain steady.
- The median sagittal plane is adjusted at right-angles to the middle of the cassette. The shoulders are rotated forward and pressed downward in contact with the cassette.
- This is achieved by placing the dorsal aspect of the hands behind and below the hips, with the elbows brought forward, or by allowing the arms to encircle the cassette.

Direction and centring of the X-ray beam

- The horizontal central beam is directed at right-angles to the cassette at the level of the eighth thoracic vertebrae (i.e. spinous process of T7), which is coincident with the lung mid-point (Unett and Carver 2001).
- The surface marking of T7 spinous process can be assessed by using the inferior angle of the scapula before the shoulders are pushed forward.
- Exposure is made in full normal arrested inspiration.
- In a number of automatic chest film-changer devices, the central beam is centred automatically to the middle of the film.

Essential image characteristics

The ideal postero-anterior chest radiograph should demonstrate the following:

- Full lung fields with the scapulae projected laterally away from the lung fields.
- The clavicles symmetrical and equidistant from the spinous processes and not obscuring the lung apices.
- The lungs well inflated, i.e. it should be possible to visualize either six ribs anteriorly or ten ribs posteriorly.
- The costophrenic angles and diaphragm outlined clearly.
- The mediastinum and heart central and defined sharply.
- The fine demarcation of the lung tissues shown from the hilum to the periphery.

Expiration technique

A radiograph may be taken on full expiration to confirm the presence of a pneumothorax. This has the effect of increasing intrapleural pressure, which results in the compression of the lung, making a pneumothorax bigger. The technique is useful in demonstrating a small pneumothorax and is also used to demonstrate the effects of air-trapping associated with an inhaled foreign body obstructing the passage of air into a segment of lung, and the extent of diaphragmatic movement.

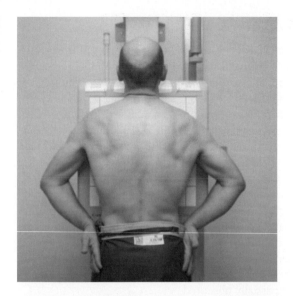

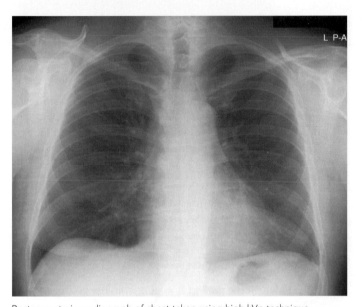

Postero-anterior radiograph of chest taken using high kVp technique

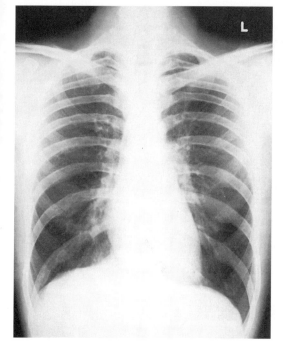

Postero-anterior radiograph of chest taken using conventional kVp technique (70 kVp)

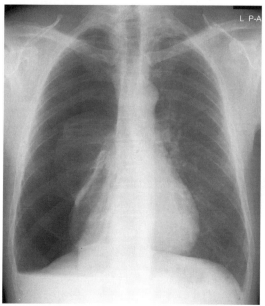

Postero-anterior radiograph of thorax showing large right pneumothorax

Postero-anterior – erect

Common faults and remedies

- The scapulae sometimes obscure the outer edges of the lung fields. If the patient is unable to adopt the basic arm position, then the arms should be allowed to encircle the vertical Bucky.
- Rotation of the patient will result in the heart not being central, thus making assessment of heart size impossible. Attention to how the patient is made to stand is essential to ensure that they are comfortable and can maintain the position. The legs should be well separated and the pelvis symmetrical in respect to the vertical Bucky.
- The lung fields sometimes are not well inflated. Explanation and rehearsal of the breathing technique before exposure is therefore essential.

Radiological considerations

- All comments in the general section apply.
- Soft tissues: in large patients, overlying soft tissue at the bases (obesity or large breasts) obscures detail of the lung bases and pleura as well as giving unnecessary radiation to the breast. This can be made worse by many of the factors outlined above. For diagnostic reasons and for dose reduction, female patients may hold their breasts out of the main field.
- In thin patients, skin folds can produce linear artefacts, which could mimic pleural fluid or even pneumothorax. Creasing of the skin against the Bucky or cassette should be avoided.

Notes

- Careful patient preparation is essential, with all radio-opaque objects removed before the examination.
- When an intravenous drip is *in situ* in the arm, care should be exercised to ensure that the drip is secured properly on a drip stand before exposure.
- Patients with underwater-seal bottles require particular care to ensure that chest tubes are not dislodged, and the bottle is not raised above the level of the chest.
- A postero-anterior clip-type marker is normally used, and the image is identified with the identification marker set to the postero-anterior position. Care should be made not to mis-diagnose a case of dextracardia.
- Long, plaited hair may cause artefacts and should be clipped out of the image field.
- Reduction in exposure is required in patients suffering from emphysema.
- For images taken in expiration, the kilovoltage is increased by five when using a conventional kilovoltage technique.

Radiation protection

The patient is provided with a waist-fitting lead-rubber apron, and the radiation beam is restricted to the size of the cassette.

Antero-posterior – erect

This projection is used as an alternative to the postero-anterior erect projection for elucidation of an opacity seen on a postero-anterior, or when the patient's shape (kyphosis) or medical condition makes it difficult or unsafe for the patient to stand or sit for the basic projection. For the latter, the patient is usually supported sitting erect on a trolley.

Position of patient and cassette

- The patient may be standing or sitting with their back against the cassette, which is supported vertically with the upper edge of the cassette above the lung apices.
- The median sagittal plane is adjusted at right-angles to the middle of the cassette.
- The shoulders are brought downward and forward, with the backs of the hands below the hips and the elbows well forward, which has the effect of projecting the scapulae clear of the lung fields.
- In the unwell patient, it may not be possible to perform this procedure, with the result that the scapulae may be rotated and superimposed on the lateral chest margins. This causes an increase in radiation absorption, making it difficulty to observe underlying lung tissue. In this situation, it is preferable that the patient's arms are rotated laterally and supported with the palms of the hands facing forward. In this position, the scapulae are superimposed on the lungs but the effect of absorption is less, and comparison of either side of the upper lateral segments of the lung is made easier.

Direction and centring of the X-ray beam

- The horizontal ray is directed first at right-angles to the cassette and towards the sternal notch.
- The central ray is then angled until it is coincident with the middle of the cassette. This has the effect of confining the radiation field to the film, thus avoiding unnecessary exposure of the eyes.
- The exposure is taken on normal full inspiration.

Notes

- The use of a lower centring point combined with a horizontal beam has the undesirable effect of projecting the clavicles above the apices of the lungs.
- The radiograph opposite is of similar appearance to that of the postero-anterior chest radiograph described on p. 206. However, this projection is valuable in elucidation of relative positions of opacities seen on a postero-anterior projection.
- Small lesions previously obscured by a rib may also be demonstrated.

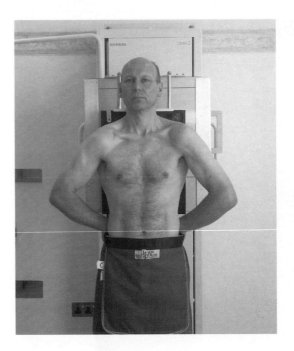

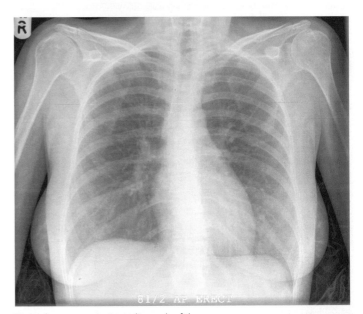

Normal antero-posterior radiograph of thorax

Radiological considerations

- This projection moves the heart away from the film plane, increasing magnification and reducing the accuracy of assessment of heart size (in this projection, a cardiothoracic ratio (CRT) of greater than 50% does not necessarily indicate cardiomegaly).

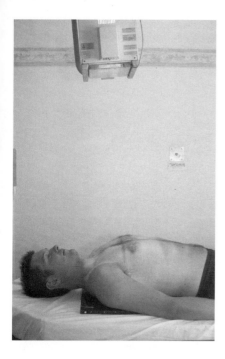

Antero-posterior – supine

This projection is selected when patients are unable to either stand or sit for the projections described previously. The patient is usually lying supine on a trolley or bed.

Position of patient and cassette

- With assistance, a cassette is carefully positioned under the patient's chest with the upper edge of the cassette above the lung apices.
- The median sagittal plane is adjusted at right-angles to the middle of the cassette, and the patient's pelvis is checked to ensure that it is not rotated.
- The arms are rotated laterally and supported by the side of the trunk. The head is supported on a pillow, with the chin slightly raised.

Direction and centring of the X-ray beam

- The central ray is directed first at right-angles and towards the sternal notch.
- The central ray is then angled until it is coincident with the middle of the film, thus avoiding unnecessary exposure to the eyes.

Notes

- The exposure is taken on full normal inspiration.
- An FFD of at least 120 cm is essential to reduce unequal magnification of intra-thoracic structures.
- In this projection, maximum lung demonstration is lost due to the absence of the gravity effect of the abdominal organs, which is present in the erect position.
- Images of heavy breasts are not readily diffused.

Radiological considerations

- Compared with the postero-anterior projection, this projection moves the heart away from the image receptor plane, increasing magnification and reducing the accuracy of assessment of heart size (in this projection, a CTR of greater than 50% does not necessarily indicate cardiomegaly).
- The normal biomechanics of blood flow are different from those in the erect position, producing relative prominence of upper-lobe vessels and mimicking the signs of heart failure.
- Pleural fluid will layer against the posterior chest wall, producing an ill-defined increase attenuation of the affected hemithorax rather than the usual blunting of the costophrenic angle; fluid levels are not seen.
- A pneumothorax, if present, will be located at the front of the chest in the supine position. Unless it is large, it will be more difficult to detect if a lateral horizontal beam image is not employed.

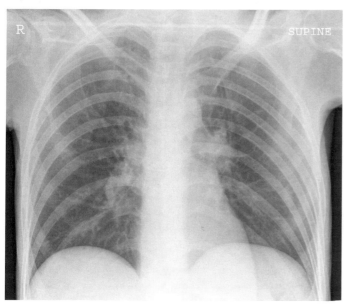

Normal supine radiograph of thorax

7 Lungs

Antero-posterior – semi-erect

This semi-recumbent position is adopted as an alternative to the antero-posterior erect projection when the patient is too ill to stand or sit erect without support.

Position of patient and cassette

- The patient is supported in a semi-recumbent position, facing the X-ray tube. The degree to which they can sit erect will depend on their medical condition.
- A cassette is supported against the back, using pillows or a large 45-degree foam pad, with its upper edge above the lung fields.
- Care should be taken to ensure that the cassette is parallel to the coronal plane.
- The median sagittal plane is adjusted at right-angles to, and in the midline of, the cassette.
- Rotation of the patient is prevented by the use of foam pads.
- The arms are rotated medially, with the shoulders brought forward to bring the scapulae clear of the lung fields.

Direction and centring of the X-ray beam

- The central ray is directed first at right-angles to the cassette and towards the sternal notch.
- The central ray is then angled until it is coincident with the middle of the film, thus avoiding unnecessary exposure to the eyes.

Notes

- Difficulties sometimes arise in positioning the cassette parallel to the coronal plane, with the resultant effect that the image of the chest is foreshortened.
- The use of a horizontal central ray is essential to demonstrate fluid levels, e.g. pleural effusion. In this situation, the patient is adjusted with the chest erect as much as possible. The horizontal central ray is directed at right-angles to the middle of the cassette. The clavicles in the resultant image will be projected above the apices.
- If the patient is unable to sit erect, fluid levels are demonstrated using a horizontal ray with the patient adopting the lateral decubitus or dorsal decubitus position.
- Sick patients may be unable to support their own head in the erect position, resulting in superimposition of the chin over the upper thorax. Care should be taken to avoid or minimize this if at all possible as apical lesions will be obscured.

Radiological considerations

An assessment of the cardiac configuration to identify individual chamber enlargement is essential, even if there is an increase in overall magnification due to shorter FFD associated with some low-powered mobiles. It is important, therefore, that the patient is not rotated.

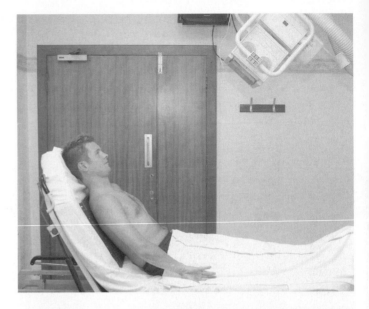

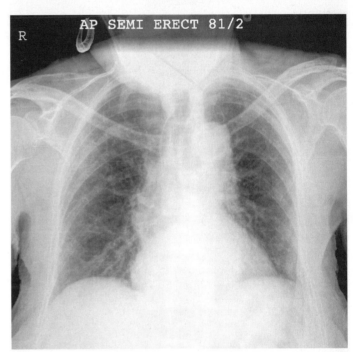

Normal semi-erect radiograph of thorax. The chin is just superimposed on the upper thorax (see notes)

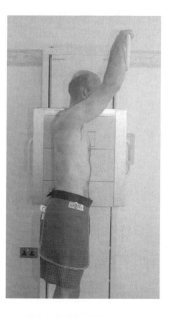
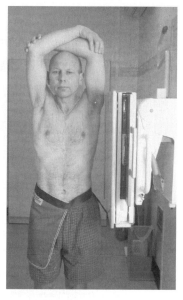

Lateral

A supplementary lateral projection may be useful in certain clinical circumstances for localizing the position of a lesion and demonstrating anterior mediastinal masses not shown on the postero-anterior projection. Lateral radiographs, however, are not taken as part of a routine examination of the lung fields, because of the additional radiation patient dose.

A moving or stationary grid may be used to prevent excess secondary radiation reaching the film. The FFD may be reduced to 150 cm to maintain a short exposure time.

Position of patient and cassette

- The patient is turned to bring the side under investigation in contact with the cassette.
- The median sagittal plane is adjusted parallel to the cassette.
- The arms are folded over the head or raised above the head to rest on a horizontal bar.
- The mid-axillary line is coincident with the middle of the film, and the cassette is adjusted to include the apices and the lower lobes to the level of the first lumbar vertebra.

Direction and centring of the X-ray beam

- Direct the horizontal central ray at right-angles to the middle of the cassette at the mid-axillary line.

Radiological considerations

- Insufficient elevation of the arms will cause the soft tissues of the upper arms to obscure the lung apices and thoracic inlet, and even the retrosternal window, leading to masses or other lesions in these areas being missed.
- Rotation will also partially obscure the retrosternal window, masking anterior mediastinal masses. It will also render the sternum less distinct, which may be important in the setting of trauma when sternal fracture may be overlooked.

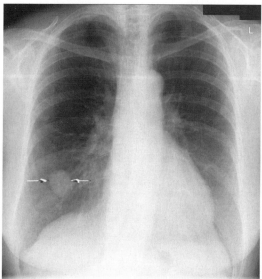

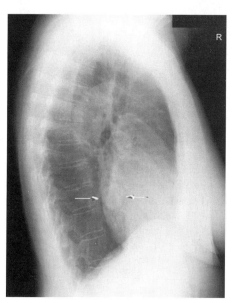

Postero-anterior and lateral radiographs of same patient showing a tumour in the right lower lobe

Apices

Opacities obscured in the apical region by overlying ribs or clavicular shadows may be demonstrated by modification of the postero-anterior and antero-posterior projections.

Direction and centring of the X-ray beam

- With the patient in the position for the postero-anterior projection, the central ray is angled 30 degrees caudally towards the seventh cervical spinous process coincident with the sternal angle.
- With the patient in the position for the antero-posterior projection, the central ray is angled 30 degrees cephalad towards the sternal angle.
- With the patient reclining, and the coronal plane at 30 degrees to the cassette, to enable the nape of the neck to rest against the upper border of the cassette, the central ray is directed at right-angles to the film towards the sternal angle. Alternatively, if the patient is unable to recline 30 degrees, the technique is adapted, with the patient reclining 15 degrees and the tube angled 15 degrees cephalad.

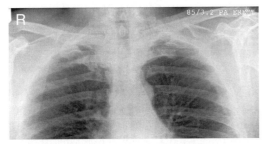

Normal postero-anterior 30 degrees caudad

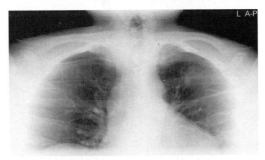

Antero-posterior 30 degrees cephalad, showing small tumour at the left apex

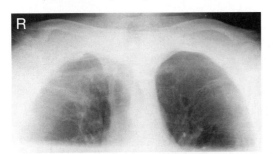

Antero-posterior: coronal plane 15 degrees, central ray 15 degrees cephalad, showing small tumour at the right apex

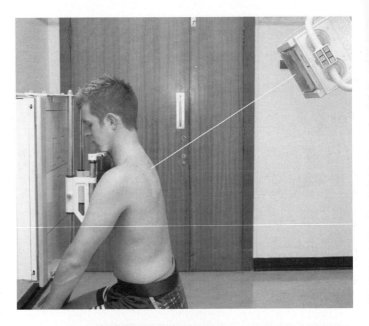

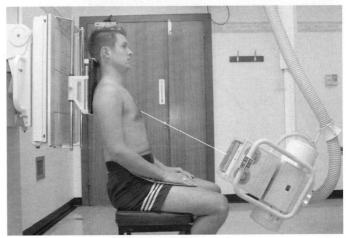

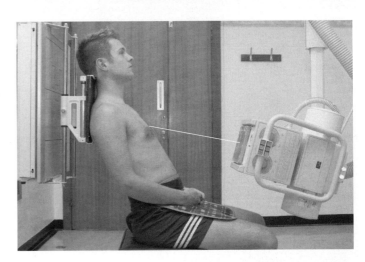

Upper anterior region – lateral

This technique may be required to demonstrate an anterior lesion and the associated relationship of the trachea.

Position of patient and cassette

- The patient is positioned with the median sagittal plane parallel to the cassette, which is centred at the level of the shoulder of the side under examination.
- Both shoulders are drawn backward and the arms extended to move the shoulders clear of the retrosternal space.
- The hands are clasped low down over the buttocks.

Direction and centring of the X-ray beam

- Direct the horizontal central ray at right-angles to the cassette to a point immediately in front of the shoulder nearest the tube.
- Collimate to the area of interest.

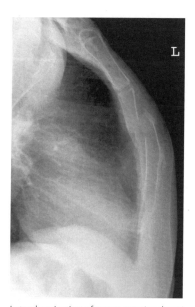

Lateral projection of upper anterior chest in a patient with a sternal fracture

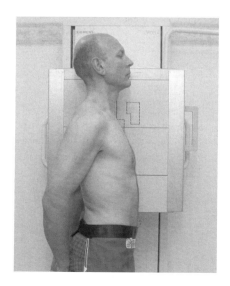

Lordotic

This technique may be used to demonstrate right middle-lobe collapse or an inter-lobar pleural effusion. The patient is positioned to bring the middle-lobe fissure horizontal.

Position of patient and cassette

- The patient is placed for the postero-anterior projection.
- Then clasping the sides of the vertical Bucky, the patient bends backwards at the waist.
- The degree of dorsiflexion varies for each subject, but in general it is about 30–40 degrees.

Direction and centring of the X-ray beam

- The horizontal ray is directed at right-angles to the cassette and towards the middle of the film.

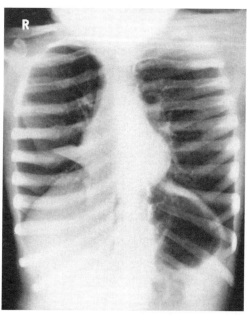

Lordotic postero-anterior radiograph showing middle lobe collapse

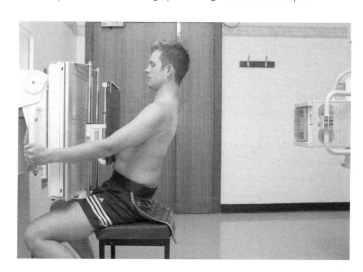

7 Heart and Aorta

Introduction

Radiography of the heart and aorta is a common examination. It is performed in the routine investigation of heart disease and to assess heart size and the gross anatomy of the major blood vessels. Examination is also performed following pacemaker insertion to determine the position of the electrode leads.

The radiographic technique used is similar to that described for the lungs, and the student is referred to this section (p. 198).

Imaging may also be performed using a variety of other modalities, notably echocardiography and radionuclide imaging, with angiography performed routinely to assess the heart chambers and coronary vessels. Multidetector CT and MRI are likely to be used increasingly in the future.

Examination is performed by means of the following projections:

Basic	Postero-anterior – erect
Supplementary	Left lateral
	Left anterior oblique
	Right anterior oblique

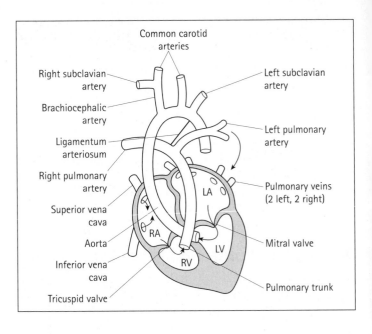

Anatomy

The heart is a hollow muscular organ that, together with the roots of the great vessels, is enclosed in a fibroserous sac, the pericardium. It is situated mainly to the left of the midline in the lower anterior part of the chest and attached to the central tendon of the diaphragm.

The heart has four chambers: the right and left atria and the right and left ventricles. The atria are separated by the interatrial septum and the ventricles are separated by the interventricular septum. Blood flows from the right atrium into the right ventricle through the tricuspid valve, and from the left atrium to the left ventricle through the mitral valve. The right ventricle outflow is via the pulmonary valve, and the left ventricle outflow is via the aortic valve. By rhythmic contractions, the heart serves as a pump to maintain the movement of blood throughout the circulatory system of blood vessels. At rest, there are approximately 60–80 beats per minute, with the average heart cycle occupying a time period of 0.8 s. The right side of the heart serves to perfuse the pulmonary circulation, while the left side perfuses the systemic circulation, the latter being a higher-pressure system.

The **aorta**, the largest of the great vessels, consists of three parts: the ascending aorta, the arch and the descending aorta, which commences at the level of the fourth thoracic vertebra.

The **superior vena cava** opens into the upper part of the right atrium, draining the upper limbs and head and neck. The **inferior vena cava** gives venous drainage from the lower limbs and abdomen, entering the inferior part of the right atrium.

Radiographically, the heart is seen as a pear-shaped structure of soft-tissue density, with its apex and inferior wall adjacent to the diaphragm and its narrower upper base overlying the spine. The size and shape of the heart vary with the build of subject, with respiration, and with the position and the clinical state of the patient.

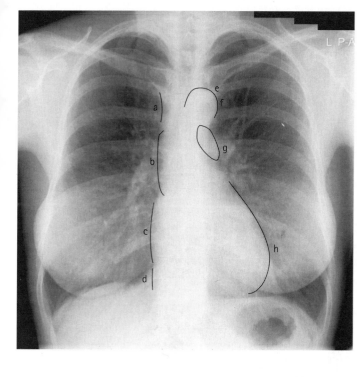

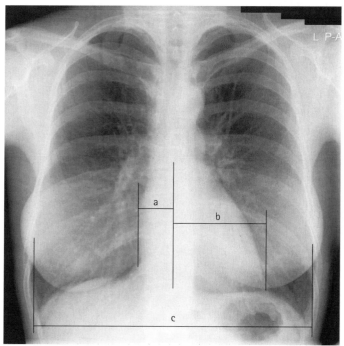

Anatomy

Radiographic anatomy

In the postero-anterior radiograph of the chest seen opposite, features of the heart and associated vessels have been outlined and labelled.

The aortic knuckle is shown as a rounded protrusion slightly to the left of the vertebrae and above the heart shadow. The prominence of the aortic knuckle depends upon the degree of dilation or unfolding of the aorta and the presence (or absence) of cardiac disease. It also alters shape as a result of deformities in the thorax, intrinsic abnormalities and with old age. Calcification in the arch, when present, is demonstrated as curvilinear opacities.

a, superior vena cava
b, ascending thoracic aorta
c, right atrium
d, inferior vena cava
e, left subclavian vein
f, aortic knuckle
g, main pulmonary artery
h, left ventricle.

Cardiothoracic ratio

The size of the heart is estimated from the postero-anterior radiograph of the chest by calculating the CRT. This is the ratio between the maximum transverse diameter of the heart and the maximum width of the thorax above the costophrenic angles, measured from the inner edges of the ribs. In adults, the normal CRT is maximally 0.5. In children, however, the CRT is usually greater.

$$\text{CRT} = \frac{(a + b)}{c}$$

where a = right heart border to midline, b = left heart border to midline, and c = maximum thoracic diameter above costophrenic angles from inner borders of ribs.

$$\text{For example, CTR} = \frac{(2.5 + 10)}{29} = 0.43.$$

Postero-anterior

A 35 × 43-cm or 35 × 35-cm cassette is selected, depending on the size of the patient. Orientation of the larger cassette will depend of the size of the patient.

Position of patient and cassette

- The patient is positioned erect, facing the cassette and with the chin extended and resting on the top of the cassette.
- The median sagittal plane is adjusted perpendicular to the middle of the cassette, with the patient's arms encircling the cassette. Alternatively, the dorsal aspects of the hands are placed behind and below the hips to allow the shoulders to be rotated forward and pressed downward in contact with the cassette.
- The thorax must be positioned symmetrically relative to the film.

Direction and centring of the X-ray beam

- The horizontal central beam is directed at right-angles to the cassette at the level of the eighth thoracic vertebrae (i.e. the spinous process of T7).
- The surface markings of the T7 spinous process can be assessed by using the inferior angle of the scapula before the shoulders are pushed forward.
- Exposure is made on arrested full inspiration.

Essential image characteristics

The ideal postero-anterior chest radiograph for the heart and aorta should demonstrate the following:

- The clavicles symmetrical and equidistant from the spinous processes.
- The mediastinum and heart central and defined sharply.
- The costo-phrenic angles and diaphragm outlined clearly.
- Full lung fields, with the scapula projected laterally away from the lung fields.

Notes

- A postero-anterior marker is normally used to identify the right or left side of the patient. Care should be made to select the correct marker so as not to misdiagnose a case of dextrocardia.
- The kilovoltage selected is adjusted to give adequate penetration, with the bodies of the thoracic vertebrae just visible through the heart (see p. 201).
- For comparison purposes, records of exposure factors used, including FFD, should be kept for follow-up examinations.
- Care should be taken with postoperative patients with underwater seals and with intravenous drips. These should not be dislodged, and the examination time should be kept to a minimum.
- Underwater-seal drain bottles must be kept below the lowest point of the patient's chest at all times to prevent the contents of the bottle being siphoned back into the chest.

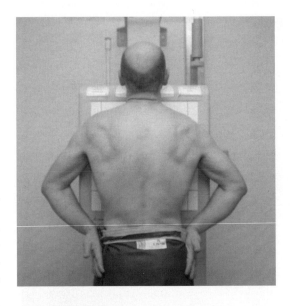

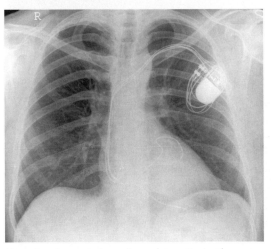

Normal postero-anterior radiograph in patient with a permanent pacemaker *in situ*

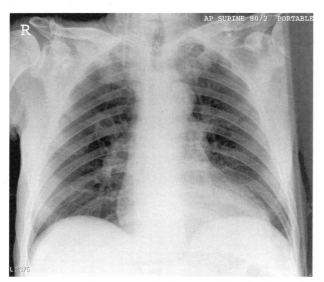

Antero-posterior supine radiograph showing artefactual enlargement of the heart due to supine posture

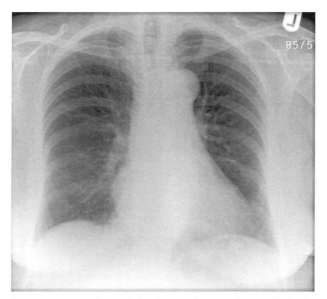

Postero-anterior radiograph showing prosthetic aortic and mitral valves

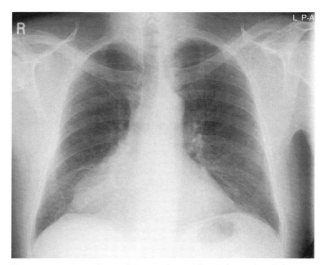

Postero-anterior radiograph in a patient with a right pericardial cyst

Radiological considerations

- An artefactual increase in the apparent size of the heart may be produced by a number of factors, including:
  - poor inspiration, as the heart rotates up into a more horizontal orientation;
  - short FFD due to geometric magnification;
  - supine posture due to a more horizontal cardiac orientation and reduced FFD.

To prevent the clinician making an erroneous diagnosis of cardiomegaly or heart failure, these factors should be avoided if possible.

- If the patient is not truly erect, there may be diversion of blood flow to the upper lobe vessels, mimicking the upper-lobe blood diversion seen in heart failure.
- Following pacemaker insertion, the clinician may wish to check that the wire is located properly and to exclude complications such as pneumothorax and pleural effusion.
- Pacemaker wires and prosthetic valves are visualized less readily on low-kVp and underexposed films. A penetrated radiograph may help to demonstrate these fully. The lateral projection is also acquired to help in localization.
- Native valve and coronary artery calcifications will be seen less well on an inadequately penetrated radiograph.

Left lateral

A left lateral image is acquired using a 35 × 43-cm cassette using a grid technique to prevent excess secondary radiation reaching the film.

Position of patient and cassette

- The patient is turned to bring the left side in contact with the cassette.
- The median sagittal plane is adjusted parallel to the cassette.
- The arms are folded over the head or raised above the head to rest on a horizontal bar.
- The mid-axillary line is coincident with the middle of the film, and the cassette is adjusted to include the apices and the inferior lobes to the level of the first lumbar vertebra.

Direction and centring of the X-ray beam

- Direct the central ray at right-angles to the middle of the cassette in the mid-axillary line.
- Exposure is made on arrested full inspiration.

Essential image characteristics

- The thoracic vertebrae and sternum should be lateral and demonstrated clearly.
- The arms should not obscure the heart and lung fields.
- The anterior and posterior mediastinum and heart are defined sharply and the lung fields are seen clearly.
- The costo-phrenic angles and diaphragm should be outlined clearly.

Radiological considerations

- A lateral radiograph may help to locate cardiac or pericardial masses, e.g. left ventricular aneurysm and pericardial cyst. These are assessed better by echocardiography or CT/MRI.
- Cardiac and pericardial calcification may be confirmed and its extent assessed more fully on a lateral chest radiograph.
- After pacemaker insertion, the lateral image confirms that the ventricular electrode lies anteriorly at the right ventricular apex.

Notes

- An FFD of 150 or 180 cm is selected.
- Patients who have recently had a permanent pacemaker implant should not raise their arms above their head. It is sufficient to raise the arms clear of the thorax, otherwise there is a risk of damage to the recently sutured tissues and possible dislodging of the pacemaker electrodes.
- Patients on trolleys may find it difficult to remain in the vertical position. A large wedge foam pad may be required to assist the patient to remain upright.

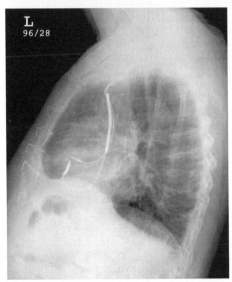

Left lateral radiograph of heart showing position of permanent pacing system

- Either a stationary or a moving grid may be employed. The kilovoltage selected is adjusted to give adequate penetration, with the bodies of the thoracic vertebrae, costo-phrenic and apical regions defined well.

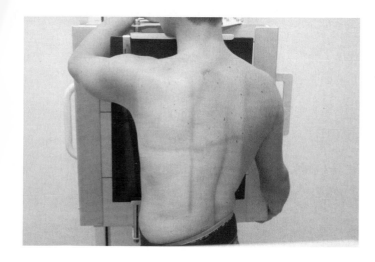

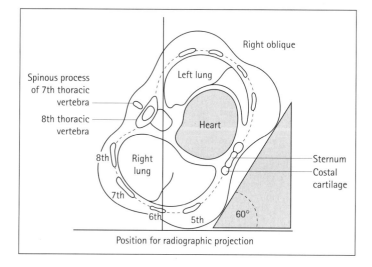

Position for radiographic projection

Right anterior oblique

This projection is used to separate the heart, aorta and vertebral column, thus enabling the path of the ascending aorta, aortic arch and descending aorta to be acquired on a 35 × 43-cm film. The projection will also demonstrate the diameter and the degree of unfolding of the aorta.

Position of patient and cassette

- The patient is initially positioned facing the cassette, which is supported vertically in the cassette holder with the upper edge above the lung apices.
- With the right side of the trunk kept in contact with the cassette, the patient is rotated to bring the left side away from the cassette, so that the coronal plane forms an angle of 60 degrees to the cassette.

Direction and centring of the X-ray beam

- Direct the horizontal central ray at right-angles to the middle of the cassette at the level of the sixth thoracic vertebrae, to show the heart, aortic arch and descending aorta.

Radiological considerations

- This projection may be a useful adjunct to the lateral in cases of doubt about dilatation or tortuosity of the aorta.
- This projection may be used in conjunction with a barium-swallow study to demonstrate enlargement of the heart or aorta, or abnormal vessels and vascular rings, which can produce abnormal impressions on the oesophagus and cause dysphagia.
- CT, MRI or angiography assess vascular rings more accurately.

Note

The FFD may be reduced to 150 cm.

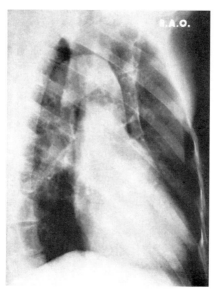

Right anterior oblique radiograph

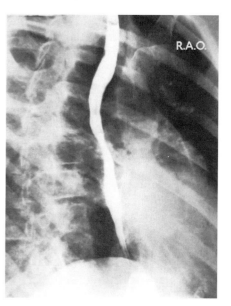

Right anterior oblique radiograph with barium outlining the oesophagus

219

7 Bones of the thorax

Introduction

The thoracic skeleton consists of the ribs and sternum (plus the thoracic spine, which is covered in Chapter 6). The ribs and sternum may be examined radiographically in the assessment of trauma, but a good postero-anterior or antero-posterior radiograph will be more important in this setting to exclude intra-thoracic complications (e.g. pneumothorax). Many centres do not perform oblique rib views for simple trauma unless a change in management will result, and an antero-posterior or postero-anterior projection will show much of the anterior and posterior ribs that are projected above the diaphragm.

The ribs may also be examined to detect other causes of chest-wall pain, e.g. rib metastases.

In cases of severe injury to the thorax, maintenance of respiratory function is of prime importance. Good postero-anterior or antero-posterior radiographs are required for full assessment of chest-wall injury, pleural changes and pulmonary damage. In cases of major trauma, damage may occur to multiple ribs, sternum, lung and thoracic spine, or any combination of these. Multiple rib and sternal fractures may result in a flail chest, where part of the chest collapses inwards during inspiration, impairing or even preventing lung ventilation. In this setting, a supine antero-posterior radiograph may be all that is attainable, and it should thus be of the highest quality possible. A pneumothorax may be obscured on a supine radiograph; in this situation, a lateral radiograph is acquired using a horizontal beam.

Injury to the lower ribs may be associated with hepatic, splenic or renal injury, and rib projections may be requested in this situation. These could be omitted if an abdominal radiograph (Section 11) is considered necessary, though ultrasound or CT may be considered more useful for assessment of possible internal organ damage.

Radiological considerations

- Pain impairs the ability of the patient to inspire deeply after rib trauma, reducing conspicuity of rib fractures and pulmonary contusion. Optimization of exposure and other factors therefore becomes more critical.
- Overexposure may allow clearer depiction of rib trauma, but it will tend to obscure associated pulmonary lesions so it should be avoided.
- Fluoroscopy may be useful to determine whether a peripheral chest lesion is real and whether it is related to a rib.

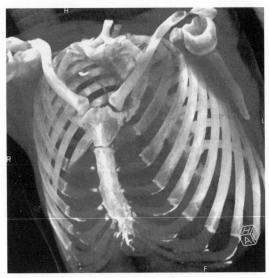

CT reconstruction of the bony thorax created using a multislice scanner

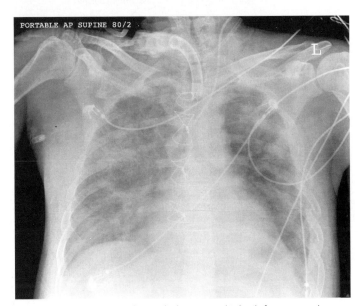

Antero-posterior supine radiograph showing multiple rib fractures and flail chest with severe pulmonary oedema

Bones of thorax	Trauma – trolley patients	Antero-posterior supine chest and lateral-horizontal beam chest; other projections of chest, abdomen, ribs, sternum, thoracic vertebrae or ATLS projections on request
Lower ribs	Trauma – non-trolley patients	Postero-anterior chest Antero-posterior (basic) Posterior oblique Other projections of chest on request
	Pathology	Antero-posterior (basic) Posterior oblique
Upper ribs	Trauma or Pathology – non-trolley patients	Postero-anterior chest Posterior oblique Antero-posterior first and second ribs on request
	Cervical ribs	Normally demonstrated on lateral and antero-posterior cervical vertebrae Postero-anterior chest Antero-posterior cervical ribs on request
Sternum	Trauma – non-trolley patients	Postero-anterior chest Anterior oblique, tube angled *or* Anterior oblique, trunk rotated Lateral
	Pathology	Anterior oblique, tube angled *or* Anterior oblique, trunk rotated Lateral CT or tomography on request, according to availability

ATLS, Advanced Trauma and Life Support; CT, computed tomography.

7 | Lower ribs

Antero-posterior (basic)

A cassette is selected that is large enough to include the whole of the right and left sides, from the level of the middle of the body of the sternum to the lower costal margin. The cassette is placed in the Bucky tray.

Position of patient and cassette

- The patient lies supine on the imaging couch, with the median sagittal plane coincident with the midline of the couch and Bucky mechanism.
- The anterior superior iliac spines should be equidistant from the couch top.
- The cassette is placed transversely, with its caudal edge positioned at a level just below the lower costal margin.

Direction and centring of the X-ray beam

- The vertical central ray is centred in the midline at the level of the lower costal margin and then angled cranially to coincide with the centre of the film.
- This centring assists in demonstrating the maximum number of ribs below the diaphragm.
- Exposure made on full expiration will also assist in this objective.

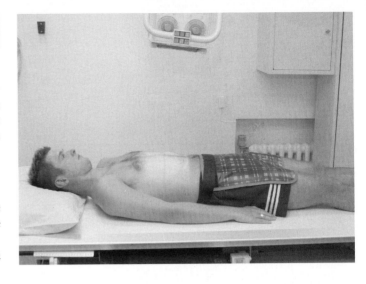

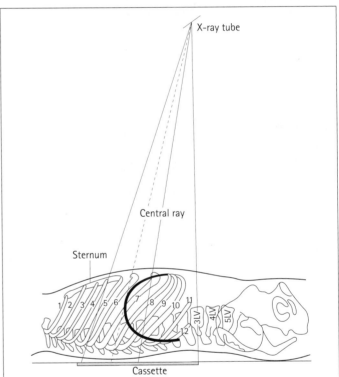

Dotted line shows diaphragm projected upwards

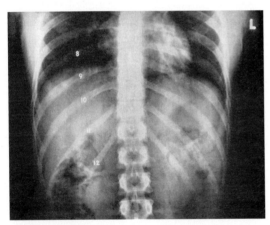

Effect of expiration

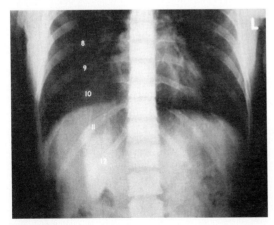

Effect of inspiration

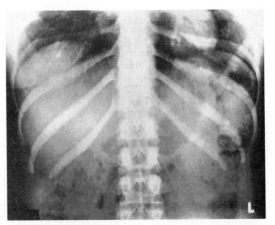

Antero-posterior radiograph showing lower ribs on both sides

Right and left posterior oblique

A 35 × 43-cm cassette is selected to include either the right or the left lower rib sides. The patient may be examined erect or supine using a Bucky grid.

Position of patient and cassette

- The patient lies supine on the Bucky table or stands erect, with the mid-clavicular line of the side under examination coincident with the midline of the Bucky grid.
- The trunk is rotated 45 degrees on to the side being examined, with the raised side supported on non-opaque pads.
- The hips and knees are flexed for comfort and to assist in maintaining patient position.
- The caudal edge of the cassette is positioned at a level just below the lower costal margin.
- The cassette should be large enough to include the ribs on the side being examined from the level of the middle of the body of the sternum to the lower costal margin.

Direction and centring of the X-ray beam

- The vertical central ray is directed to the midline of the anterior surface of the patient, at the level of the lower costal margin.
- From this position, the central ray is then angled cranially to coincide with the centre of the cassette.
- Exposure is made on arrested full expiration.

Notes

- The patient may find it difficult to maintain this position if they are in a great deal of pain.
- Selection of a short exposure time and rehearsal of the breathing technique may be necessary to reduce the risk of movement unsharpness.

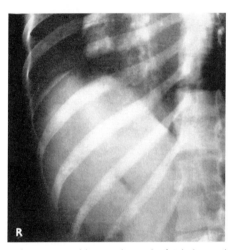

Right posterior oblique radiograph of right lower ribs

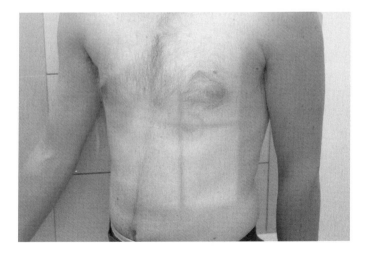

Upper ribs

Right and left posterior oblique

Radiography may be conducted with the patient erect or supine.

A cassette is selected that is large enough to include the whole of the ribs on the side being examined from the level of the seventh cervical vertebra to the lower costal margin.

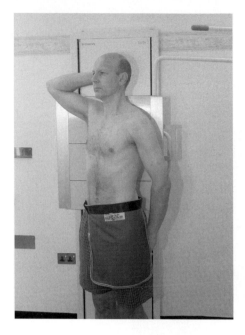

Position of patient and cassette

- The patient sits or stands with the posterior aspect of the trunk against the vertical Bucky. Alternatively, the patient lies supine on the Bucky table.
- The mid-clavicular line of the side under examination should coincide with the central line of the Bucky or table.
- The trunk is rotated 45 degrees towards the side being examined and, if supine, is supported on non-opaque pads.
- If the condition of the patient permits, the hands should be clasped behind the head, otherwise the arms should be held clear of the trunk.
- The cranial edge of the cassette should be positioned at a level just above the spinous process of the seventh cervical vertebra.

Direction and centring of the X-ray beam

- Initially, direct the central ray perpendicular to the cassette and towards the sternal angle.
- Then angle the beam caudally so that the central ray coincides with the centre of the cassette. This assists in demonstrating the maximum number of ribs above the diaphragm.
- Exposure made on arrested full inspiration will also assist in maximizing the number of ribs demonstrated.

Note

The kVp should be sufficient to reduce the difference in subject contrast between the lung fields and the heart to a more uniform radiographic contrast so that the ribs are visualized adequately in both these areas.

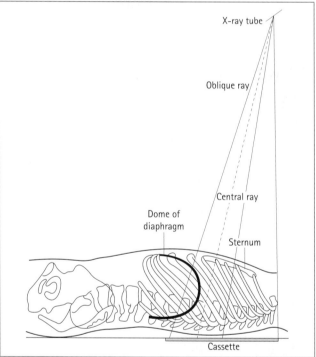

Dotted line shows diaphragm projected downwards

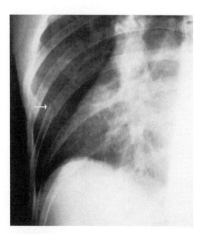

Radiograph of right lower ribs showing acute fracture

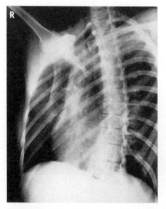

Right posterior oblique

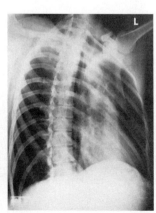

Left posterior oblique

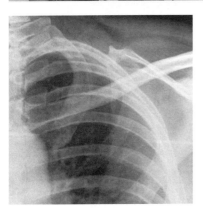

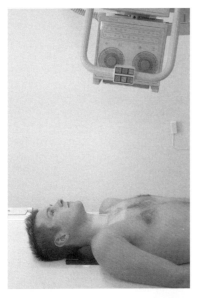

First and second – antero-posterior

The first and second ribs are often superimposed upon each other. Occasionally, a separate projection may be necessary to demonstrate them adequately.

An 18 × 24-cm or 24 × 30-cm cassette fitted with standard-speed screens is selected.

Position of patient and cassette

- The patient lies supine on the table or stands with the posterior aspect of the trunk against a cassette.
- When the patient is erect, the cassette is placed in a cassette holder attachment.
- The median sagittal plane is adjusted at right-angles to the cassette.
- The cassette is centred to the junction of the medial and middle thirds of the clavicle.

Direction and centring of the X-ray beam

- Direct the central ray perpendicular to the cassette and towards the junction of the medial and middle thirds of the clavicle.

Collimated antero-posterior radiograph of left first and second ribs

Cervical – antero-posterior

Cervical ribs are normally demonstrated adequately on an antero-posterior cervical vertebrae or postero-anterior chest projection. However, occasionally a separate projection may be necessary.

A 24 × 30-cm cassette is place transversely on the Bucky tray.

Position of patient and cassette

- The patient sits or stands, with the posterior aspect of the trunk against a vertical Bucky. Alternatively, the patient lies supine on the Bucky table.
- The median sagittal plane should be at right-angles to the cassette and coincident with the midline of the table or Bucky.
- The cassette is positioned transversely in the cassette tray and should be large enough to include the fifth cervical to the fifth thoracic vertebrae

Direction and centring of the X-ray beam

- The central ray is angled 10 degrees cranially from the perpendicular and is directed towards the sternal notch.

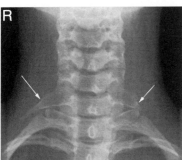

Rudimentary bilateral cervical ribs

Anterior oblique – tube angled

This projection may be performed with the patient prone or erect, with the sternum at a minimal distance from the image receptor to reduce geometric unsharpness. However, if the patient has sustained a major injury to the sternum, then they may not be able to adopt the prone position due to pain.

A 24 × 30-cm grid cassette fitted with standard-speed screens is selected.

Position of patient and cassette

- The patient stands or sits facing the vertical Bucky or lies prone on the table.
- The medial sagittal plane should be at right-angles to, and centred to, the cassette.
- As the central ray is to be angled across the table, the cassette is placed transversely to avoid grid cut-off.
- If the Bucky is to be used on the table, the patient should lie on a trolley positioned at right-angles to the table, with the thorax resting on the Bucky table.
- The cassette is centred at the level of the fifth thoracic vertebra.
- Immobilization will be assisted if it is possible to use an immobilization band.

Direction and centring of the X-ray beam

- The perpendicular central ray is centred initially to the axilla of either side at the level of the fifth thoracic vertebra.
- The central ray is then angled transversely so that the central ray is directed to a point 7.5 cm lateral to the midline on the same side.

Notes

- The patient is allowed to breathe gently during an exposure time of several seconds using a low mA.
- This technique diffuses the lung and rib shadows, which otherwise tend to obscure the sternum.

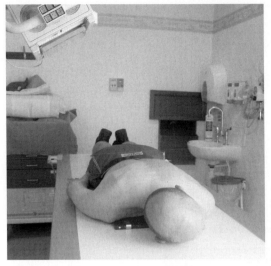

Left anterior oblique

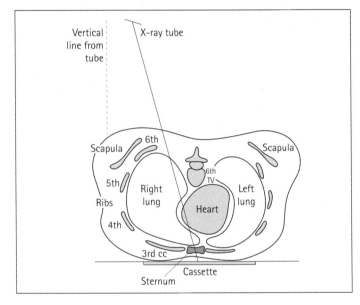

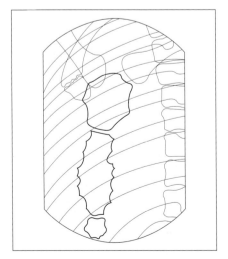

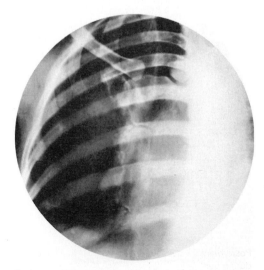

Postero-anterior oblique radiograph of sternum taken during gentle respiration

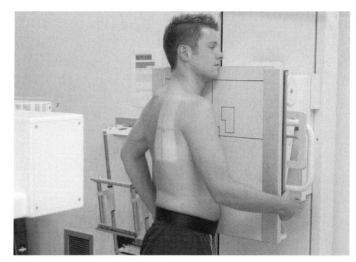

Right anterior oblique

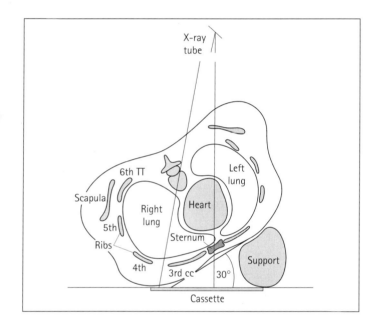

Anterior oblique – trunk rotated

A 24 × 30-cm cassette is selected for use in the Bucky mechanism. Alternatively, a grid cassette may be used in the vertical cassette holder.

Position of patient and cassette

- The patient initially sits or stands facing the vertical Bucky or lies prone on the Bucky table with the median sagittal plane at right-angles to, and centred to, the cassette.
- The patient is then rotated approximately 20–30 degrees, with the right side raised to adopt the left anterior oblique position, which will ensure that less heart shadow obscures the sternum.
- The patient is supported in position with non-opaque pads and an immobilization band where possible.
- The cassette is centred at the level of the fifth thoracic vertebra.

Direction and centring of the X-ray beam

- Direct the central ray perpendicular to the cassette and towards a point 7.5 cm lateral to the fifth thoracic vertebra on the side nearest the X-ray tube.

Note

The patient is allowed to breathe gently during an exposure time of several seconds using a low mA, provided that immobilization is adequate.

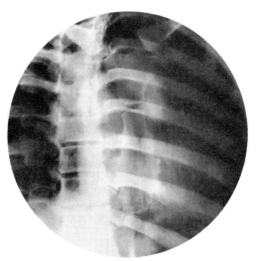

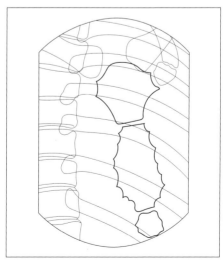

Postero-anterior oblique radiograph of sternum taken during gentle respiration

227

Lateral

A 24 × 30-cm grid cassette fitted with standard-speed screens is selected. Alternatively a cassette may be used in the vertical Bucky.

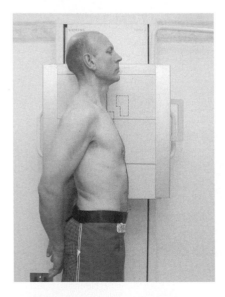

Position of patient and cassette

- The patient sits or stands, with either shoulder against a vertical Bucky or cassette stand.
- The median sagittal plane of the trunk is adjusted parallel to the cassette.
- The sternum is centred to the cassette or Bucky.
- The patient's hands are clasped behind the back and the shoulders are pulled well back.
- The cassette is centred at a level 2.5 cm below the sternal angle.

Direction and centring of the X-ray beam

- Direct the horizontal central ray towards a point 2.5 cm below the sternal angle.
- Exposure is made on arrested full inspiration.

Notes

- Immediately before exposure, the patient is asked to pull back the shoulders.
- If the patient is standing, the feet should be separated to aid stability.
- An FFD of 120 or 150 cm is selected.

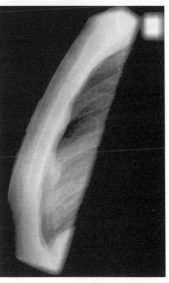

Normal lateral radiograph of sternum

Radiological considerations

- The lateral sternal projection can be confusing, especially in elderly patients, who often have heavily calcified costal cartilages.
- Interpretation of the lateral projection is much easier when the sternum is truly lateral and at right-angles to the image receptor, with corresponding superimposition of ribs and cartilage.
- It is important to remember that the initial interpretation is often done in the emergency department by inexperienced observers; therefore, care should be exercised to ensure that the sternum is projected in the true lateral position.
- Sternal fracture, especially when there is overlap of the bone ends, may be associated with compression (wedge) fracture of the fourth to sixth thoracic vertebrae. It is appropriate to image the thoracic spine if this is suspected.

Reference

Unett EM, Carver BJ (2001). The chest X-ray: centring points and central rays – can we stop confusing our students and ourselves? *Synergy* **November**:16.

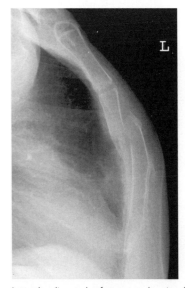

Lateral radiograph of sternum showing fracture of the body with overlap of bone ends

Section 8

The Skull

CONTENTS

INTRODUCTION 230
Interpretation of skull images 230
Anatomical terminology 230
Radiographic anatomy for positioning 231
Equipment 233
Positioning terminology 234
Patient preparation 236

GUIDE TO SKULL TECHNIQUE:
RECOMMENDED TECHNIQUE 237

CRANIUM: NON-ISOCENTRIC
TECHNIQUE 238
Lateral – supine with horizontal beam 238
Lateral – erect 239
Occipito-frontal 240
Fronto-occipital 242
Half-axial, fronto-occipital 30 degrees
    caudad – Towne's projection 243
Occipito-frontal 30-degree cranial
    angulation – reverse Towne's projection 245
Submento-vertical 246

Sella turcica: lateral 247
Optic foramina and jugular foramina 248
Optic foramina: postero-anterior
    oblique 248
Jugular foramina: submento-vertical
    20 degrees caudad 249
Temporal bones 250
Frontal-occipital 35 degrees caudad 250
Submento-vertical 251
Mastoid – lateral oblique 25 degrees
    caudad 252
Mastoid – profile 253
Petrous bone: anterior oblique
(Stenver's) 254

CRANIUM: ISOCENTRIC SKULL
TECHNIQUE 255
Introduction 255
Basic principles of use 255
Basic position 256
Occipito-frontal projection 257
Half-axial, reverse Towne's projection 257
Lateral 257

The importance of plain radiography of the skull has diminished in recent years due to the widespread availability of imaging modalities such as computed tomography (CT) and magnetic resonance imaging (MRI). These play a much more significant role in the management of a patient with a suspected intracranial pathology and either one would usually be the modality of choice if such a pathology were suspected. Plain radiography does, however, still play a significant role in the management of patients with certain skeletal conditions and, to a limited extent, in trauma, e.g. when a depressed or penetrating injury is suspected or if the patient is difficult to assess. Consequently, a significant number of referrals are still received from the accident and emergency department.

In order to produce high-quality images of the cranium and minimize risk for the patient, the radiographer must have a good understanding of the relevant anatomy, positioning landmarks and equipment used for imaging. This should be coupled with an ability to assess the patient's ability and thus apply the correct technique in any given situation.

This chapter will enable the radiographer to balance the technical factors with individual patient needs in order to maximize diagnostic outcome.

Interpretation of skull images

Skull films are recognized to be among the most difficult to interpret due to the complexity of the bony construction (numerous bones joined by sutures) and arterial and venous markings in the diploe, all of which may mimic fracture. Anteriorly, the complex facial skeleton is superimposed over the lower part of the skull vault; the dense petrous temporal bone also obscures detail. Fractures of the skull base are important because of the risk of cerebrospinal fluid (CSF) leak and spread of infection to the intracranial contents, but they are hard to demonstrate due to the thin, flat nature of the bones and superimposition of the facial skeleton and petrous bone.

Superimposition of other unwanted structures, including ponytails, hair clips, and hair matted with blood, can cause confusion. Surgical clips used for wound closure should not cause confusion, and they may help by marking the site of injury.

The initial interpretation of a skull film series will often be done by a clinician who is relatively inexperienced in trauma radiology. They will need the highest-quality examination possible.

Anatomical terminology

All radiography of the skull is undertaken with reference to a series of palpable landmarks and recognized lines or planes of the skull. It is vital that the radiographer possesses a good understanding of these before undertaking any positioning.

Landmarks

- **Outer canthus of the eye:** the point where the upper and lower eyelids meet laterally.
- **Infra-orbital margin/point:** the inferior rim of the orbit, with the point being located at its lowest point.
- **Nasion:** the articulation between the nasal and frontal bones.
- **Glabella:** a bony prominence found on the frontal bone immediately superior to the nasion.
- **Vertex:** the highest point of the skull in the median sagittal plane.
- **External occipital protuberance (inion):** a bony prominence found on the occipital bone, usually coincident with the median sagittal plane.
- **External auditory meatus:** the opening within the ear that leads into the external auditory canal.

Lines

- **Inter-orbital (inter-pupillary) line:** joins the centre of the two orbits or the centre of the two pupils when the eyes are looking straight forward.
- **Infra-orbital line:** joints the two infra-orbital points.
- **Anthropological baseline:** passes from the infra-orbital point to the upper border of the external auditory meatus (also known as the Frankfurter line).
- **Orbito-meatal base line (radiographic baseline):** extends from the outer canthus of the eye to the centre of the external auditory meatus. This line is angled approximately 10 degrees to the anthropological baseline.

Planes

- **Median sagittal plane:** divides the skull into right and left halves. Landmarks on this plane are the nasion anteriorly and the external occipital protuberance (inion) posteriorly.
- **Coronal planes:** these are at right-angles to the median sagittal plane and divide the head into anterior and posterior parts.
- **Anthropological plane:** a horizontal plane containing the two anthropological baselines and the infra-orbital line. It is an example of an axial plane. Axial planes are parallel with this plane.
- **Auricular plane:** perpendicular to the anthropological plane. Passes through the centre of the two external auditory meatuses. It is an example of a coronal plane.

The median sagittal, anthropological and coronal planes are mutually at right-angles.

Radiographic anatomy for positioning

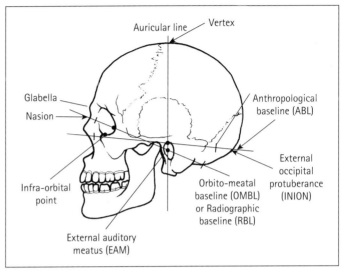

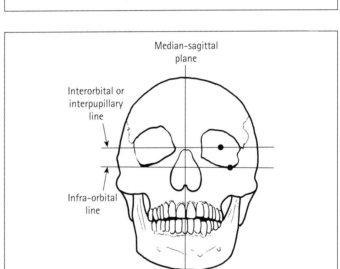

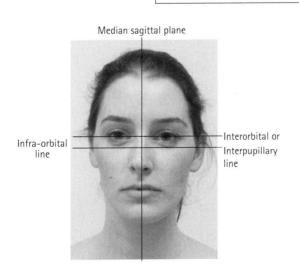

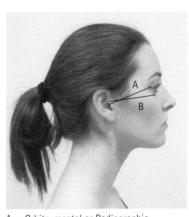

A = Orbito-meatal or Radiographic baseline (RBL)
B = Anthropological baseline

Radiographic anatomy for positioning (*contd*)

In order to evaluate radiographs successfully, it is important to be aware of a range of anatomical features. This will enable a judgement to be made in relation to the quality of the radiograph with respect to positioning.

The radiographs below show a range of features that are used in image evaluation and will be referred to regularly in the remainder of this chapter.

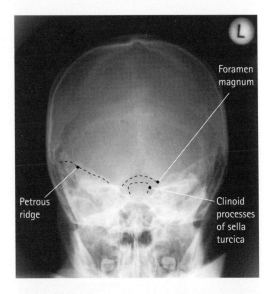

Foramen magnum

Petrous ridge

Clinoid processes of sella turcica

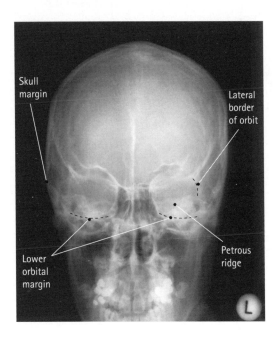

Skull margin

Lateral border of orbit

Lower orbital margin

Petrous ridge

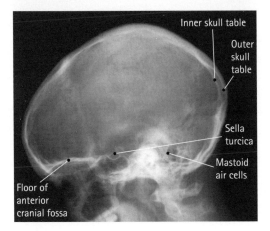

Inner skull table

Outer skull table

Sella turcica

Mastoid air cells

Floor of anterior cranial fossa

Radiography of the skull can be carried out using a specialized skull unit, or with an ordinary Bucky, or simply with a stationary grid and tube. Each method has specific advantages and disadvantages in any given situation, and these will be considered later. Problems arise for the radiographer, as the different methods use slightly different imaging techniques, which in turn utilize different planes and beam angulations to achieve the same projection. It is important for the radiographer to be fully aware of each technique in order to maximize the diagnostic outcome for their patients.

Skull units

Images taken on skull units yield the highest-quality skull images. All aspects of tube and tube support design have been optimized for skull radiography. Their use is to be recommended when undertaking skull radiography, provided that the patient's condition will allow them to be moved on to the table.

Advantages include:

- reduction in distortion;
- high-resolution images resulting from a grid with a large number of gridlines per unit length (grid lattice) and very fine focal spot on the tube anode (typically 0.3–0.4 mm^2);
- projections that are accurate and consistent as the patient is placed in one or a limited number of positions and the tube is then positioned around the head once this position is achieved;
- it can be more comfortable for the patient, as only one position has to be achieved;
- purpose-designed circular collimators allow close collimation to the head, reducing the dose and minimizing secondary radiation.

Disadvantages include:

- the table on which the patient lies is often quite narrow and difficult to get on to; this may make it unsuitable for patients who are unable to cooperate, since they may fall off;
- most units are accompanied by their own technique manual requiring the radiographer to acquire a set of skills unique to one piece of equipment;
- units are expensive;
- units can be lacking in versatility for sick patients and patients with conditions such as thoracic kyphosis.

Types of skull unit include the following:

- **Isocentric skull unit:** this is the most widely available unit and will produce the highest-quality images. This is achieved by the design of the equipment, which ensures that the image-receptor plate and primary beam are always perpendicular to each other, thus eliminating distortion. Note that the point around which the tube pivots is always adjusted so that it is at the centre of the object of interest. The technique used by each manufacturer will vary slightly, but all use the anthropological baseline rather than the radiographic baseline when describing projections.
- **Lysholm skull unit:** this differs from the isocentric skull unit in that the point around which the tube pivots is always in the same plane as the film. This has the potential to produce distorted images if large angulations are used. The techniques used to operate these units are very similar to those for skull radiography carried out with a simple tube and Bucky and utilize the radiographic baseline when describing techniques. This type of skull unit is not used widely in modern imaging departments.

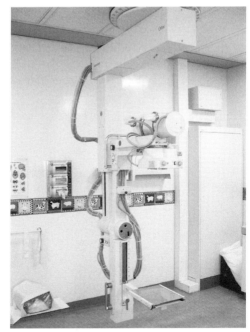

Isocentric skull unit

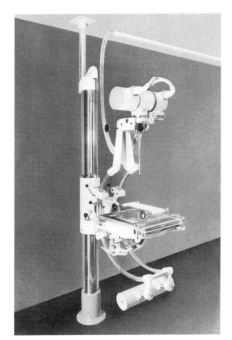

Lysholm skull unit

Positioning terminology

To describe a skull projection, it is necessary to state the relative positions of the skull planes to the image receptor and the central ray relative to skull planes/image receptor and to give a centring point or area to be included within the beam.

Traditionally, a centring point has always been given, but this may not always be appropriate. This is because some centring points will lead to the irradiation of a large number of radiosensitive structures that are of no diagnostic interest. Rather than focusing entirely on centring points, it is often better for the radiographer to be mindful of the anatomy that needs to be demonstrated for a diagnosis to be made and to ensure that this is included within the primary beam, whilst ensuring that it is not obscured by other structures.

Occipito-frontal projections

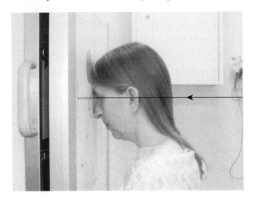

Projections in which the central ray is parallel to the sagittal plane are named according to the direction of the central ray. In the photograph above, the central ray enters the skull through the occipital bone and exits through the frontal bone. This is therefore an occipto-frontal (OF) projection.

Fronto-occipital projections

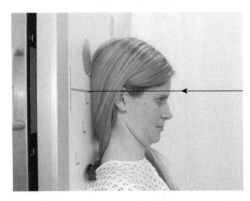

Again, the central ray is parallel to the sagittal plane, except that the central ray now enters the skull through the frontal bone and exits through the occipital bone. This is a fronto-occipital (FO) projection.

Beam angulation

Many occipto-frontal and front-occipital projections will require the central ray to pass along the sagittal plane at some angle to the orbital-meatal plane. In these cases, the degree of angulation is stated after the name of the projection. The direction of angulation is also given. Caudo-cranial angulation (usually shortened to cranial angulation) involves the beam pointing up the body towards the head (written in short form as ↑). If the beam is angled towards the feet, the beam is then said to be angled cranio-caudally (usually shortened to caudal angulation, and written in short form as ↓).

The photograph below shows a fronto-occipital 30-degree caudal projection (FO30° ↓).

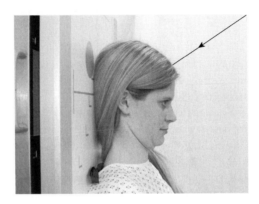

Lateral

For the lateral projection, the central ray passes along a coronal plane at right-angles to the median sagittal plane. It is named according to the side of the head nearer to the image receptor. In the example below, the beam enters the head on the left side, passes along a coronal plane, and exits the head on the right side, where the image receptor is located. This is, therefore, a right lateral.

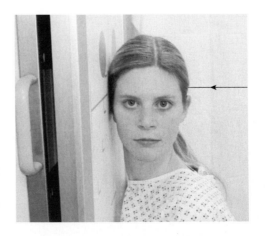

Lateral with angulation

If the central ray passes along a coronal plane at some angle to the median sagittal plane, then the degree of angulation is stated. The photograph below shows a right lateral with 30-degree caudal angulation (R Lat 30°↓).

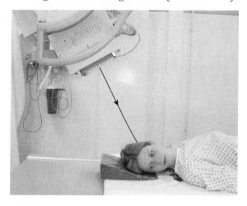

Oblique projections

As can be seen in the photograph, an oblique projection is obtained when the central ray is at some angle to the median sagittal plane and the coronal plane. How the projection is named will depend on two factors: first whether the anterior or posterior portion of the head is in contact with the cassette and second whether the left or right side of the head is in contact with the cassette.

Forty-degree left anterior oblique

In this example, the head is rotated to the right, such that the median sagittal plane is at 40 degrees to the cassette and the left side of the head is in contact with the cassette (40°LAO).

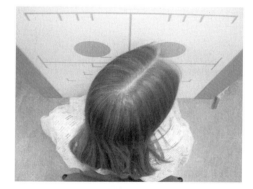

Complex oblique projections

Oblique projections may become more complex when there is an additional caudal or cranial angle added in relation to a specified baseline. This additional angle is usually achieved by raising or lowering the chin, such that the relevant baseline makes the required angle to the cassette. Alternatively, the tube can be angled or a combination of both approaches may be useful if the patient has limited mobility. The photograph on the top right is an example of one such projection used for plain imaging of the optic foramina.

Fifty-five-degree left anterior oblique with 35 degree caudal angulation

The head has been rotated, such that the right side of the face is in contact with the cassette and the median sagittal plane makes

an angle of 55 degrees to the Bucky. In the example below, the central ray has a 35-degree caudal angulation. Alternatively, this angulation may be achieved by raising the orbito-meatal plane by 35 degrees whilst using a horizontal beam (55°LAO35°↓).

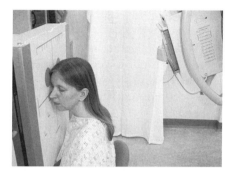

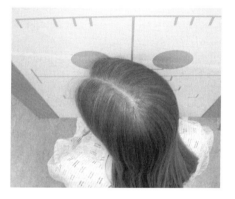

The photograph below shows how the same projection has been achieved with a combination of tube and orbital-meatal plane angulation. In this case, the plane has been raised 20 degrees and the tube has been given a 15-degree caudal angulation, in effect producing a total beam angulation of 35 degrees to the orbital-meatal plane.

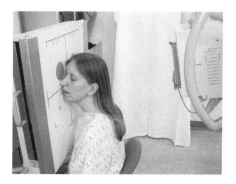

Warning

When undertaking oblique skull radiography, always ensure that the beam is angled in the same direction as the grid lattice, i.e. parallel to the grid lines. If any angulation is applied such that beam is angled across the grid lines, i.e. perpendicular to their direction of travel, then a grid cut-off artefact will result and the image will need to be repeated.

Patient preparation

Before undertaking skull radiography, the following specific considerations should be made:

- Ensure that all metal objects are removed from the patient, e.g. hair clips and hairpins.
- Bunches of hair often produce artefacts and thus should be untied.
- If the area of interest includes the mouth, then false teeth containing metal and metal dental bridges should be removed.
- The patient should be provided with a clear explanation of any movements and film positions associated with the normal operation of the skull unit.

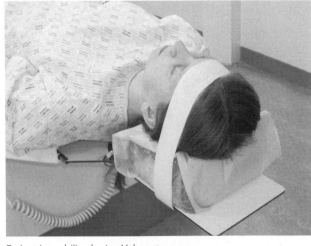

Patient immobilized using Velcro straps

Useful accessories

- The usefulness of foam pads as an aid to immobilization cannot be overstated. The photograph opposite shows a specially designed pad for skull radiography. It is available in a range of sizes to accommodate different age groups.
- Forty-five-degree triangular pads are extremely useful for immobilizing children. They can be held by the parent and support the head without the parent placing their hands in the primary beam.
- Individual side markers are essential for skull radiography, as the clip-type side markers are easily lost in the collimation, particularly when using a skull unit.
- Velcro straps are of great use when immobilizing a patient on a skull unit.

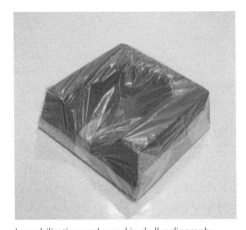

Immobilization pads used in skull radiography

General image quality guidelines and radiation protection considerations

The European Guidelines on Quality Criteria for Diagnostic Images describe various criteria by which images should be assessed. Many of these criteria are included with the specific projection descriptions and in the introduction to this chapter, but some more general points and other considerations are included below:

- Images should have a visually sharp reproduction of all structures, such as outer and inner lamina of the cranial vault, the trabecular structure of the cranium, the various sinuses and sutures where visible, vascular channels, petrous part of the temporal bone and the pituitary fossa.
- Important image details should be in the 0.3–0.5 mm range.
- A 400 (regular) speed imaging system is recommended (regular conventional film/screen combination).
- Use 70–85 kV tube voltage.
- Whenever possible, use an occipito-frontal (postero-anterior) rather than a fronto-occipital (antero-posterior) technique, since this vastly reduces the dose to the eyes.
- 24 × 30-cm cassettes are generally used for plain skull radiography.

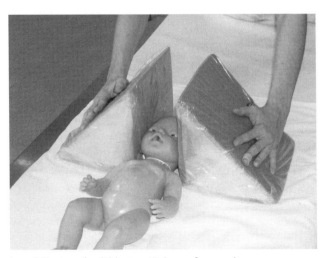

Immobilization of a child using 45-degree foam pads

The flowchart below can be used as a guide to help select the correct skull technique in any given clinical situation. The choice of projections will vary from department to department, depending on local protocols.

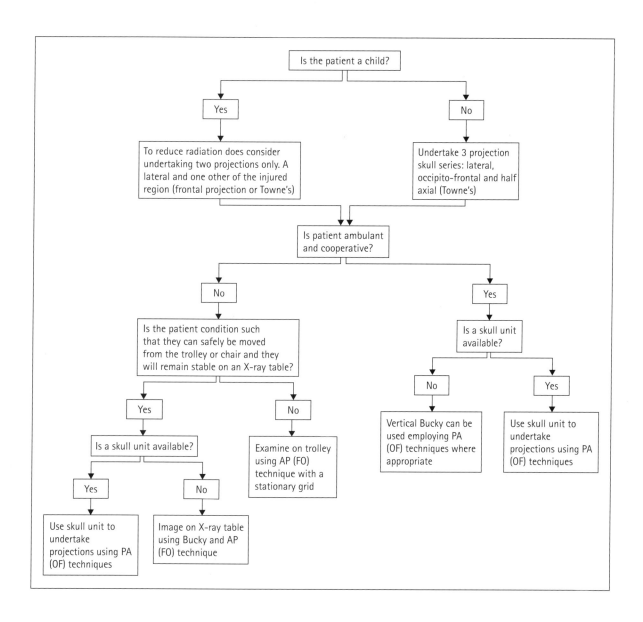

8 Cranium: non-isocentric technique

Non-isocentric skull technique should be undertaken when there is no isocentric skull unit available or the patient's condition will not allow them to be transferred on to the skull unit table. Images are acquired using a 24 × 30-cm cassette. Grid cassettes are used when it is impossible to use a Bucky grid system.

Lateral – supine with horizontal beam

Position of patient and cassette

- The patient lies supine, with the head raised and immobilized on a non-opaque skull pad. This will ensure that the occipital region is included on the final image.
- The head is adjusted, such that the median sagittal plane is perpendicular to the table/trolley and the interorbital line is perpendicular to the cassette.
- Support the grid cassette vertically against the lateral aspect of the head parallel to the median sagittal plane, with its long edge 5 cm above the vertex of the skull.

Direction and centring of the X-ray beam

- The horizontal central ray is directed parallel to the interorbital line, such that it is at right-angles to the median sagittal plane.
- Centre midway between the glabella and the external occipital protuberance to a point approximately 5 cm superior to the external auditory meatus.
- The long axis of the cassette should be coincident with the long axis of the skull.

Essential image characteristics

- The image should contain all of the cranial bones and the first cervical vertebra. Both the inner and outer skull tables should be included.
- A true lateral will result in perfect superimposition of the lateral portions of the floors of the anterior cranial fossa and those of the posterior cranial fossa. The clinoid processes of the sella turcica should also be superimposed (see p. 232).

Radiological considerations

- This projection is performed as part of the Advanced Trauma and Life Support (ATLS) primary screen.
- Skull-base fractures are potentially life-threatening due to the risk of intracranial infection and are often very difficult to detect. Lateral skull projections taken supine with a horizontal beam may reveal sinus fluid levels, which may be a marker of skull-base injury. They may also help to confirm the presence of free intracranial air, which is another sign of breach of the integrity of the cranium.

Common faults and remedies

- Failure to include the occipital region as a result of not using a pad that ensures the head is raised far enough from the table/trolley surface.
- Poor superimposition of the lateral floors of the cranial fossa. Always ensure that the inter-orbital line is perpendicular to the film and that the median sagittal plane is exactly perpendicular to the table/trolley top.

Notes

- The choice of lateral will depend on the site of the suspected pathology.
- If the suspected pathology is to the left side of the head, then a left lateral should be undertaken with the cassette supported on the left side of the patient, and vice versa. This will ensure that the pathology is shown at the maximum possible resolution due to the minimization of geometric unsharpness.
- This is the projection of choice for the majority of trauma cases on a trolley.

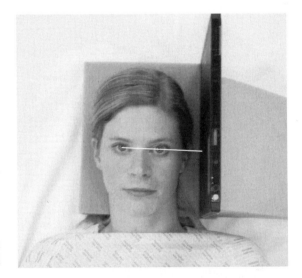

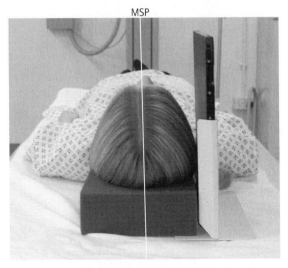

MSP

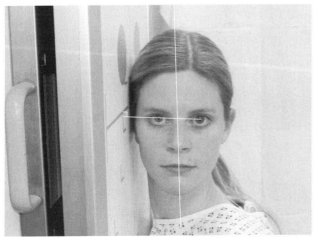

Lateral – erect

This position may be used for a cooperative patient. Variations from the supine horizontal beam technique are noted below, but all other imaging criteria remain the same.

Position of patient and cassette

- The patient sits facing the erect Bucky and the head is then rotated, such that the median sagittal plane is parallel to the Bucky and the inter-orbital line is perpendicular to it.
- The shoulders may be rotated slightly to allow the correct position to be attained. The patient may grip the Bucky for stability.
- Position the cassette transversely in the erect Bucky, such that its upper border is 5 cm above the vertex of the skull.
- A radiolucent pad may be placed under the chin for support.

Direction and centring of the X-ray beam

- The X-ray tube should have been centred previously to the Bucky.
- Adjust the height of the Bucky/tube so that the patient is comfortable (NB: do not decentre the tube from the Bucky at this point).
- Centre midway between the glabella and the external occipital protuberance to a point approximately 5 cm superior to the external auditory meatus.

Common faults and remedies

This is not an easy position for the patient to maintain. Check the position of all planes immediately before exposure, as the patient probably will have moved.

Notes

- This projection can also be performed with the patient prone on a floating-top table.
- The projection may be performed usefully on babies in the supine position, with the head rotated to either side.
- An air/fluid level in the sphenoid sinus (an indicator for a base-of-skull fracture) will not be visible if the patient is imaged with a vertical central ray. This is not relevant in young babies, as the sinus is not developed fully.

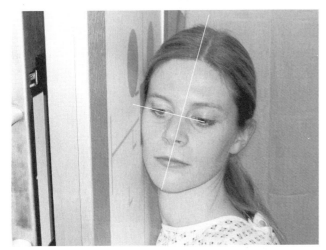

Correct positioning

Incorrect positioning

Occipito-frontal

Occipito-frontal projections can be employed with different degrees of beam angulation. The choice of projection will depend upon departmental protocol and the anatomy that needs to be demonstrated.

Position of patient and cassette

- This projection may be undertaken erect or in the prone position. The erect projection will be described, as the prone projection is uncomfortable for the patient and will usually be carried out only in the absence of a vertical Bucky.
- The patient is seated facing the erect Bucky, so that the median sagittal plane is coincident with the midline of the Bucky and is also perpendicular to it.
- The neck is flexed so that the orbito-meatal base line is perpendicular to the Bucky. This can usually be achieved by ensuring that the nose and forehead are in contact with the Bucky.
- Ensure that the mid-part of the frontal bone is positioned in the centre of the Bucky.
- The patient may place the palms of each hand either side of the head (out of the primary beam) for stability.
- A 24 × 30-cm cassette is placed longitudinally in the Bucky tray. Ensure that the lead name blocker will not interfere with the final image.

Direction and centring of the X-ray beam

Occipito-frontal

- The central ray is directed perpendicular to the Bucky along the median sagittal plane.
- A collimation field should be set to include the vertex of the skull superiorly, the region immediately below the base of the occipital bone inferiorly, and the lateral skin margins. It is important to ensure that the tube is centred to the middle of the Bucky.

Occipito-frontal caudal angulation: 10, 15 and 20 degrees

- The technique used for these three projections is similar to that employed for the occipito-frontal projection, except that a caudal angulation is applied. The degree of angulation will depend on the technique, e.g. for an OF20°↓ projection, a 20-degree caudal angulation will be employed.
- Ensure that the central ray is always centred to the middle of the Bucky once the tube angulation has been applied and not before.

Essential image characteristics

- All the cranial bones should be included within the image, including the skin margins.
- It is important to ensure that the skull is not rotated. This can be assessed by measuring the distance from a point in the midline of the skull to the lateral margin. If this is the same on both sides of the skull, then it is not rotated.

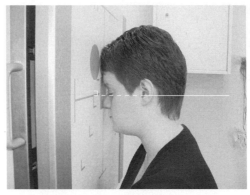

Positioning for occipito-frontal skull projection

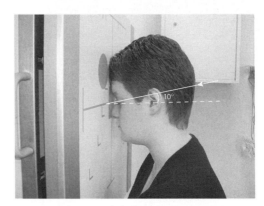

Positioning for OF10°↓ skull projection

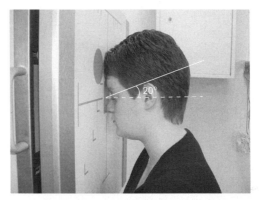

Positioning for OF20°↓ skull projection

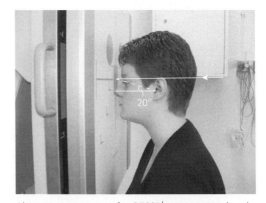

Alternative positioning for OF20°↓ using a straight tube with the orbito-meatal baseline raised 20 degrees

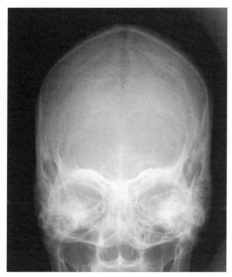

OF

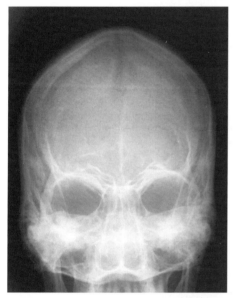

OF10°↓

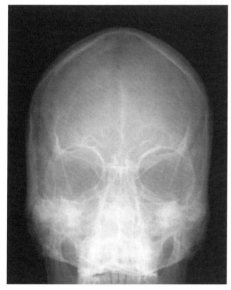

OF20°↓

Occipito-frontal

- The degree of beam angulation can be evaluated from an assessment of the position of the petrous ridges within the orbit:
  - **Occipito-frontal:** the petrous ridges should be completely superimposed within the orbit, with their upper borders coincident with the upper third of the orbit.
  - **OF10°↓:** the petrous ridges appear in the middle third of the orbit.
  - **OF15°↓:** the petrous ridges appear in the lower third of the orbit.
  - **OF20°↓:** the petrous ridges appear just below the inferior orbital margin.

Radiological considerations

- Asymmetry of projection of the squamo-parietal suture due to rotation increases the risk of it being mistaken for a fracture.
- As the beam angle increases, more of the orbital region is demonstrated and less of the upper part of the frontal bone anterior parietal bones is shown. Thus, the site of the suspected pathology should be considered when selecting the beam angle, e.g. an injury to the upper orbital region is best evaluated with an OF20°↓ projection.

Common faults and remedies

- **Rotation:** ensure that the patient's head is straight immediately before the exposure is made.
- **Incorrect beam angulation:** it is worth remembering that greater beam angulations will result in the petrous ridges appearing further down the orbit. If an OF20°↓ is undertaken and the petrous bones appear in the middle third of the orbit, then a greater angle should have been applied, in this case a further 10 degrees.

Notes: alternative technique

- Patients often find it difficult to maintain their orbito-meatal baseline perpendicular to the film, as this is an unnatural position and they are likely to move.
- Instead of angling the beam to achieve the desired position of the petrous ridge within the orbit, a **vertical** central ray, i.e. perpendicular to the film, can be used. The desired angulation for the projection can then be achieved by raising the orbito-meatal baseline by the desired angle, e.g. for an OF20°↓, the chin can be raised such that the orbito-meatal baseline will be at an angle of 20 degrees to the horizontal (see photograph). Similarly, for an OF10°↓, the orbito-meatal line will be raised by 10 degrees.

Fronto-occipital

Fronto-occipital projections of the skull will demonstrate the same anatomy as occipito-frontal projections. The orbits and frontal bone, however, will be magnified, since they are positioned further from the image receptor.

Such projections should be carried out only when the patient cannot be moved and must be imaged supine. These projections result in increased eye dose and loss of resolution of anterior skull structures due to increased object-to-film distance (OFD).

Position of patient and cassette

- The patient lies supine on a trolley or Bucky table, or with the posterior aspect of the skull resting on a grid cassette.
- The head is adjusted to bring the median sagittal plane at right-angles to the film and coincident with its midline. In this position, the external auditory meatuses are equidistant from the cassette.
- The orbito-meatal baseline should be perpendicular to the cassette.

Direction and centring of the X-ray beam

All angulations for fronto-occipital projections are made cranially.

Fronto-occipital

- The central ray is directed perpendicular to the cassette or Bucky along the median sagittal plane.
- A collimation field should be set to include the vertex of the skull superiorly, the base of the occipital bone inferiorly, and the lateral skin margins. It is important to ensure that all of the tube is centred to the middle of the Bucky.

Fronto-occipital caudal angulation: 10, 15 and 20 degrees

- The technique used for these three projections is similar to that employed for the occipito-frontal, except that a cranial angulation is applied. The degree of angulation will depend on the projection required.
- Remember that the cassette or Bucky must be displaced superiorly to allow for the tube angulation, otherwise the area of interest will be projected off the film. For a 20-degree angle, the top of the cassette will need to be 5 cm above the skull vertex.

Essential image characteristics and radiological considerations

See occipito-frontal projections (p. 240).

Common faults and remedies

See occipito-frontal projections (p. 241).

- Remember that increasing the degree of cranial angulation will project the petrous ridges further down the orbits.

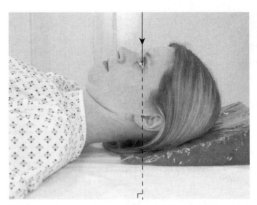
FO projection

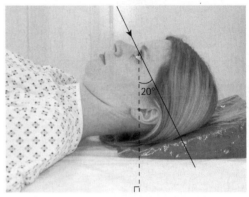
FO20°↑ projection

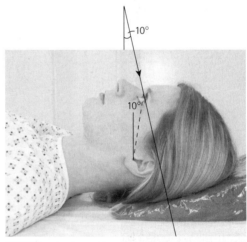
FO20°↑ projection achieved with 10° tube angle and RBL raised 10°

Notes: alternative technique

See occipito-frontal projections (p. 241).

- In the example given below, an FO20°↓ projection is required, but the patient can only maintain their orbito-meatal base line in a position 10 degrees back from perpendicular (i.e. with the chin raised slightly). In order to achieve an overall 20-degree angle, a ten-degree cranial angulation will need to be applied to the tube.
- Similarly, if the patient's chin was raised such that the baseline was 20 degrees to the perpendicular, then an FO20°↓ projection could be achieved by using a straight tube perpendicular to the film.

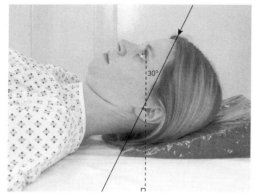

FO 30°↑ 'Towne's projection'

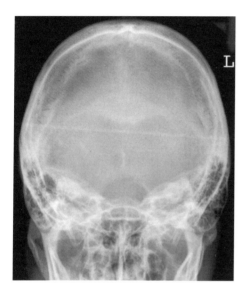

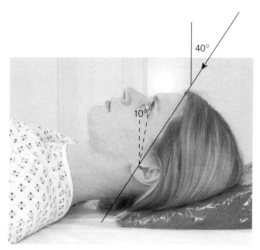

The chin is raised, such that the baseline makes an angle of 10 degrees to the perpendicular and therefore a 40-degree tube angle must be employed to ensure a 30-degree angle to the orbito-meatal plane

Half-axial, fronto-occipital 30 degrees caudad – Towne's projection

Position of patient and cassette

- The patient lies supine on a trolley or Bucky table, with the posterior aspect of the skull resting on a grid cassette.
- The head is adjusted to bring the median sagittal plane at right-angles to the cassette and so it is coincident with its midline.
- The orbito-meatal base line should be perpendicular to the film.

Direction and centring of the X-ray beam

- The central ray is angled caudally so it makes an angle of 30 degrees to the orbito-meatal plane.
- Centre in the midline such that the beam passes midway between the external auditory meatuses. This is to a point approximately 5 cm above the glabella.
- The top of the cassette should be positioned adjacent to the vertex of the skull to ensure that the beam angulation does not project the area of interest off the bottom of the image.

Essential image characteristics

- The sella turcica of the sphenoid bone is projected within the foramen magnum.
- The image must include all of the occipital bone and the posterior parts of the parietal bone, and the lambdoidal suture should be visualized clearly.
- The skull should not be rotated. This can also be assessed by ensuring that the sella turcica appears in the middle of the foramen magnum.

Radiological considerations

- The foramen magnum should be seen clearly on this projection. The margins may be obscured by incorrect angulation, thus hiding important fractures.
- The zygoma may be seen well on this projection. If fractured, this gives a clue to the presence of associated facial injury.

Common faults and remedies

- Under-angulation: the foramen magnum is not demonstrated clearly above the petrous ridges. This is probably the most common fault, as the patient may find it difficult to maintain the baseline perpendicular to the film.
- If the patient's chin cannot be depressed sufficiently to bring the orbito-meatal baseline perpendicular to the film, then it will be necessary to increase the angle of the tube more than 30 degrees to the vertical. A 30-degree angle to the orbito-meatal plane must be maintained (see figure).
- Over-angulation: the posterior arch of the atlas bone (C1) is visible within the foramen magnum.

(contd)

Half-axial, fronto-occipital 30 degrees caudad – Towne's projection (*contd*)

- The large tube angle introduces a significant degree of distortion in the final image. This is eliminated using the isocentric skull unit technique.
- Some patients, particularly those with an increased thoracic kyphosis, may have difficulties in positioning the back of their head against the Bucky. This can be overcome somewhat by angling the Bucky table as shown in the photograph.

Notes: alternative technique

- Some or all of the 30-degree angle required for this projection can be applied by using a skull board. If a 30-degree board is used and the patient's orbito-meatal baseline is perpendicular to the top of the board, then a vertical central ray should be employed. If a 15-degree board is used, then a 15-degree caudal angulation must be applied.
- If a skull board with a 20-degree angle is used, then a 10-degree caudal angulation will be required to give the correct overall beam angulation.

Modified half axial

Denton (1998) has suggested an alternative projection that avoids irradiating the eyes and thyroid.

- The central ray is angled caudally so it makes an angle of 25 degrees to the orbito-meatal plane.
- Instead of using a centring point, a collimation field is set. The lower border of this field should be limited immediately above the supraorbital ridges at their highest point. The upper border of the light beam should just include the vertex of the skull at its highest point. Collimate laterally to include the skin margins within the field.

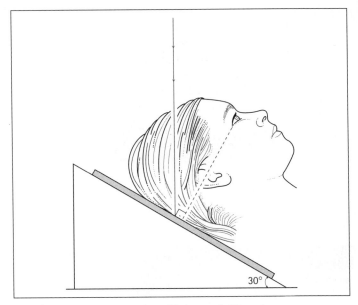

F030°↓ Towne's projection using a 30-degree skull board

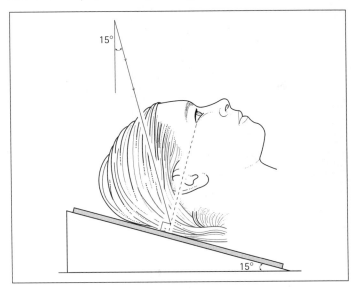

F030°↓ Towne's projection using a 15-degree skull board

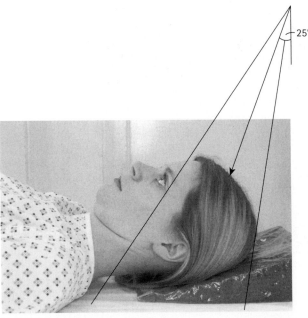

Modified half axial

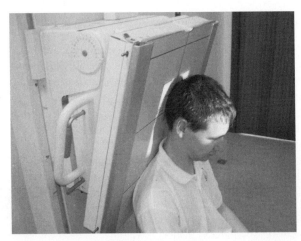

The Bucky can be tilted for kyphotic patients

Occipito-frontal 30-degree cranial angulation – reverse Towne's projection

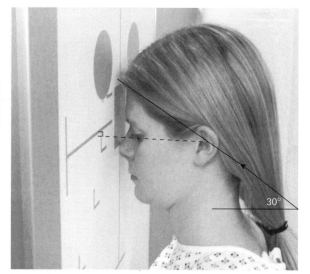

Reverse Towne's

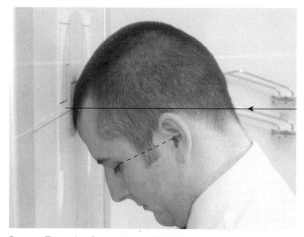

Reverse Towne's, alternative positioning

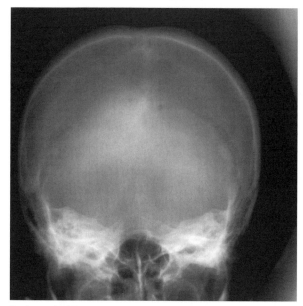

Under angled Towne's

Position of patient and cassette

- This projection is usually undertaken with the patient in the erect position and facing the erect Bucky, although it may be performed prone.
- Initially, the patient is asked to place their nose and forehead on the Bucky table. The head is adjusted to bring the median sagittal plane at right-angles to the cassette and so it is coincident with its midline.
- The orbito-meatal baseline should be perpendicular to the cassette.
- The patient may place their hands on the Bucky for stability.

Direction and centring of the X-ray beam

- The central ray is angled cranially so its makes an angle of 30 degrees to the orbito-meatal plane.
- Adjust the collimation field, such that the whole of the occipital bone and the parietal bones up to the vertex are included within the field. Avoid including the eyes in the primary beam. Laterally, the skin margins should also be included within the field.

Essential image characteristics

- The sella turcica of the sphenoid bone is projected within the foramen magnum.
- The image must include all of the occipital bone and the posterior parts of the parietal bone, and the lambdoidal suture should be visualized clearly.
- The skull should not be rotated. This can also be assessed by ensuring that the sella turcica appears in the middle of the foramen magnum.

Radiological considerations

- The foramen magnum should be seen clearly on this projection. The margins may be obscured by incorrect angulation, thus hiding important fractures.
- The zygoma may be seen well on this projection. If fractured, this gives a clue to the presence of associated facial injury.

Common faults and remedies

See Half-axial, fronto-occipital 30 degrees caudad – Towne's projection (p. 244).

Notes

- This projection will carry a lower radiation dose to sensitive structures than the equivalent antero-posterior projection.
- Positioning may be easier to undertake on patients who find it difficult to achieve the position required for the equivalent antero-posterior half-axial projections.

Submento-vertical

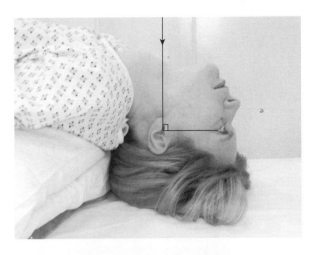

Position of patient and cassette

The patient may be imaged erect or supine. If the patient is unsteady, then a supine technique is advisable.

Supine

- The patient's shoulders are raised and the neck is hyperextended to bring the vertex of the skull in contact with the grid cassette or table.
- The head is adjusted to bring the external auditory meatuses equidistant from the cassette.
- The median sagittal plane should be at right-angles to the cassette along its midline.
- The orbito-meatal plane should be as near as possible parallel to the cassette.

Erect

- The patient sits a short distance away from a vertical Bucky.
- The neck is hyperextended to allow the head to fall back until the vertex of the skull makes contact with the centre of the vertical Bucky.
- The remainder of the positioning is as described for the supine technique.

Direction and centring of the X-ray beam

- The central ray is directed at right-angles to the orbito-meatal plane and centred midway between the external auditory meatuses.

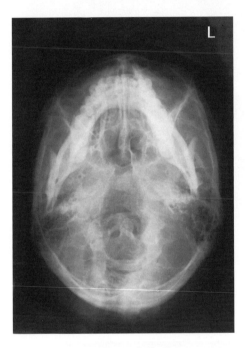

Essential image characteristics

- A correct projection will show the angles of the mandible clear of the petrous portions of the temporal bone.
- The foramina of the middle cranial fossa should be seen symmetrically either side of the midline.

Radiological considerations

- Erosion of the bony margins of the skull-base foramina is an important indicator of destruction by tumour. Under-tilt, over-tilt and rotation reduce the visibility of these foramina.
- This is now an uncommon projection, as CT demonstrates more completely the bony detail of the skull base in axial and coronal planes. MRI offers multiplanar imaging with superb detail of the soft tissues as well as the skull base.

Common faults and remedies

- This projection involves positioning that is very uncomfortable for the patient. It is well worth ensuring that the equipment is prepared fully before commencing the examination, so that the patient need maintain the position for only a minimum period.
- The position is achieved much more easily if a skull unit is used, since the object table and tube can be adjusted to minimize hyperextension of the neck.

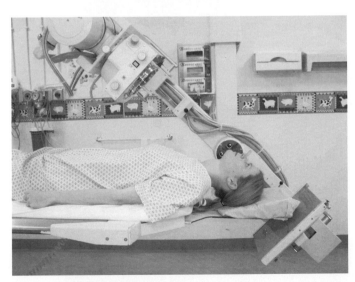

Submento-vertical (SMV) using skull unit

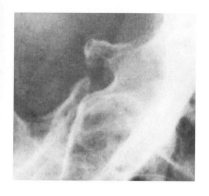

Sella turcica: lateral

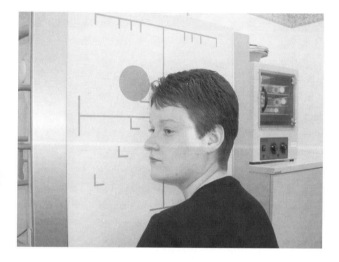

Position of patient and cassette

- The patient sits facing the erect Bucky and the head is then rotated, such that the median sagittal plane is parallel to the Bucky and the inter-orbital line is perpendicular to the Bucky.
- The shoulders may be rotated slightly to allow the correct position to be attained. The patient may grip the Bucky for stability.
- The head and Bucky heights are adjusted so that the centre of the Bucky is 2.5 cm vertically above a point 2.5 cm along the baseline from the external auditory meatus
- A radiolucent pad may be placed under the chin and face for support.

Direction and centring of the X-ray beam

- A well-collimated beam is centred to a point 2.5 cm vertically above a point 2.5 cm along the baseline from the auditory meatus nearer the X-ray tube.

Radiological considerations

This examination is increasingly uncommon, as in the presence of good clinical or biochemical evidence of a pituitary tumour MRI or CT will be the test of choice. If these modalities are unavailable, then evidence of sella expansion by a large lesion may be obtained from plain image radiography. A double floor to the sella turcica may be a sign of smaller intra-pituitary tumour, but it can also be a normal variant due to a slope of the sella floor; this may be resolved by use of a well-collimated OF20°↓ projection.

8 Cranium

Optic foramina and jugular foramina

The main indication for imaging these foramina is detection of tumour (e.g. glomus jugulare tumour, optic nerve glioma), which currently requires imaging by CT and/or MRI for full evaluation.

Optic foramina: postero-anterior oblique

The optic canal opens into the rear of the bony orbit at the optic foramen. The canal passes forwards and laterally at approximately 35 degrees to the median sagittal plane and downwards at approximately 35 degrees to the orbito-meatal plane. This is the path that the central ray must take to demonstrate the foramen.

Both sides are usually imaged separately for comparison by undertaking postero-anterior oblique projections of the cranium.

Position of patient and cassette

- The patient lies prone or, more commonly, erect with the nose, cheek and chin of the side being examined in contact with the Bucky or cassette table.
- The centre of the orbit of the side under examination should coincide with the centre of the Bucky or cassette table.
- The median sagittal plane is adjusted to make an angle of 35 degrees to the vertical (55 degrees to the table).
- The orbito-meatal base line is raised 35 degrees from the horizontal.

Direction and centring of the X-ray beam

- With the beam collimated well, the horizontal central ray should be centred to the middle of the Bucky. This is to a point 7.5 cm above and 7.5 cm behind the uppermost external auditory meatus, so that the central ray emerges from the centre of the orbit in contact with the table.
- A small lead side-marker can be placed above the superior orbital margin.

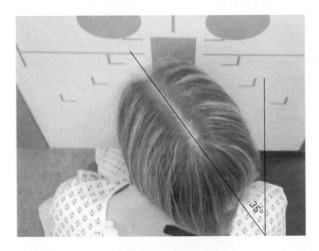

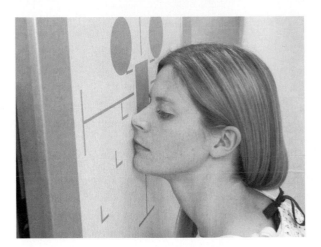

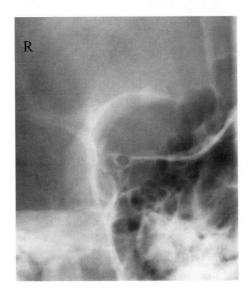

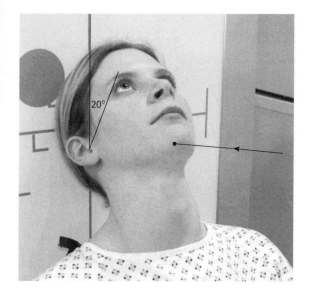

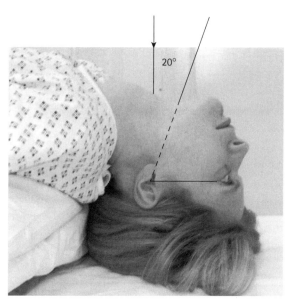

Jugular foramina: submento-vertical 20 degrees caudad

The jugular foramina lie in the posterior cranial fossa between the petrous temporal and occipital bones on each side of the foramen magnum. Both sides are imaged simultaneously on a single image by undertaking a submento-vertical (SMV) 20 degrees caudad projection.

Position of patient and cassette

- As per the SMV projection described previously (p. 246).

Direction and centring of the X-ray beam

- Using a well-collimated beam, the central ray is angled caudally so that it makes an angle of 70 degrees to the orbito-meatal plane and centred in the midline to pass midway between the external auditory meatuses.

Notes: alternative technique

- With the patient's neck less extended, the head can be positioned with the orbito-meatal plane at an angle of 20 degrees to the Bucky, in which case a horizontal central ray will make the required angle of 70 degrees to the base plane (see photograph).

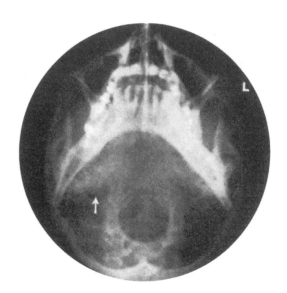

8 Cranium

Temporal bones

These projections are traditionally difficult to perform. They are also difficult to interpret, especially if the examination is not of the highest quality. Modern CT with direct coronal imaging affords exquisite demonstration of temporal bone detail and has largely obviated the need for these projections.

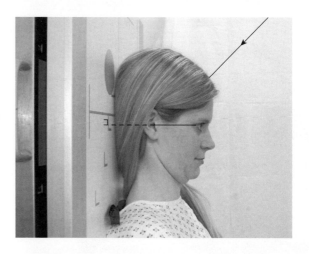

Frontal-occipital 35 degrees caudad

Position of patient and cassette

- The patient may be supine in the midline of the table or erect with their back to an erect Bucky.
- The head is adjusted to bring the external auditory meatuses equidistant from the table, so that the median sagittal plane is at right-angles to, and in the midline of, the table.
- The chin is depressed so that the orbito-meatal line is at right-angles to the table.
- A small (24 × 30-cm) cassette is placed transversely in the cassette tray and is centred to coincide with the angled central ray.

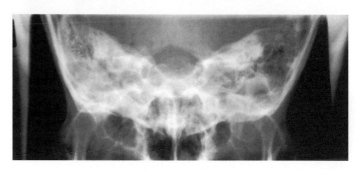

Direction and centring of the X-ray beam

- A caudal angulation is employed, such that it makes an angle of 35 degrees to the orbito-meatal plane.
- The beam is centred midway between the external auditory meatuses.
- Collimate laterally to include the lateral margins of the skull and supra-inferiorly to include the mastoid and petrous parts of the temporal bone. The mastoid process can be palpated easily behind the ear.

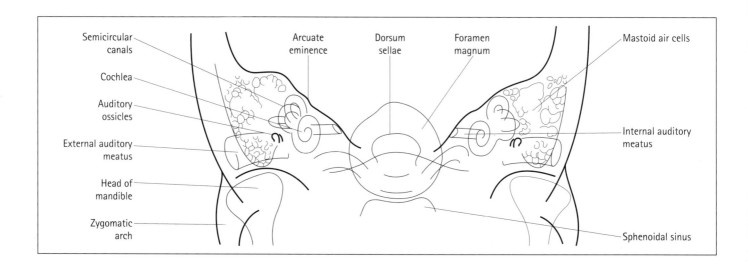

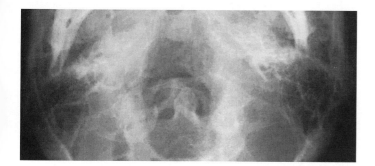

Frontal-occipital 35 degrees caudad

Essential image characteristics

- The sella turcica of the sphenoid bone should be projected within the foramen magnum.
- The skull should not be rotated. This can also be assessed by ensuring that the sella turcica appears in the middle of the foramen magnum.
- All of the anatomy included on the radiograph opposite and line diagram below should be included.

Common faults and remedies

- Under-angulation: the foramen magnum is not demonstrated clearly above the petrous ridges. This is probably the most common fault, since the patient may find it difficult to maintain the baseline perpendicular to the film.
- If the patient's chin cannot be depressed sufficiently to bring the orbito-meatal base line perpendicular to the film, then it will be necessary to increase the angle of the tube more than 35 degrees to the vertical. A 35-degree angle to the orbito-meatal plane must be maintained.

Submento-vertical

As an alternative, an SMV projection (see p. 246 for details) collimated down to include only the petrous and mastoid parts of the temporal bone is a further projection that has been employed to demonstrate the anatomy of this region.

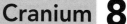

Patient positioned for SMV projection

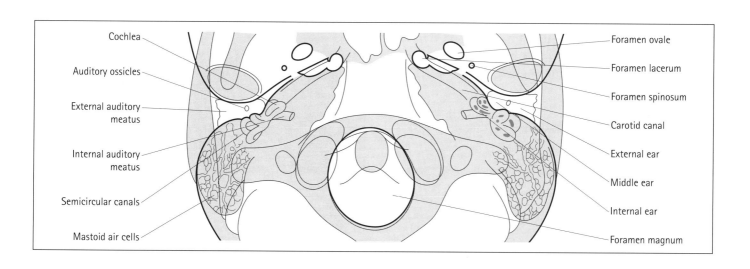

Cochlea
Auditory ossicles
External auditory meatus
Internal auditory meatus
Semicircular canals
Mastoid air cells

Foramen ovale
Foramen lacerum
Foramen spinosum
Carotid canal
External ear
Middle ear
Internal ear
Foramen magnum

Mastoid – lateral oblique 25 degrees caudad

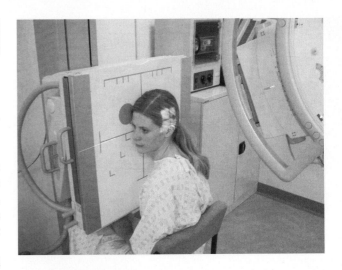

Position of patient and cassette

- The patient sits facing the erect Bucky. The head is then rotated, such that the median sagittal plane is parallel to the Bucky and the inter-orbital line is perpendicular to the Bucky.
- The shoulders may be rotated slightly to allow the correct position to be attained. The patient may grip the Bucky for stability.
- The auricle of the ear adjacent to the table is folded forward to ensure that its soft-tissue outline is not superimposed over the region of interest.
- Position the mastoid process in the middle of the Bucky.
- An 18 × 24-cm cassette is positioned longitudinally in the Bucky and is centred to coincide with the central ray and mastoid process.

Direction and centring of the X-ray beam

- A 25-degree caudal angulation is employed and centred 5 cm above and 2.5 cm behind the external auditory meatus remote from the cassette.
- Collimate to the area under examination.

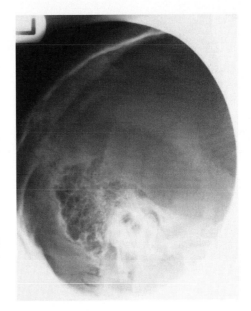

Essential image characteristics

- Ensure that all of the mastoid air cells have been included within the image. The size of these structures can vary greatly from individual to individual.

Common faults and remedies

- Failure to centre far enough posteriorly might exclude part of the mastoid air cells from the image if these structures are very well developed.
- Failure to ensure that the auricle of the ear is folded forward will result in a soft-tissue artefact. Check that the ear is in the correct position just before the exposure is undertaken.

Note

Examine both sides for comparison.

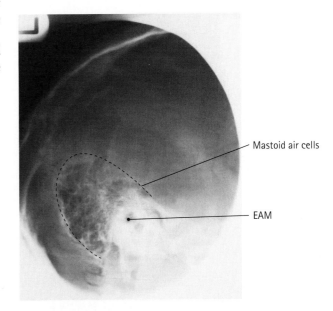

Mastoid air cells

EAM

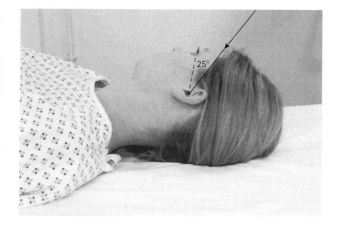

Mastoid – profile

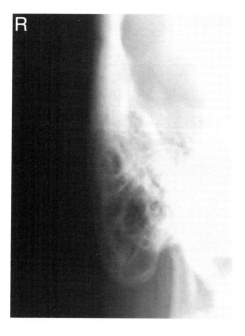

Position of patient and cassette

- The patient lies supine on the table, with the orbito-meatal baseline perpendicular to the table top.
- From a position with the median sagittal plane perpendicular to the table, the head is rotated through an angle of 35 degrees away from the side under examination, such that the median sagittal plane now makes an angle of 55 degrees to the table.
- The vertical tangent to the skull should now be at the level of the middle of the mastoid process under examination, so that the mastoid process is in profile.
- Finally, the head is moved transversely across the table so that the mastoid process being examined is in the midline of the table.

Direction and centring of the X-ray beam

- The central ray is angled caudally so that it makes an angle of 25 degrees to the orbito-meatal plane and is centred to the middle of the mastoid process on the side under examination.
- Collimate tightly around the mastoid process.

Notes

- Both sides are often imaged for comparison.
- A small lead side-marker should be included within the collimation field.

Petrous bone: anterior oblique (Stenver's)

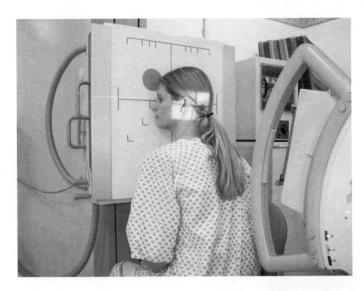

Position of patient and cassette

- The patient may be prone or may be more comfortable being examined erect and facing a vertical Bucky.
- The middle of the supra-orbital margin on the side being examined is centred to the middle of the Bucky.
- The neck is flexed so that the nose and forehead are in contact with the table and the orbito-meatal line is perpendicular to the table.
- From a position where the median sagittal plane is perpendicular to the table, the head is rotated toward the side under examination, such that the median sagittal plane is now at an angle of 45 degrees to the table. This brings the petrous part of the temporal bone parallel to the cassette.
- The neck is extended so that the orbito-meatal line is raised five degrees from horizontal.
- An 18 × 24-cm cassette is placed transversely in the Bucky and is centred at a level to coincide with the central ray.

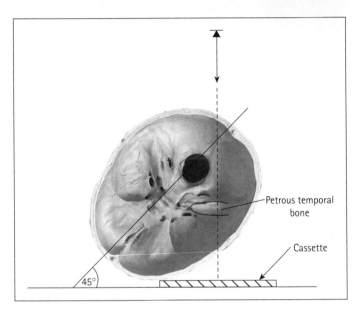

Direction and centring of the X-ray beam

- A 12-degree cephalad beam angulation is employed, i.e. at an angle of seven degrees to the orbito-meatal plane, to separate the occiput from the petrous bone.
- Centre midway between the external occipital protuberance and the external auditory meatus furthest from the cassette.
- Collimate to the mastoid and petrous parts of the temporal bone under examination.

Note

This projection is now more or less redundant due to the superior diagnostic capabilities of CT.

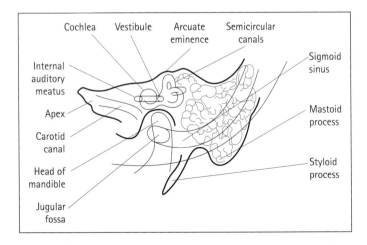

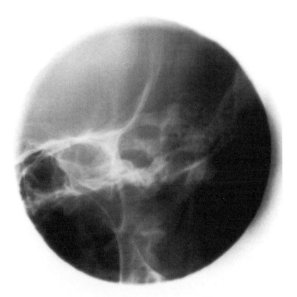

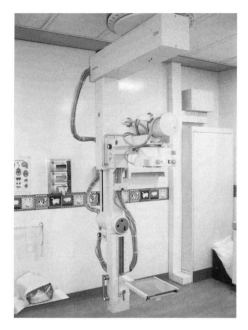

Introduction

The use of the isocentric technique offers considerable advantages over the techniques described previously and will produce images of much higher quality than those produced with just a tube and Bucky or stationary grid. The reasons for this are as follows:

- The central ray and cassette are always perpendicular to each other, thus eliminating distortion.
- The patient is always supine, thus increasing comfort and efficiency of immobilization.
- The patient's head needs to be placed in only one or a limited number of positions. Positioning is then achieved by moving only the skull unit. Again, this increases patient comfort.
- Skull unit movements are very precise and the constant position of the patient's head facilitates accurate corrections to inadequately positioned radiographs.
- It is easier to reproduce images when follow-up projections are requested or to correct errors if an image needs to be repeated.

The Orbix skull unit is one of the most widely used skull units, and the descriptions of technique that follow will be based on this unit. Other manufacturers produce units with slightly different designs, and the reader is advised to consult the handbook supplied with the individual unit. It is worth noting, however, that many of the basic principles used in positioning are very similar, regardless of which unit is employed.

Basic principles of use

All positioning and tube movement is described using the following planes and lines:

- median sagittal plane;
- anthropological plane;
- anthropological baseline;
- auricular plane.

As can be seen from the pictures opposite, the skull unit consists of a tube and cassette holder mounted on an arm (known as the tube arm). This is attached via another arm, which is fastened to the ceiling (the ceiling arm). The table upon which the patient rests can also be moved, allowing a third plane of movement.

An imaginary pivot point about which the tube arm and ceiling arm rotate is known as the isocentre. When positioning, the height of the tube arm and the patient table are arranged in such a way that the isocentre sits in the middle of the anatomical area of interest. The isocentre will then remain in this position, regardless of what angulation is applied to either the tube or the ceiling arm.

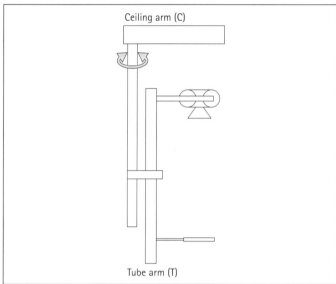

Ceiling arm (C)

Tube arm (T)

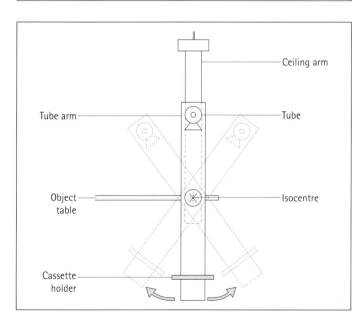

Ceiling arm

Tube arm — Tube

Object table — Isocentre

Cassette holder

8 Cranium: isocentric skull technique

Basic position

One of the advantages of isocentric skull radiography is that the positioning for the various projections undertaken is achieved from one starting position. This is known as the basic position. Once this has been achieved, the patient will remain stationary and the desired projection can be achieved simply by moving the tube arm, ceiling arm and table.

To achieve the basic position, the various tube arm and table movements are used in conjunction with the unit-centring lights to achieve the following:

- The patient lies supine on the skull unit table, with the vertex of the skull close to the top of the table. The median sagittal plane should approximate to the middle of the table. The head should rest on a dedicated foam pad skull support.
- Both the tube arm and the ceiling arm are positioned by the side of the patient, such that they are perpendicular to the median sagittal plane (see photograph). The tube arm angulation should be set to zero.
- The table is moved so that the patient's median sagittal plane is coincident with the vertical line of the cross of positioning light on the light beam diaphragm (A on photograph).
- The patient's infra-orbital plane should be perpendicular to the tabletop and will coincide with the vertical beam of the cross light found on the axis of the tube arm. It may be necessary to move the table along its longitudinal axis in order to achieve this. Immobilize with Velcro headbands once in this position.
- The table height may have to be raised (perhaps in conjunction with the height of the tube arm) to ensure that the centre of the cross light found on the axis of the tube arm is positioned over the external auditory meatus (B on the photograph). The table is usually used at its maximum height.
- Finally, once the above position is achieved, the millimetre positioning scales that measure table movements should be set to zero.

Once the basic position has been achieved, a basic skull series can be undertaken by making the following modifications to the basic position:

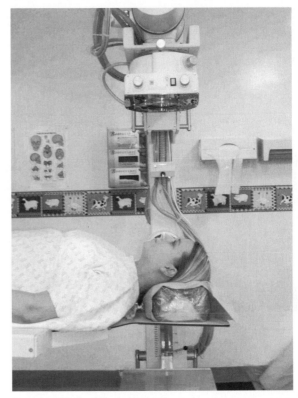

Position of skull unit for basic position

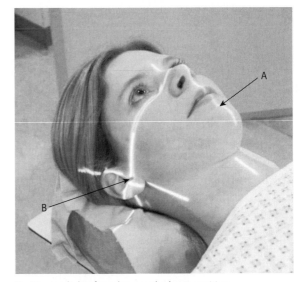

Positioning lights for achieving the basic position

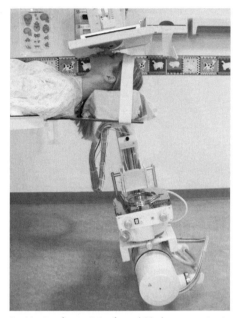

Positioning for occipito-frontal 20-degree projection

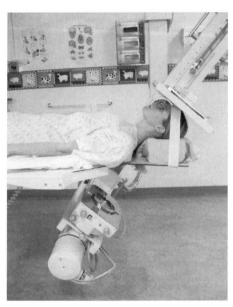

Positioning for half-axial Towne's projection

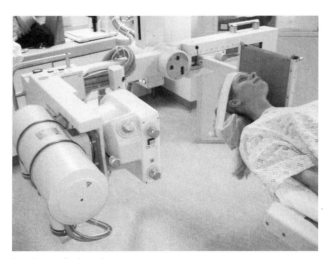

Positioning for lateral projection

Occipito-frontal projection

- From the basic position the table is moved down 40–60 mm (depending on the head size) along its longitudinal axis, such that the positions of cross lights on the light beam diaphragm move superiorly in relation to the patient's head.
- Confine the beam to the size of the head using the iris collimator.
- The tube is now positioned under the patient's head in the postero-anterior position. To achieve this, the ceiling arm will have to be moved so that it is parallel to the median sagittal plane. This allows the tube arm to swing round into the correct position. Once this has been achieved, the ceiling arm is returned to its original position by the right side of the patient.
- A 10-degree caudal angulation will be applied for an 20-degree occipito-frontal projection, zero-degree caudal angulation will be used for a 10-degree occipito-frontal projection, and a 10-degree cranial angulation will be used for an occipito-frontal projection. (Remember that the anthropological baseline is used in isocentric skull radiography. This is deviated from the orbito-meatal base line by 10 degrees.)

Half-axial, reverse Towne's projection

- Position as above, except that a 40-degree cranial angulation is applied with the tube arm in the postero-anterior position.
- The resulting image will be free from the distortion evident when using non-isocentric techniques.

Lateral

- From the basic position, the table is moved down 40–60 mm (depending on the head size) along its longitudinal axis, such that the positions of cross lights on the light beam diaphragm move superiorly in relation the patient's head.
- Swing the ceiling arm round through 90 degrees, such that it is parallel with the median sagittal plane.
- The tube arm is now moved 90 degrees, such that the central ray will be perpendicular to the median sagittal plane. It can be rotated in either direction, so a left or right lateral can be obtained. It is preferable, however, to arrange the cassette on the side of the patient's head that is closest to the injury.
- Confine the beam to the size of the head using the iris collimator.

In all of the projections described, ensure that the cassette holder is moved as close as possible to the patient's head before exposure. This will minimize magnification (unless a degree of magnification is desired).

References

Denton BK (1998). Improving plain radiography of the skull: the half-axial projection re-described. *Synergy* **August**: 9–11.

European Commission (1996). *European Guidelines on Quality Criteria for Diagnostic Radiography Images*. EUR 16260. Luxembourg: Office for Official Publications of the European Communities.

Section 9

The Facial Bones and Sinuses

CONTENTS

INTRODUCTION	260	Orbits: occipito-mental (modified)	269
Radiographic anatomy for positioning	260	Nasal bones: lateral	270
Equipment	262	Mandible: lateral 30 degrees cephalad	271
Recommended projections	262	Mandible: postero-anterior	272
Preparation of patient and immobilization	262	Mandible: postero-anterior oblique	273
		Temporal-mandibular joints: lateral	
FACIAL BONES	263	25 degrees caudad	274
Occipito-mental	263		
Modified mento-occipital	264	PARANASAL SINUSES	275
Occipito-mental 30 degrees caudad	265	Introduction	275
Modified reverse occipito-mental		Recommended projections	275
30 degrees for the severely injured		Anatomy	275
patient	266	Occipito-mental	276
Lateral	267	Occipito-frontal 15 degrees caudad	277
Zygomatic arches: infero-superior	268	Lateral	278

Radiographic anatomy for positioning

The facial bones are a series of irregular bones that are attached collectively to the antro-inferior aspect of the skull. Within these bones, and some of the bones forming the cranium, are a series of air-filled cavities known as the paranasal air sinuses. These communicate with the nasal cavity and appear of higher radiographic density than surrounding tissues, since the air offers little attenuation to the X-ray beam. If the sinuses become filled with fluid due to pathology (e.g. blood in trauma), this results in a decrease in density. The sinuses are therefore best imaged by using a horizontal beam, usually with the patient in the erect position, thus demonstrating levels resulting from any fluid collection.

The following comprise the paranasal air sinuses:

- **Maxillary sinuses (maxillary antra):** paired, pyramidal-shaped structures located within the maxillary bone either side of the nasal cavity. They are the largest of the sinuses.
- **Frontal sinuses:** paired structures located within the frontal bone adjacent to the fronto-nasal articulation. They are very variable in size, and in some individuals they may be absent.
- **Sphenoid sinuses:** structures that lie immediately beneath the sella turcica and posterior to the ethmoid sinuses.
- **Ethmoid sinuses:** a labyrinth of small air spaces that collectively form part of the medial wall of the orbit and the upper lateral walls of the nasal cavity.

Radiological considerations

- The facial bones and sinuses are complicated structures, and the radiographer must be aware of their location and radiographic appearances in order to assess the diagnostic suitability of an image. The accompanying diagrams and radiographs outline the position of the major structures and landmarks used for image assessment.
- Facial projections must demonstrate clearly the likely sites of facial fracture, especially in the mid-facial area. These include the orbital floor, lateral orbital wall and zygomatico-frontal suture, lateral antral wall, and zygomatic arch.
- The signs of fracture in these areas may be subtle, but if they form part of a complex facial fracture they will be very important.
- Facial fractures may be bilateral and symmetrical.

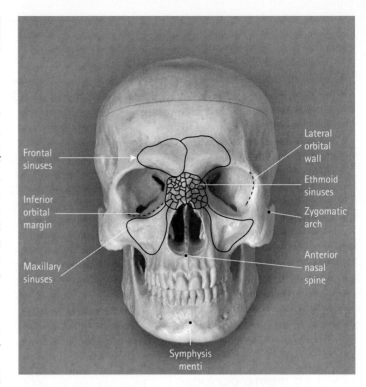

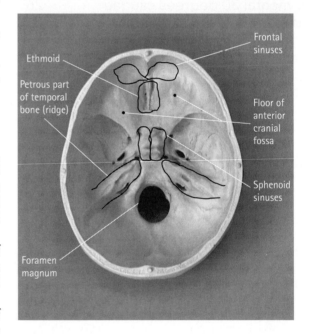

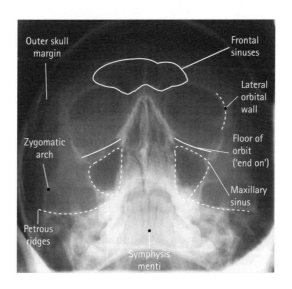

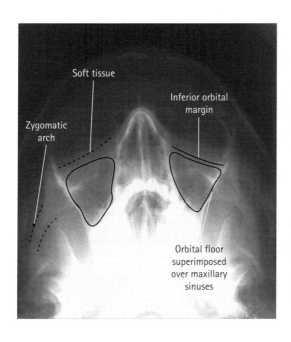

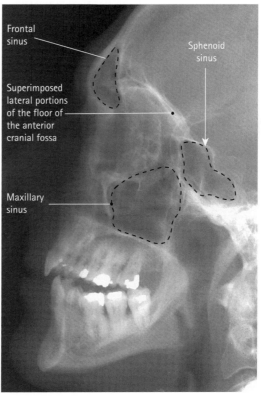

Equipment

Given the subtle pathologies often encountered in this region, resolution is an important consideration. The highest-quality images will be obtained using a skull unit with the cassette holder in the vertical position. The facility to tilt the object table offers considerable advantages for positioning, patient comfort and immobilization.

If no skull unit is available, then a vertical tilting Bucky or stationary grids can be used. A high grid lattice with more than 40 grid lines per centimetre will give far superior results in terms of resolution, and their use is to be recommended.

Cassette size

Since the sinuses are grouped close together, 18 × 24-cm cassettes will provide enough space to visualize the region. A 24 × 30-cm cassette may be required to provide enough coverage for entire facial region.

Collimation

It is essential to use a small field of radiation to exclude all structures except those immediately adjacent to the sinuses, thereby reducing scatter to a minimum and improving image quality. A slightly larger field will be required if all of the facial bones need to be included. Certain skull units offer the advantage of using a circular field collimator, which is more suited to this region.

Opaque legends

Given the tight collimation required, the clip-type side-marker will often be excluded from the field. Therefore, individual side markers that can be attached directly to the cassette face should be available.

Screens

Cassettes with a high-speed intensifying screen/receptor should be employed due to the radiosensitivity of the eyes and other adjacent structures. The loss of resolution is compensated for by gains from using the skull unit, appropriate grid selection and small focal spot size.

Preparation of patient and immobilization

Patient preparation

It is important to remove all items likely to cause artefacts on the final image. These may include metal dentures, spectacles, earrings, hair clips, hair bunches/buns and necklaces. Hearing aids should be removed after full instructions have been given to and understood by the patient.

Immobilization

Short exposure times attainable on modern equipment have led to immobilization not being used in many cases. It should be noted that errors often occur as the patient may move between being positioned and the radiographer walking back to the control panel. If the patient appears to be unstable in any way, it is recommended that the head is immobilized using Velcro straps or other appropriate devices.

Recommended projections

Trauma and pathology	Occipito-mental
	Occipito-mental 30°↓
	(Basic series)
Gross trauma	Basic series; consider lateral
Suspected depressed zygomatic fracture	Basic series; consider modified infero-superior for zygomatic arches
Nasal injury	Collimated occipito-mental may be indicated
Foreign body in eye	Modified occipito-mental for orbits
Mandible trauma	Postero-anterior mandible plus either tomography (orthopantomography) or lateral obliques
	Anterior oblique for symphysis menti injury
TMJ pathology	Tomography; consider lateral 25°↓
TMJ trauma	Tomography; consider lateral oblique mandible or postero-anterior mandible 10-degree cephalad

TMJ, temporo-mandibular joint.

This projection shows the floor of the orbits in profile, the nasal region, the maxillae, the inferior parts of the frontal bone and the zygomatic bone. The zygomatic arches can be seen, but they are visualized end-on, with their entire length superimposed over a small part of the image.

The occipito-mental (OM) projection is designed to project the petrous parts of the temporal bone (which overlie the region and would cause unwanted noise on a facial bone image) below the inferior part of the maxilla.

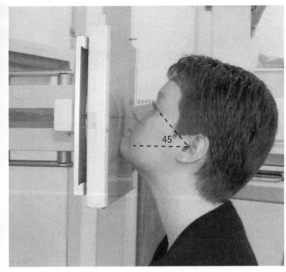

Occipito-mental projection using skull unit

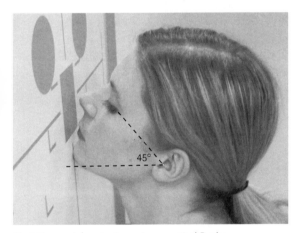

Occipito-mental projection using a vertical Bucky

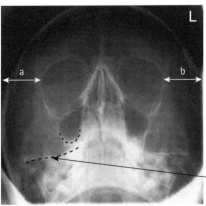

Petrous ridges just below inferior margin of maxillary sinus

Position of patient and cassette

- The projection is best performed with the patient seated facing the skull unit cassette holder or vertical Bucky.
- The patient's nose and chin are placed in contact with the midline of the cassette holder. The head is then adjusted to bring the orbito-meatal baseline to a 45-degree angle to the cassette holder.
- The horizontal central line of the Bucky/cassette holder should be at the level of the lower orbital margins.
- Ensure that the median sagittal plane is at right-angles to the Bucky/cassette holder by checking the outer canthi of the eyes and that the external auditory meatuses are equidistant.

Direction and centring of the X-ray beam

- The central ray of the skull unit should be perpendicular to the cassette holder. By design, it will be centred to the middle of the cassette holder. If this is the case and the above positioning is performed accurately, then the beam will already be centred.
- If using a Bucky, the tube should be centred to the Bucky using a horizontal beam before positioning is undertaken. Again, if the above positioning is performed accurately, and the Bucky height is not altered, then the beam will already be centred.
- To check that the beam is centred properly, the cross-lines on the Bucky or cassette holder should coincide with the patient's anterior nasal spine.

Essential image characteristics

- The petrous ridges must appear below the floors of the maxillary sinuses.
- There should be no rotation. This can be checked by ensuring that the distance from the lateral orbital wall to the outer skull margins is equidistant on both sides (marked a and b on the image opposite).

Common faults and remedies

- Petrous ridges superimposed over the inferior part of the maxillary sinuses: in this case, several errors may have occurred. The orbito-meatal baseline may not have been positioned at 45 degrees to the film: a five- to ten-degree caudal angulation could be applied to the tube to compensate for this.
- As this is an uncomfortable position to maintain, patients often let the angle of the baseline reduce between positioning and exposure. Always check the baseline angle immediately before exposure.

9 Facial bones

Modified mento-occipital

Patients who have sustained trauma will often present supine on a trolley, in a neck brace, and with the radiographic baseline in a fixed position. Modifications in technique will therefore be required by imaging the patient in the antero-posterior position and adjusting the beam angle to ensure that the petrous bones are projected away from the facial bones.

Position of patient and cassette

- The patient will be supine on the trolley and should not be moved. If it is possible to place a cassette and grid under the patient's head without moving the neck, then this should be undertaken. If this is not possible, then place the cassette and grid in the cassette tray under the patient.
- The top of the cassette should be at least 5 cm above the top of the head to allow for any cranial beam angulation.
- A 24 × 30-cm cassette is recommended.

Direction and centring of the X-ray beam

- The patient should be assessed for position (angle) of the orbito-meatal line in relation to the cassette.
- If the baseline makes an angle of 45 degrees back from the vertical (chin raised), then a perpendicular beam can be employed centred to the midline at the level of the lower orbital margins.
- If the orbito-meatal baseline makes an angle of less than 45 degrees with the cassette because of the neck brace, then the difference between the measured angle and 45 degrees should be added to the beam in the form of a cranial angulation. The centring point remains the same.
- For example, if the orbito-meatal baseline was estimated to be 20 degrees from the vertical as the chin was raised, then a 25-degree cranial angulation would need to be applied to the tube to maintain the required angle (see diagram).

Notes

- As the cranial angulation increases, the top of the cassette should be displaced further from the top of the head.
- These images suffer greatly from poor resolution resulting from magnification and distortion from the cranial angulation. It may be worth considering postponing the examination until any spinal injury can be ruled out and the patient can be examined without the neck brace or moved on to a skull unit if other injuries will allow.

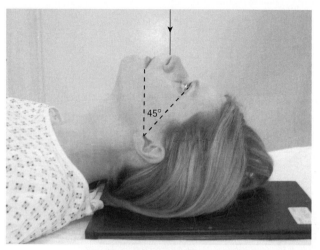
Patient imaged supine with 45-degree baseline

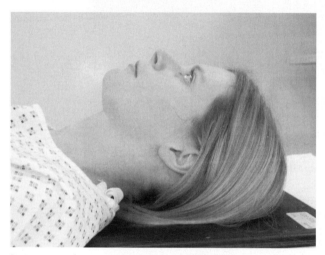
Patient imaged supine with 20-degree baseline and 25-degree cranial angulation

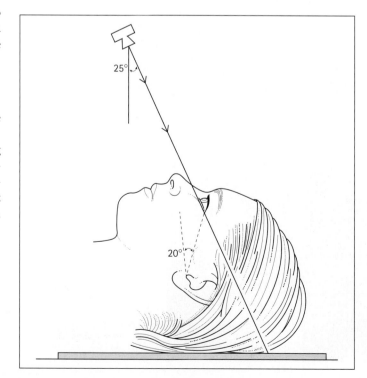

Occipito-mental 30 degrees caudad

This projection demonstrates the lower orbital margins and the orbital floors en face. The zygomatic arches are opened out compared with the occipito-mental projection but they are still foreshortened.

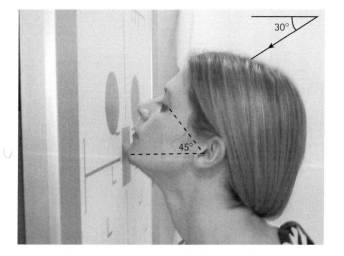

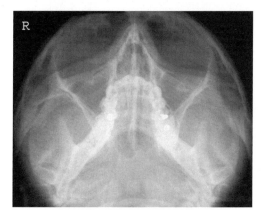

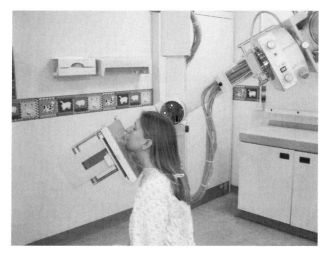

Position of patient and cassette

- The projection is best performed with the patient seated facing the skull unit cassette holder or vertical Bucky.
- The patient's nose and chin are placed in contact with the midline of the cassette holder. The head then is adjusted to bring the orbito-meatal baseline to a 45-degree angle to the cassette holder.
- The horizontal central line of the Bucky or cassette holder should be at the level of the symphysis menti.
- Ensure that the median sagittal plane is at right-angles to the Bucky or cassette holder by checking that the outer canthi of the eyes and the external auditory meatuses are equidistant.

Direction and centring of the X-ray beam

- The tube is angled 30 degrees caudally and centred along the midline, such that the central ray exits at the level of the lower orbital margins.
- To check that the beam is centred properly, the cross-lines on the Bucky or cassette holder should coincide approximately with the upper symphysis menti region (this will vary with anatomical differences between patients).

Essential image characteristics

- The floors of the orbit will be clearly visible through the maxillary sinuses, and the lower orbital margin should be demonstrated clearly.
- There should be no rotation. This can be checked by ensuring that the distance from the lateral orbital wall to the outer skull margins is equidistant on both sides.

Common faults and remedies

- Failure to demonstrate the whole of the orbital floor due to under-angulation and failure to maintain the orbito-meatal baseline at 45 degrees. For the patient who finds difficulty in achieving the latter, a greater caudal tube angle may be required.

Note

On many skull units, the tube and cassette holder are fixed permanently, such that the tube is perpendicular to the cassette. This presents a problem for this projection, as the baseline should be 45 degrees to the cassette. This would not be the case when the 30-degree tube angle is applied. The patient must therefore be positioned with their orbito-meatal line positioned at 45 degrees to an imaginary vertical line from the floor (see image opposite). Although such an arrangement makes positioning and immobilization more difficult, it does have the advantage of producing an image that is free of distortion.

9 | Facial bones

Modified reverse occipito-mental 30 degrees for the severely injured patient

It is possible to undertake a reverse OM30°↓(i.e. an MO30°↑) with the patient supine on a trolley, provided that the patient can raise their orbito-meatal baseline to 45 degrees. Problems arise when the baseline is less than 45 degrees, as additional cranial angulation causes severe distortion in the resultant image. This results from the additional cranial angulation that must be applied to the tube. Clements and Ponsford (1991) have proposed an effective solution to this problem, which is described below.

Position of patient and cassette

- The patient is supine on the trolley with the head adjusted, such that the median sagittal plane and orbito-meatal baseline are perpendicular to the trolley top.
- A gridded cassette is positioned vertically against the vertex of the skull and supported with foam pads and sandbags, such that it is perpendicular to the median sagittal plane.

Direction and centring of the X-ray beam

- The tube is angled 20 degrees to the horizontal (towards the floor) and centred to the symphysis menti in the midline.
- A 100-cm focus-to-film distance (FFD) is used, but it may be necessary to increase this for obese or large patients, as the tube will be positioned close to the chest. Remember to increase the exposure if the FFD is increased.

Essential image characteristics

- The floors of the orbit will be visible clearly through the maxillary sinuses, and the lower orbital margin should be demonstrated clearly.
- There should be no rotation. This can be checked by ensuring that the distance from the lateral orbital wall to the outer skull margins is equidistant on both sides.

Note

If the orbito-meatal baseline is raised by any degree, then there will have to be a corresponding correction of the tube angle to compensate. This may be required if the patient is in a rigid neck brace, when the neck must not be moved.

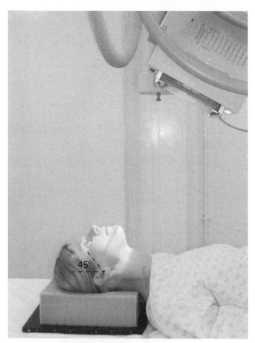

Positioning for reverse OM30; this will result in image distortion

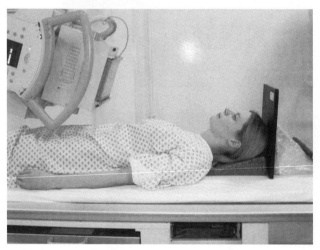

Positioning for modified projection

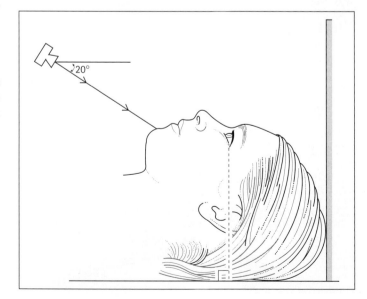

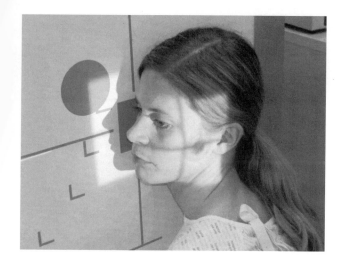

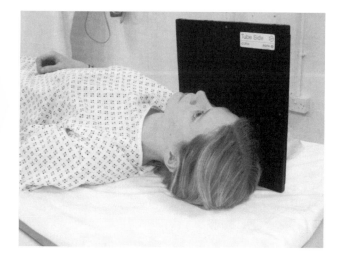

Lateral

In cases of injury, this projection should be taken using a horizontal beam in order to demonstrate any fluid levels in the paranasal sinuses. The patient may be positioned erect or supine.

Position of patient and cassette

Erect

- The patient sits facing the vertical Bucky or cassette holder of the skull unit. The head is rotated, such that the side under examination is in contact with the Bucky or cassette holder.
- The arm on the same side is extended comfortably by the trunk, whilst the other arm may be used to grip the Bucky for stability. The Bucky height is altered, such that its centre is 2.5 cm inferior to the outer canthus of the eye.

Supine

- The patient lies on the trolley, with the arms extended by the sides and the median sagittal plane vertical to the trolley top.
- A gridded cassette is supported vertically against the side under examination, so that the centre of the cassette is 2.5 cm inferior to the outer canthus of the eye.

Notes

In either case, the median sagittal plane is brought parallel to the cassette by ensuring that the inter-orbital line is at right-angles to the cassette and the nasion and external occipital protuberance are equidistant from it.

Direction and centring of the X-ray beam

- Centre the horizontal central ray to a point 2.5 cm inferior to the outer canthus of the eye.

Essential image characteristics

- The image should contain all of the facial bones sinuses, including the frontal sinus and posteriorly to the anterior border of the cervical spine.
- A true lateral will have been obtained if the lateral portions of the floor of the anterior cranial fossa are superimposed.

Notes

- This projection is often reserved for gross trauma, as the facial structures are superimposed.
- If a lateral is undertaken for a suspected foreign body in the eye, then additional collimation and alteration in the centring point will be required.

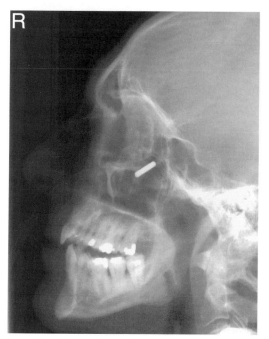

Lateral facial bones showing foreign body

Facial bones

Zygomatic arches: infero-superior

This projection is essentially a modified submento-vertical (SMV) projection. It is often referred to as the 'jug-handle projection', as the whole length of the zygomatic arch is demonstrated in profile against the side of the skull and facial bones.

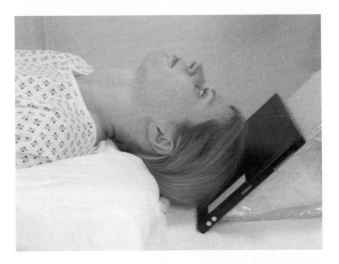

Position of patient and cassette

- The patient lies supine, with one or two pillows under the shoulders to allow the neck to be extended fully.
- An 18 × 24-cm cassette is placed against the vertex of the skull, such that its long axis is parallel with the axial plane of the body. It should be supported in this position with foam pads and sandbags.
- The flexion of the neck is now adjusted to bring the long axis of the zygomatic arch parallel to the cassette.
- The head in now tilted five to ten degrees away from the side under examination. This allows the zygomatic arch under examination to be projected on to the film without superimposition of the skull vault or facial bones.

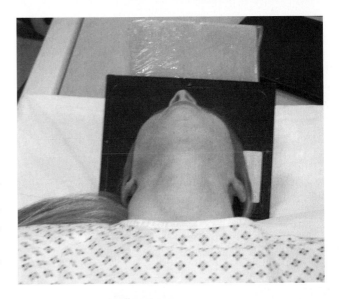

Direction and centring of the X-ray beam

- The central ray should be perpendicular to the cassette and long axis of the zygomatic arch.
- A centring point should be located such that the central ray passes through the space between the midpoint of the zygomatic arch and the lateral border of the facial bones.
- Tight collimation can be applied to reduce scatter and to avoid irradiating the eyes.

Essential image characteristics

- The whole length of the zygomatic arch should be demonstrated clear of the skull. If this has not been achieved, then it may be necessary to repeat the examination and alter the degree of head tilt to try and bring the zygomatic arch clear of the skull.

Radiological considerations

Depressed fracture of the zygoma can be missed clinically due to soft-tissue swelling, making the bony defect less obvious. Radiography has an important role in ensuring that potentially disfiguring depression of the cheekbones is not missed.

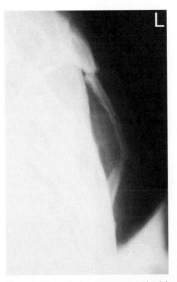

Zygomatic arch demonstrating double fracture

Notes

- Both sides may be examined on one cassette using two exposures.
- It is important for the radiographer to have a good understanding of anatomy to correctly locate the position of the zygomatic arch and thus allow for accurate positioning and collimation.
- In some individuals, variations in anatomy may not allow the arch to be projected clear of the skull.

Orbits: occipito-mental (modified)

This is a frequently undertaken projection used to assess injuries to the orbital region (e.g. blow-out fracture of the orbital floor) and to exclude the presence of metallic foreign bodies in the eyes before magnetic resonance imaging (MRI) investigations. The projection is essentially an under-tilted occipito-mental with the orbito-meatal baseline raised 10 degrees less than in the standard occipito-mental projection.

Position of patient and cassette

- The projection is best performed with the patient seated facing the skull unit cassette holder or vertical Bucky.
- The patient's nose and chin are placed in contact with the midline of the cassette holder. The head is then adjusted to bring the orbito-meatal baseline to a 35-degree angle to the cassette holder.
- The horizontal central line of the vertical Bucky or cassette holder should be at the level of the midpoint of the orbits.
- Ensure that the median sagittal plane is at right-angles to the Bucky or cassette holder by checking that the outer canthi of the eyes and the external auditory meatuses are equidistant.

Direction and centring of the X-ray beam

- The central ray of the skull unit should be perpendicular to the cassette holder and by design will be centred to the middle of the image receptor. If this is the case and the above positioning is performed accurately, then the beam will already be centred.
- If using a Bucky, the tube should be centred to the Bucky using a horizontal beam before positioning is undertaken. Again, if the above positioning is performed accurately and the Bucky height is not altered, then the beam will already be centred.
- To check that the beam is centred properly, the cross-lines on the Bucky or cassette holder should coincide with the midline at the level of the mid-orbital region.

Essential image characteristics

- The orbits should be roughly circular in appearance (they will be more oval in the occipito-mental projection).
- The petrous ridges should appear in the lower third of the maxillary sinuses.
- There should be no rotation. This can be checked by ensuring that the distance from the lateral orbital wall to the outer skull margins is equidistant on both sides.

Notes

- If the examination is purely to exclude foreign bodies in the eye, then tight 'letter-box' collimation to the orbital region should be applied.
- A dedicated cassette should be used for foreign bodies This should be cleaned regularly to avoid small artefacts on the screens being confused with foreign bodies.
- If a foreign body is suspected, then a second projection may be undertaken, with the eyes in a different position to differentiate this from an image artefact. The initial exposure could be taken with the eyes pointing up and the second with the eyes pointing down.

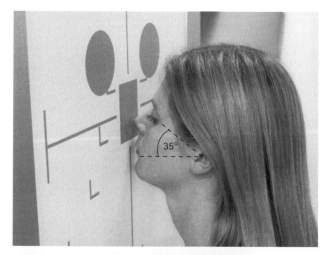

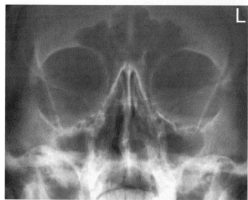

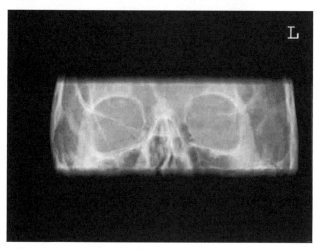

Collimation used for foreign-body projection

9 Facial bones

Nasal bones: lateral

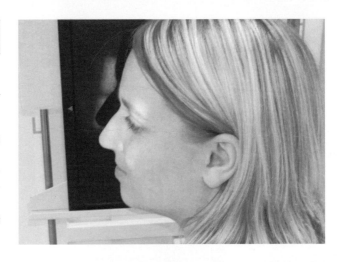

Position of patient and cassette

- The patient sits facing an 18 × 24-cm cassette supported in the cassette stand of a vertical Bucky.
- The head is turned so that the median sagittal plane is parallel with the cassette and the inter-pupillary line is perpendicular to the cassette.
- The nose should be roughly coincident with the centre of the cassette.

Direction and centring of the X-ray beam

- A horizontal central ray is directed through the centre of the nasal bones and collimated to include the nose.

Radiological considerations

Nasal fracture can usually be detected clinically and is rarely treated actively. If a fracture causes nasal deformity or breathing difficulty, then it may be straightened, but lateral projections will not help. Considering the dose of radiation to the eye, this projection should be avoided in most instances.

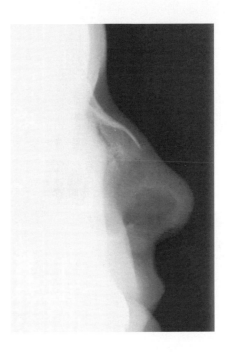

Notes

- A high-resolution cassette may be used if detail is required.
- This projection may be useful for foreign bodies in the nose. In this case, a soft-tissue exposure should be employed.
- In the majority of cases, severe nasal injuries will require only an occipito-mental projection to assess the nasal septum and surrounding structures.
- The projection can also be undertaken with the patient supine and the cassette supported against the side of the head.

Mandible: lateral 30 degrees cephalad

Position of patient and cassette

- The patient lies in the supine position. The trunk is rotated slightly and then supported with pads to allow the side of the face being examined to come into contact with the cassette, which will be lying on the tabletop.

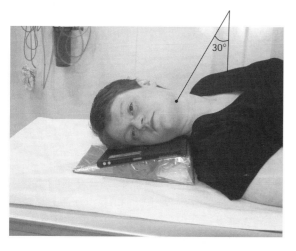

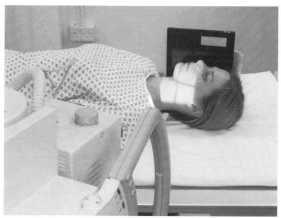

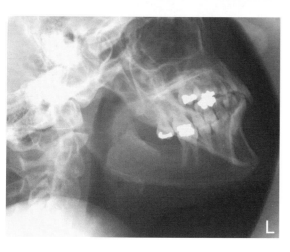

- The median sagittal plane should be parallel with the cassette and the inter-pupillary line perpendicular.
- The neck may be flexed slightly to clear the mandible from the spine.
- The cassette and head can now be adjusted and supported so the above position is maintained but is comfortable for the patient.
- The long axis of the cassette should be parallel with the long axis of the mandible and the lower border positioned 2 cm below the lower border of the mandible.
- The projection may also be performed with a horizontal beam in trauma cases when the patient cannot be moved.
- In this case, the patient will be supine with the median sagittal plane at right-angles to the tabletop. The cassette is supported vertically against the side under examination.

Direction and centring of the X-ray beam

- The central ray is angled 30 degrees cranially at an angle of 60 degrees to the cassette and is centred 5 cm inferior to the angle of the mandible remote from the cassette.
- Collimate to include the whole of the mandible and temporo-mandibular joint (TMJ) (include the external auditory meatus (EAM) at the edge of the collimation field).

Essential image characteristics

- The body and ramus of each side of the mandible should not be superimposed.
- The image should include the whole of the mandible, from the TMJ to the symphysis menti.

Radiological considerations

Do not mistake the mandibular canal, which transmits the inferior alveolar nerve, for a fracture.

Common faults and remedies

- Superimposition of the mandibular bodies will result if the angle applied to the tube is less than 30 degrees or if the centring point is too high.
- If the shoulder is obscuring the region of interest in the horizontal beam projection, then a slight angulation towards the floor may have to be applied, or, if the patient's condition will allow, tilt the head towards the side under examination.

Notes

- In cases of injury, both sides should be examined to demonstrate a possible contre-coup fracture.
- Tilting the head towards the side being examined may aid positioning if the shoulder is interfering with the primary beam.

Mandible: postero-anterior

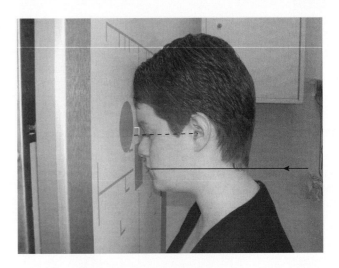

Position of patient and cassette

- The patient sits facing the vertical Bucky or skull unit cassette holder. Alternatively, in the case of trauma, the projection may be supine on a trolley, giving an antero-posterior projection.
- The patient's median sagittal plane should be coincident with the midline of the Bucky or cassette holder. The head is then adjusted to bring the orbito-meatal baseline perpendicular to the Bucky or cassette holder.
- The median sagittal plane should be perpendicular to the cassette. Check that the external auditory meatuses are equidistant from the cassette.
- The cassette should be positioned such that the middle of an 18 × 24-cm cassette, when placed longitudinally in the Bucky or cassette holder, is centred at the level of the angles of the mandible.

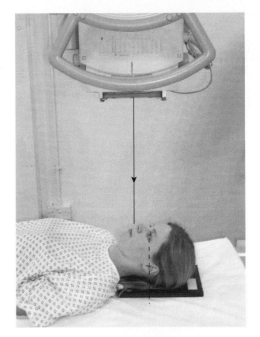

Direction and centring of the X-ray beam

- The central ray is directed perpendicular to the cassette and centred in the midline at the levels of the angles of the mandible.

Essential image characteristics

- The whole of the mandible from the lower portions of the TMJs to the symphysis menti should be included in the image.
- There should be no rotation evident.

Radiological considerations

- This projection demonstrates the body and rami of the mandible and may show transverse or oblique fractures not evident on other projections or dental panoramic tomography (DPT) (orthopantomography, OPT).
- The region of the symphysis menti is superimposed over the cervical vertebra and will be seen more clearly when using the anterior oblique projection.

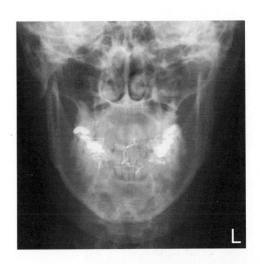

Common faults and remedies

Superimposition of the upper parts of the mandible over the temporal bone will result if the orbito-meatal baseline is not perpendicular to the cassette.

Note

A 10-degree cephalad angulation of the beam may be required to demonstrate the mandibular condyles and temporal mandibular joints.

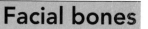

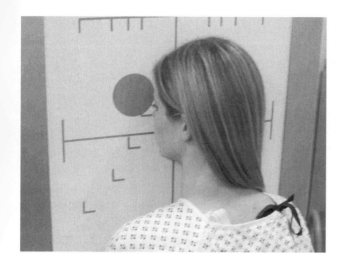

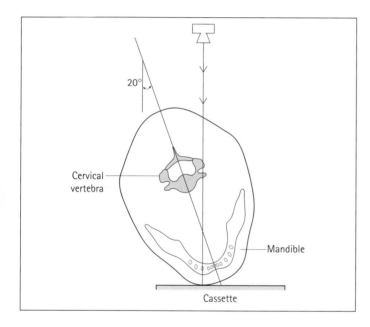

Mandible: postero-anterior oblique

This projection demonstrates the region of the symphysis menti.

Position of patient and cassette

- The patient sits facing the vertical Bucky or skull unit cassette holder. Alternatively, in the case of trauma, the projection may be supine on a trolley, giving an antero-posterior projection.
- The patient's median sagittal plane should be coincident with the midline of the Bucky or cassette holder. The head is then adjusted to bring the orbito-meatal baseline perpendicular to the Bucky or cassette holder.
- From a position with the median sagittal plane perpendicular to the cassette, the head is rotated 20 degrees to either side, so that the cervical vertebra will be projected clear of the symphysis menti.
- The head is now repositioned so the region of the symphysis menti is coincident with the middle of the cassette.
- The cassette should be positioned such that the middle of an 18 × 24-cm cassette, when placed longitudinally in the Bucky or cassette holder, is centred at the level of the angles of the mandible.

Direction and centring of the X-ray beam

- The central ray is directed perpendicular to the cassette and centred 5 cm from the midline, away from the side being examined, at the level of the angles of the mandible.

Essential image characteristics

- The symphysis menti should demonstrated without any superimposition of the cervical vertebra.

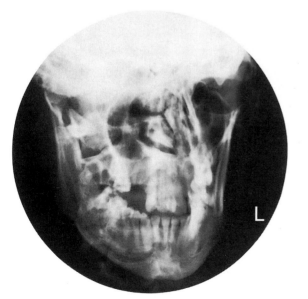

Temporal-mandibular joints: lateral 25 degrees caudad

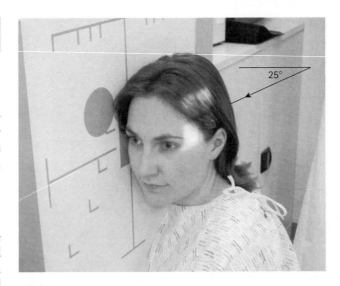

It is usual to examine both temporal-mandibular joints. For each side, a projection is obtained with the mouth open as far as possible and then another projection with the mouth closed. An additional projection may be required with the teeth clenched.

Position of patient and cassette

- The patient sits facing the vertical Bucky or skull unit cassette holder or lies prone on the Bucky table. In all cases, the head is rotated to bring the side of the head under examination in contact with the table. The shoulders may also be rotated slightly to help the patient achieve this position.
- The head and Bucky or cassette holder level is adjusted so the centre cross-lines are positioned to coincide with a point 1 cm along the orbito-meatal baseline anterior to the external auditory meatus.
- The median sagittal plane is brought parallel to the cassette by ensuring that the inter-pupillary line is at right-angles to the table top and the nasion and external occipital protuberance are equidistant from it.
- The cassette is placed longitudinally in the cassette holder, such that two exposures can be made without superimposition of the images.

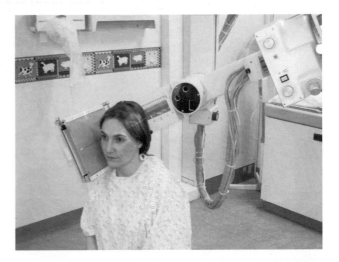

Direction and centring of the X-ray beam

- Using a well-collimated beam or an extension cone, the central ray is angled 25 degrees caudally and will be centred to a point 5 cm superior to the joint remote from the cassette so the central ray passes through the joint nearer the cassette.

Radiological considerations

TMJ images are useful in assessing joint dysfunction by demonstrating erosive and degenerative changes. Open- and closed-mouth projections can be very helpful in assessing whether normal anterior gliding movement of the mandibular condyle occurs on jaw opening. MRI promises greater accuracy, since it also demonstrates the articular cartilages and fibrocartilage discs and how they behave during joint movement.

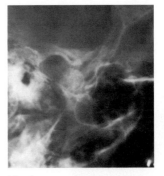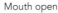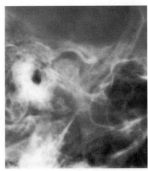

Mouth open   Mouth closed

Notes

- The image should include the correct side-marker and labels to indicate the position of the mouth when the exposure was taken (open, closed, etc.).
- If using a skull unit in which the tube cannot be angled independently of the cassette holder, the inter-pupillary line is at right-angles to an imaginary vertical line drawn from the floor.
- This projection may supplement DPT (OPT) images of the TMJs. Postero-anterior projections may be undertaken by modifying the technique described for the postero-anterior mandible on p. 272.

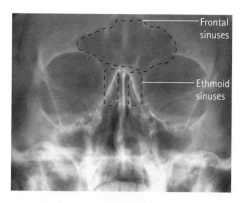

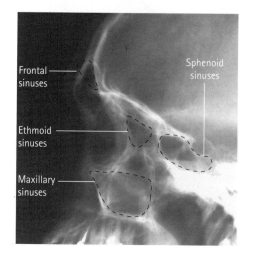

Introduction

Plain images of the sinuses are unreliable for diagnosis of inflammatory sinus disease, since many asymptomatic people will have sinus opacification and sinus symptoms may be present in the absence of gross sinus opacification. Acute sinusitis (especially infective) may manifest radiologically as fluid levels in the maxillary antrum, but it is questionable as to whether this alters clinical management. Malignant sinus disease requires more comprehensive imaging by computed tomography (CT) and/or MRI. Some radiology departments will no longer perform plain sinus radiographs.

Recommended projections

Referral	Projection
General sinus survey (GP referral)	Occipito-mental (with open mouth)
Consultant referral (specific projections will vary according to local needs)	Occipito-mental (with open mouth) Occipito-frontal 15 degrees caudad (Lateral)

Anatomy

As mentioned in the introduction to this chapter, the sinuses collectively consist of the following structures (outlined on the radiographs opposite):

- **Maxillary sinuses (maxillary antra):** paired, pyramidal-shaped structures located within the maxillary bone either side of the nasal cavity. They are the largest of the sinuses.
- **Frontal sinuses:** paired structures located within the frontal bone adjacent to the fronto-nasal articulation. They are very variable in size, and in some individuals they may be absent.
- **Sphenoid sinuses:** structures lying immediately beneath the sella turcica and posterior to the ethmoid sinuses.
- **Ethmoid sinuses:** a labyrinth of small air spaces that collectively form part of the medial wall of the orbit and the upper lateral walls of the nasal cavity.

9 Paranasal sinuses

Occipito-mental

This projection is designed to project the petrous part of the temporal bone below the floor of the maxillary sinuses so that fluid levels or pathological changes in the lower part of the sinuses can be visualized clearly.

Position of patient and cassette

- The projection is best performed with the patient seated facing the skull unit cassette holder or vertical Bucky.
- The patient's nose and chin are placed in contact with the midline of the cassette holder. The head is then adjusted to bring the orbito-meatal baseline to a 45-degree angle to the cassette holder.
- The horizontal central line of the Bucky or cassette holder should be at the level of the lower orbital margins.
- Ensure that the median sagittal plane is at right-angles to the Bucky or cassette holder by checking that the outer canthi of the eyes and the external auditory meatuses are equidistant.
- The patient should open the mouth as wide as possible before exposure. This will allow the posterior part of the sphenoid sinuses to be projected through the mouth.

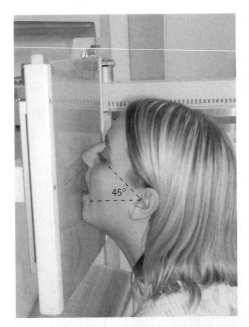

Direction and centring of the X-ray beam

- The central ray of the skull unit should be perpendicular to the cassette holder and by design will be centred to the middle of the image receptor. If this is the case and the above positioning is performed accurately, then the beam will already be centred.
- If using a Bucky, the tube should be centred to the Bucky using a horizontal beam before positioning is undertaken. If the above positioning is performed accurately and the Bucky height is not altered, then the beam will already be centred.
- To check the beam is centred properly, the cross-lines on the Bucky or cassette holder should coincide with the patient's anterior nasal spine.
- Collimate to include all of the sinuses.

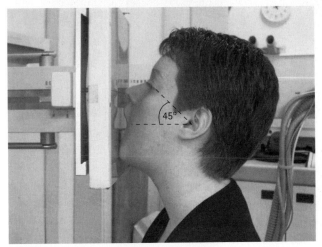

Essential image characteristics

- The petrous ridges must appear below the floors of the maxillary sinuses.
- There should be no rotation. This can be checked by ensuring that the distance from the lateral orbital wall to the outer skull margins is equidistant on both sides.

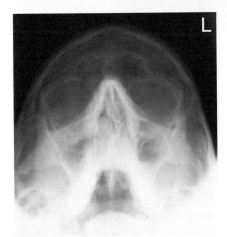

OM radiograph for sinuses demonstrating a polyp in the right maxillary sinus

Common faults and remedies

- Petrous ridges appearing over the inferior part of the maxillary sinuses: in this case, several things may have occurred. The orbito-meatal baseline was not positioned at 45 degrees to the film or a five- to ten-degree caudal angulation may be applied to the tube to compensate. As this is an uncomfortable position to maintain, patients often let the angle of the baseline reduce between positioning and exposure. Therefore, always check the baseline angle immediately before exposure.

Note

To distinguish a fluid level from mucosal thickening, an additional projection may be undertaken with the head tilted, such that a transverse plane makes an angle of about 20 degrees to the floor.

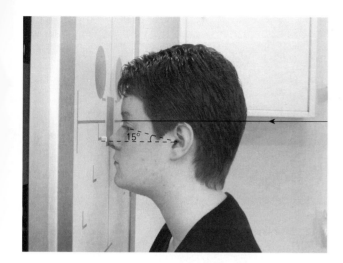

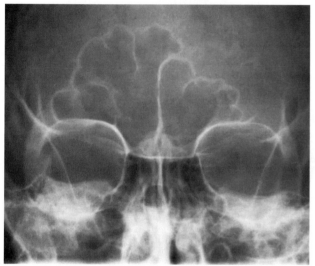

OF 15°↓

Occipito-frontal 15 degrees caudad

This projection is used to demonstrate the frontal and ethmoid sinuses.

Position of patient and cassette

- The patient is seated facing the vertical Bucky or skull unit cassette holder so the median sagittal plane is coincident with the midline of the Bucky and is also perpendicular to it.
- The head is positioned so that the orbito-meatal baseline is raised 15 degrees to the horizontal.
- Ensure that the nasion is positioned in the centre of the Bucky.
- The patient may place the palms of each hand either side of the head (out of the primary beam) for stability.
- An 18 × 24-cm cassette is placed longitudinally in the Bucky tray. The lead name blocker must not interfere with the final image.

Direction and centring of the X-ray beam

- The central ray is directed perpendicular to the vertical Bucky along the median sagittal plane so the beam exits at the nasion.
- A collimation field or extension cone should be set to include the ethmoidal and frontal sinuses. The size of the frontal sinuses can vary drastically from one individual to another.

Essential image characteristics

- All the relevant sinuses should be included within the image.
- The petrous ridges should be projected just above the lower orbital margin.
- It is important to ensure that the skull is not rotated. This can be assessed by measuring the distance from a point in the midline of the skull to the lateral orbital margins. If this is the same on both sides of the skull, then it is not rotated.

Notes

- The degree of angulation may vary according to local preferences. Some departments may prefer to use an OF20°↓ projection. In this case, the orbito-meatal baseline is then raised to the angle required by the projection, i.e. 20 degrees. Alternatively a 20-degree caudal angulation could be employed with the orbito-meatal baseline perpendicular to the image receptor.
- An OF10°↓ or occipito-frontal projection would not be suitable for demonstration of the ethmoid sinuses, as the petrous ridges would obscure the region of interest.

Lateral

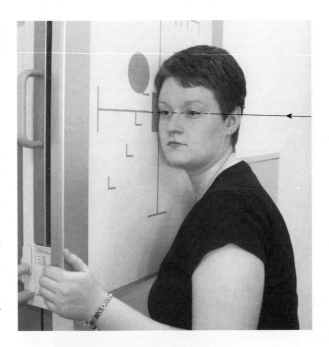

Position of patient and cassette

- The patient sits facing the vertical Bucky or skull unit cassette holder. The head is then rotated, such that the median sagittal plane is parallel to the Bucky and the inter-orbital line is perpendicular to the Bucky.
- The shoulders may be rotated slightly to allow the correct position to be attained. The patient may grip the Bucky for stability.
- The head and Bucky heights are adjusted so that the centre of the Bucky is 2.5 cm along the orbito-meatal line from the outer canthus of the eye.
- Position an 18 × 24-cm cassette longitudinally in the erect Bucky, such that its lower border is 2.5 cm below the level of the upper teeth.
- A radiolucent pad may be placed under the chin for support.

Direction and centring of the X-ray beam

- A horizontal central ray should be employed to demonstrate fluid levels.
- The tube should have been centred previously to the Bucky, such that the central ray will now be centred to a point 2.5 cm posterior to the outer canthus of the eye.

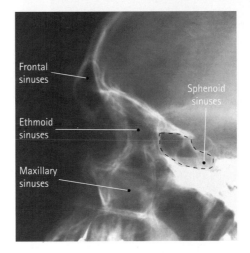

Frontal sinuses

Ethmoid sinuses

Maxillary sinuses

Sphenoid sinuses

Common faults and remedies

This is not an easy position for the patient to maintain. Check the position of all planes immediately before exposure, as the patient probably will have moved.

Essential image characteristics

- A true lateral will have been achieved if the lateral portions of the floors of the anterior cranial fossa are superimposed.

Note

This projection may also be undertaken with the patient supine and the cassette supported vertically against the side of the face. Again, a horizontal beam is used to demonstrate fluid levels.

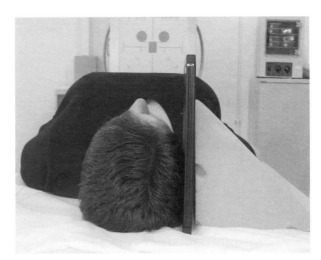

Reference

Clements R, Ponsford A (1991). A modified view of the facial bones in the seriously injured. *Radiography Today* **57**:10–12.

CONTENTS

INTRODUCTION	280
Intra-oral radiography	280
Extra-oral radiography	280
The dentition	281
Dental formulae	282
Palmer notation	282
Fédération Dentaire International notation	283
Terminology	284
Occlusal planes	284
X-ray equipment features	285
Image receptors	286
Image acquisition	288
Film mounting and identification of intra-oral films	289
Radiation protection	290
Cross-infection control	290
Film processing	290
Principles for optimal image geometry	291
BITEWING RADIOGRAPHY	292
Quality standards for bitewing radiography	294
PERIAPICAL RADIOGRAPHY	295
Bisecting angle technique	295
Paralleling technique	300
Third molar region	304
Complete mouth survey or full mouth survey	305
OCCLUSAL RADIOGRAPHY	306
Terminology	306
Recommended projections	306

Radiological considerations	306
Vertex occlusal of the maxilla	307
True occlusal of the mandible	308
Oblique occlusal of the maxilla	310
Oblique occlusal of the mandible	312
LATERAL OBLIQUE OF THE MANDIBLE AND MAXILLA	314
General imaging principles	314
Lateral oblique of the body of the mandible and maxilla	314
Lateral oblique of the ramus of the mandible	316
DENTAL PANORAMIC TOMOGRAPHY	318
Principles of panoramic image formation	318
Image acquisition	319
Problems with panoramic radiography	323
CEPHALOMETRY	325
X-ray equipment features	325
Lateral projection	326
Postero-anterior projection	328
REFERENCES	329
Specialized textbooks on dental radiography	329
ACKNOWLEDGEMENTS	329

10 Introduction

Dental radiography is the most common radiographic examination, comprising 33% of all medical examinations (Tanner *et al.* 2000). Radiographs are used in dentistry for many reasons, summarized below:

- To detect pathology associated with teeth and their supporting structures, such as caries, periodontal disease and periapical pathology.
- To detect anomalies/injuries associated with the teeth, their supporting structures, the maxilla and the mandible.
- To determine the presence/absence of teeth and to localize unerupted teeth.
- To measure the length of the roots of teeth before endodontic therapy.
- To detect the presence/absence of radio-opaque salivary calculi and foreign bodies.
- To detect anomalies/injuries/pathology of adjacent facial structures.
- To evaluate skeletal and/or soft tissues before orthodontic treatment.
- To monitor the progression of orthodontic treatment and dental disease.
- To enable a preoperative assessment of skeletal and soft tissue patterns before orthognathic surgery.
- To assess bony healing and effectiveness of surgical treatment of the patient postoperatively.

Dental radiography involves techniques in which the film is placed either inside the mouth (intra-oral radiography) or outside the mouth (extra-oral radiography).

Intra-oral radiography

The most frequently requested intra-oral projections are bitewing radiography, periapical radiography and occlusal radiography.

Bitewing radiography is a lateral view of the posterior regions of the jaws. The view demonstrates the crowns of the teeth and the alveolar crestal bone of the premolar and molar regions of both the maxilla and mandible.

Periapical radiography is a lateral projection displaying both the crown and the root of the tooth and the surrounding bone.

Occlusal radiography comprises a number of views in which the film is positioned in the occlusal plane.

Extra-oral radiography

The most frequently requested extra-oral projections are dental panoramic radiography, oblique lateral radiography and cephalometry.

Dental panoramic radiography is a projection that produces an image of both jaws and their respective dentitions on a single extra-oral film.

Oblique lateral radiography demonstrates large areas of the maxilla and mandible, with the region imaged dependent on the technique chosen.

Cephalometry employs techniques to produce standardized and reproducible films of the facial bones for use in orthodontic, orthognathic and implant treatment.

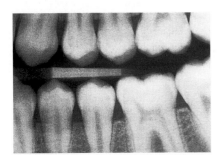

Left horizontal adult bitewing radiograph

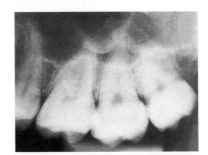

Periapical radiograph of the left maxillary premolar/molar region

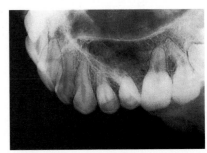

Upper left posterior oblique occlusal radiograph

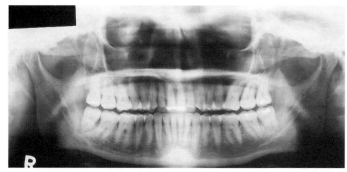

Dental panoramic tomograph of an adult dentate patient

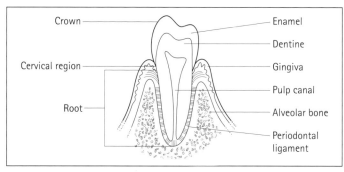

Schematic view of the basic components of the tooth and its supporting tissue

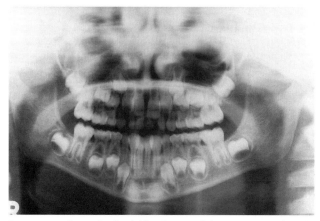

Panoramic radiograph of a child in the mixed-dentition stage of tooth development

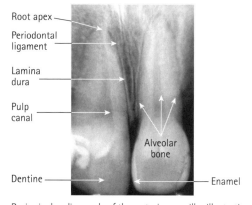

Periapical radiograph of the anterior maxilla, illustrating normal radiographic anatomy of the tooth and supporting structures

The primary or deciduous dentition comprises 20 teeth, with five in each quadrant of the jaws. These are replaced from six years onwards by a permanent dentition of 32 teeth. With eruption of all 32 permanent teeth, there will be eight permanent teeth in each quadrant. Some teeth may fail to develop or erupt, a complication most commonly affecting the third permanent molars (the wisdom teeth).

From the midline moving posteriorly, the teeth in the anterior part of the jaws comprise the central incisor, the lateral incisor and the canine (cuspid). This terminology is used in both deciduous and permanent dentitions. In the permanent dentition posterior to the canine, there are a first and a second premolar (bicuspid) followed by a first, a second and, if they develop, a third permanent molar. The deciduous dentition differs in that there are only two teeth posterior to the deciduous canine, a first and a second deciduous molar.

Each tooth consists of a variety of hard, mineralized tissues with a central area, the pulp chamber and canal, consisting of blood vessels and nerves supported by loose connective tissue. The part of the tooth that projects above the gingiva (gum) and is evident in the mouth is the crown; the portion embedded within the jaw is known as the root. The constriction between the crown and the root is known as the cervical region.

The outer surface of the crown of the tooth comprises enamel with a less mineralized tissue, dentine, below it. The enamel, containing 96% by weight of inorganic material, is radiographically distinguishable from the dentine, which is 70% mineralized with hydroxyapatite. Enamel is limited to the crown of the tooth, whereas dentine encircles the pulp chamber in the crown of the tooth and extends into the root of the tooth, enveloping the pulp canal. Cementum is a thin layer of bone-like material (50% mineralized with hydroxyapatite) covering the dentine of the root and forming the periphery of the root surface. It is not possible to distinguish radiographically between cementum and dentine. Nerves and nutrient vessels enter the pulp through the root apex.

The tooth, depending on its position in the mouth, may have one or several roots. In the anterior regions of the jaws, in both dentitions, the incisor and canine teeth are single-rooted. The molar teeth, in both dentitions, have several roots. As a generality, in the upper jaw the molar teeth have three roots, whilst in the lower jaw two-rooted molars are the norm. The roots associated with the third permanent molar in both jaws may vary in their number and complexity.

The tooth is supported in its alveolar socket by a periodontal ligament, the fibres of which are embedded in the cementum of the root surface and the surrounding alveolar bone. A thin layer of dense bone encircles the tooth socket. Radiographically, this appears as a linear radio-opacity and is referred to as the lamina dura. The periodontal ligament appears as a uniform (0.4–1.9 mm), linear radio-lucency around the root. In the absence of periodontal disease, the alveolar bone should extend to a point 1.5 mm below the cemento-enamel junction.

Dental formulae

There are several internationally recognized methods of identifying the teeth that require radiography. In those cases in which a patient is edentulous (i.e. no teeth visible within the dental arches), a clinician will continue to use the dental formula to denote the part of the oral cavity requiring radiography.

The two most commonly used methods of notation are:

- Palmer notation; and
- Fédération Dentaire International (FDI) notation.

Palmer notation

This technique is known also by the names Zsigmondy–Palmer system, chevron system and the set square system.

Each dental quadrant extends from the midline of the oral cavity posteriorly and, individually, corresponds to the upper left and right quadrants in the maxilla and the lower left and right quadrants in the mandible.

The Palmer notation is depicted schematically, with a vertical line between the central maxillary and mandibular incisors and a horizontal line between the maxilla and mandible, dividing the oral cavity into quadrants. The clinician requesting intraoral radiography uses these vertical and horizontal lines to denote the quadrant to which the tooth/teeth to be radiographed belong.

To avoid confusion between the permanent and deciduous dentition, the following convention is observed:

- **For the deciduous dentition:** five teeth in each quadrant are assigned the letters A–E, from the central deciduous incisor to the second deciduous molar, respectively.
- **For the permanent dentition:** eight teeth in each quadrant are assigned the numbers 1–8, from the central incisor to the third permanent molar, respectively.

The number or letter of the tooth to be radiographed is then added to complete the notation.

Examples of requests for dental examinations using this system are:

C⌋ – upper right deciduous canine.

⌈78 – lower left second and third molars.

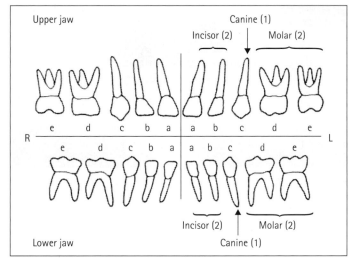

Deciduous teeth

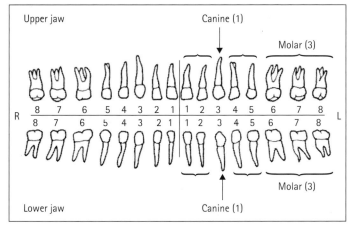

Permanent teeth

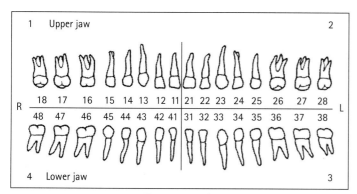

Deciduous teeth

Permanent teeth

Fédération Dentaire International notation

The formula devised by the FDI identifies each tooth using two digits. This method of notation is preferred by some clinicians to avoid the typographical errors that can sometimes affect the Palmer system.

The dentition is again divided into four quadrants. These are assigned the numbers 1–4 for the permanent teeth and the numbers 5–8 for the deciduous dentition. In both dentitions, the quadrants follow on numerically, starting from the upper right, to the upper left, to the lower left and, finally, to the lower right. The number of the quadrant precedes the number of the tooth to be radiographed.

The convention is for individual teeth in either dentition to be numbered sequentially from 1 (for the central incisor) to the most distal molar, i.e. 1–8 in each quadrant in the permanent dentition and 1–5 for the deciduous dentition.

Examples of requests for dental examinations using this formula are:

53 – upper right deciduous canine.
37, 38 – lower left second and third molars.

Terminology

Dentists use the following terms to describe the tooth surfaces:

- **Mesial** represents that surface of the tooth adjacent to the median plane following the curvature of the dental arch.
- **Distal** represents that surface of the tooth furthest away from the median plane following the curvature of the dental arch.
- **Lingual** or **palatal** refers to the inner aspect of the teeth or dental arches adjacent to the tongue or palate, respectively.
- **Buccal** or **labial** refers to the outer aspect of the teeth or dental arches adjacent to the cheeks or lips, respectively.
- **Occlusal** refers to the biting surface of both premolar and molar teeth.
- **Incisal** refers to the horizontal flat surface of the incisor teeth.

Occlusal planes

The occlusal plane is the plane that passes through the opposing biting surfaces of the teeth. The terms **upper occlusal plane** and **lower occlusal plane** are used in radiographic positioning when carrying out intra-oral radiography.

It is necessary to adjust the position of the patient's head before intra-oral radiography to ensure that the appropriate occlusal plane is horizontal and the median plane is vertical. Common radiographic centring points are used to achieve these aims with the patient seated and the head supported adequately.

With the mouth open, the upper occlusal plane lies 4 cm below and parallel to a line joining the tragus of the ear to the ala of the nose.

The lower occlusal plane lies 2 cm below and parallel to a line joining the tragus of the ear to the angle of the mouth with the mouth open.

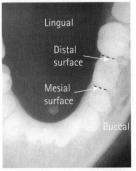

True occlusal radiograph of the mandible

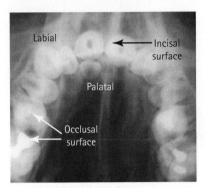

Vertex occlusal radiograph

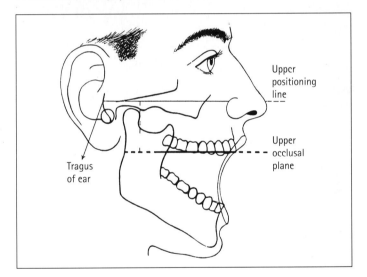

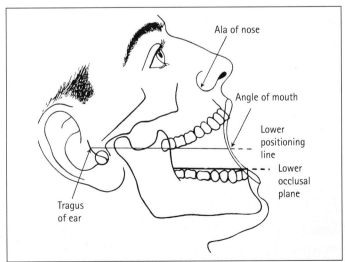

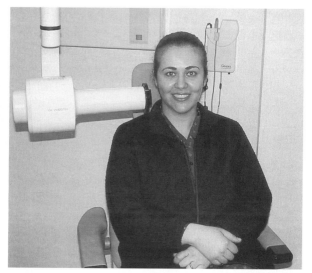

Patient sitting in dental chair with adjacent intra-oral X-ray. X-ray equipment is fitted with a long, open-ended spacer cone (beam-indicating device)

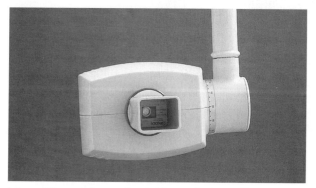

Intra-oral X-ray equipment fitted with metallic rectangular spacer cone

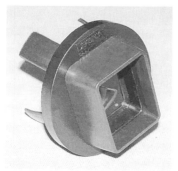

Example of a removable collimator (Dentsply Rinn® Universal collimator)

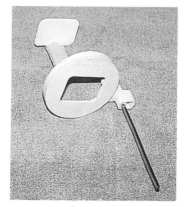

Dentsply Rinn® stainless steel collimator attached by tabs to a Dentsply Rinn XCP® film holder

X-ray equipment features

Dental equipment for intra-oral radiography is designed in order to comply with radiation protection legislation and to ensure that the patient dose is minimized. Such equipment will have the following features:

- **X-ray tube potential:**
  - nominal tube potential not lower than 50 kVp;
  - recommended operating range of 60–70 kVp.
- **X-ray tube filtration:**
  - 1.5 mm aluminium equivalent for dental units up to 70 kVp;
  - 2.5 mm aluminium equivalent (of which 1.5 mm should be permanent) for dental units over 70 kVp.
- **X-ray beam dimensions:**
  - beam diameter at the patient's skin not greater than 60 mm;
  - rectangular collimation to be provided on new equipment and retro-fitted to existing equipment.
- **Minimum focus-to-skin distance:**
  - 200 mm for dental units of 60 kVp or greater;
  - 100 mm for dental units less than 60 kVp.

Recommended kilovoltage operating range

The use of a higher kilovoltage (60–70 kVp) in dental radiography represents a prudent compromise between minimizing surface dose to the patient and obtaining sufficient contrast to allow radiological diagnosis of dental and bony tissue.

Rectangular collimation

The use of rectangular collimation for intra-oral dental radiography (see figure) has been shown to reduce patient dose by up to 50% compared with a 6-cm round beam.

Rectangular collimation is available as:

- manufactured component of the X-ray tube head;
- 'removable' universal fitting to open-ended cylinder type of equipment;
- additional component of some types of film holders.

Film-holding devices

The use of a film holder, incorporating an extra-oral aiming arm to ensure accurate alignment of the X-ray tube relative to the intra-oral film, is mandatory when using rectangular collimation in order to prevent 'cone-cut' (see p. 290).

Image quality is improved when employing rectangular collimation and longer focus-to-film distance (FFD) by reducing the amount of scattered radiation and reducing the penumbra effect, respectively.

Image receptors

The following types of image receptors are used in dental radiography:

- **Intra-oral radiography:**
  - direct or non-screen film;
  - digital receptors.
- **Extra-oral radiography:**
  - film-screen (usually rare-earth);
  - digital receptors: storage phosphor and solid-state.

Direct or non-screen film

Dental radiography uses direct film. For the dental clinician, direct (or packet) film has the advantage of producing a high-resolution image that provides the fine detail needed to assess pathological changes.

The contents of the film packet consist of the following:

- Outer plastic wrapper to prevent moisture contamination. The reverse side of the outer wrapper has a two-toned appearance to differentiate it as the non-imaging side of the film packet.
- Black paper that is wrapped around the film to protect it from light ingress and damage during handling.
- Lead foil with an embossed pattern is positioned at the back of the film to reduce film fogging from scattered radiation. If the packet is inadvertently positioned back-to-front, the foil pattern is evident on the processed film, identifying the cause of underexposure.
- A single sheet of film comprising a plastic base with emulsion adherent to both surfaces.

Intra-oral film sizes

Several film sizes are available:

- **Size 0 – 22 × 35 mm:** used for small children and anterior periapicals using the paralleling technique.
- **Size 1 – 24 × 40 mm:** used for bitewings in small children and also for anterior projections in adults. Not available routinely in the UK.
- **Size 2 – 31 × 41 mm:** used for bitewings in adults and older (generally six years plus) children and periapical projections. Can be used for occlusal views in young children.
- **Size 4 – 57 × 76 mm:** used for occlusal projections of the maxilla and mandible.

Intra-oral film is available in some sizes as double film packets. This enables the practitioner to forward one to, for instance, the insurer funding the treatment whilst retaining the other within the patient's records.

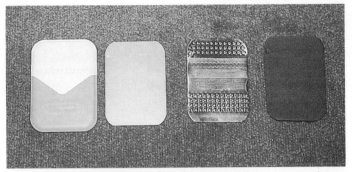

The contents of a film packet. From left to right: the outer plastic wrapper, the film, the sheet of lead foil and the black paper

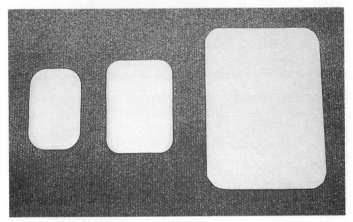

Intra-oral film sizes. From left to right: small periapical/bitewing film (size 0), large periapical/bitewing film (size 2) and an occlusal film (size 4)

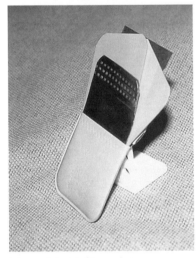

Intra-oral double film packet

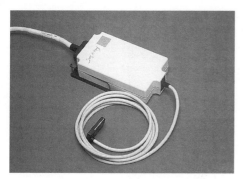

Intra-oral charge-coupled device/complementary metal oxide semiconductor sensor of the Regam Medical Sens-A-Ray® system

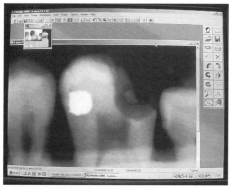

Monitor display of Dentsply's VisualixUSB system

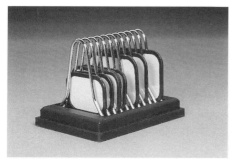

Imaging plates of the Soredex Digora® photostimulable phosphor digital imaging system

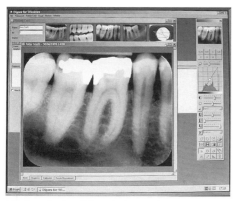

Monitor display of Soredex Digora® system

Image receptors

Digital receptors

Many manufacturers are now producing digital imaging systems specifically for dental radiography. The two methods of image capture used are solid-state and storage phosphor:

- **Solid state:** manufacturers employ a range of electronic sensor technology within digital imaging systems. These include charge-coupled device (CCD)-, charge-injection device (CID)- and complementary metal oxide semiconductor (CMOS)-based sensors. The sensor is linked directly to the computer via a cable. There is an instantaneous image display with these systems.
- **Storage phosphor:** these systems are commonly found in general radiography departments and may be referred to as computed radiography (CR). Other terms used to describe the technique are photostimulable phosphor radiography (PPR), storage phosphor radiography (SPR) and photostimulable phosphor (PSP). The PSP imaging plates consist of europium-activated barium fluorohalide. When exposed to X-rays, the energy of the incident X-ray beam is stored in valency traps in the phosphor. This latent image of stored energy is released as light following scanning of the exposed plate by a laser beam. The pattern of light released is received and then amplified by a CCD and photomultiplier, respectively. The image is displayed on a monitor.

The advantages of solid-state and storage phosphor systems are:

- instant image in the case of solid-state systems;
- almost instant images with storage phosphors. There is a negligible delay of 20 s as the plate is read by the laser;
- image manipulation.

The advantages of storage phosphor are:

- very wide exposure latitude;
- sensors are identical in size and thickness to the film and are tolerated well by patients.

Disadvantages of solid-state and storage phosphor systems are:

- cost;
- in some solid-state systems, the sensor may have a smaller sensitive area than the film, requiring more exposures to the cover area of interest;
- solid-state sensors are bulky and have an attached cable;
- some imaging systems provide insubstantial intra-oral positioning devices.

Although intra-oral digital dental equipment is becoming more generally available, this chapter will continue to refer to film in the technique sections, since film remains the most frequently used type of image receptor in dental radiography.

Image acquisition

Film-holding instruments and film-holding beam-alignment instruments

These devices have been developed in order to simplify intra-oral (bitewing and periapical) radiography for both the operator and the patient. Although bitewing and periapical radiography may be carried out without these devices, research has shown that they noticeably reduce technical errors (Rushton and Horner, 1994; Kaffe *et al.*, 1981).

The devices available are:

- **Film-holding instrument:** localizes the film intra-orally.
- **Film-holding beam-alignment instrument:** localizes the film intra-orally and aligns the X-ray tube relative to the film.

The term 'film holder' is a generic term applied to both instrument types. An ideal film holder must incorporate the following features:

- a bite block to stabilize and locate the device correctly;
- a rigid backing to prevent bending;
- an extra-oral arm (or extension) to ensure correct angulation.

Film-holding beam-alignment instruments are, in most cases, designed with an aiming ring attached to an external indicator rod. This type of device has the advantage of accurate localization. The ring must be positioned in contact with the skin surface to achieve the correct focal spot-to-skin distance.

Specialized film holders

Specialized film holders are available for use in or with:

- endodontic practice;
- periodontal practice;
- digital equipment.

During endodontic treatment, the film-holding beam-aiming instrument allows a working length calculation or enables length determination of a master cone. This is achieved by replacing the dense bite block with an open 'basket' design.

The specialized periodontal film-holding beam-alignment instrument allows assessment of bone loss in advanced periodontal disease by stabilizing the intra-oral film with its long axis vertically.

Various manufacturers have produced modified film-holding instruments/film-holding beam-alignment instruments to accommodate bulkier intra-oral digital sensors.

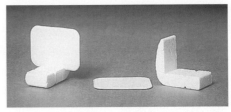

Rinn Greene Stabe® intra-oral film holder with and without film in position

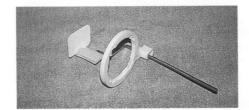

Rinn XCP® posterior film holder

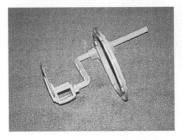

Lateral view of the Rinn Endoray®

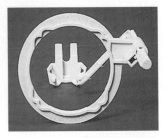

Antero-posterior view of the Rinn Endoray®, showing open 'basket' arrangement to accommodate endodontic instruments

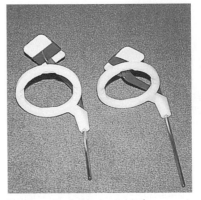

Rinn bitewing holders suitable for (from left to right) a horizontal bitewing and a vertical bitewing. The latter is appropriate in patients with advanced periodontal disease

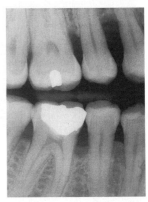

Adult right vertical bitewing of the right premolar/molar region

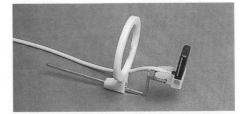

Intra-oral charge-coupled device/complementary metal oxide semiconductor sensor of the Regam Medical Sens-A-Ray® system positioned in a specially designed Rinn XCP® anterior film holder. Note the modification to the bite block to accommodate the bulky sensor. The sensor is always covered by a moisture-proof barrier envelope before being placed in the oral cavity

Film mounting and identification of intra-oral films

The embossed dot at one corner of the front of the film packet allows correct film orientation by denoting the front of the film. The radiographer should adopt a working practice of positioning the dental film with this dot towards the crown of the tooth, so that it will not obscure pathology within areas of interest.

Orientation of radiographs of edentulous patients is made easier by adopting the convention of positioning the embossed dot towards the anterior part of the mouth. This technique is also helpful when soft-tissue views have been requested.

Films are mounted with the (embossed) dot towards the radiographer and as though the operator was looking at the patient. This ensures that the mounted films exactly match the dental charting.

- Arrange all films to be mounted on the viewing box.
- Arrange films as to whether they were taken in the maxilla or mandible followed by region, i.e. anterior and posterior. Use anatomical landmarks for guidance as well as root formation.
- Arrange the films of the maxillary teeth by placing the crowns of the teeth towards the bottom of the viewer.
- Arrange the films of the mandibular teeth with the crowns of the teeth towards the top of the viewer.
- When maxillary and mandibular teeth have been identified, radiographs are then arranged as belonging to either the right or left side of the patient.

Radiographs of the anterior incisors are placed in the centre of the mount. The radiographs of the lateral and canine teeth (positioned correctly, according to side) are placed adjacent to them. This is repeated successively for premolars and molar films to complete film mounting in both dental arches.

General comments

Most dental radiographic examinations require the patient to be seated with the head supported and usually with the occlusal plane horizontally positioned and parallel to the floor.

Prior to the examination, the patient's spectacles, orthodontic appliances and partial/full dentures should be removed. Removal of other jewellery such as earrings, necklaces, tongue bars, nose rings, etc., may also be necessary for certain views.

Dental radiography examinations of the mouth may be complicated by a variety of factors, including:

- the patient's medical and dental condition;
- the degree of patient cooperation;
- anatomical factors, e.g. large tongue, shallow palate, narrow dental arches.

Careful film placement, explanation of the procedure and reassuring the patient will reduce the need for repeat radiographs.

Small children often find the equipment very intimidating and need careful reassurance. Elderly patients may find difficulty in maintaining the position for dental radiography, and movement during the exposure may be a problem. Both groups of individuals often benefit from a clear explanation of the procedure and the use of short exposure times.

The X-ray request form should be checked to ensure that the examination has been justified and that the correct film type and equipment are available.

Exposure factors should be set before the examination.

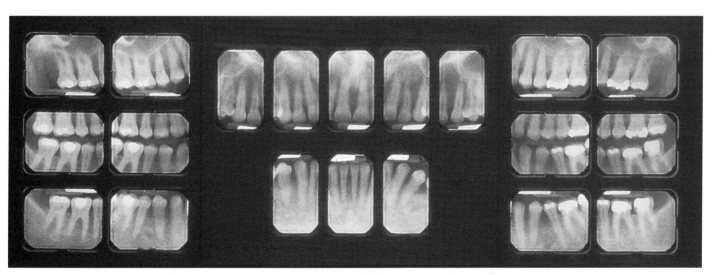

Complete mouth survey taken using the paralleling technique. Both periapical and bitewing radiographs are shown

Radiation protection

Dental radiography is a low-dose but high-volume technique. The following comprise the basic requirements of radiation protection legislation, as it relates to dental radiography, which has been adopted for dental practice within the UK (National Radiological Protection Board, 2001):

- Each request for dental radiography must be justified.
- Radiographers must never position themselves in the direction of the primary beam.
- Controlled areas are determined in consultation with the Radiation Protection Adviser.
- The radiographer must never support a film inside the patient's mouth.
- Film holders should be used routinely for intra-oral radiography.
- Quality assurance procedures must be adopted.
- The use of a higher kilovoltage (60–70 kVp) in dental radiography represents a prudent compromise between minimizing surface dose to the patient and obtaining sufficient contrast to allow radiological diagnosis of dental and bony tissue.
- The use of rectangular collimation for intra-oral dental radiography has been shown to reduce patient dose by up to 50% compared with a 6-cm round beam.
- The use of a film holder incorporating an extra-oral aiming arm to ensure accurate alignment of the X-ray tube relative to the intra-oral film is mandatory when using rectangular collimation in order to prevent 'cone-cut'.
- Image quality is improved when employing rectangular collimation and longer FFD by reducing the amount of scattered radiation and reducing the penumbra effect, respectively.
- There is no indication for the routine use of lead aprons in dental radiography. It is well recognized that lead protection for the patient has no demonstrable effect against internal scatter and provides only a practicable degree of protection in the case of the very infrequently used vertex occlusal projection. In this case, the use of a lead apron could only be regarded as prudent for a female patient who is, or may be, pregnant (National Radiological Protection Board, 2001).

Cross-infection control

Dental radiography is not an invasive procedure and is generally considered low-risk for the operator, except when blood is present, e.g. post-extraction, post-trauma.

Since saliva and/or blood can contaminate films and radiographic equipment, meticulous cross-infection control is important:

- The radiographer should wash his/her hands before and after each examination within sight of the patient.
- If the operator has any open wounds on the hands, these should be covered with a dressing.
- Hospital policies vary on the need for gloves to be worn routinely during intra-oral radiography.
- Barrier envelopes for intra-oral films significantly reduce the risk of microbial contamination by saliva and/or blood.
- If barrier envelopes are not available, then exposed film packets should be disinfected before they are handled and processed.
- The use of a disposable tray system containing film packets and film holders significantly reduces contamination of work surfaces.
- Contaminated empty film packets, barrier envelopes, gloves, cotton-wool rolls and disposable tray should be discarded as clinical waste.
- Intra-oral film-holding devices should be sterilized according to the manufacturer's guidelines. Most manufacturers recommend rinsing and steam autoclaving after use. Some film-holding devices are disposable.
- Surface disinfectants should be used on all work surfaces, the dental chair, cassettes, the control panel, the X-ray tube head and the exposure switch after each patient.
- Manufacturers of panoramic equipment may provide individual bite blocks or disposable bite-block covers for each patient. The former are sterilized, whilst the latter are discarded after exposure. Chin rests and head-positioning guides should be cleaned between patients.
- Manufacturers provide disposable barrier envelopes for the sensor in digital imaging systems. The mouse and the keyboard of computers are a potential weak spot in cross-infection control. If you feel that there is a risk from oral fluids, then you should protect these items.

Film processing

Films may be processed both manually and automatically in specially adapted processing machines.

The operator should pay particular attention to careful handling of the film and should ensure that the processing and darkroom techniques employed result in:

- no pressure marks on the film and no emulsion scratches;
- no roller marks (automatic processing only);
- no evidence of film fog;
- no chemical streaks/splashes/contamination;
- no evidence of inadequate fixation/washing.

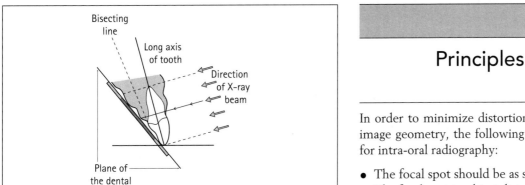

Principles for optimal image geometry

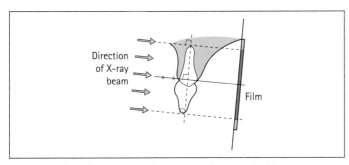

Diagram to show the theoretical basis of the bisecting angle technique

Diagram to show the geometrical relationship between the X-ray beam, tooth and film in the paralleling technique

In order to minimize distortion effects and to achieve optimal image geometry, the following principles have been advocated for intra-oral radiography:

- The focal spot should be as small as possible.
- The focal spot-to-object distance should be as great as possible.
- The object-to-film distance (OFD) should be as small as possible.
- The film should be parallel to the plane of the object.
- The central ray should be perpendicular to both the object and the film.

Both bitewing and periapical radiography benefit from an accurate and stable position of the image receptor.

Bitewing radiography requires that the beam, in the horizontal plane, meets the teeth and the film at right-angles and passes through all the contact areas.

For periapical radiography, the ideal principles for optimal image geometry cannot be satisfied in all patients, due to a variety of factors. To overcome these problems, two techniques have been developed:

- **Bisecting angle technique:** this is based upon the geometric theorem of isometry. It requires the central ray of the X-ray beam to pass through the root of the tooth at right-angles to a plane that is the bisector of the angle formed by the long axis of the tooth and the plane of the film.
- **Paralleling technique:** this requires that the X-ray film is positioned parallel with the long axes of the teeth or tooth to be imaged. This enables the central ray of the X-ray beam to pass at right-angles, i.e. perpendicular, to the beam to the long axes of the teeth and the plane of the film.

10 Bitewing radiography

Bitewing radiography is used for:

- the detection of dental caries in the upper and lower pre-molar and molar teeth;
- monitoring the progression of dental caries;
- assessment of existing restorations;
- assessment of the periodontal condition.

Three methods are available to position the film intra-orally:

- **Bitewing tab:** a heavy-duty paper tab attached to an intra-oral film. The attachment can be either by an adhesive backing to the tab or by a bitewing loop with an attached tab for the patient to bite on.
- **Film-holding instrument:** a simple device to localize the film, comprising a bite block and a film-positioning slot.
- **Film-holding beam-alignment instrument:** a device with a bite block, rigid backing and an extra-oral arm to correctly position the tube relative to the film.

Irrespective of the method used to position the film intra-orally, the front aspect (or imaging surface) of the film must be positioned facing the X-ray tube.

Radiological considerations

It is important to use the correct-sized film for the patient:

- In an adult, a size 2 film (31 × 41 mm) is usual.
- In adults with erupted third molars and in patients with larger jaws, two size 2 films may be needed.
- For younger children, the convention is to use a size 0 film (22 × 35 mm).
- In older children, a common-sense approach will determine when to upgrade from a size 0 to a size 2 film to obtain adequate coverage.

When using bitewing tabs:

- Correct position and angulation of the X-ray tube is needed to ensure adequate film coverage without evidence of coning off.
- Incorrect vertical angulation of the X-ray tube causes distortion of the image.
- Incorrect horizontal placement of the X-ray tube results in horizontal overlap of the contact points of the teeth, reducing the diagnostic yield for the clinician.

When using a bitewing film-holding beam-alignment instrument:

- Young children often find these devices uncomfortable.
- If the patient clinically exhibits periodontal bone loss of more than 6 mm, then two vertically positioned films (i.e. with the narrower length positioned parallel to the floor of the mouth) are required to enable the bone of the periodontium to be imaged (see section on specialized film holders, p. 288).

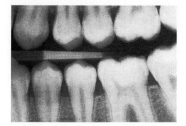

Left horizontal adult bitewing radiograph

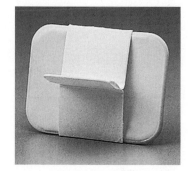

Intra-oral film packet with tab attached

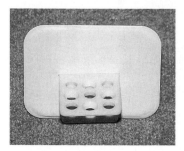

Twix® film holder with intra-oral film packet positioned in localizing slot

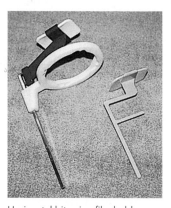

Horizontal bitewing film holders. From left to right: Rinn bitewing holder and Hawe-Neos Kwikbite with beam-aiming rod

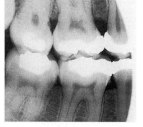

Right horizontal adult bitewing radiograph, showing coning off or cone cutting

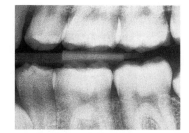

Left horizontal adult bitewing radiograph, showing incorrect horizontal angulation of the X-ray tube head

Note

Access to previous radiographs may reveal the need for vertical bitewings.

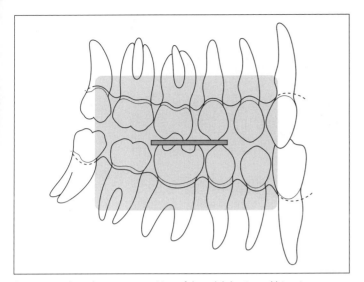

Diagram to show the correct position of the adult horizontal bitewing

Position of patient and film using a bitewing tab attached to the packet

- The correct film size is chosen and the bitewing tab is attached.
- The patient's head must be supported adequately, with the medial plane vertical and the occlusal plane horizontal.
- Hold the tab between thumb and forefinger.
- Place the film in the lingual sulcus.
- The anterior edge of the film should be located opposite to the distal aspect of the lower canine.
- The tab rests on the occlusal surface of the lower teeth.
- The patient is told to bite gently on the tab and, when the teeth are almost in contact, the operator pulls the tab laterally to ensure that there is good contact between the film and the teeth.
- The operator releases their hold on the tab and concomitantly informs the patient to continue biting on the tab.

Direction and centring of the X-ray beam

- The tube is angled five to eight degrees downward (caudad) with the central ray at the level of the occlusal plane and perpendicular to the contact points of the teeth.

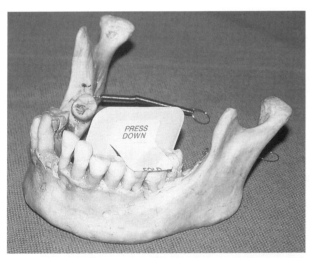

Ideal position for a left adult horizontal bitewing using a bitewing tab

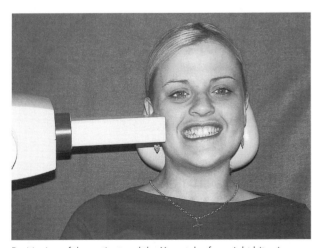

Positioning of the patient and the X-ray tube for a right bitewing radiograph using a bitewing tab

10 Bitewing radiography

Position of patient and film using a bitewing film-holding/beam-alignment instrument

- The correct film size is chosen and placed in the film holder.
- The film holder is introduced into the mouth, rotated over the tongue and positioned in the lingual sulcus.
- The anterior edge of the film should be located opposite to the distal edge of the lower canine.
- The bite block rests on the occlusal surface of the lower teeth.
- The patient is told to bite gently on the bite block. At the same time, the operator ensures that there is good contact between the image receptor and the teeth.
- Ask the patient to continue biting on the bite block to position securely the film holder.

Direction and centring of the X-ray beam

- As directed by the extra-oral aiming device of the holder.

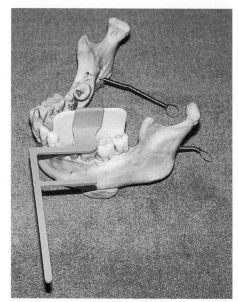
Lateral view of a Hawe-Neos Kwikbite film holder positioned for a left bitewing radiograph on a dried mandible

Quality standards for bitewing radiography

Evidence of optimal image geometry

- There should be no evidence of bending of the image of the teeth on the image.
- There should be no foreshortening or elongation of the teeth.
- Ideally, there should be no horizontal overlap.

If overlap is present, it should not obscure more than one-half the enamel thickness. This may be unavoidable due to anatomical factors (e.g. overcrowding, shape of dental arch), necessitating an additional bitewing or periapical radiograph.

Correct coverage

- The film should cover the distal surfaces of the canine teeth and the mesial surfaces of the most posterior erupted teeth.
- The periodontal bone level should be visible and imaged equally in the maxilla/mandible, confirming ideal centring.

Good density and contrast

There should be good density and adequate contrast between the enamel and the dentine.

Adequate number of films

When the third molars are erupted or partially erupted and impacted, and all the other teeth are present, two films may be needed on each side to evaluate the dentition.

Extreme curvature of the arch may impact on the number of films required.

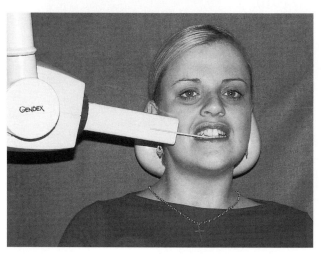
Positioning of the patient and the X-ray tube for a right bitewing radiograph using a Hawe-Neos Kwikbite film holder and rectangular collimation of the X-ray tube

Adequate processing and dark room techniques

- No pressure marks on film, no emulsion scratches.
- No roller marks (automatic processing only).
- No evidence of film fog.
- No chemical streaks/splashes/contamination.
- No evidence of inadequate fixation/washing.

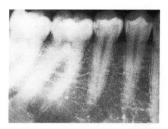

Periapical radiograph of the right mandibular molar region

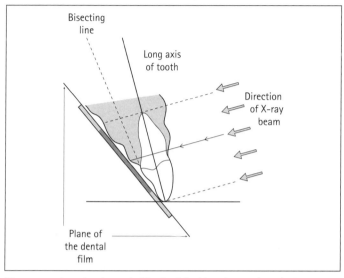

Diagram to show the theoretical basis of the bisecting angle technique

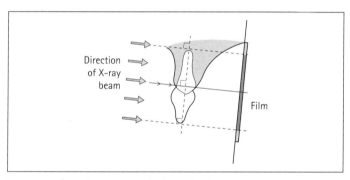

Diagram to show the geometrical relationship between the X-ray beam, tooth and film in the paralleling technique

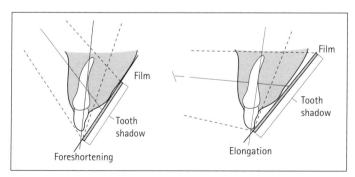

Left: diagram to show the geometric foreshortening of the image by using too steep a vertical angulation of the X-ray tube. Right: diagram to show the geometric elongation of the image by using too shallow a vertical angulation of the X-ray tube

Periapical radiography provides an image of the teeth, the surrounding periodontal tissues and the alveolar bone.

There are many clinical indications for periapical radiography:

- Assessment of the periodontium encompassing the periapical and the periodontal status.
- Assessment of apical pathology and other lesions situated within alveolar bone.
- Pre- and postoperative assessment of alveolar surgery.
- Following trauma to teeth and alveolar bone.
- Localization of teeth and presence/absence of teeth.
- Before extraction to assess root morphology and the relationship of roots to vital structures, i.e. the inferior dental canal, the maxillary antrum.
- During endodontic therapy.
- Pre- and postoperative assessment of implants.

The two available techniques are:

- bisecting angle technique;
- paralleling technique.

Irrespective of the technique used, the front aspect (or imaging surface) of the film must be positioned facing the X-ray tube.

Bisecting angle technique

This technique is based upon the geometric theorem of isometry. It requires the central ray of the X-ray beam to pass through the root of the tooth at right-angles to a plane that is the bisector of the angle formed by the long axis of the tooth and the plane of the film.

With the bisecting angle technique, positioning is relatively simple but there are many variables in the technique.

Two methods are employed to stabilize the film intra-orally:

- the patient's finger;
- a film-holding instrument.

The use of a film-holding instrument is preferred, as it reduces distortion due to film bending and stabilizes the film, ensuring better patient cooperation. However, the resulting X-ray may exhibit image shape distortion as a result of incorrect vertical angulation of the tube.

Bisecting angle technique (*contd*)

The convention for intra-oral film placement is as follows:

- Anterior teeth (incisors and canines): long axis of film vertical.
- Posterior teeth (premolars and molars): long axis of film horizontal.

Position of patient and film

- The patient's head must be supported adequately with the medial plane vertical and the occlusal plane horizontal (i.e. upper occlusal plane and lower occlusal plane for maxillary and mandibular radiography, respectively).

If a film holder is used:

- The correct film size is chosen and placed in the film holder.
- Position the film holder intra-orally adjacent to the lingual/palatal aspects of the tooth/teeth to be imaged.
- Insert a cotton-wool roll between the opposing teeth and the bite block.
- Ask the patient to close together slowly to allow gradual accommodation of the film holder intra-orally.
- Tell the patient to continue biting on the bite block to position the film holder securely.

If the patient's finger is used:

- The correct film size is chosen and positioned intra-orally.
- Ensure that the tooth/teeth being examined are in the middle of the film.
- 2 mm of the film packet should extend beyond the incisal or occlusal margin to ensure that the entire tooth is imaged.
- Instruct the patient to gently support the film using either their index finger or thumb.
- Apply the patient's finger/thumb solely to the area of film that overlies the crown and gingival tissues of the teeth. This reduces the possibility of distortion by bending of the film covering the root and periapical tissues.

Direction and centring of the X-ray beam

- The X-ray beam should be centred vertically on the midpoint of the tooth to be examined.
- Look at the tooth, the film, and the bisecting angle between the two. This achieves the correct vertical angulation of the tube.
- It is important to remember that proclined teeth will require more angulation, whilst retroclined teeth will need less angulation.
- The X-ray tube must be positioned so that the beam is at right-angles to the labial or buccal surfaces of the teeth to prevent horizontal overlap.

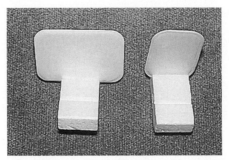

Rinn Greene Stabe® film holder with (from left to right) horizontal film placement for the premolars and molars and vertical film placement for the incisors and canines

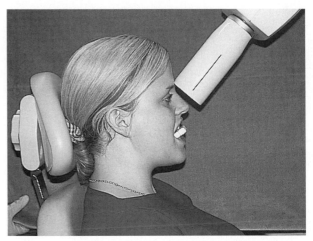

Positioning of the patient and the X-ray tube for a periapical radiograph of the maxillary incisors using the Rinn Greene Stabe® film holder

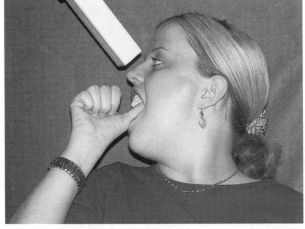

Positioning of the patient and the X-ray tube for a periapical radiograph of the maxillary incisors, using the thumb for support

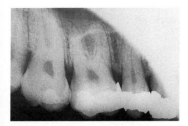

Coning off or cone cutting occurs when the X-ray tube is positioned incorrectly. The X-ray tube head was positioned too far posteriorly so the anterior region of the periapical radiograph was not exposed

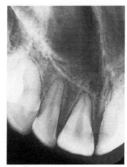

Foreshortened image due to the vertical angle being too steep

Notes

- Correct positioning and angulation of the X-ray tube are needed to ensure adequate film coverage without evidence of coning off.
- Incorrect vertical angulation of the X-ray tube causes distortion of the image and may result in inaccuracies in diagnosis.
- The image can be distorted due to incorrect placement of film and/or the patient's finger.
- Inaccurate vertical angulation of the X-ray tube results in misrepresentation of the alveolar bone levels.
- Incorrect horizontal placement of the X-ray tube results in horizontal overlap of the contact point of the teeth.
- The image of the zygomatic bone frequently overlies the roots of upper molars.

Imaging considerations

Conventionally, the technique uses a short tube-to-film distance and the object distance is reduced by close approximation of the film to the palatal or lingual aspect of the alveolar ridge.

With the occlusal plane horizontal, the X-ray tube is positioned vertically by an assessment of the bisected plane for each individual patient. This technique is preferred to the use of the standardized vertical tube angulations (see tables on p. 298) as it allows for anatomical variations.

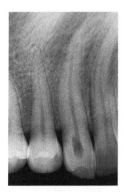

Excessive pressure when stabilizing the film or incorrect placement of the film in the mouth results in bending of the film packet during exposure

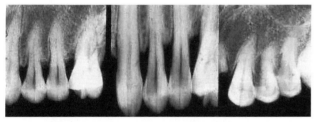

The effect of beam angulation on periodontal bone levels. A steep vertical angle (extreme right) masks bone loss, whilst too shallow an angle (centre) amplifies the extent of bone loss. The image on the extreme left of this dried skull series represents the correct geometry and accurate bone levels

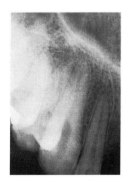

Superimposition of structures due to incorrect horizontal angulation of the tube

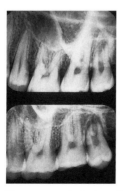

The upper periapical was taken using the bisecting angle technique, resulting in dense radio-opacity of the zygomatic buttress overlying and obscuring the apices of the upper molar teeth. In the lower image, taken using the paralleling technique, the shadow of the buttress is well above the apices as it is a true lateral image

Bisecting angle technique (*contd*)

Angulations and centring points for the bisecting angle technique in the maxilla

Region	Centring point	Vertical angulation (degrees)
Incisor: central	Midline through tip of nose	50–60 (average 50)
Incisor: lateral	Ala of nose, 1 cm from midline	50–60 (average 50)
Canine	Ala of nose	45–50
Premolar	On the cheek: at the point of intersection of a line down from the midpoint of the inner and outer canthus of the eye and the ala-tragus line	35–40
Molar	On the cheek: at the point of intersection of a line down from a point 1 cm posterior to the outer canthus of the eye and the ala-tragus line	20–30

Angulations and centring points for the bisecting angle technique in the mandible (negative angle indicates upward (cephalad) angulation of the tube)

Region	Centring point	Vertical angulation (degrees)
Incisors	Midline, 1 cm above the lower border of the mandible	−20 to −30
Canine	Vertical line down from the outer aspect of the ala of nose, centring 1 cm above the lower border of the mandible	−20 to −30
Premolar	Vertical line down from the midpoint between the inner and outer canthus of the eye, centring 1 cm above the lower border of the mandible	−10 to −15
Molar	Vertical line down from a point 1 cm posterior to the outer canthus of the eye, centring 1 cm above the lower border of the mandible	0 to −10

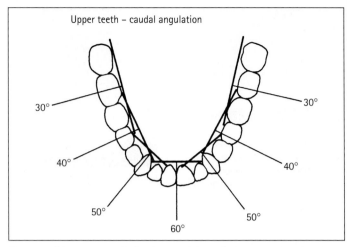

Diagram of the upper teeth showing caudal angulations

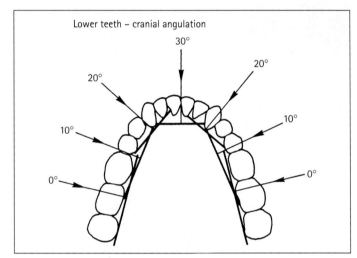

Diagram of the lower teeth showing cranial angulations

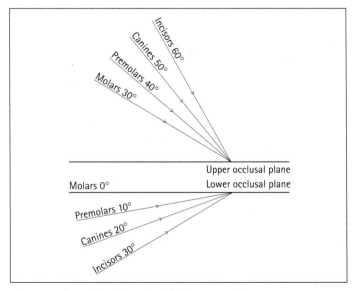

Schematic of angulations to upper and lower occlusal planes

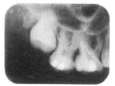

Standard size films may replace smaller films for incisor and canine regions

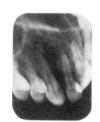

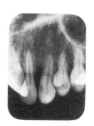

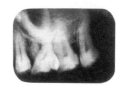

Unerupted wisdom

Zygomatic bone obscuring apices of upper left 1st and 2nd molar teeth

3rd molar · 2nd molar · 1st molar · 2nd premolar

1st molar · 2nd premolar · 1st premolar · Canine · Lateral incisor

1st premolar · Canine · Lateral incisor

Central incisors

Central incisor · Lateral incisor · Canine

Lateral incisor · Canine · 1st premolar · 2nd premolar · 1st molar

2nd premolar · 1st molar · 2nd molar · 3rd molar

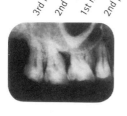

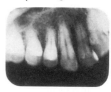

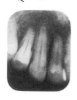

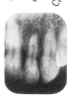

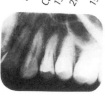

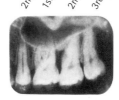

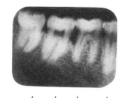

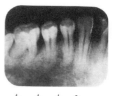

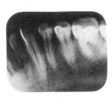

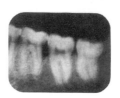

3rd molar · 2nd molar · 1st molar · 2nd premolar

1st molar · 2nd premolar · 1st premolar · Canine

1st premolar · Canine · Lateral incisor · Central incisors

Lateral incisor · Central incisors · Lateral incisor

Lateral incisor · Canine · 1st premolar

Lateral incisor · Canine · 1st premolar · 2nd premolar · 1st molar

1st molar · 2nd molar · 3rd molar

Unerupted wisdom

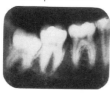

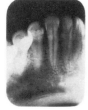

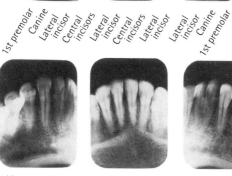

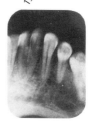

Standard size films may replace smaller films for incisor and canine regions

Examples of adult full mouth radiography (upper and lower jaw)

10 Periapical radiography

Paralleling technique

The paralleling technique requires that the X-ray film is positioned parallel with the long axes of the teeth. The central ray of the X-ray beam passes at right-angles, i.e. perpendicular, to the tooth.

In order to minimize magnification of the image and subsequent loss of image sharpness, the technique uses an increased focal spot-to-object distance, ensuring that a more parallel X-ray beam is incident to the object and image receptor.

Adopting the paralleling technique has many benefits for both the operator and the patient:

- Minimal elongation/foreshortening/distortion.
- Increased focus-to-skin distance (FSD) reduces surface dose.
- Increased FSD improves image quality by reducing the penumbra effect.
- Reduction in distortion effects due to bending of the film/image receptor.

Disadvantages of the paralleling technique include:

- The paralleling technique can be used when using X-ray equipment with a short FFD (less than 20 cm) providing the operator accepts increased magnification.
- Anatomical limitations, such as a shallow palate, principally in the maxillary molar and anterior regions, preclude true parallel placement of the film relative to the tooth.

Radiological considerations

- The use of the paralleling technique along with film-holding beam-alignment instruments allows the operator to obtain images that have reproducibility and standardization. This allows the clinician to study longitudinal disease progression and to assess accurately treatment outcomes.
- Provided the film position does not diverge from the long axis (or axes) of the tooth by more than 20 degrees, the image will demonstrate no evidence of longitudinal distortion.
- In endodontic treatment, it may be necessary to separate superimposed root canals using two radiographs at different horizontal angles. Obtain one 'normal' film and one with a 20-degree oblique horizontal beam angle for all molars and maxillary first premolars.
- Assessment of some horizontally impacted mandibular third molars may require two films to image the apex. Obtain one 'normal' film and one with a more posterior 20-degree oblique horizontal beam angle.

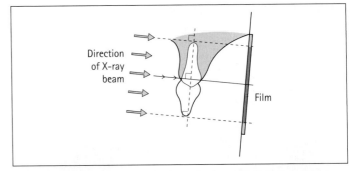

Diagram to show the geometrical relationship between X-ray beam, tooth and film in the paralleling technique

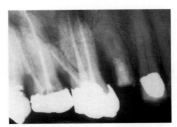

Paralleling periapical radiograph of upper right molar region. Endodontic treatment has been carried out on each of the molar teeth

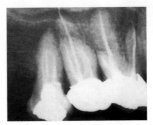

Second paralleling periapical radiograph of the same region as above, but using a 20-degree posterior horizontal tube shift. This has the effect of identifying and separating the root canals of the upper right first molar

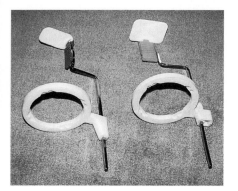

The Rinn XCP® film holder: from left to right the anterior and posterior devices with size 0 and size 2 films respectively

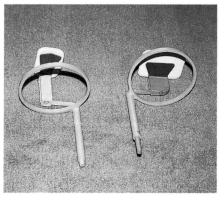

The Hawe-Neos Super Bite® film holder: from left to right the anterior and posterior devices with size 0 and size 2 films respectively

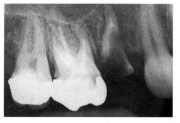

A posterior periapical of the right maxilla taken using the paralleling technique

Paralleling technique

Film-holding beam-alignment instruments

Most devices require the use of different sized films in the anterior and posterior regions of the oral cavity. The usual convention for film use is:

- Anterior teeth (incisors and canines): size 0 (or size 1) film with long axis of film vertical. The alternative use of a size 1 film is governed solely by operator preference.
- Posterior teeth (premolars and molars): size 2 film (31 × 41 mm) with long axis of film horizontal.
- Some operators use size 0 (or size 1) for premolars.
- Adopting these techniques limits longitudinal distortion and ensures patient comfort.

Essential image characteristics

- There should be no evidence of bending of the teeth and the periapical region of interest on the image.
- There should be no foreshortening or elongation of the teeth.
- Ideally, there should be no horizontal overlap. If overlap is present, then it must not obscure the pulp/root canals.
- The film should demonstrate all the tooth/teeth of interest (i.e. crown and root(s)).
- There should be 3 mm of periapical bone visible to enable an assessment of apical anatomy.
- There should be good density and adequate contrast between the enamel and dentine.
- There should be no pressure marks on the film and no emulsion scratches.
- There should be no roller marks (automatic processing only).
- There should be no evidence of film fog.
- There should be no chemical streaks/splashes/contamination.
- There should be no evidence of inadequate fixation/washing.

10 Periapical radiography

Paralleling technique (*contd*)

Position of patient and film

- The appropriate film holder and periapical film are selected and assembled.
- Place the bite block in contact with the edge of the tooth to be imaged. Ensure that the film covers the particular tooth/teeth to be examined.
- **Maxilla:**
  - For the incisor, canine, premolar and molar regions, the film holder must be positioned some distance from the tooth to achieve parallelism. This requires using the entire horizontal length of the bite block with the film holder occupying the highest part of the palate.
- **Mandible:**
  - For the lower incisor teeth, position the film holder in the plane of an imaginary line intersecting the first mandibular premolars or as posterior as anatomy will allow.
  - For the mandibular premolars and molars, position the film holder in the lingual sulcus adjacent to the teeth selected for imaging.
- Insert a cotton-wool roll between the opposing teeth and the bite block.
- Ask the patient to close together slowly to allow gradual accommodation of the film holder intra-orally.
- As the patient closes together, rotate the bite block in an upward/downward direction (as appropriate).
- Instruct the patient to close firmly on the bite block and to continue biting until the examination is completed.
- Slide the aiming ring down the indicator rod to approximate the skin surface.

Direction and centring of the X-ray beam

- Correctly align the X-ray tube adjacent to the indicator rod and aiming ring in both vertical and horizontal planes.

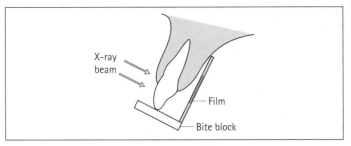

Diagram showing the correct position of the film in the film holder bite block relative to an anterior tooth in the maxilla

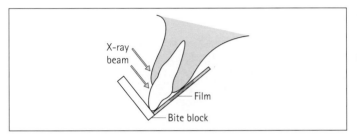

Diagram showing the incorrect position of the film in the film holder bite block. When the holder is positioned adjacent to the tooth (mimicking the set-up for the bisecting technique), true parallelism cannot be achieved and the holder is extremely uncomfortable for the patient

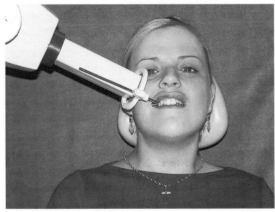

Positioning of the patient and the X-ray tube for a periapical radiograph of the maxillary molar region using the Rinn XCP® posterior film holder

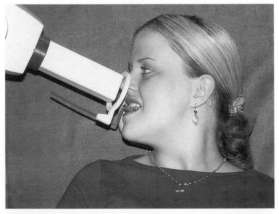

Positioning of the patient and the X-ray tube for a periapical radiograph of the maxillary central incisors using the Rinn XCP® anterior film holder

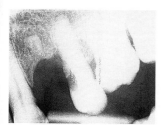

Radiograph of the upper left maxilla shows the bite block being trapped against the upper left canine due to the adjacent edentulous region. This has the effect of 'propping' open the bite

Paralleling technique

Common faults and remedies

- Care must be taken in the partially dentate patient, as edentulous areas can displace the holder and prop open the bite.
- Cotton wool rolls used as a support in the edentulous area often overcome the problem.
- Ensure that the patient understands that they must continue to bite on the bite block. Failure to do this results in loss of apices from the resultant image.
- In edentulous patients, the bisecting technique is preferred.

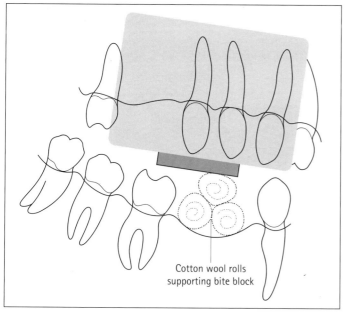

Cotton wool rolls supporting bite block

Use of cotton wool rolls to stabilize the bite block in an edentulous area

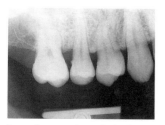

Loss of apices due to lack of continuous biting pressure

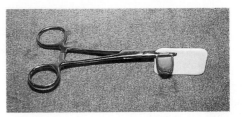

Modified surgical haemostats with soldered bite block

Third molar region

Positioning of the film using conventional film holders can be uncomfortable for the patient in the third molar region. To overcome these problems, the following techniques should be adopted:

Imaging mandibular third molars

Surgical haemostats/needle holders can be used to stabilize the film. One beak of the device is modified into a bite block by soldering a semi-circular stainless wire on to the needle holder and covering it with heavy-duty autoclavable plastic. This simple addition significantly reduces the problem of the patient inadvertently moving the holder.

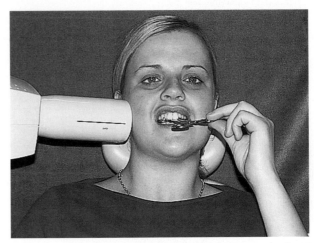

Positioning of the patient and the X-ray tube for a periapical radiograph of the mandibular third molar. The holder is stabilized by the patient's hand

Position of patient and film

- The upper leading anterior edge of a size 2 film is attached securely to the beaks of the needle holder, ensuring that the front aspect (or imaging surface) will face the X-ray tube when positioned intra-orally.
- The film is positioned in the lingual sulcus as far posteriorly as possible.
- The patient is instructed to bring their teeth together slowly. This has the effect of lowering of the floor of the mouth, thereby providing more space to accommodate the film.
- Simultaneously, the operator positions the film holder so that the leading edge of the film lies adjacent to the mesial aspect of the mandibular first molar. It is important to do this gradually to reduce discomfort for the patient.
- The patient is instructed to hold the handles of the needle holder.

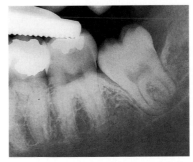

Periapical radiograph of the lower left third molar showing a complex root form and close approximation of root apices to the mandibular canal

Direction and centring of the X-ray beam

- The tube is centred and angulated as outlined in the table on p. 298 for the mandibular molar region.
- The X-ray tube must be positioned so that the beam is at right-angles to the labial or buccal surfaces of the teeth to prevent horizontal overlap, and the film is exposed.

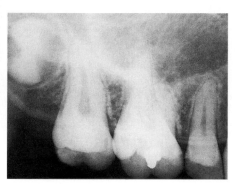

Periapical of the right molar region showing a developing third maxillary molar

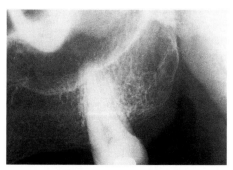

Periapical of the left molar region showing normal anatomy of the tuberosity, the antral floor and the inferior aspect of the zygoma

Third molar region

Imaging maxillary third molars

The use of a film holder in this region is dependent on the patient's ability to tolerate the device. If the use of a film holder is impossible, then the bisecting angle technique is adopted.

Position of patient and film

- The patient's head must be supported adequately with the medial plane vertical and the maxillary occlusal plane horizontal.
- Position the film intra-orally so that the front aspect (or imaging surface) will face the X-ray tube.
- The film is positioned far enough posteriorly to cover the third molar region, with the anterior border just covering the second premolar.
- The film is supported by the patient's index finger or thumb. It is positioned with 2 mm of film packet extending beyond the occlusal plane to ensure that the entire tooth is imaged. The image plane must be flat to reduce the distortion effects of bending.

Direction and centring of the X-ray beam

- The X-ray tube is centred and angulated as outlined in the table on p. 298 for the maxillary molar region.
- The X-ray tube must be positioned so that the beam is at right-angles to the labial or buccal surfaces of the teeth to prevent horizontal overlap, and the film is exposed.

Complete mouth survey or full mouth survey

The complete mouth survey or full mouth survey is composed of a series of individual periapical films covering all the teeth and the tooth-bearing alveolar bone of the dental arches. Most patients require 14 periapical films to fulfil these requirements. Careful technique is essential to reduce the need for repeat examinations.

10 Occlusal radiography

Occlusal projections are used to image relatively large areas of the dental arches. Their main uses are as follows:

- To localize accurately unerupted teeth, supernumeraries, retained roots, odontomes, foreign bodies, radio-opaque salivary calculi, etc. in regions of the oral cavity where the occlusal view provides a plan view of the jaw.
- To localize accurately unerupted teeth, supernumeraries, retained roots, odontomes and foreign bodies using parallax when combined with another film of the region taken using a different vertical angulation.
- To evaluate a patient with severe trismus or who cannot tolerate periapical radiography.
- To evaluate patients in cases of trauma, when information is required on the extent and location of fractures to the teeth and the maxillary and mandibular bones.
- To evaluate the medial-lateral extent of pathology, e.g. cysts, tumours, malignancy, osteodystrophies.

Terminology

There is a diversity of terminology used to describe the various types of occlusal projections. The terminology used reflects beam angulation or the anatomical region in which the tube is positioned.

In this section, alternative but synonymous nomenclature appears in brackets to ensure a common understanding amongst the wider readership of the text.

Recommended projections

The occlusal projections that are necessary for full examination of the dental arches can be seen below. These are presented as true and oblique projections.

Radiological considerations

The clinician should ensure that their request for certain occlusal projections (i.e. true occlusal) should indicate the tooth over which the beam is centred.

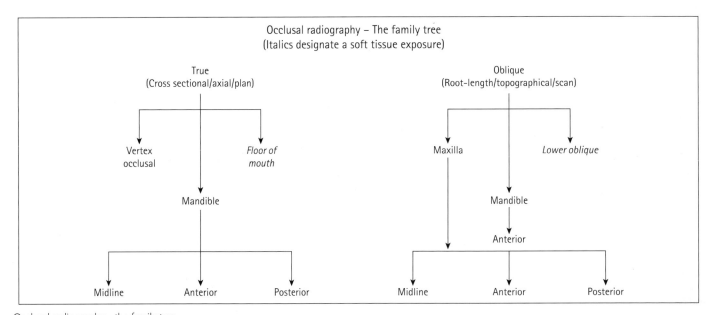

Occlusal radiography – the family tree

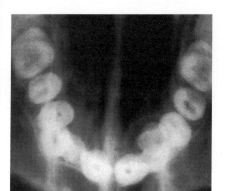

A vertex occlusal radiograph

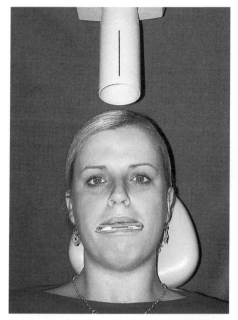

Positioning of the patient and the X-ray tube for a vertex occlusal

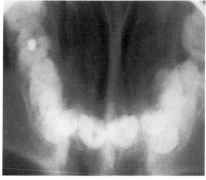

A vertex occlusal radiograph showing buccally positioned left canine and palatally positioned left second premolar

Vertex occlusal of the maxilla

This projection shows a plan view of the maxillary teeth and is used to demonstrate the bucco-palatal relationship of unerupted teeth in the dental arch.

The vertex occlusal is a projection that is requested infrequently now. Because of the density of tissue through which the beam must pass, it requires the use of an intra-oral cassette with rare-earth intensifying screens to reduce the dose to the patient. If these screens are not available routinely, then existing rare-earth screens can easily be cut down to size to fit the intra-oral cassette.

The loaded cassette, pre-labelled with a lead letter to designate the side, is placed inside a small plastic bag to prevent salivary contamination. Statutory requirements require the use of a lead apron for this projection [see Radiation protection, p. 290).

Position of patient and cassette

- The patient sits comfortably, with the head supported. The median plane is vertical and the occlusal plane is horizontal.
- The occlusal cassette is positioned with its long axis anteroposteriorly (i.e. parallel to the median plane) within the oral cavity.
- The cassette should be placed flat in the patient's mouth, adjacent to the occlusal surface of the lower teeth.
- Position the cassette as far back as possible, at least to the level of the first permanent molars.
- The patient should bite together gently to stabilize the cassette intra-orally.

Direction and centring of the X-ray beam

- The tube is positioned over the vertex of the skull, and the central ray is directed along the median plane downward (caudad) through the long axis of the upper central incisor teeth.

Note

It is important to remember that the beam is not at right-angles to the occlusal plane.

True occlusal of the mandible

Synonyms: submental occlusal, lower true occlusal, occlusal plan view of the lower jaw, cross-sectional mandibular occlusal projection.

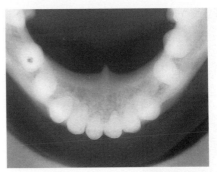

A true occlusal radiograph of the mandible

Midline

This projection shows a plan view of the mandible, with the teeth and the lingual and buccal cortices seen in cross-section.

Position of patient and film

- The occlusal film should be placed as far back in the mouth as the patient will tolerate, with the film resting on the occlusal surfaces of the lower teeth. The tube side of the film faces the floor of the mouth with the long axis of film extending across the oral cavity (i.e. perpendicular to the sagittal plane).
- The anterior leading edge of the film should extend 1 cm beyond the labial aspects of the mandible incisor teeth.
- The patient is instructed to extend their head backwards so that the ala-tragus line is almost perpendicular to the floor. The head is then supported adequately in this position.
- The patient should bite together gently to avoid pressure marks on the film.

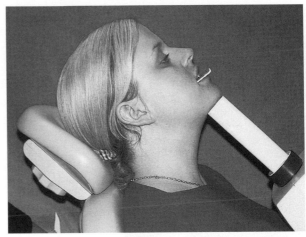

Positioning of the patient and the X-ray tube for a true occlusal radiograph of the mandible

Direction and centring of the X-ray beam

- The tube is placed well down below the patient's chin and directed vertically at 90 degrees to the occlusal plane and the film.
- Centre the tube in the midline at 90 degrees to an imaginary line joining the first permanent molars (i.e. ≅3 cm distal to the midline of the chin).

Anterior

This projection is designed to image the anterior regions of the mandible.

The only modification to the technique described for the midline true occlusal is that the tube is centred on the symphysis menti, with the beam positioned so that the central ray passes through the root canals of the lower central incisors.

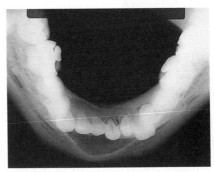

A true occlusal radiograph of the mandible showing a cystic lesion in the anterior region of the jaw

True occlusal of the mandible

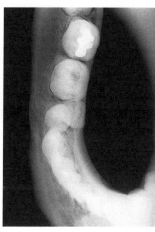

Posterior true occlusal radiograph of right mandible

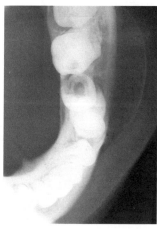

Posterior true occlusal radiograph of the left mandible. A cystic lesion is apparent in the premolar region

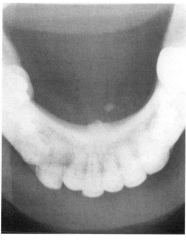

True occlusal (with soft tissue exposure) showing a discrete salivary calculus in the midline, adjacent to the left submandibular duct orifice

Posterior

If pathology is related to only one side of the mandible, then the posterior view is used.

To achieve this projection, some modifications of the technique outlined for the midline true occlusal are needed:

- The film is positioned with its long axis antero-posteriorly (i.e. parallel with the sagittal plane) on the side of interest.
- The lateral aspect of the film extends $\cong 1$ cm buccally to the dental arch but remains parallel to the buccal surfaces of the posterior teeth.
- The tube is centred below the body of the mandible on the side of interest ($\cong 3$ cm distal to the antero-lateral aspect of the chin) at 90 degrees to the film.

Floor of mouth

This projection is performed to image radio-opaque calculi in the anterior aspect of the floor of the mouth and to identify effectively fragments of fractured tooth and radio-opaque foreign bodies embedded within the lower lip.

- Positioning of the patient, along with film and tube placement, are identical to those described previously for the midline true occlusal.
- Exposure is reduced by a factor of $\cong 50\%$ to that used to produce an image of the teeth and mandible.

Radiological considerations

More than one-third (35%) of submandibular calculi are found at the hilum of the gland. While the true occlusal of the mandible (see p. 308 opposite) images the anterior aspects of the submandibular duct adequately, the posterior portion is obscured by the image of the lingual cortex of the mandible. The posterior oblique occlusal (see p. 313) overcomes the problem.

Notes

Other radiographic projections are available to image calculi in this region, including true lateral with floor of mouth depressed and panoramic view.

Oblique occlusal of the maxilla

Midline occlusal

Synonyms: upper standard occlusal, standard occlusal, 70-degree maxillary occlusal.

The projection is used to show the anterior maxilla.

Position of patient and film

- The patient sits comfortably with the head supported. The median plane is vertical and the occlusal plane is horizontal.
- An occlusal film is placed flat in the patient's mouth, resting on the occlusal surfaces of the lower teeth, with the tube side of the film facing the vault of the palate.
- The convention for positioning the film in the mouth is:
  - **Adults:** long axis of film extending across the oral cavity (i.e. perpendicular to the sagittal plane).
  - **Children:** long axis of film positioned antero-posteriorly in the oral cavity (i.e. parallel to the sagittal plane). NB: in younger children with small mouths, a periapical film can be substituted effectively.
- The anterior leading edge of the film should extend 1 cm beyond the labial aspects of the maxillary incisor teeth.
- The film should be placed as far back as the patient will tolerate.
- The patient should bite together gently to avoid pressure marks on the film.

Direction and centring of the X-ray beam

- The tube is positioned above the patient in the midline and angled downwards (caudad) at 65–70 degrees, the central ray passing through the bridge of the nose towards the centre of the film.

Modifications of the technique

Using a soft-tissue exposure, this projection is effective in identifying fragments of tooth and/or radio-opaque foreign bodies within the upper lip following trauma.

Another useful projection to identify radio-opaque structures embedded within the lips is the true lateral. The patient holds the occlusal film parallel to the sagittal plane using the thumb to support the lower edge and the fingers to stabilize the film against the cheek.

This projection is taken using soft-tissue settings. Unless the object is confirmed clinically to be solitary and situated in the midline, then the true lateral must be supplemented by other projections (i.e. at right-angles to it) to enable accurate localization.

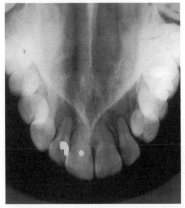

Upper standard oblique occlusal radiograph

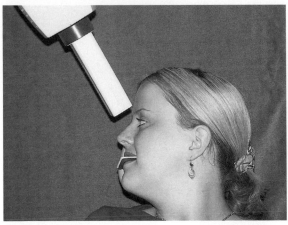

Positioning of the patient and the X-ray tube (from the side) for an upper standard oblique occlusal radiograph

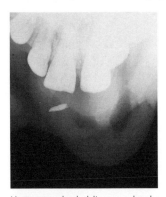

Upper standard oblique occlusal radiograph (with soft tissue exposure) showing fractured tooth fragment localized to soft tissues of upper lip

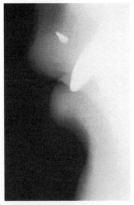

True lateral projection of the case illustrated above. Embedded tooth fragment is clearly seen

Anterior oblique occlusal

This projection is used to image the anterior region of the maxilla. The tube is centred over the lateral/canine region and is commonly

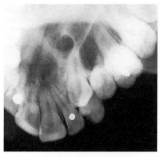

Anterior oblique occlusal of the left maxilla showing an unerupted left canine

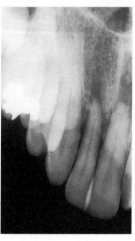

Anterior oblique occlusal of the right maxilla. The region has sustained trauma. The upper right central and lateral incisors are partially extruded

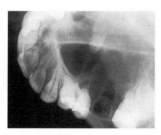

An upper left posterior oblique occlusal. During the extraction of the first permanent molar, the palatal root has been displaced into the maxillary antrum. It is clearly seen overlying the floor of the nasal fossa

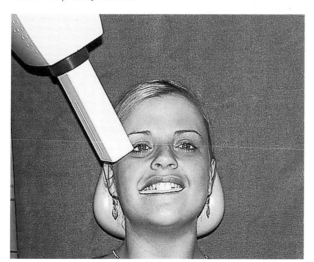

Positioning of the patient and the X-ray tube for the right upper posterior oblique occlusal

used combined with a periapical film of this region to assist in localization of supernumerary teeth, unerupted canines, etc.

Position of patient and film

- Positioning is identical to the standard, except that film coverage is restricted to the anterior region of interest.

Direction and centring of the X-ray beam

- The centring point is the bridge of the nose with downward (caudal) angulation of 60 degrees.

Posterior oblique occlusal

Synonyms: upper oblique occlusal, oblique maxillary occlusal, oblique occlusal of the upper jaw, lateral maxillary occlusal projection.

This projection demonstrates the posterior quadrant of the maxillary arch, the teeth, the alveolar bone and part of the maxillary antrum, the floor of the antrum and the zygomatic process of the maxilla superimposed over the roots and crowns of the molar teeth.

Position of patient and film

- The patient sits comfortably, with the head supported. The median plane is vertical and the occlusal plane is horizontal.
- An occlusal film is placed flat in the patient's mouth on the side of interest.
- The film lies on the occlusal surfaces of the lower teeth, with the tube side of the film facing the vault of the palate. The convention for positioning the film is that the long axis of the film lies antero-posteriorly in the oral cavity (i.e. parallel to the median plane).
- The edge of the film adjacent to the cheek should extend 1 cm lateral to the buccal surfaces of the posterior teeth to be imaged.
- It should be positioned as far back as the patient will tolerate.
- The patient should bite together gently to avoid pressure marks on the film.

Direction and centring of the X-ray beam

- The X-ray tube is positioned towards the side of the face where pathology is suspected and angled downwards (caudad) at 65–70 degrees through the cheek.
- The centring point is medial to the outer canthus of the eye but level with the pupil. It is important to ensure that the central ray is at right-angles to the dental arch.

Notes

- It is important not to position the tube more laterally than the centring point outlined above, otherwise the body of the zygoma will obscure important detail in the area of interest.
- This is a technically demanding view when using rectangular collimation.

Oblique occlusal of the mandible

Anterior oblique occlusal

Synonyms: lower anterior occlusal, lower midline oblique occlusal, oblique mandibular occlusal, anterior mandibular occlusal projection.

This projection shows the anterior teeth and the inferior cortical border.

Position of patient and film

- The patient sits comfortably, with the head supported. The median plane is vertical.
- An occlusal film is placed flat in the patient's mouth, resting on the occlusal surfaces of the lower teeth. The film should be placed with the tube side of the film facing the floor of the mouth.
- The long axis of film is positioned so that it extends across the oral cavity (i.e. perpendicular to the sagittal plane).
- The anterior leading edge of the film should extend 1 cm beyond the labial aspects of the mandibular incisor teeth.
- The patient should bite together gently to avoid pressure marks on the film.
- The patient is instructed to extend their head backwards so that the occlusal plane is 35 degrees to the horizontal. This allows the tube to be more easily positioned adjacent to the chin. The head is supported adequately in this position.

Direction and centring of the X-ray beam

- The tube is positioned in the midline achieving an upward angle of ten degrees (i.e. an overall upward angulation of 45 degrees) to the plane of the film, centring through the midpoint of the chin.

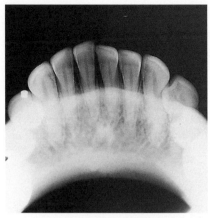

Anterior oblique occlusal of the mandible

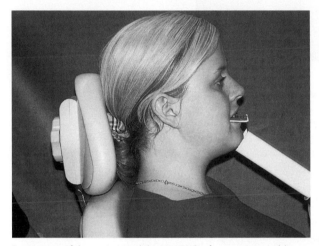

Positioning of the patient and the X-ray tube for an anterior oblique occlusal of the mandible

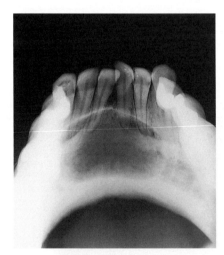

An anterior oblique occlusal showing a large unilocular radiolucency in the midline region

Oblique occlusal of the mandible

Lower oblique occlusal

Synonym: oblique occlusal.

This projection demonstrates the soft tissues of the middle and posterior aspects of the floor of the mouth.

Position of patient and film

- The patient sits comfortably, with the head supported. The median plane is vertical and the occlusal plane is horizontal.
- An occlusal film is placed flat in the patient's mouth on the side of interest.
- The film lies on the occlusal surfaces of the lower teeth, with the tube side of the film facing the floor of the mouth. The convention for positioning the film is that the long axis of film lies antero-posteriorly in the oral cavity (i.e. parallel with the sagittal plane).
- The edge of the film adjacent to the cheek should extend 1 cm lateral to the buccal surfaces of the posterior teeth to be imaged.
- The film must be positioned as far back as the patient will tolerate and the patient should bite together gently to avoid pressure marks on the film.
- The operator then supports the patient's head and rotates it away from the side of interest and, simultaneously, elevates the chin.
- This rotation and elevation allows the X-ray tube to be positioned below the angle of the mandible.

Direction and centring of the X-ray beam

- The X-ray tube is positioned 2 cm below and behind the angle of the mandible.
- The centring point is the angle of the mandible with an upward angle (cephalad) to the plane of the film of 115 degrees.
- It is important to ensure that the beam is parallel to the lingual plate of the mandible.

Alternative technique

Elderly or short-necked patients can be difficult to image with this technique, but an effective modification has been devised (Semple and Gibb, 1982):

- The patient is seated adjacent to a flat surface (i.e. table or work surface). With the film positioned intra-orally, the head is tipped over so that the forehead and nose are in contact with the table, and the head is rotated with the affected side 20 degrees away from the table.
- The X-ray tube is positioned above and behind the patient's shoulder. Use identical centring points as detailed above, with the tube position 25 degrees from the vertical.

Modifications of the technique

Using a soft-tissue exposure, this projection is employed primarily to detect radio-opaque calculi in the proximal regions of the submandibular duct as it crosses the free edge of the mylohyoid muscle. This modification is also referred to as the posterior oblique occlusal and postero-anterior lower occlusal.

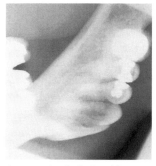

An example of a lower oblique occlusal

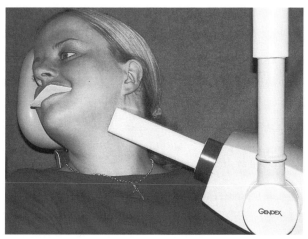

Positioning of the patient and the X-ray tube for a lower oblique occlusal of the mandible

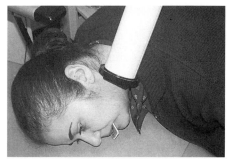

Alternative positioning of the patient and the X-ray tube for a lower oblique occlusal of the mandible

10 Lateral oblique of the mandible and maxilla

The lateral oblique radiograph is an extra-oral projection produced using conventional intra-oral X-ray equipment that reveals a larger area of the jaws than intra-oral radiography. It can also be produced using a skull unit.

Despite the growth of panoramic radiography, lateral oblique radiography remains a valid technique.

Although intra-oral radiography remains the obvious imaging modality for the majority of dental patients, there will be a relatively small number of dental/oral conditions that, because of their size and/or location, cannot be adequately imaged using intra-oral techniques. These are outlined as follows:

- Assessment of the presence/absence of teeth and also the position of unerupted teeth (especially third molars).
- Detection and assessment of fractures of the mandible.
- Assessment of large pathological lesions (e.g. cysts, tumours, osteodystrophies).
- When intra-oral radiography is impossible (e.g. trismus, severe gagging).
- Patients with physical and/or medical conditions in which large coverage and a rapid imaging technique is needed.

As a variety of different lateral oblique projections are carried out, the exact positioning of each of these views depends on the area or region of the jaws under examination.

This section will confine itself to describing the two most commonly requested lateral oblique projections:

- A lateral oblique projection imaging the body of the mandible and the maxilla.
- A lateral oblique projection imaging the ascending ramus of the mandible.

Radiographers requiring a fuller description of the range of oblique lateral projections are referred to the specialist textbooks on dental radiography listed at the end of this chapter.

General imaging principles

- The head is rotated to ensure that the area under examination is parallel to the film.
- The film and the median plane are not parallel.
- To avoid superimposition of the opposite side of the jaws, the combined angulation of the angle between the median plane and the film plus the angulation of the X-ray beam must not be less than 20 degrees.
- The central ray is perpendicular to the film but oblique to the median plane.

Lateral oblique of the body of the mandible and maxilla

This projection shows the dentition in the premolar/molar region of the maxilla and mandible, the inferior cortex of the mandible, and the angle and ascending ramus of the mandible.

Position of patient and cassette

- The patient sits comfortably, with the head supported. The median plane is vertical.
- A 13 × 18-cm cassette is used with a removable film marker attached to designate the side of the mandible to be imaged.
- The cassette is positioned against the patient's cheek overlying the region of the mandible under investigation, with the lower border parallel to the inferior border of the mandible but lying at least 2 cm below it.
- The positioning achieves a 10-degree angle of separation between the median sagittal plane and the film.
- The patient is instructed to stabilize the cassette in this position.
- The patient's head is rotated to the side of interest. This positions the contralateral ascending ramus forwards and increases the area between the neck and the shoulder to provide space for the X-ray tube.
- The chin is raised slightly to increase the space between the posterior aspect of the mandible and the cervical spine.
- The patient is asked to protrude the mandible.

Direction and centring of the X-ray beam

- Direct the central ray at a point 2 cm below and behind the angle of the contralateral side of the mandible (see figure).
- Positioning of the tube is dependent upon the area of clinical interest, i.e.:
  - third molar region for assessment of the position of third molars and possible pathology in this region;
  - premolar region for assessment of the developing dentition;
  - lower canine region if there is evidence of mandibular fracture or other pathology.
- The choice of beam angulation varies between 10 degrees upward and 10 degrees downward (see p. 315).
- The central ray is perpendicular to the plane of the film.

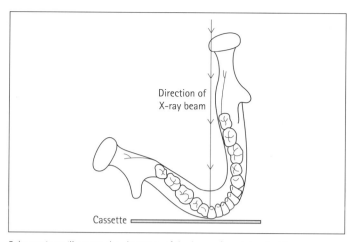

Schematic to illustrate the direction of the beam for a lateral oblique radiograph of the body of the mandible and maxilla

Lateral oblique of the body of the mandible and maxilla

Modification of the projection

- The choice of a downward beam angulation is related to the (clinical) need to avoid superimposition of the hyoid bone on the body of the mandible.
- To image the maxillary and mandibular canine/incisor region requires further rotation of the head to a point where the patient's nose is flattened against the cassette.
- It is important to ensure that the area of interest is parallel to the film. This technique reduces the angle of separation between the median sagittal plane and the film to five degrees.

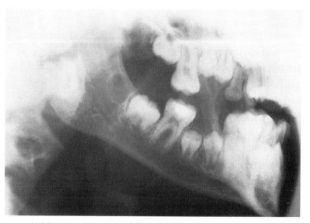

Lateral oblique radiograph of the body of the mandible and maxilla of a child in the mixed dentition

Cassette and the X-ray tube positions for a right lateral oblique radiograph of the body of the mandible and maxilla. Note the rotation of the head with flattening of the nose against the cassette

10 Lateral oblique of the mandible and maxilla

Lateral oblique of the ramus of the mandible

This projection gives an image of the ramus from the angle of the mandible to the condyle.

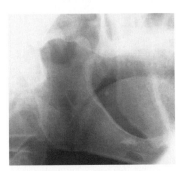

Lateral oblique radiograph of the ramus of the mandible

Position of patient and cassette

- The patient sits comfortably, with the head supported. The median plane is vertical.
- A 13 × 18-cm cassette is used with a removable film marker attached to designate the side of the mandible to be imaged.
- The cassette is positioned against the patient's cheek overlying the ascending ramus and the posterior aspect of the condyle of the mandible under investigation.
- The cassette is positioned so that its lower border is parallel with the inferior border of the mandible but lies at least 2 cm below it.
- The positioning achieves a 10-degree angle of separation between the median sagittal plane and the film.
- The patient is instructed to support the cassette in this position.
- The mandible is extended as far as possible.
- Limit rotation of head (≅ 10 degrees) towards the cassette.

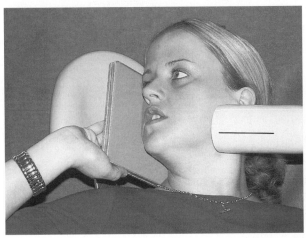

Cassette and the X-ray tube positions for a right lateral oblique radiograph of the ramus of the mandible

Direction and centring of the X-ray beam

- The central ray is directed posteriorly with upward angulation (cephalad) of 10 degrees towards the centre of the ramus of the mandible on the side of interest.
- The centring position of the tube is the contralateral side of the mandible at a point 2 cm below the inferior border in the region of the first/second permanent molar.

Note

Some operators prefer a slight (≅ 10 degrees) downward (caudad) angulation of the tube to prevent the image of the hyoid bone being superimposed on the body of the mandible.

Essential image characteristics

- There should be no removable metallic foreign bodies.
- There should be no motion artefacts.
- There should be no antero-posterior positioning errors.
- There should be no evidence of excessive elongation.
- There should be no evidence of incorrect horizontal angulation.
- There should be minimal superimposition of the hyoid bone on the region of (clinical) interest.
- There should be good density and adequate contrast between the enamel and the dentine.
- There should be no pressure marks on the film and no emulsion scratches.

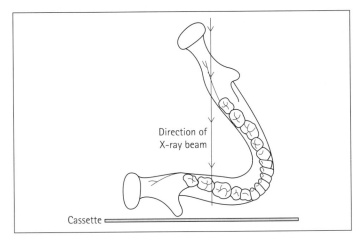

Schematic to illustrate the direction of the beam for a lateral oblique radiograph of the ramus of the mandible

- There should be no roller marks (automatic processing only).
- There should be no evidence of film fog.
- There should be no chemical streaks/splashes/contamination.
- There should be no evidence of inadequate fixation/washing.
- The name/date/left or right marker should be legible.

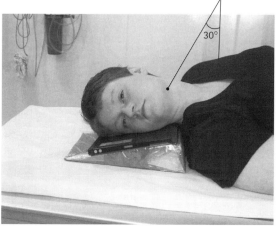

Patient lying supine on the X-ray couch and positioned for a right lateral oblique

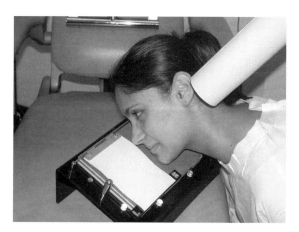

Patient positioned on an angle board for a right lateral oblique

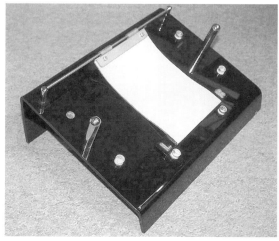

An angle board

Lateral oblique of the ramus of the mandible

Modification of the projection – patient supine

In a general department, the most convenient method of achieving the lateral oblique projection is with the patient supine on the X-ray couch.

Position of patient and cassette

- Use a 10-degree wedge-shaped foam pad to achieve separation of one side of the mandible from the other.
- Attach a removable film marker to the cassette to designate the side of the mandible to be imaged.
- With the cassette on the pad, the patient's head is rotated so the side of the jaw to be examined is parallel to the film, with the median sagittal plane parallel to the cassette.
- The head is tilted back on the spine to achieve further extension of the contralateral mandible away from the region of interest.

Direction and centring of the X-ray beam

- The central ray is angled 30 degrees cranially at an angle of 60 degrees to the cassette and is centred 5 cm inferior to the angle of the mandible remote from the cassette.

Using an angle board

An angle board is a device incorporating an incline to help separate the sides of the mandible.

Position of patient and cassette

- The head is positioned parallel to the angle board and cassette, but with the sagittal plane inclined to the vertical by the degree of angulation set by the device.
- Some angle boards incorporate ear rods to ensure accurate localization of the patient.
- A small forward tilt of the chin avoids superimposition of the cervical vertebrae on the ramus.

Direction and centring of the X-ray beam

- The tube is positioned below the angle of the mandible, remote from the film, and the central ray is directed towards the vertex.
- To avoid superimposition of the opposite side of the face, there must be an effective separation of 20 degrees.
- For example, with a sagittal plane angled at 15 degrees by the angle board, the central ray must be angled five degrees to the vertex to achieve the required separation of 20 degrees.

Bimolar projection

This technique is used in orthodontic practice. It shows both left and right oblique lateral views on one film. The technique incorporates a hinged lead shield to prevent exposure of the other side of the film.

10 Dental panoramic tomography

Synonyms: rotational panoramic radiography, orthopantomography (OPT), dental panoramic tomography (DPT), panoral.

Dental panoramic radiography is an extra-oral radiographic technique that produces an image of both jaws and their respective dentitions on a single film.

Panoramic radiography has supplanted lateral oblique radiography in that it is most useful in those patients who require an imaging modality providing a wide coverage of the jaws, such as:

- orthodontic assessment of the presence/absence of teeth;
- detection and assessment of fractures of the mandible;
- assessment of large pathological lesions (e.g. cysts, tumours, osteodystrophies);
- when intra-oral radiography is impossible (e.g. trismus, severe gagging);
- assessment of third molars before surgical removal.

Principles of panoramic image formation

Panoramic equipment is based upon a simultaneous rotational movement of the tube head and film cassette/carriage in equal but opposite directions around the patient's head, which remains stationary. The technique employs a slit-collimated vertical X-ray beam, with an eight-degree upward inclination, in association with a similar collimation slit in front of the film cassette/carriage to receive the image.

Improvements in image production have centred upon refining the rotational movement and determining the 'correct' form of the image layer. Manufacturers vary in the methods employed to produce the panoramic image. However, irrespective of the type of rotational movement involved, the result is the production of an elliptical image layer with three-dimensional form (i.e. height and width) in the shape of the dental arch. This image layer is referred to as the focal trough.

Within the different types of panoramic equipment, there are noticeable variations in the width of this image layer. This variability is much more apparent in equipment employing a continuous moving rotational centre, resulting in a narrow anterior layer compared with the lateral aspects of the focal trough.

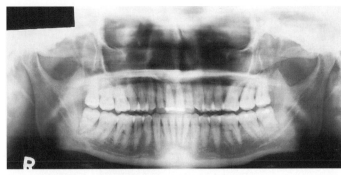

A dental panoramic tomograph of an adult dentate patient

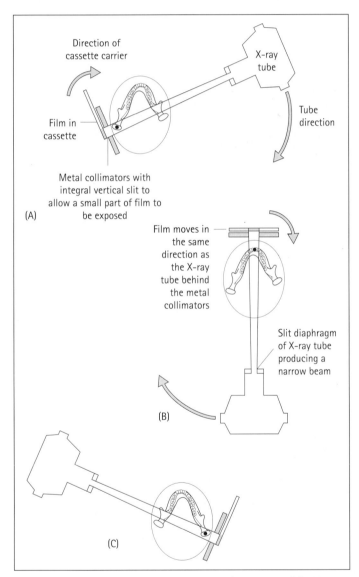

The schematic illustrates the relative positions and movement of the X-ray tubehead, cassette carrier and film during three stages of the exposure cycle of a continuous mode panoramic unit. The stages shown are: A, start of the exposure; B, intermediate stage of panoramic exposure; C, end of exposure. Throughout the exposure, a different part of the film is exposed as illustrated

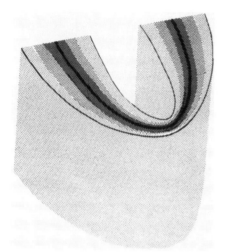

The focal trough

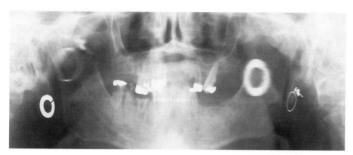

Patient position too close to the film with very obvious reduction in the width of the anterior teeth. The patient is also wearing earrings (of different design) and their ghost shadow appears at a higher level on the contralateral side of the image

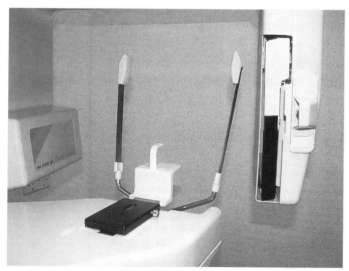

Patient-positioning devices on the Planmeca PM2002® panoramic unit: bite-peg, chin and temporal supports

Image acquisition

There are a number of factors inherent to panoramic radiography that reduce the diagnostic quality of the final image. These factors are:

- magnification variation;
- tomographic blur;
- overlap of adjacent teeth;
- superimposition of soft tissue and secondary shadows;
- limitations of resolution imposed by the image receptor, exposure parameters and processing conditions.

Magnification variation

While all types of radiographic projections exhibit a degree of magnification, the type associated with panoramic radiography is more complex. The individualized movement patterns, variations in the width of the beam, differing focus/object/film relationships, and the position/shape of the image layer chosen by the manufacturer can produce variations in magnification ranging from 10 to 30% between units.

Horizontal and vertical magnifications are only equal for structures at the centre of the focal plane. Within panoramic images, the degree of horizontal magnification varies considerably, depending upon the relationship of the structure to the image layer. Objects lying closer to the X-ray source (i.e. situated inside the focal trough) will display a greater degree of horizontal magnification. The situation is the reverse for those objects lying closer to the cassette (i.e. objects outside the focal trough), as they will be imaged with a relatively diminished horizontal magnification while the vertical shape remains virtually the same. This variability in horizontal shape is apparent by examining the appearance of anatomical structures within the focal trough (the tongue, hyoid bone) and those outside it (the zygomatic arch).

Minor inaccuracies in the antero-posterior positioning of the patient can easily lead to discrepancies between the vertical and horizontal magnification of teeth, with consequent distortions of tooth shape. These errors are most marked in the anterior regions of the jaws, where the focal plane is narrower.

Correct patient positioning is therefore essential for good image production. To achieve this, panoramic equipment employs various positioning aids to assist the operator. These include a system of light localizers (light beams diaphragm) to correctly position the patient, along with combinations of some or all of the following: chin rest, bite block, and two or more head supports.

Image acquisition (*contd*)

Tomographic blur

Panoramic radiography is known as a modified form of tomography, but only when tomography is described in the most general terms as a 'layer-forming imaging system'. The majority of panoramic systems have only one pre-designated rotational movement, resulting in one fixed form of image layer. The parameters of that image layer have been chosen to enable radiography of the 'average' jaw. Therefore, accurate patient positioning is always necessary to consistently accommodate the tooth-bearing regions of the maxilla and diagnostic quality. If a patient presents with a gross skeletal abnormality of one jaw relative to another, then two panoramic films may be required. If there are gross discrepancies within a single jaw, then the limitation of the imaging modality is obvious and has to be accepted.

Overlap of adjacent teeth

Although different movement patterns of the beam are adopted in different units, the aim of the manufacturer is to produce a beam of radiation that is perpendicular to the average arch. The maximum deviation from the ideal orthoradial (i.e. 90 degrees) projection occurs in the canine/premolar region, resulting in a variable amount of overlap of contact points, reducing caries diagnosis in these areas.

Superimposition of soft tissue and secondary shadows

Panoramic images are degraded further, to a variable degree, by shadows of soft tissues and surrounding air. Whilst many of these shadows are on the periphery of the image, the presence of air between the dorsum of the tongue and the hard palate leads to a band of relative overexposure of the roots of the maxillary teeth and associated alveolar bone. Elimination of this shadow is accomplished easily by positioning the tongue against the palate during radiography.

Secondary images of the spine and mandible reduce diagnostic quality further. In some panoramic equipment, compensation is made for the density of the cervical spine by stepping up the kVp or mA as the anterior structures are imaged. Whilst this technique is successful, it cannot compensate for incorrect positioning of the patient, which can result in the spine being imaged as a dense radio-opacity in the midline of the image. The same principles apply to the secondary imaging of the mandible, with these images becoming apparent and intrusive when careful patient positioning is not achieved.

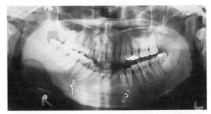

Patient suffers from hemifacial hypoplasia affecting the right side of the face. This has resulted in a marked reduction in the size of the bones on this side affecting correct positioning of the patient in the focal trough

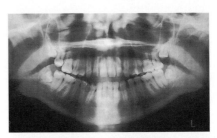

The problems of overlap in the premolar/molar region

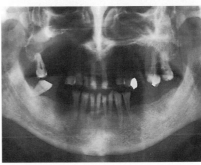

The presence of air between the dorsum of the tongue and the hard palate. This produces a band of relative overexposure of the roots of the maxillary teeth and the alveolar bone

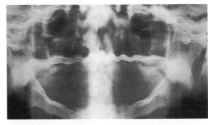

Incorrect positioning of the patient resulting in the presence of the dense radio-opacity of the spine in the midline of the panoramic image. The patient has moved throughout the exposure in a vertical direction. This is evidenced by the undulating outline of the lower border of the mandible and that of the hard and soft palate

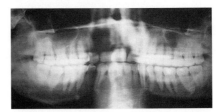

Patient positioned too far from the film resulting in the horizontal magnification of the anterior teeth and also blurring of the teeth. Incorrect positioning has also resulted in the production of secondary images of the mandible. These are seen as dense radio-opacities overlying the posterior maxillary and mandibular teeth

Essential image characteristics

- Edge-to-edge incisors.
- No removable metallic foreign bodies.
- No motion artefacts.
- Tongue against roof of mouth.
- Minimization of spine shadow.
- No antero-posterior positioning errors.
- No mid-sagittal plane positioning errors.
- No occlusal plane positioning errors.
- Correct positioning of spinal column.
- There should be good density and adequate contrast between the enamel and the dentine. (Use of a wide-latitude film is recommended.)
- Name/date/left or right marker all legible.
- Correct anatomical coverage, depending upon clinical application, i.e. limit area covered to clinical needs.
- No cassette/screen problems.
- Adequate processing techniques.
- No pressure marks on film.
- No roller marks (automatic processing only).
- No evidence of film fog.
- No chemical streaks/splashes/contamination.
- No evidence of inadequate fixation/washing.
- Name/date/left or right markers all legible.

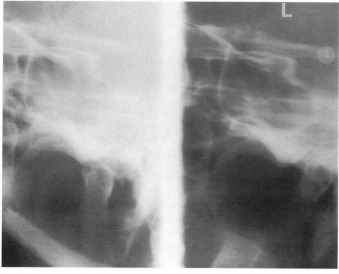

Sectional image of the left temporo-mandibular joint region

Limitations of resolution imposed by the image receptor, exposure parameters and processing conditions

There is an inevitable reduction in resolution when using screen film. In addition, the exposure factors and processing conditions profoundly influence the perception of detail.

The quality of panoramic films is heavily dependent upon careful attention to technique and processing. Failure to observe these principles has been reported in a recent study (Rushton et al. 1999), which found that one-third of all panoramic films taken were diagnostically unacceptable.

Dose reduction in panoramic radiography

Newer panoramic equipment incorporates improved methods of X-ray generation, such as direct current generators. It also employs field limitation, which enables the operator to image selected areas of designated interest, thereby reducing the dose to the patient. Further dose reduction is achieved by the provision of a variable mA and kVp facility, allowing the equipment to be used with faster film/screen combinations.

Recent advances in panoramic imaging

Newer panoramic equipment, combined with linear tomography, offers greater versatility for the clinician. Most manufacturers provide field-size limitation as standard. These programmes may include some or all of the following: jaws, maxillary sinuses, temporo-mandibular joint (TMJ) programmes, and a child programme. Some manufacturers offer digital sensors as an alternative to film/screen combinations.

Many panoramic machines now include an optional cephalometric facility. These combined machines may have a separate cephalometric tube head, or the machine is converted rapidly from panoramic to cephalometric mode with a simple switch.

Image acquisition (*contd*)

Patient preparation

- If the patient is wearing a bulky coat, then they should be asked to remove it as it can interfere with the rotational movement of the panoramic equipment.
- The patient should remove all radio-opaque objects from the head and neck areas. These include spectacles, metallic hair clips at the neckline on the back or side of head, hearing aids, earrings, tongue studs, nose jewellery and necklaces. This instruction also includes intra-oral devices, such as complete/partial dentures and removable orthodontic appliances. High-necked sweaters with metal zippers/fasteners should also be removed. Chewing gum appears as a radio-opaque mass on the image and should be disposed of before imaging.
- If the patient is unable to remove earrings from the lobule of the ear, then the lobule and attached earring should be folded inwardly on the anti-tragus and taped to the helix/anti-helix of the external ear. The use of this technique ensures that the ghost images of the earrings will not appear on the final image.

General comments

- The unit should be readied in the start position and raised sufficiently to allow the patient to walk into the equipment.
- Depending on the type of equipment used, the examination can be carried out with the patient either standing or seated.
- Careful explanation of the procedure must be given to the patient, as the exposure times vary from 12 to 20 s.
- In view of the exposure time involved, this technique should not be used to image the following patients:
  - children unable to remain motionless for the duration of the 12–20-s exposure;
  - patients suffering from medical conditions resulting in uncontrollable involuntary movement and lack of coordination.

Position of patient and cassette

- A 15 × 30-cm cassette should be inserted in the cassette carrier.
- Position a bite block on the machine (or chin rest if this is all that is available).
- Ask the patient to walk straight into the machine, gripping the handles if available, and ask them to adopt an upright stance, the so-called 'ski position'. Often patients are afraid of the equipment and hence enter tentatively, with their neck craning forward.

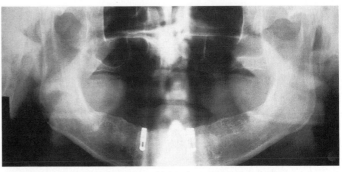

Ghost shadow of radio-opaque necklace obscuring the mandible

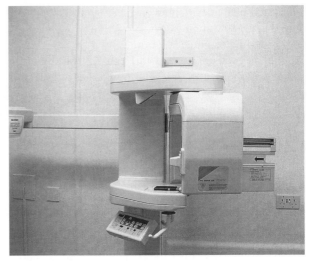

Panoramic unit in start position

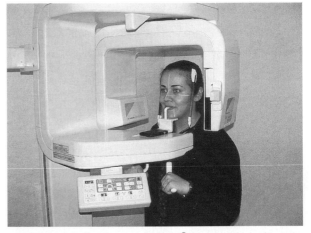

Patient positioned in Planmeca PM2002®. The bite block, chin rest and temporal supports and the light beam marker lines ensure correct positioning

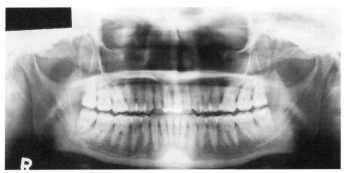

A dental panoramic tomograph of an adult dentate patient

Image acquisition

- The patient's head should be tilted down towards the floor, so that the Frankfort plane is parallel to floor. In this position, ala-tragus is five degrees caudad.
- Turn on the positioning lights:
  - the sagittal plane light should be down the middle of the face;
  - the Frankfort plane should be five degrees down from the ala-tragus line;
  - the antero-posterior light should be centred distal to the upper lateral incisor (i.e. the lateral/canine inter-proximal space).
- Adjust the height of the machine to the patient, not vice versa.
- Ask the patient to bite into the bite block groove. Check that the upper and lower incisors are both in the groove. In patients with a prominent mandible relative to the maxilla (i.e. class III patients), at least ensure that the upper incisors are in the groove.
- Have the patient rest their chin on the chin rest. If the chin is not on the support, or if the cassette is too far below the mandible, then adjust to prevent the image being positioned too high with consequent loss of the upper portion of the image.
- Stand behind the patient and check the symmetry of position. Adjust if needed by holding the shoulders.
- Close the head restraints.
- Make any fine adjustments at this point.
- Ask the patient to close their lips and press their tongue to the roof of their mouth. The latter instruction is particularly important, since if it is not done a dark radiolucent shadow of the air space above the tongue will obscure the apices of the maxillary teeth. Closing the lips around the bite block reduces the air shadow, which can be mistaken for caries where it overlies the dentition in the premolar region.
- Explain again that the patient must stay absolutely still for about 20 s.
- Make the exposure.

Problems with panoramic radiography

This technique is plagued with problems relating to positioning errors. The more common positioning errors and those related to movement are outlined in the table on the next page.

Problems with panoramic radiography

Common panoramic film faults and how to correct them

Panoramic film fault	Appearance of fault	Remedy
Anterior teeth positioning errors Head too far forward, i.e. dental arch positioned anterior to focal trough	Narrow unsharp image of anterior teeth present; spine overlaps the rami	Ensure occlusal plane is tilted downward slightly and the teeth are biting in the grooves on the bite block, as outlined in procedures
Head too far back, i.e. dental arch positioned posterior to focal trough	Wide unsharp image of anterior teeth present; TMJ region not evident	
Mid-sagittal plane positioning errors Head off-centre Tilting of the head Twisted position of patient	Mid-sagittal plane off-centre, rami and posterior teeth unequally magnified; side tilted towards X-ray tube enlarged; side closer towards the film looks smaller	Ensure correct sagittal position of the patient Ensure interpupillary (interorbital) line is parallel
Occlusal plane positioning errors Excessive downward angulation (patient's chin too far down)	Severe curvature of the occlusal plane; lack of definition of the lower incisors	Ensure correct position of occlusal plane
Upward over-angulation (patient's chin too far up)	Flattening of occlusal plane, superimposition of apices of maxillary teeth on hard palate; image of anterior teeth unsharp	
Spinal column positioning error	Underexposed region in midline of image due to excessive attenuation of energy of beam by spinal column; appears as dense radio-opacity	Ensure patient adopts 'ski position'; operator must correct position before exposure if patient slumps forward
Patient's shoulder interfering with movement of cassette	Slows cassette, resulting in dark band due to prolonged exposure in region where obstruction occurred	Patient usually has short neck, elevate chin until ala-tragus line is parallel to floor; positioning cassette 1 cm higher may also help

TMJ, temporo-mandibular joint.

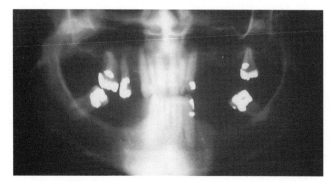

Panoramic radiograph with the patient's chin too far down

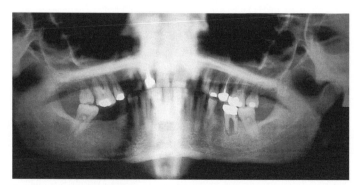

Panoramic radiograph with the patient's chin too far up

Cephalometric radiography ensures standardization and reproducibility of the images taken.

Lateral and postero-anterior projections are used as part of the initial evaluation of patients who are being considered for orthodontic treatment and/or orthognathic surgery. The technique is also used in the assessment of dentofacial abnormalities.

X-ray equipment features

The equipment can be stand-alone (i.e. existing X-ray equipment employed with a separate cephalostat). More commonly, however, the equipment is an integral component of a panoramic unit. The cephalostat (or craniostat) provides the mechanism by which the projection is standardized. It consists of two Perspex arms with attached ear pieces/rods to position the patient accurately.

Stand-alone equipment uses a fixed FFD of 200 cm, whilst that employed in combined panoramic/cephalometric equipment is about 150 cm. Whichever method is used, the longer FFD ensures that the beam is parallel, thereby minimizing magnification in the image. It is important that the X-ray equipment used has sufficient output to produce a final image exhibiting adequate penetration.

A filter attenuates the beam in the anterior regions so that the soft tissues of the face can also be demonstrated on one film. Pre-patient image enhancement is obtained when the filter is attached to the tube head covering the anterior part of the emerging beam. Post-patient image enhancement is achieved by placing a filter between the patient and the anterior part of the cassette. The former technique is preferable, as, in this position, the filter leaves no line of demarcation on the film and also provides dose reduction. A beam collimator must be incorporated at the tube head to limit the beam to those areas containing the main cephalometric points (British Society for the Study of Orthodontics and the British Society of Dental and Maxillofacial Radiology, 1985; Isaacson and Thom, 2001).

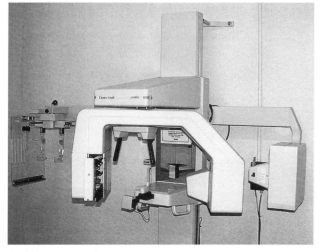

Cephalometric attachment to a panoramic unit

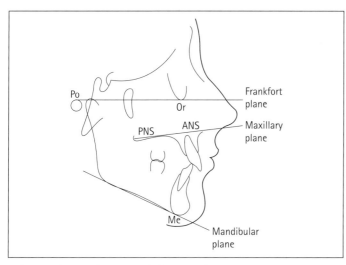

A diagram showing the main cephalometric planes

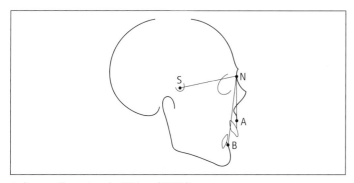

A diagram illustrating the SNA and SNB lines

Lateral projection

The projection is a standardized true lateral projection of the skull.

Position of patient and cassette

- The patient sits or stands inside the cephalometric unit, with the sagittal plane vertical and parallel to the cassette.
- The Frankfort plane should be horizontal.
- The head is immobilized by guiding the ear pieces carefully into the external auditory meati. Metal circular markers within the ear pieces allow the operator to rapidly recognize off-centring of the cephalostat.
- The nose support is positioned against the nasion.
- A wedge-shaped filter is positioned so that it will be superimposed on the face, with its thick edge placed anteriorly.
- The patient is instructed to close their mouth and to bite together on their back teeth (i.e. in centric occlusion). Some children find this difficult to do, so it is worth checking before exposing the radiograph.
- The lips should be relaxed.

Direction and centring of the X-ray beam

- The direction and centring of the X-ray beam will normally be fixed. The horizontal beam is centred on the external auditory meati.

Essential image characteristics

- No removable metallic foreign bodies.
- No distortion due to movement.
- Frankfort plane perpendicular to the film.
- No anterior-posterior positioning errors.
- No sagittal plane positioning errors.
- No occlusal plane positioning errors.
- Teeth in centric occlusion (stable and natural intercuspation).
- Lips relaxed.
- Exact matching of external auditory meati with positioning devices.
- Visibility of all cephalometric tracing points required for analysis.
- Visibility of all anterior skeletal and soft tissue structures.
- Good density and contrast.
- No cassette/screen problems.
- No pressure marks on film.
- No roller marks (automatic processing only).
- No evidence of film fog.
- No chemical streaks/splashes/contamination.
- No evidence of inadequate fixation/washing.
- Name and date legible.

Radiological considerations

The use of beam collimation has dramatically reduced the dose to patients whilst adequately imaging the patient without loss of the information that is necessary for orthodontic or orthognathic

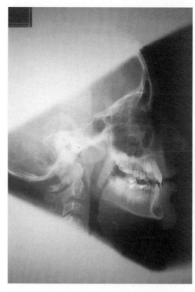

True cephalometric lateral skull radiograph. Images of metal ear rods are superimposed over one another and image displays optimal collimation

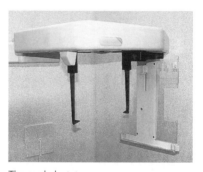

The cephalostat

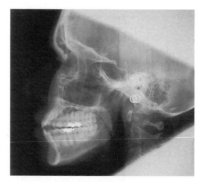

True cephalometric lateral skull radiograph with images of metal ear rods separated indicating 'off centring'

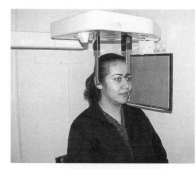

Positioning for the true cephalometric lateral skull radiograph

diagnosis (British Society for the Study of Orthodontics and the British Society of Dental and Maxillofacial Radiology, 1985). The wedge collimation limits the dose to the superior aspects of the calvarium above the orbits and to the lower aspects of the cervical spine. Unfortunately, when using modern panoramic equipment, it is impossible with some models to access the tube head to add the additional wedge collimation.

Cephalometric analysis

Cephalometric analysis uses reference lines and points to evaluate underlying skeletal developmental discrepancies. The analysis involves the identification of certain hard and soft tissue landmarks evident on a standardized true lateral projection of the skull. These are subsequently either traced manually from the radiograph onto an overlying sheet of paper or digitally recorded. The latter technique has simplified the process and also provides the clinician with a range of cephalometric analysis packages (i.e. Eastman, Rickett, McNamara etc.) as standard within the software. Using either technique results in the clinician obtaining quantitative measurements with which to evaluate the patient.

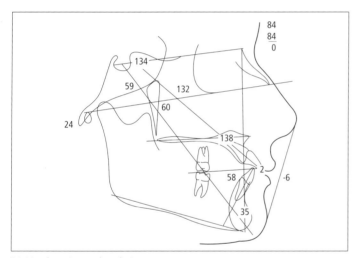

Digitized tracing and analysis

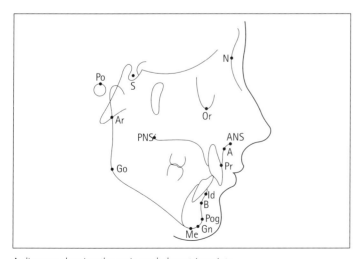

A diagram showing the main cephalometric points

Lateral projection

The main cephalometric points are listed below in alphabetical order and are shown in the lower figure opposite:

Anterior nasal spine (ANS): The point or tip of the bony nasal spine.
Articulare (Ar): The point of intersection of the projection of the surface of the neck of the condyle and the inferior surface of the basi-occiput.
Gnathion (Gn): The most anterior and inferior point on the bony symphysis of the mandible. It is equidistant from the pogonion and the menton.
Gonion (Go): The most posterior and inferior point on the angle of the mandible.
Infradentale (Id): The most anterior point of the alveolar crest between the lower incisors.
Menton (Me): The lowest point on the mandibular symphysis.
Nasion (N): The most anterior point on the frontonasal suture.
Orbitale (Or): The most inferior point on the infra-orbital margin.
Pogonion (Pog): The most anterior point of the bony chin.
Point A or Subspinale (A): This is the deepest point on the maxillary profile between the anterior nasal spine and the alveolar crest.
Point B or Supramentale (B): This is the deepest point on the concavity of the mandible between the point of the chin and the alveolar crest.
Porion (Po): The highest point on the bony external acoustic meatus. It has been suggested that one takes the highest point of the earpieces of the cephalostat.
Posterior nasal spine (PNS): The point or tip of the posterior spine of the palatine bone of the hard palate.
Prosthion (Pr): The most anterior point of the alveolar crest in the pre-maxilla.
Sella (S): The mid point of the sella turcica.

The main cephalometric planes and angles are listed below and are outlined in the two figures on p. 325.

Frankfort plane: A plane transversing the skull and represented by a line joining the porion and the orbitale.
Mandibular plane: This line causes confusion as a variety of definitions have been applied to describe it. The simplest way to locate the mandibular line is to draw a line from the menton tangential to the lower border of the mandible at the angle. Other definitions include:

- A line joining the gnathion and gonion.
- A line joining the menton and gonion.

Maxillary plane: A line joining the anterior and posterior nasal spines.
SN plane: A line joining the sella and the nasion.
SNA: This relates the antero-posterior position of the maxilla, represented by the A point, to the cranial base.
SNB: This relates the antero-posterior position of the mandible, represented by the B point, to the cranial base.

Postero-anterior projection

Most cephalometric equipment has the facility to allow this projection to be taken. It is an important view in assessing patients with facial asymmetry.

Position of patient and cassette

- The equipment is rotated through 90 degrees.
- The patient is set up as for a postero-anterior projection of the mandible.
- The orbito-meatal baseline is parallel to the floor.
- The head is immobilized using ear pieces inserted into the external auditory meati.

Direction and centring of the X-ray beam

- The horizontal X-ray beam is fixed.
- The central beam is centred through the cervical spine at the level of the rami.

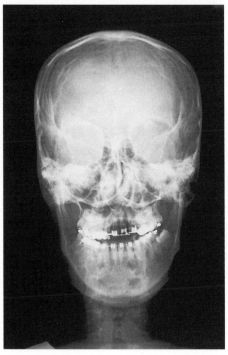

A cephalometric postero-anterior jaws

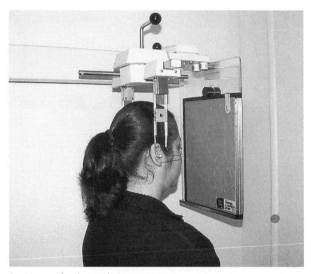

Positioning for the cephalometric postero-anterior jaws projection

References

British Society for the Study of Orthodontics and the British Society of Dental and Maxillofacial Radiology (1985). Report of a Joint Working Party for the British Society for the Study of Orthodontics and the British Society of Dental and Maxillofacial Radiology. The reduction of the dose to patients during lateral cephalometric radiography. *British Journal of Orthodontics* **12**:176–178.

Isaacson KG, Thom AR (eds) (2001). *Guidelines for the Use of Radiographs in Clinical Orthodontics*, 2nd edn. London: British Orthodontic Society.

Kaffe I, Littner MM, Tamse A, Serebro L (1981). Clinical evaluation of a bitewing film holder. *Quintessence International* **12**:935–938.

National Radiological Protection Board (2001). *Guidance Notes for Dental Practitioners on the Safe Use of X-ray Equipment.* London: Department of Health.

Rushton VE and Horner K (1994). A comparative study of five periapical radiographic techniques in general dental practice. *Dentomaxillofacial Radiology* **23**:37–45, 96.

Rushton VE, Horner K, Worthington H (1999). The quality of panoramic radiographs in a sample of general dental practices. *British Dental Journal* **186**:630–633.

Semple J, Gibb D (1982). The postero-anterior lower occlusal view – a routine projection for the submandibular gland. *Radiography* **48**:122–124.

Tanner RJ, Wall BF, Shrimpton PC, Hart D, Bungay DR (2000). *Frequency of Medical and Dental X-ray Examinations in the UK – 1997/98.* Chilton: National Radiological Protection Board – R320.

The quality standards used in the text are derived from: Radiation Protection: European Guidelines on Radiation Protection in Dental Radiology. Luxembourg: European Commission. Also available as a download PDF file at: http://europa.eu.int/comm/energy/nuclear/radioprotection/publication_en.htm.

Specialized textbooks on dental radiography

Whaites E (2002). *Essentials of Dental Radiography and Radiology*, 3rd edn. Edinburgh: Churchill Livingstone.

White SC, Pharoah MJ (2004). *Oral Radiology – Principles and Interpretation*, 5th edn. St Louis: Mosby.

Acknowledgements

The author is indebted to Michael Rushton for the majority of the photography in this section. James Peacop was responsible for the new schematics and line drawings, which are a testament to his artistic skills. Professor Keith Horner, Angela Carson, Di Whitfield, Sue Wilson, Christine Rowley, Corinne Niman, Pamela Coates and Ian Triffitt at the X-ray Unit, University Dental Hospital of Manchester, provided me with help, advice and encouragement during the writing of this text. Mr Peter Hirschmann, Consultant in Dental and Maxillofacial Radiology at Leeds Dental Institute, gave valuable and constructive comments as well as providing a great deal of valuable technical and editorial advice. Finally to Sue Lea and Zina Ismael, I extend my thanks for their unflagging enthusiasm during the many hours that they spent as photographic models.

The Abdomen and Pelvic Cavity

CONTENTS

INTRODUCTION   332
Planes and regions   332
Most common referral criteria   334
Typical imaging protocols   334
Recommended projections   334
Image parameters   335
Radiological considerations   336

ABDOMEN AND PELVIC CAVITY   338
Antero-posterior – supine   338
Antero-posterior – erect   340
Antero-posterior – erect (patient sitting)   341
Antero-posterior – left lateral decubitus   342
Lateral dorsal decubitus (supine)   342

LIVER AND DIAPHRAGM   343
Antero-posterior technique   343

DIAPHRAGMATIC MOVEMENT DURING
RESPIRATION   344

URINARY TRACT   345
Antero-posterior   345
Right posterior oblique   346
Lateral   346

URINARY BLADDER   347
Antero-posterior 15 degrees caudad   347
Right or left posterior oblique   347

BILIARY SYSTEM   348
Left anterior oblique   348
Right posterior oblique   349

This chapter deals only with plain radiography of the abdomen and pelvic contents. Examinations including the introduction of contrast media will be found in Whitley *et al.* (1999).

Planes and regions

The abdominal cavity extends from the undersurface of the diaphragm above to the pelvic inlet below and is contained by the muscles of the abdominal walls.

To mark the surface anatomy of the viscera, the abdomen is divided into nine regions by two transverse planes and two parasagittal (or vertical) planes.

The upper transverse plane, called the transpyloric plane, is midway between the suprasternal notch and the symphysis pubis, approximately midway between the upper border of the xiphisternum and the umbilicus. Posteriorly, it passes through the body of the first lumbar vertebra near its lower border; anteriorly, it passes through the tips of the right and left ninth costal cartilages.

The lower transverse plane, called the transtubercular plane, is at the level of the tubercles of the iliac crest anteriorly and near the upper border of the fifth lumbar vertebra posteriorly.

The two parasagittal planes are at right-angles to the two transverse planes. They run vertically, passing through a point midway between the anterior superior iliac spine and the symphysis pubis on each side.

These planes divide the abdomen into nine regions centrally from above to below epigastric, umbilical and hypogastric regions and laterally from above to below right and left hypochondriac, lumbar and iliac regions.

The pelvic cavity is continuous with the abdominal cavity at the pelvic inlet, extends inferiorly to the muscles of the pelvic floor, and is contained within the bony pelvis.

Although viscera are said to occupy certain regions of the abdomen, and surface markings can be stated, it must be remembered that surface markings of viscera are variable, particularly those organs that are suspended by a mesentery. The main factors affecting the position and surface markings of organs are: (a) body build, (b) phase of respiration, (c) posture (erect or recumbent), (d) loss of tone of abdominal muscles, which may occur with age, (e) change of size due to pathology, (f) quantity of contents of hollow viscera, (g) the presence of an abnormal mass, and (h) normal variants within the population.

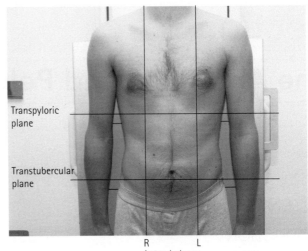

Lateral planes

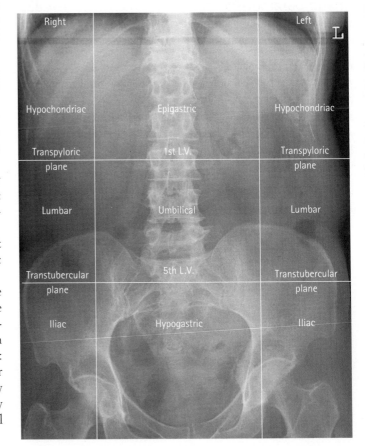

Planes and regions

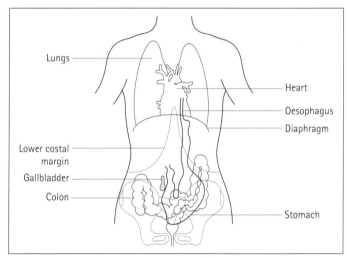

Hypersthenic

Asthenic

Individuals have been classified, according to body build, into four types: hypersthenic, sthenic, hyposthenic and asthenic. The shape and position of organs tend to follow a particular pattern typifying each type.

Hypersthenic – massively built. The dome of the diaphragm is high and the lower costal margin is at a high level with a wide angle, resulting in the widest part of the abdomen being its upper part. The stomach and transverse colon are in the upper part of the abdomen. The fundus of the gallbladder is pushed upwards so that the gallbladder lies horizontally in the abdomen well away from the midline.

Asthenic – thin and slender. The elongated narrow thorax with a narrow costal angle is associated with a low position of the dome of the diaphragm. The abdominal cavity is shallow, being widest in its lowest region. The pylorus of the stomach is low and the long stomach may reach well below the iliac crests, while the transverse colon can loop down into the pelvic cavity. The gallbladder lies vertically close to the midline, with the fundus below the level of the iliac crests.

Between these two extremes of body build are the **sthenic** (tending towards hypersthenic, but not as broad in proportion to height) and the **hyposthenic** (tending towards asthenic, but not as thin and slender).

For any given body type, abdominal viscera occupy a lower position:

- in inspiration compared with expiration;
- in the erect position compared with the recumbent position;
- with age and the associated loss of muscle tone.

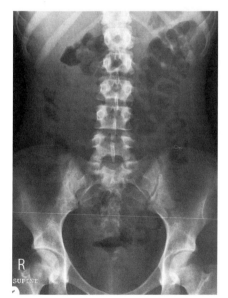

Asthenic

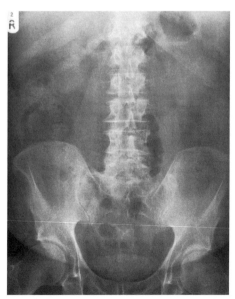

Hypersthenic

It may be possible to fit the whole of an asthenic abdomen on one image whereas hypersthenic body habitus will usually necessitate two transverse cassettes for full imaging of the abdomen. Note that in the right hand image only the lower half of the abdomen has been demonstrated

333

11 Introduction

Most common referral criteria

Radiographic examination of the abdomen and pelvic cavity is performed for a variety of reasons, including:

- obstruction of the bowel;
- perforation;
- renal pathology;
- acute abdomen (with no clear clinical diagnosis);
- foreign body localization (see also Section 14);
- toxic megacolon;
- aortic aneurysm;
- prior to the introduction of a contrast medium, e.g. intra-venous urography (IVU) to demonstrate the presence of radio-opaque renal or gallstones and to assess the adequacy of bowel preparation;
- to detect calcification or abnormal gas collections, e.g. abscess;
- alimentary studies using barium preparations.

Typical imaging protocols

The following table illustrates projections used to diagnose common clinical conditions (see also Royal College of Radiologists, 2003).

Recommended projections

Examination is performed by means of the following:

Basic	• Antero-superior – supine
Alternatively	• Postero-anterior – prone
Supplementary	• Antero-posterior – erect
	• Antero-posterior or postero-anterior – left lateral decubitus
	• Lateral – dorsal decubitus
	• Posterior obliques

Condition	Supine abdomen	Additional projections
Obstruction	Yes	• Erect abdomen
Perforation	If indicated by local protocol	• Erect postero-anterior or antero-posterior chest
		• Antero-posterior or postero-anterior – left lateral decubitus
		• Lateral – dorsal decubitus
Renal pathology	Yes	• Supine on inspiration
		• Right or left posterior oblique
Acute abdomen	Yes	• Erect postero-anterior or antero-posterior chest
Foreign body (FB)		
• Swallowed	Not indicated unless FB is potentially poisonous, sharp, unusually large (risk of impaction), or obstruction is suspected e.g. in a child with abdominal pain	• Lateral soft tissue neck
		• Erect postero-anterior or antero-posterior chest
• Inhaled	No	• Erect postero-anterior or antero-posterior chest to include soft tissue neck
• Penetrating	Yes	• Lateral
• Other	Yes	• Lateral rectum or lateral bladder
Toxic megacolon	Yes	• Erect abdomen
Aortic aneurism	Yes	• Lateral
	NB: The preferred examination is CT or ultrasound if available	• Erect postero-anterior or antero-posterior chest

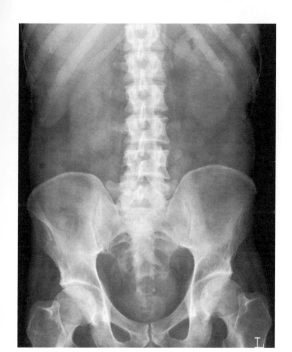

Correctly exposed image showing well defined renal outlines

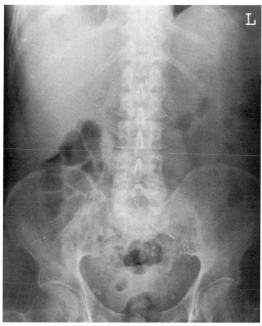

Poor quality 'flat' image with ill-defined margins due to too high kVp. Note artefact from an elasticized band of an undergarment

Image parameters

Although the radiographic technique used will depend on the condition of the patient, there are a number of requirements common to any plain radiography of the abdomen and pelvic cavity. Maximum image sharpness and contrast must be obtained so that adjacent soft tissues can be differentiated.

Radiography is normally performed using a standard imaging table with a moving grid. However, depending on the condition of the patient, imaging may be performed using a stationary grid either on a patient transport trolley or on the ward using a mobile X-ray machine.

The patient should be immobilized, and exposure is made on arrested respiration, usually after full expiration.

The following table illustrates the parameters necessary to provide optimum and consistent image resolution and contrast for the antero-posterior supine abdomen projection.

Item	Comment
Focus spot size	≤1.3 mm
Total filtration	3.00 mm Al equivalent
Anti-scatter grid	R = 10 (8); 40/cm
Film/screen combination	Speed class 400–800
FFD	115 (100–150) cm
Radiographic voltage	75–90 kVp
Automatic exposure control	Chamber(s) selected – central or central and right upper lateral
Exposure time	Less than 200 ms

Note

By choosing both chambers, this avoids the risk of underexposure due to the beam passing through regions containing mainly bowel gas.

Essential image characteristics

- Coverage of the whole abdomen to include diaphragm to symphysis pubis and lateral properitoneal fat stripe for the acute abdomen.
- Visualization of the whole of the urinary tract (kidneys, ureters and bladder – KUB).
- Visually sharp reproduction of the bones and the interface between air-filled bowel and surrounding soft tissues with no overlying artefacts, e.g. clothing.
- In calculus disease, good tissue differentiation is essential to visualize small or low-opacity stones.

Radiation protection

- The 'pregnancy rule' should be observed unless it has been decided to ignore it in the case of an emergency.
- Gonad shielding can be used, but not when there is a possibility that important radiological signs may be hidden.
- By following a well-planned procedure, the necessity to repeat the examination is avoided, thus limiting the radiation dose to the patient.

Radiological considerations

General observations

The abdominal radiograph is a vital first-line investigation in a range of acute abdominal pathologies. Interpretation can be very difficult and is often performed initially by a relatively inexperienced doctor. High-quality examination is important but may be difficult to achieve as these patients are often in pain and may be very distended with gas.

Selection of the appropriate strategy for imaging the acute abdomen depends largely upon the clinical indication for the investigation. The following is a discussion of possible indications for this investigation, some of the signs that may be demonstrated, and the role of other modalities.

Calculi

Acute renal colic is a severe, sharp, intermittent pain on one side of the abdomen, often radiating to the groin or testicle. Frequently the patient has some degree of haematuria. Calculi may be visible on plain radiographs, depending on their chemical composition, in up to 90% of cases. Visible calculi appear as foci of increased attenuation, often tiny, and more often oval than round. Some chemical types are relatively low density, and even when calcified are hard to see if very small, especially when obscured by overlying gas, faeces or bone. Larger calculi appear more round, and very large calculi may assume the shape of the calyceal system (stag-horn calculi).

The radiographic examination is a single supine abdominal radiograph, which must cover from the top of the highest kidney to the symphysis pubis (the KUB: kidneys, ureters and bladder). On larger patients, separate renal and bladder area images may be required. Breath-hold is vital as very slight movement unsharpness will obscure small calculi and larger calculi of lower visibility. The area where calculi are most often overlooked is the sacrum and sacro-iliac joints, where the background is most complex.

IVU is the most frequently used investigation to confirm that an opacity is truly within the urinary tract, and to detect lucent calculi, although computed tomography (CT) scanning is increasingly used where it is available. The role of ultrasound is very limited, as it cannot visualize the ureters. Nuclear medicine can demonstrate the presence and level of ureteric obstruction, but not the cause.

Intestinal obstruction

Intestinal obstruction may have many causes, but the commonest is adhesions due to previous disease or surgery. Tumours (especially in the colon), hernias and Crohn's disease (especially in the small bowel) are other common causes. The patient may have a previous history, and typically presents with colicky abdominal pain and distension. The bowel sounds on auscultation are said to be high-pitched and 'tinkling'. The supine plain

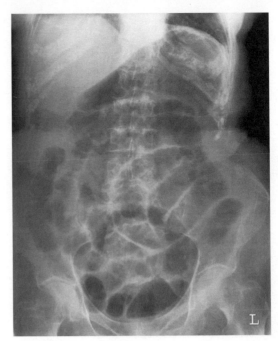

Antero-posterior supine radiograph of the abdomen showing small bowel obstruction

radiograph typically shows abnormally distended bowel loops containing excessive gas. Not infrequently the typical signs are absent, especially if the bowel contains predominantly fluid; an erect image may then show fluid levels that confirm the diagnosis (in the appropriate clinical setting). Air fluid levels also occur in a range of conditions, including those not requiring surgery, such as gastroenteritis and jejunal diverticulosis.

Obstruction of the large bowel is differentiated from that of the small bowel mainly by the mucosal pattern of the affected bowel (requiring optimum radiographic technique) and its distribution within the abdomen (requiring full coverage of the abdomen).

Gastric outlet obstruction may be seen on supine images (if gas-filled) or erect chest or abdomen images if there is more fluid.

CT may demonstrate intestinal obstruction and will often show the cause. Ultrasound can also detect obstruction but less often the cause, and is not the primary imaging modality.

Fluid collections

Extensive ascites may be seen as a medium opacity band in the paracolic gutters, loss of clarity of the liver edge, and medial displacement of the ascending and descending colon or small bowel loops. Ultrasound is far more sensitive and specific than plain radiography and will be used for confirmation in cases of clinical doubt. Loculated fluid collections such as abscess or cyst will have the appearance of a soft tissue mass, displacing bowel loops. If an abscess contains gas, then an air fluid level may be seen on the erect image. The exact appearance will depend on the location and the underlying cause.

Perforation

Perforation of a hollow abdominal viscus releases free gas into the peritoneal cavity. This can be detected sensitively by horizontal-beam radiography. As little as 1 ml can be detected under ideal circumstances (Miller 1973). Common causes are perforated

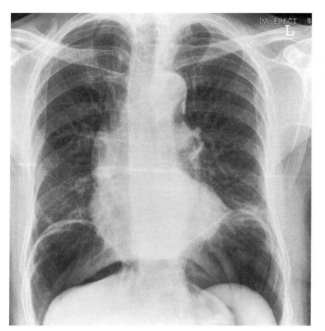

Postero-anterior erect chest and upper abdomen showing large perforation of the abdominal cavity

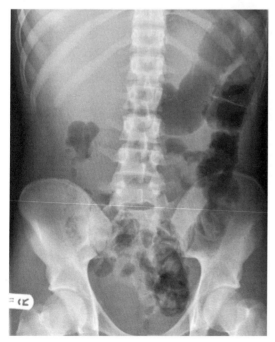

Antero-posterior supine radiograph of the abdomen showing the effect of right renal trauma with the loss of right psoas muscle and renal outlines

diverticular disease and perforated peptic ulcer. The best investigation is an erect chest radiograph, which will show free gas under one hemi-diaphragm, especially above the liver on the right. If this is not possible, then an antero-posterior left lateral decubitus projection (right side raised) is a suitable alternative, or a lateral dorsal decubitus (supine) can be obtained. Whichever projection is used, the patient should be left for 20 minutes in that position to allow the air to rise, otherwise the diagnosis may be missed. The outcome is an image showing a crescent or bubble of gas in the most non-dependent part of the peritoneal cavity.

On supine images, free gas may be seen in about 50% of patients by the presence of a double wall sign due to visualization of the outside of the bowel wall.

Intraperitoneal air may be demonstrable in over 60% of cases for over three weeks after abdominal surgery.

Aortic aneurysm

Abdominal aortic aneurysm may be detected by plain radiography only if there is significant calcification in the wall of the aneurysm. A non-calcified aneurysm may appear as a posterior central soft tissue mass. A lateral projection is used to confirm the calcification and the pre-vertebral location of a mass.

Aneurysms are normally diagnosed and followed up by ultrasound. In the event of a patient presenting with suspected rupture of a previously unknown aneurysm, plain images may be vital to confirm the diagnosis if ultrasound is not immediately available. CT is used to determine the extent of the aneurysm and its relationship to the renal arteries, and in some circumstances for assessment of possible rupture.

Retroperitoneal disease

Masses may be seen incidentally on plain images, displacing other structures (especially stomach and bowel) or as lack of clarity of the psoas muscle outline. Loss of the psoas outline may also occur in psoas abscess or haematoma, but it is also common in normal people so this is a poor test for any of these conditions. CT and magnetic resonance imaging (MRI) are the preferred techniques, as ultrasound access is too often obstructed by bowel gas.

Constipation

This is normally a clinical diagnosis based on frequency and consistency of the stool, change in bowel habit, and clinical examination. Radiography is required rarely, except to assess secondary obstruction or to determine the residual faecal load (usually in chronic constipation states).

Use in children

As this is a high-dose examination, its use in children should be avoided if possible. Radiological indications are discussed in Section 14.

Antero-posterior – supine

A 35 × 43-cm cassette is selected. In the case of a large patient, an additional projection using a 35 × 43-cm cassette placed at right-angles to the spine of the upper abdomen may be necessary to include the upper abdomen.

Position of patient and cassette

- The patient lies supine on the imaging table, with the median sagittal plane at right-angles and coincident with the midline of the table.
- The pelvis is adjusted so that the anterior superior iliac spines are equidistant from the tabletop.
- The cassette is placed longitudinally in the cassette tray and positioned so that the symphysis pubis is included on the lower part of the film, bearing in mind that the oblique rays will project the symphysis pubis downwards.
- The centre of the cassette will be approximately at the level of a point located 1 cm below the line joining the iliac crests. This will ensure that the symphysis pubis is included on the image.

Direction and centring of the X-ray beam

- The vertical central ray is directed to the centre of the cassette.
- Using a short exposure time, the exposure is made on arrested respiration.

Notes

- In the case of a large abdomen, an immobilization band may be applied to compress the soft tissue and reduce the effects of scatter.
- The beam is collimated to the size of the cassette selected and adjusted to ensure that it does not extend beyond the lateral edges of the abdomen.
- Ensure that position and anatomical markers are included on the cassette.
- When using the automatic exposure control (AEC) device, the central and right chambers may be selected simultaneously to avoid the risk of underexposure due to the beam passing through regions containing mainly bowel gas.
- If the patient is too ill to be moved onto the X-ray table (e.g. multiple trauma or acute pain), the image can be acquired using a stationary grid and cassette placed in the tray under the patient transport trolley. Care must be taken to use the correct FFD and to centre to the middle of the cassette to avoid grid cut off. A piece of lead rubber is placed under the cassette to reduce 'back scatter' and improve image contrast.

Essential image characteristics

- The bowel pattern should be demonstrated with minimal unsharpness.

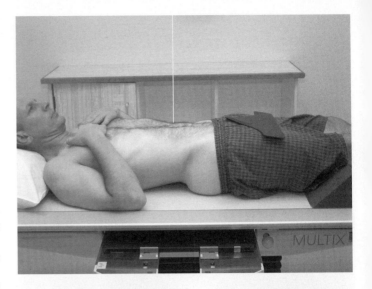

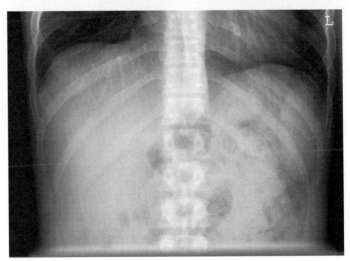

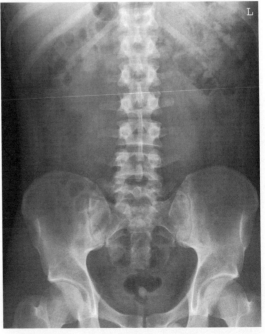

Two radiographs used to give full coverage of the abdomen

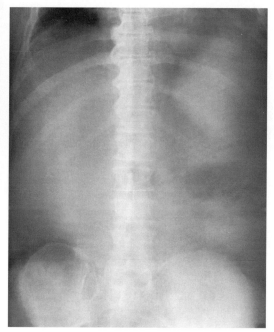

Poor quality image showing movement unsharpness due to incorrect exposure factors

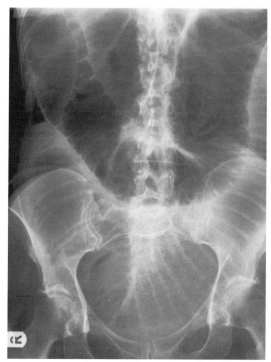

Antero-posterior supine radiograph of the abdomen showing distal ileum obstruction

Antero-posterior – supine

Common faults and remedies

- Failure to include symphysis pubis and diaphragm on the same image. This may be due to patient size, in which case two images are acquired with the second across the upper abdomen using a 35 × 43-cm cassette oriented horizontally.
- Failure to visualize the lateral extent of the abdominal cavity may be due to patient size or poor positioning.
- Respiratory movement unsharpness. Rehearsal of the breathing technique prior to exposure may help to reduce this, together with selection of the shortest exposure time.
- Patient rotation, especially when the patient is examined in bed.
- Underexposure may be caused by patient size or incorrect selection of AEC.
- Presence of artefacts such as buttons or contents of pockets if the patient remains clothed for the examination.
- Grid cut off, associated with trolley or ward radiography can be prevented by ensuring that the vertical central beam is perpendicular and centred to the middle of the grid cassette.
- Poor image contrast is often associated with selection of too high kVp, poor collimation, using a stationary grid for trolley examination with a low grid ratio and failing to use abdominal compression with very large patients. Optimum adjustment of all of these factors will improve image quality.

Radiological considerations

- Any cause of movement unsharpness may render small or even medium-sized renal and ureteric calculi invisible.
- Some radiologists assert that the erect abdomen is rarely if ever needed to diagnose intestinal obstruction, as subtle signs will nearly always be present on a supine image. In the acute setting, however, the erect image can be very valuable to surgical staff who do not have immediate access to an experienced radiologist.
- Blunt trauma injury may be associated with the loss of the psoas muscle outline and loss of renal outline due to tissue damage and haematoma.

Radiation protection

- Strict application of the 'pregnancy rule' or the 'ten-day rule' is important in females of childbearing age.
- For males, the correct size of gonad protection should be selected and applied carefully so the gonads are shielded and the pelvic region not obscured with lead.

Antero-posterior – erect

If possible, the patient is examined standing against a vertical Bucky. Alternatively, they may be examined on a tilting table with a C-arm using a large image intensifier/X-ray tube assembly. If necessary, the patient may be examined whilst sitting on a trolley or a chair using a stationary grid/cassette.

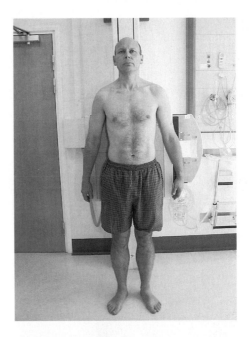

Position of patient and cassette (patient standing)

- The patient stands with their back against the vertical Bucky.
- The patient's legs are placed well apart so that a comfortable and steady position is adopted.
- The median sagittal plane is adjusted at right-angles and coincident with the midline of the table.
- The pelvis is adjusted so that the anterior superior iliac spines are equidistant from the imaging tabletop.
- A 35 × 43-cm cassette is placed in the Bucky tray with its upper edge at the level of the middle of the body of the sternum so that the diaphragms are included.

NB: diverging rays will displace the diaphragms superiorly.

Direction and centring of the X-ray beam

- The horizontal ray is directed so that it is coincident with the centre of the cassette in the midline.
- An exposure is taken on normal full expiration.

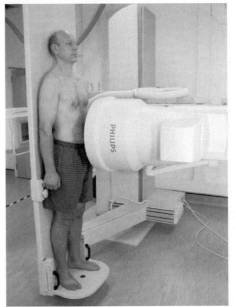

Position of patient and cassette (tilting table)

This may be undertaken using a tilting table with a C-arm assembly with a large image intensifier and the X-ray tube in an over-couch position. It is used when undertaking barium examinations of the alimentary tract and other studies requiring an erect image, e.g. IVU, to show the site of obstruction.

- The patient lies supine on the tilting table, with the feet firmly against the step. The table is moved slowly towards the vertical position until the patient is erect.
- If necessary, immobilization bands are tightened across the knees and chest to prevent the patient from collapsing when the table is moved towards the vertical position. However, it is not recommended that this procedure should be undertaken if the patient is unwell and unable to stand unaided.
- The upper edge of the image intensifier is adjusted so that it is at the level of the middle of the body of the sternum in order to include the diaphragms.
- The X-ray tube/C-arm assembly is positioned so that the central ray is horizontal.
- The exposure is made as soon as table movement is stopped. This is preferably when the table is vertical, but how near the vertical will depend on the condition of the patient.
- As soon as the exposure has been made, the X-ray tube is moved away and the table moved back into the horizontal position.

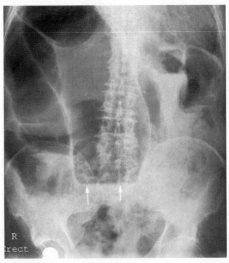

Antero-posterior erect radiograph of the abdomen showing dilated bowel with small fluid levels (arrows)

Antero-posterior – erect (patient sitting)

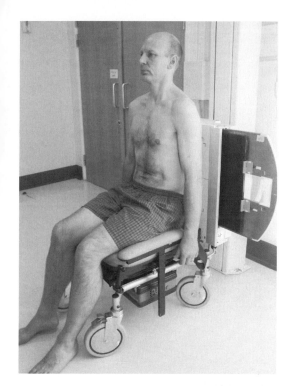

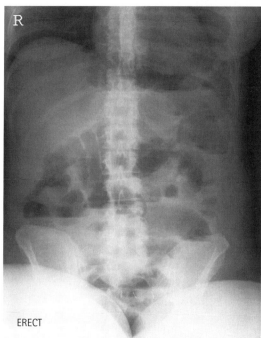

Antero-posterior erect radiograph of the abdomen in sitting position showing postoperative small bowel obstruction (note lower abdominal clips on transverse incision). NB: If the legs are not abducted details of the pelvis are obscured, as in this example

Notes

- Exposure factors are set using a high mA and short exposure time and an increase of 7–10 kVp over that required with the patient supine.
- In a case of suspected perforation, the patient should be kept erect, ideally for 20 minutes prior to the exposure, to allow any free gas to rise. The appropriate image in this situation would be erect chest, or an antero-posterior left lateral decubitus abdomen, or as a last resort a lateral dorsal decubitus.

This method of obtaining a horizontal beam projection of the abdomen can be used with the patient sitting on a trolley with their legs over the side of the trolley, using a vertical Bucky/cassette holder, or with the patient in a wheelchair with the back of the wheelchair removed, again using a vertical Bucky, or with the patient on a trolley with the backrest raised in the vertical position, using a grid cassette.

Patients requiring this technique are usually very ill and the technique is performed to confirm an obstruction.

Position of patient and cassette

- Having set the exposure factors and positioned the X-ray tube so that a horizontal central ray will be approximately at the correct height, the patient, already erect, is turned through 90 degrees so that they are facing the X-ray tube.
- Care should be exercised to abduct the legs to avoid superimposing soft tissue of the thighs over the pelvic cavity.
- The median sagittal plane is adjusted at right-angles and coincident with the midline of the vertical Bucky or grid cassette.
- The patient is supported in this position with a 35 × 43-cm cassette in the Bucky or a grid cassette supported vertically against the patient's back, with its upper edge not lower than mid-sternum.
- Alternatively, depending on the patient's condition, the patient may sit on a stool or wheelchair with the back removed and with their back against a vertical Bucky. If necessary, the patient may also be examined with the backrest of the trolley raised to the vertical position.

Direction and centring of the X-ray beam

- Final adjustment is made to the position of the X-ray tube so that the horizontal central ray will be directed to the anterior aspect of the patient to the centre of the cassette at the correct focus-to-film distance (FFD).
- The exposure is made on arrested expiration, after which the patient is returned to the supine position.

Essential image characteristics

- The acquired image must include both domes of the diaphragm to ensure that any free air in the peritoneal cavity is demonstrated.

Radiological considerations

- Fluid levels on an erect film do not necessarily indicate obstruction, as a variety of other conditions may produce fluid levels, e.g. severe gastroenteritis, jejunal diverticulosis.
- Suspected intestinal obstruction is the usual indication for this request, but it may also be useful for confirming the presence of a gas-containing abscess.

Antero-posterior – left lateral decubitus

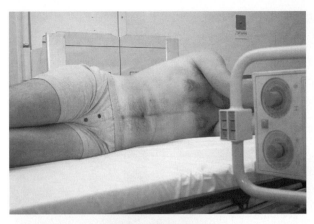

This projection is used if the patient cannot be positioned erect or sitting to confirm the presence of subdiaphragmatic gas suspected seen on the antero-posterior supine projection. It is also used for confirming obstruction.

With the patient lying on the left side, free gas will rise, to be located between the lateral margin of the liver and the right lateral abdominal wall. To allow time for the gas to collect there, the patient should remain lying on the left side for 20 minutes before the exposure is made.

Position of patient and cassette

- The patient lies on the left side, with the elbows and arms flexed so that the hands can rest near the patient's head.
- A 35 × 43-cm cassette is positioned transversely in the vertical Bucky or alternatively a grid cassette is placed vertically against the posterior aspect of the trunk, with its upper border high enough to project above the right lateral abdominal and thoracic walls.
- A small region of the lung above the diaphragm should be included on the film.
- The patient's position is adjusted to bring the median sagittal plane at right-angles to the cassette.

Direction and centring of the X-ray beam

- The horizontal central ray is directed to the posterior aspect of the patient and centred to the centre of the film.

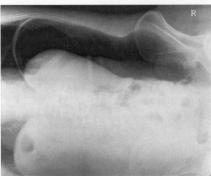

Antero-posterior left lateral decubitus image of the abdomen showing free air in the abdominal cavity

Lateral dorsal decubitus (supine)

Occasionally, the patient cannot sit or even be rolled on to the side, in which case the patient remains supine and a lateral projection is taken using a horizontal central ray.

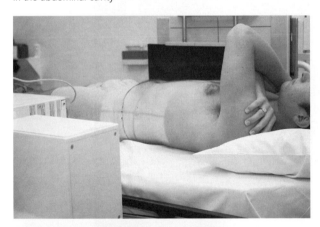

Position of patient and cassette

- The patient lies supine, with the arms raised away from the abdomen and thorax.
- A grid cassette is supported vertically against the patient's side, to include the thorax to the level of mid-sternum and as much of the abdomen as possible. Care should be taken that the anterior wall of the trunk is not projected off the film.
- Alternatively, when using a trolley, the patient may be positioned against a vertical Bucky.

Direction and centring of the X-ray beam

- The horizontal central ray is directed to the lateral aspect of the trunk so that it is at right-angles to the cassette and centred to it.
- The exposure is made on arrested expiration.

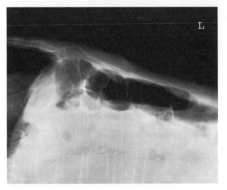

Lateral dorsal decubitus (supine) image of the abdomen

Note

Use of a wedge filter will enable both the lateral abdominal wall and the bowel to be seen for the same exposure.

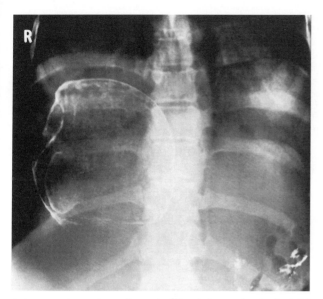

Antero-superior supine radiograph of the abdomen showing hydatid cyst of the liver

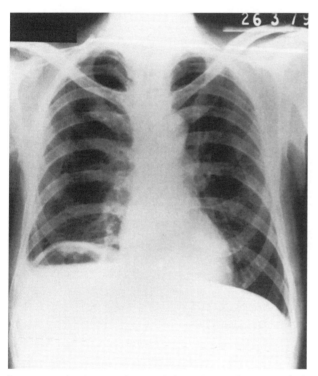

Postero-anterior thorax and upper abdomen image showing a subphrenic abscess below the right hemidiaphragm

The liver is best demonstrated using ultrasound, CT or MRI, but in certain conditions conventional radiography can be used to provide a diagnosis, e.g. abnormal calcification in the liver due to hydatid cysts.

Antero-posterior technique

Calcification

- To demonstrate abnormal calcifications, a cassette large enough to include the whole of the liver area is used (43 × 53 cm).
- With the patient supine on the table, the cassette is placed transversely in the Potter Bucky tray so that its lower margin is at the level of the upper part of the iliac crests; its upper border should be not lower than mid-sternum, to ensure that the full upper surface of the diaphragm is included on the image.
- With the vertical central ray centred to the middle of the cassette, the exposure is made on arrested expiration.

Intra-hepatic and subphrenic abscess

Horizontal beam projections are required to demonstrate an air fluid level under the right hemidiaphragm.

- An antero-posterior (or postero-anterior) projection is taken using a horizontal central ray with the patient erect, standing or sitting, and also in the left lateral decubitus position (patient lying on the left side) in the same way as that described to demonstrate abdominal fluid levels.
- Pathology in this region may cause elevation of the right side of the diaphragm; therefore care must be taken that the cassette is positioned high enough to include the upper abdomen, diaphragm and lower part of the thorax.
- Ultrasound or fluoroscopy may be used to demonstrate diaphragmatic movement during respiration. If neither of these is available, then the double exposure technique described later may be employed.

11 Diaphragmatic movement during respiration

On the chest radiograph, the right hemidiaphragm is normally about 2.5 cm higher than the left. On fluoroscopy, both sides of the diaphragm can be seen to fall on inspiration and rise on expiration, the full movement being about two intercostal spaces.

Pathology below the diaphragm, e.g. subphrenic abscess or a space-occupying lesion of the liver, or pathology above the diaphragm, e.g. collapse of the right lower lobe or paralysis of the diaphragm, can cause the normal position of the diaphragm and its excursion during respiration to be changed.

Ultrasound or fluoroscopy may be used to study the movement of the diaphragm during various respiratory manoeuvres, but an alternative could be to acquire postero-anterior chest images taken in inspiration and expiration to assess diaphragmatic excursion.

Imaging procedure

- The procedure may involve taking two separate radiographs or alternatively making two exposures, one on inspiration and one on expiration on the one film, each exposure being half that used for normal chest radiography.
- Care should be taken that the patient does not move between exposures.
- The outline of the diaphragm might be obscured by increased opacity due to inflammatory processes in the lung, in which case additional kilovoltage can be used to provide the required penetration.

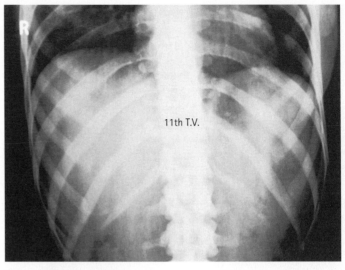

Inspiration

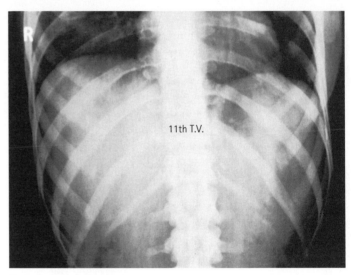

Expiration

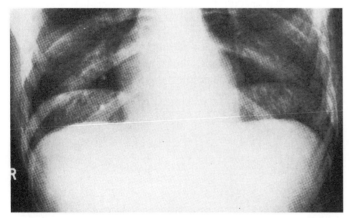

Double exposure

Antero-posterior

Plain radiography of the abdominal and pelvic cavity is carried out to visualize:

- outline of the kidneys, surrounded by their perirenal fat;
- the lateral border of the psoas muscle;
- opaque stones in the kidney area, in the line of the ureters and in the region of the bladder;
- calcifications within the kidney or in the bladder wall;
- the presence of gas within the urinary tract.

Radiation protection

The 'pregnancy rule' should be observed unless permission has been given to ignore it in the case of emergency. If the whole of the renal tract including bladder is to be visualized, then no gonad shielding is possible for females; for males, a lead sheet can be placed over the lower edge of the symphysis pubis to protect the testes. If the bladder and lower ureters are not to be included on the image, then females can also be given gonad protection by placing a lead-rubber sheet over the lower abdomen to protect the ovaries. Other methods discussed previously that reduce radiation dose to the patient should be followed.

Preparation of the patient

If possible, the patient should have a low-residue diet and laxatives during the 48 hours prior to the examination to clear the bowel of gas and faecal matter that might overlie the renal tract. In the case of emergency radiography, no bowel preparation is possible. The patient wears a clean gown.

Position of patient and cassette

- The patient lies supine on the X-ray table, with the median sagittal plane of the body at right-angles to and in the midline of the table.
- The hands may be placed high on the chest, or the arms may be by the patient's side and slightly away from the trunk.
- The size of cassette used should be large enough to cover the region from above the upper poles of the kidneys to the symphysis pubis (e.g. a 35 × 43-cm cassette).
- The cassette is placed in the Bucky tray and positioned so that the symphysis pubis is included on the lower part of the film, bearing in mind that the oblique rays will project the symphysis downwards.
- The centre of the cassette will be approximately at the level of a point located 1 cm below the line joining the iliac crests. This will ensure that the symphysis pubis is included on the image.
- A wide immobilization band is applied to the patient's abdomen and, depending on the patient's condition, compression is applied. This compression is more effective if a long pad is placed along the midline under the compression band before tightening the band.

Direction and centring of the X-ray beam

- The vertical central ray is directed to the centre of the cassette, which is in the midline about the level of the lower costal margin in the mid-axillary line. The X-ray beam is collimated to just within the margins of the cassette.
- Using a high mA and a short exposure time, the exposure is made on arrested respiration after full expiration.

Notes

- Small opacities overlying the kidney may be inside or outside the kidney substance. A further radiograph taken on arrested respiration after full inspiration might show a difference in extent and direction of movement of the kidney and calcification lying outside the kidney.
- In some cases it may be necessary to include a collimated kidney area if the superior renal borders are excluded in the full-length film.

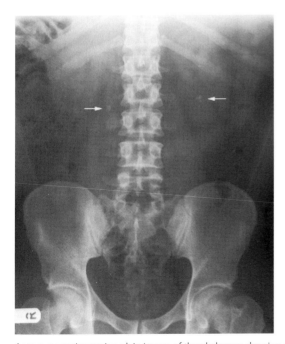

Antero-posterior supine plain image of the abdomen showing a left lower pole renal calculus and a calculus in the upper right ureter

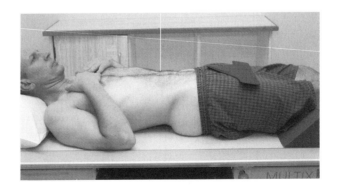

11 | Urinary tract

Additional information about the relationship of opacities to the renal tract may be obtained with posterior oblique projections. The right posterior oblique projection shows the right kidney and collecting system in profile and the left kidney *en face*. Similarly, the left posterior oblique projection shows the left kidney in profile and the right kidney *en face*.

A lateral projection may be necessary to confirm or otherwise the presence of opacities anterior to the renal tract, which will be seen superimposed on the antero-posterior projection.

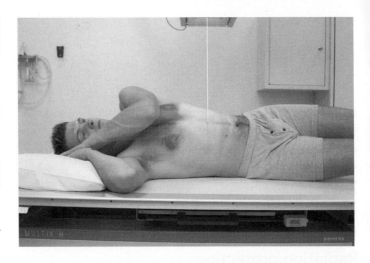

Right posterior oblique

Position of patient and cassette

- The patient lies supine on the table. The left side of the trunk and thorax is raised until the coronal plane is at an angle of 15–20 degrees to the table.
- The patient is moved across the table until the vertebral column is slightly to the left side of the midline of the table; then the patient is immobilized in this position.
- For the kidney area alone, a 24 × 30-cm cassette is placed transversely in the Bucky tray and centred to a level midway between the sterno-xiphisternal joint and umbilicus.
- For the whole of the renal tract, a 35 × 43-cm cassette might be required; this is centred at the level of the lower costal margin.

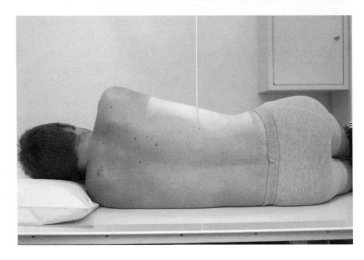

Direction and centring of the X-ray beam

- The vertical central ray is directed to the centre of the cassette.

Note

Excessive rotation of the patient will show the right kidney projected over the spine.

Lateral

Position of patient and cassette

- The patient is turned on to the side under examination, with the hands resting near the head. The hips and knees are flexed to aid stability.
- With the median sagittal plane parallel to the table, the vertebral column (about 8 cm anterior to the posterior skin surface) is positioned over the midline of the table and an immobilization band applied.
- The cassette is placed in the tray and, for the kidney area, is centred to LV1/2, about 5 cm superior to the lower costal margin.

Direction and centring of the X-ray beam

- The vertical central ray is directed to the centre of the cassette and the exposure made on arrested expiration.

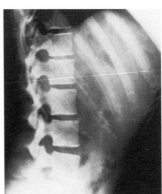
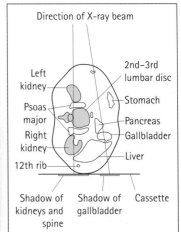

Lateral radiograph of abdomen

346

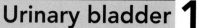

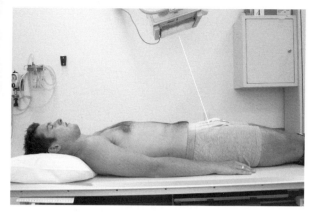

Calculi within the urinary bladder can move freely, particularly if the bladder is full, whereas calcification and calculi outside the bladder, e.g. prostatic calculi, are immobile. Antero-posterior and oblique projections can be taken to show change in the relative position of calculi and bladder. To examine the bladder region, caudal angulation is required to allow for the shape of the bony pelvis and to project the symphysis below the bladder.

Antero-posterior 15 degrees caudad

Position of patient and cassette

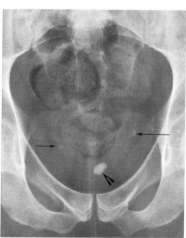

- The patient lies supine on the table, with the median sagittal plane at right-angles to and in the midline of the table.
- An 18 × 24-cm cassette is commonly used, placed longitudinally in the tray with its lower border 5 cm below the symphysis pubis to ensure that the symphysis is not projected off the film.

Direction and centring of the X-ray beam

- The central ray is directed 15 degrees caudally and centred in the midline 5 cm above the upper border of the symphysis pubis. (e.g. midway between the anterior superior iliac spines and upper border of the symphysis pubis).

Antero-posterior 15 degrees caudad image of the lower abdomen showing a bladder calculus (large arrowhead) and small pelvic phleboliths having lucent centres (arrows)

Right or left posterior oblique

Position of patient and cassette

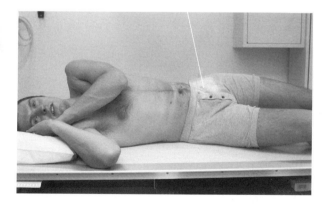

- From the supine position, one side is raised so that the median sagittal plane is rotated through 35 degrees.
- To help stability, the knee in contact with the table is flexed and the raised side supported using a non-opaque pad.
- The patient's position is adjusted so that the midpoint between the symphysis pubis and the anterior superior iliac spine on the raised side is over the midline of the table.
- A 30 × 24-cm cassette is placed longitudinally in the tray with its upper border at the level of the anterior superior iliac spines.

Direction and centring of the X-ray beam

- The vertical central ray is directed to a point 2.5 cm above the symphysis pubis.
- Alternatively, a caudal angulation of 15 degrees can be used with a higher centring point and the cassette displaced downwards to accommodate the angulation.

Note

The right posterior oblique, i.e. left side raised, will show the right vesico-ureteric junction, a common place for small ureteric calculi to lodge.

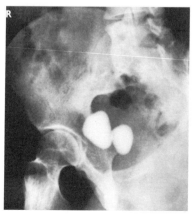

Right posterior oblique image of the lower abdomen showing large calculi in the bladder

11 Biliary system

Ultrasound imaging is normally undertaken to demonstrate the biliary system. However, plain radiographs of the biliary system may be taken to demonstrate opacities, including calcifications, in the region of the gallbladder and biliary tree.

Laxatives and a low-residue diet may be taken during the two days before the examination to clear overlying faeces and bowel gas. In order to be able to differentiate soft tissues in the region, the radiographic image must be sharp and have the maximum possible contrast.

Immobilization, compression, collimation, and short exposure time with high mA and a low kilovoltage (70 kVp) are all used to give maximum image quality.

The position of the gallbladder, although in the middle of the inferior liver margin, will be very variable, low and near to the vertebral column in thin patients, and high and lateral in patients of stocky build.

For a general survey of the region, a left anterior oblique projection is taken. Alternatively, a right posterior oblique projection may also be taken.

Left anterior oblique

The cassette size is chosen such that a large region of the right side of the abdomen is included.

Position of patient and cassette

- The patient lies prone on the X-ray table. The right side is raised, rotating the median sagittal plane through an angle of 20 degrees; the coronal plane is now at an angle of 20 degrees to the table.
- The arm on the raised side is flexed so that the right hand rests near the patient's head, while the left arm lies alongside and behind the trunk.
- The patient is moved across the table until the raised right side is over the centre of the table, and a compression band is applied.
- A 24 × 30-cm cassette is placed longitudinally in the Bucky tray with its centre 2.5 cm above the lower costal margin to include the top of the iliac crest.

Direction and centring of the X-ray beam

- The vertical central ray is directed to a point 7.5 cm to the right of the spinous processes and 2.5 cm above the lower costal margin and to the centre of the cassette.
- The exposure is made on arrested respiration after full expiration.

Note

An additional image can be taken on arrested respiration after full inspiration to show the relative movement of the gallbladder and overlying calcifications that are suspected to be outside the gallbladder, e.g. within costal cartilages.

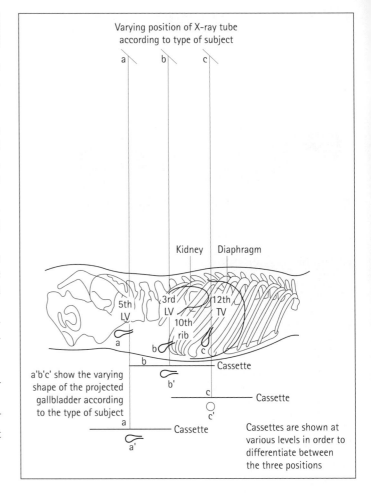

Varying position of X-ray tube according to type of subject

a'b'c' show the varying shape of the projected gallbladder according to the type of subject

Cassettes are shown at various levels in order to differentiate between the three positions

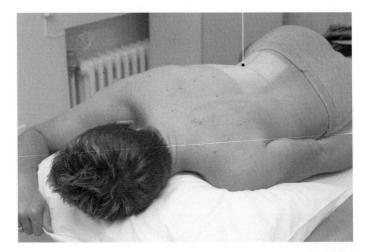

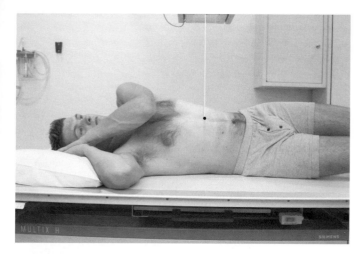

Position of patient and cassette

- The patient lies supine on the X-ray table. The left side is raised, rotating the median sagittal plane through 20 degrees; the coronal plane is now at an angle of 20 degrees to the table and the trunk is supported in this position using a non-opaque pad.
- The patient is moved across the table so that the right side of the abdomen is over the centre of the table. The elbows and shoulders are flexed so that the patient can rest the hands behind the head.
- An immobilization band helps to compress the abdomen.
- A 24 × 30-cm cassette is placed longitudinally in the Bucky tray, with its centre 2.5 cm above the lower costal margin.

Direction and centring of the X-ray beam

- The vertical central ray is directed to a point midway between the midline and the right abdominal wall 2.5 cm above the lower costal margin, and to the centre of the cassette.
- Exposure is made on arrested respiration after full expiration.

Radiological considerations

- Not all gallstones are radio-opaque. The pattern of calcification is variable, from an amorphous solid appearance to a concentric laminar structure.
- Calcified stones tend to gather in the most dependent part of the gallbladder, which will usually be the fundus in the prone position. Cholesterol stones in particular are lighter than bile and tend to float, but they are not usually radio-opaque.
- Air in the biliary tree may be seen after instrumentation (e.g. sphincterotomy), after passage of calculi, or in a normal elderly person with a patulous sphincter of Oddi.

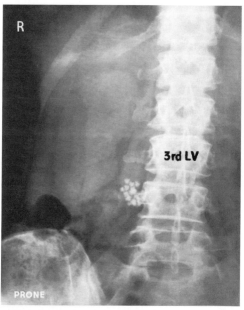

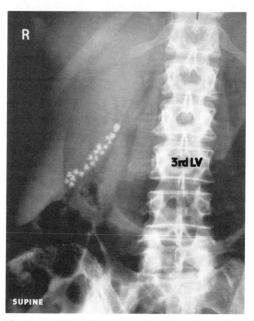

The images above demonstrate the change in position of the stone-filled gallbladder when the patient is moved from the prone (b) to the supine position (c)

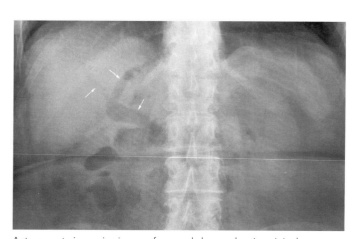

Antero-posterior supine image of upper abdomen showing air in the biliary tree

11 References

Miller RE (1973). The technical approach to the acute abdomen. *Semin Roentgenol* 8:267–9.

Royal College of Radiologists (2003). *Making the Best Use of a Department of Clinical Radiology: Guidelines for Doctors*, 5th edn. London: Royal College of Radiologists.

Whitley AS, Alsop CW, Moore AD (1999). *Clark's Special Procedures in Diagnostic Imaging*. London: Butterworth-Heinemann.

Section 12

Ward Radiography

CONTENTS

INTRODUCTION	352
General comments	352
Radiation protection	352
Control of infection	353
Accessory equipment	353
X-ray equipment	353
HEART AND LUNGS	354
Antero-posterior	354
HEART AND LUNGS – FLUID LEVELS	355
Postero-anterior or antero-posterior (lateral decubitus)	355
Lateral (dorsal decubitus)	355
HEART AND LUNGS – TEMPORARY PACEMAKER	356
Mobile image intensifier	356
HEART AND LUNGS – POSTOPERATIVE RADIOGRAPHY	357
Endotracheal tube	357
Central venous pressure line	357
Chest drain insertions	357
ABDOMEN	358
Recommended projections	358
Antero-posterior – supine	358
Antero-posterior – erect	359
Antero-posterior (left lateral decubitus)	359
Lateral dorsal decubitus – supine	360
CERVICAL SPINE	361
Lateral supine	361
FRACTURED LOWER LIMBS AND PELVIS	362
Antero-posterior	362
FRACTURED FEMUR	363
Lateral	363
Arthroplasty postoperative radiography	363
FRACTURED FEMUR – PAEDIATRIC (GALLOWS TRACTION)	364
Antero-posterior	364
Lateral	364
HEART AND LUNGS – SPECIAL CARE BABY UNIT	365
Antero-posterior	365

12 Introduction

Ward radiography should be restricted to the patient whose medical condition is such that it is impossible for them to be moved to the X-ray department without seriously affecting their medical treatment and nursing care. Such patients may be found in surgical and medical ward environments and in the following areas:

- coronary care unit;
- medical assessment unit;
- surgical assessment unit;
- cardiac surgery unit;
- intensive care unit (ICU);
- high dependency unit;
- special care baby unit;
- orthopaedic ward;
- accident and emergency ward.

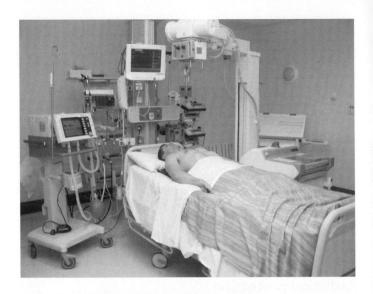

General comments

Examinations are normally complicated by a variety of situations: the patient's medical condition; degree of consciousness and cooperation; the patient's treatment; restrictions due to life-support system, drips, and chest or abdominal drains; location of electrocardiogram (ECG) leads; traction apparatus; physical restrictions due to room size and layout of monitoring and life-support equipment; adequate power supply; and the shape, size and ability to move mobile or portable X-ray equipment in confined spaces.

The radiographer must be able to assume total control of the situation, and should enlist the help, cooperation and advice of nursing and medical staff before embarking on an examination.

Any X-ray requests should be checked first to ensure that the examination on the ward is necessary, and that the correct equipment and cassettes are obtained for transfer to the wards.

The patient should be correctly identified and cassettes used clearly marked to avoid double exposure if more than one patient needs examining on the ward.

A thorough examination of the location of, or knowledge of, the ward is necessary in order that any problems or difficulties can be resolved with the minimum of fuss.

Advice regarding the patient's medical condition should be sought first, before moving or disturbing the patient. Any disturbance of traction, ECG leads or drains should be undertaken only with the permission of the medical staff. Positioning of cassettes and movement or lifting of seriously ill patients should be undertaken with supervision from nursing staff.

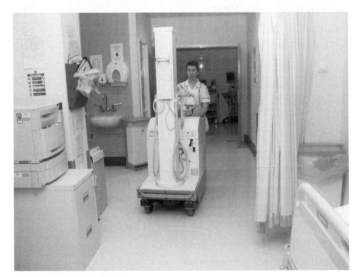

Radiation protection

- This is of paramount importance in the ward situation. The radiographer is responsible for ensuring that nobody enters the controlled area during exposure of the patient.

- The radiographer must liaise clearly with the ward staff on their arrival on the ward and issue verbal instructions in a clear and distinct manner to staff and patients to avoid accidental exposure to radiation.
- The radiographer, and anyone assisting in an examination, must be protected adequately from scatter radiation by the use of a lead-rubber apron.
- Use of the inverse square law, with staff standing as far away as possible from the unit and outside the radiation field, should be made when making an exposure. The patient should also receive appropriate radiation protection.
- Lead protective shields may be used as backstops when using a horizontal beam to limit the radiation field, e.g. when the absorption nature of room-dividing walls is unknown.
- Exposure factors used for the examination should be recorded, enabling optimum results to be repeated. Patients tend to be X-rayed frequently when under intensive care.

Control of infection

The control of infection plays an important role in the management of all patients, especially following surgery and in the nursing of premature babies.

To prevent the spread of infection, local established protocols should be adhered to by staff coming into contact with patients, e.g. hand-washing between patients and the cleanliness of equipment used for radiographic examination.

Patients with a known highly contagious infection, and those with a compromised immune system and at high risk of infection, will be barrier-nursed. In such circumstances, it is important that local protocols associated with the prevention of spread of infection are followed.

The X-ray equipment used in ICU, cardiac surgery units and special care baby units should, ideally, be dedicated units and kept on site. Failing this, they should be cleaned with antiseptic solution before being moved into infection-controlled units. Equipment is wheeled over dust-absorbent mats at the entrance of such units. Radiographers should wear gowns or disposable plastic aprons, facemasks and over-shoes before entering these areas. Cassettes should be cleaned and covered with plastic sheets or clean pillowcases/towels before use. After use, cassettes and all equipment should be cleaned with antiseptic solution. Disposable gloves are worn when touching the patient.

Methicillin-resistant *Staphylococcus aureus* (MRSA) is a bacterial infection that is resistant to methicillin and many other antibiotics. MRSA is a particular threat to vulnerable patients and can cause many symptoms, including fever, wound and skin infections, inflammation and pneumonia. The bacteria can be spread readily from an infected patient to others. MRSA is spread mainly from person to person by hand. When healthcare workers deal with MRSA-infected patients, the bacteria may transfer to their hands and can then be passed on to a vulnerable patient.

MRSA patients are usually barrier-nursed. Controls such as effective hand-washing, wearing of gloves and aprons, and the cleaning of the environment and equipment are necessary to prevent spread of the bacteria.

When undertaking radiography on more than one barrier-nursed patient on a ward or ICU, it is important that disposable aprons are changed between patients as well as ensuring that the hands of the operators are washed between patients to prevent the spread of infection. A number of speciality wards use differently coloured aprons per patient bay as a prompt to confine the use of aprons to a specific patient.

Accessory equipment

- Various aids are available that can assist in positioning both the patient and cassette. These include foam pads of different sizes and shapes, such as cassette pads that support the patient and allow the cassette to be inserted in a groove in the pad, cassette tunnels and cassette holders. The correct accessories should be selected as part of the equipment needed for the radiographic procedure.
- Selection of a low-ratio 6 : 1 30 lines per cm parallel stationary grid will reduce the risk of grid cut-off when undertaking conventional radiography.

X-ray equipment

Units fall broadly into two groups – portable and mobile, the broad distinction between the two being the difference in power output and the ability to transfer equipment.

- Portable sets have relatively low mA settings and normally can be dismantled for transfer. Mobile sets have higher power output, are much heavier, and need to be motorized or pushed between locations.
- Mobile X-ray units can be either mains-independent or mains-dependent. These types of machines are very heavy and may be battery-driven to aid transportation around the hospital.
- Older mobile sets, with conventionally powered X-ray generators, require the need of a separate 30-A supply and are connected to socket outlets marked 'X-ray only'. Patients requiring radiography with such machines should be nursed in beds that are within reach of these sockets.
- Capacitor discharge (CD) units require the use of a 13-A supply to generator X-ray exposure. Their use in special care baby units or similar high dependency units is not recommended because of the risk of disconnection of the wrong electrical plug when many electrical devices are employed.
- Mains-independent machines such as medium-/high-frequency can be operated from a standard 13-A supply. These are designed with high-powered battery packs to generate the electrical power for X-ray exposure. Therefore, these units can be moved to areas without electrical mains power or in wards where there is a restriction of mains sockets. They require only access to a 13-A power supply for battery recharging during storage.
- In radiography of the chest and abdomen, the use of short exposure times is essential to reduce the risk of movement unsharpness. For such examinations, the choice of equipment is therefore restricted to the higher-output mobile sets.

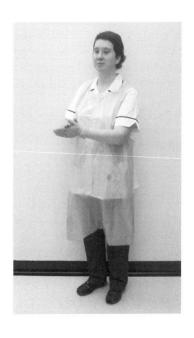

12 | Heart and lungs

Patients suffering from dyspnoea and severe chest pain are often assessed on the ward. Radiographs are requested to aid in diagnosis. Common conditions include congestive heart failure, coronary heart disease, left ventricular failure, pulmonary oedema, pulmonary embolus, pneumothorax and pleural effusion and pneumonia. Postoperative chest radiography is also often required.

As a general rule, ward radiography should be performed only when it is not possible to move the patient to the X-ray department and when medical intervention is dependent on the diagnosis confirmed on the radiograph.

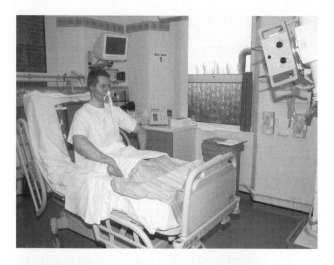

Antero-posterior

Position of patient and cassette

- Where possible, the patient should be X-rayed sitting erect and facing the X-ray tube. The cassette is supported against the back, using pillows or a large wedge-shaped foam pad, with its upper edge above the lung fields.
- If this is not possible, the patient may be positioned supine. The semi-recumbent position is not favoured as the degree of recumbence is not reproducible across a series of images.
- The median sagittal plane is adjusted at right-angles to, and in the midline of, the cassette.
- Rotation of the patient is prevented by the use of foam pads. Rotation produces a range of artefacts (see p. 205) and must be avoided or minimized. If possible, the arms are rotated medially, with the shoulders brought forward to bring the scapulae clear of the lung fields.

Direction and centring of the X-ray beam

- Assuming the patient can sit fully erect, the central ray is directed first at right-angles to the cassette and towards the sternal angle.
- The central ray is then angled until it is coincident with the middle of the film, thus avoiding unnecessary exposure to the eyes.
- The use of a horizontal central ray, however, is essential to demonstrate fluid, e.g. pleural effusion or any air under the diaphragm. If the patient is able to sit erect, direct the central ray at right-angles to the middle of the cassette. The clavicles in the resultant radiograph, however, will be projected above the apices.
- If the patient is unable to sit erect, fluid levels are demonstrated using a horizontal ray with the patient lying down in the positions (described on p. 355 opposite).

Notes

- Where possible, a high-powered mobile is used to enable a 180-cm focus-to-film distance (FFD) for erect positioning of the patient.
- For supine images, the FFD may be restricted due to the height of the bed and the height limitations of the X-ray tube column. The FFD should be higher than 120 cm, otherwise image magnification will increase disproportionately.

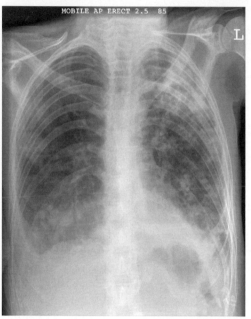

Antero-posterior erect radiograph showing bilateral consolidation with a right pleural effusion (in this case due to tuberculosis)

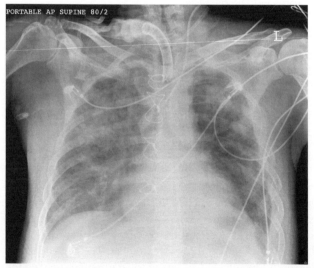

Antero-posterior supine radiograph showing extensive pulmonary oedema and haemorrhage after trauma, with multiple left-sided rib fractures. Sternal wires indicate previous cardiac surgery. Note left jugular central line and tracheostomy. It is not possible to exclude pleural effusion or pneumothorax on an antero-posterior supine image

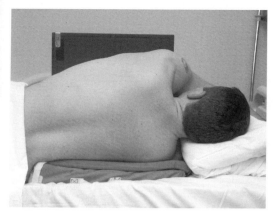

Patient positioned for postero-anterior chest (lateral decubitus) projection

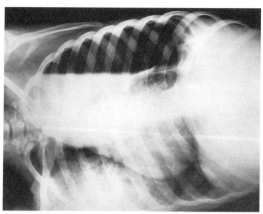

Postero-anterior radiograph in lateral decubitus position showing pleural effusion with pneumothorax

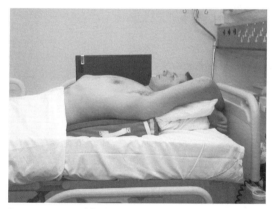

Patient positioned for lateral chest (dorsal decubitus) projection

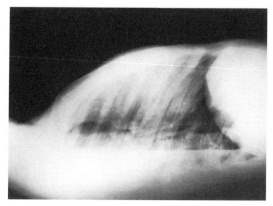

Lateral radiograph in dorsal decubitus position showing pleural effusion with pneumothorax

Patients who are too ill to sit erect may be examined whilst lying down. The use of a horizontal central ray is essential to demonstrate fluid levels, e.g. hydropneumothorax.

Postero-anterior or antero-posterior (lateral decubitus)

This projection is used to confirm the presence of fluid. Moving the patient into a different position causes movement of free fluid, so that loculation is also detected. It may also be used to demonstrate the lateral chest wall of the affected side clear of fluid, and to unmask any underlying lung pathology.

Position of patient and cassette

- The patient is turned on to the unaffected side and, if possible, raised on to a supporting foam pad.
- A cassette is supported vertically against the anterior chest wall, and the median sagittal plane is adjusted at right-angles to the cassette.
- The patient's arms are raised and folded over the head to clear the chest wall.

Direction and centring of the X-ray beam

- Centre to the level of the eighth thoracic vertebra, with the central ray horizontal and directed at right-angles to the cassette.

Alternatively, an antero-posterior projection may be taken, with the cassette supported against the posterior aspect of the patient.

Lateral (dorsal decubitus)

This projection will show as much as possible of the lung fields, clear of a fluid level, when the patient is unable to turn on their side.

Position of patient and cassette

- The patient lies supine and, if possible, is raised off the bed on a supporting foam pad.
- The arms are extended and supported above the head.
- A cassette is supported vertically against the lateral aspect of the chest of the affected side and adjusted parallel to the median sagittal plane.

Direction and centring of the X-ray beam

- Centre to the axilla, with the central ray horizontal and directed at right-angles to the cassette.

Notes

- Further projections may be taken with the patient lying on the affected side or in the prone position to disclose further aspects of the lung fields not obscured by fluid.
- A grid cassette may have to be used if the width of the thorax is likely to produce an unacceptable amount of secondary radiation.

12 Heart and lungs – temporary pacemaker

Patients suffering from heart block are often treated with an electrical pacemaker, which regulates the heart rate. A temporary cardiac electrode is used consisting of a bipolar wire 100-cm long, covered in Teflon, and terminating in a platinum tip electrode separated from a second electrode, which encircles the wire. At the other end, two wires are connected to a battery pacemaker.

The electrode is usually passed into the right subclavian vein and directed into the right ventricle, where the tip is lodged against the endocardial surface near the lower part of the interventricular septum. An electrical impulse is generated across the endocardial surface and adjusted to the required heart rate.

This procedure may be performed in a cardiac catheter laboratory, if available, or in a side ward or dedicated pacing room adjacent to a coronary care facility.

The procedure described below, using a mobile image intensifier, is typical of an insertion of a temporary pacemaker in a side ward dedicated for this procedure.

Mobile image intensifier

- A mobile image intensifier (23 or 31 cm) is selected. As insertion of the electrodes may be prolonged, it is important that the set is equipped with 'last image hold' and pulsed fluoroscopy in order to reduce patient and staff dose.
- The patient lies on a trolley or bed with a radiolucent top, which can accommodate the C-arm of the intensifier.
- The intensifier is positioned on the opposite side of the operating position, with the long axis of the machine at right-angles to the bed or trolley and with the intensifier face above and parallel to the patient's upper thorax.
- The wheels of the image intensifier are rotated in order to allow free longitudinal movement of the device, with the cross-arm brakes released to facilitate movement across the patient.
- During the procedure, the image intensifier is 'panned' so that the advancement and direction of the tip are observed until the tip of the electrode is located correctly within the right ventricle.
- Control of the screening factors, screening time and radiation protection is the responsibility of the radiographer.
- As the procedure is performed under aseptic conditions, a sterile protective cover is normally secured to the image intensifier housing.

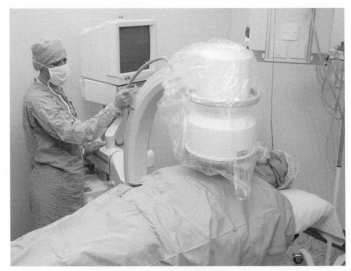

Radiographer positioning the image intensifier prior to pacemaker wire insertion via the left subclavian vein approach

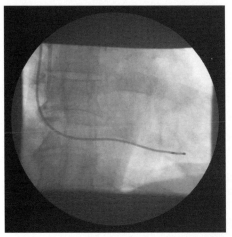

Fluoroscopic image showing location of pacemaker wire

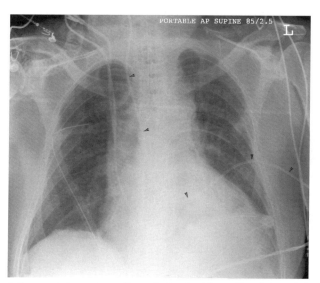

PORTABLE AP SUPINE 85/2.5

Antero-posterior supine radiograph showing bilateral basal chest drains, endotracheal tube, right jugular central venous catheter and a pulmonary artery catheter (in this case unusually passing to the left pulmonary artery rather than the right). Note: to avoid confusion the extracorporeal part of the pulmonary artery catheter (arrowheads) should have been positioned out of the field of view

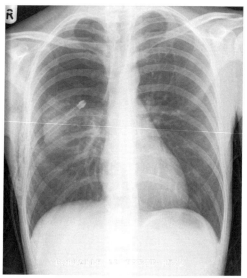

Erect antero-posterior radiograph of chest showing intercostal drain *in situ* for pneumothorax

Heart and lungs – 12
postoperative radiography

Patients who have undergone major cardiac or thoracic surgery are invariably nursed intensively in either a cardiac surgery unit or ICU, depending on the type of surgery performed. Such patients can be connected to an assortment of catheters and tubes for monitoring purposes and chest drainage, e.g. following post-cardiac or -thoracic surgery for drainage of the thoracic cavity of fluid and connections to underwater seals may be necessary to keep the lungs inflated. Strict control of infection procedures must be followed to ensure that the patient is not exposed to infection. A series of radiographs may be required during postoperative care, the first shortly after surgery. The first radiograph, and for a few days until the patient is fit to sit erect, is usually taken with the patient supine. The same principles of consistent radiographic positioning and exposure are applied to enable accurate comparisons of radiographs over a period of time. The positioning of the patient should be carried out using a rehearsed lifting procedure to reduce patient movement and undue back strain for everyone involved in handling the patient. Care should also be taken to expose on full inspiration when the patient is connected to a ventilator.

Endotracheal tube

The position of an endotracheal tube can be assessed from an antero-posterior projection of the chest, which must be exposed with enough penetration to show the trachea and carina. The position of the tube is checked to ensure that its distal end is not lying in the right bronchus.

Central venous pressure line

A fine catheter is positioned in the superior vena cava in seriously ill patients as a means of measuring central venous pressure and injecting drugs. The catheter may be introduced via one of the jugular or subclavian veins, or a peripheral vein. The position of a catheter or line can be assessed from the antero-posterior projection of the chest exposed with enough kilovoltage to penetrate the mediastinum. The position of the catheter is checked to ensure that its distal end has not been directed into the right internal jugular vein or the right atrium of the heart. The root of the neck should be included on the radiograph. There is a risk of inducing a pneumothorax with this procedure and therefore it is important that the chest image includes the apex of the lung.

Chest drain insertions

Chest drains are used for drainage of pneumothorax or pleural effusion, either spontaneous or following cardiac or thoracic surgery. If the drain is connected to an underwater seal chamber, care must be taken not to elevate the chamber above the level of the drain, or water may siphon back into the thorax. An antero-posterior erect image is required to show the position of the tube and to show any residual air within the thorax.

357

Mobile radiography is often required in cases of acute abdominal pain or following surgery, when the patient is unstable, to determine whether any of the following are present:

- gaseous distension of any part of the gastrointestinal tract;
- free gas or fluid in the peritoneal cavity;
- fluid levels in the intestines;
- localization of radio-opaque foreign bodies;
- evidence of aortic aneurysm.

Recommended projections

Typical imaging protocols are described in Section 11. Below is a summary of some of projections used for the conditions listed.

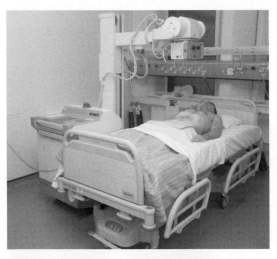

Gaseous distension	Antero-posterior abdomen, patient supine
Free gas in the peritoneal cavity	Antero-posterior chest, patient erect Antero-posterior abdomen, patient supine Antero-posterior/postero-anterior left lateral decubitus
Fluid levels	Antero-posterior abdomen, patient erect
Radio-opaque foreign bodies	Antero-posterior abdomen, patient supine
Aortic aneurysm	Antero-posterior abdomen, patient supine Lateral (dorsal decubitus)

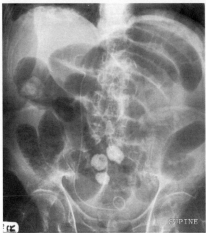

Supine portable radiograph of abdomen showing small bowel obstruction. Also note the right ureteric pigtail stent as patient had transitional cell carcinoma of the bladder

Antero-posterior – supine

Position of patient and cassette

- With the patient supine, a grid cassette is carefully positioned under the abdomen. The patient may be lifted by using a well-rehearsed and safe lifting technique whilst a cassette is slipped beneath them. Care should be exercised to avoid hurting the patient by forcing a cassette into position, or using a cold cassette, which might shock the patient.
- The grid cassette should be positioned to include the symphysis pubis on the lower edge of the image. The cassette should also be in a horizontal position on the bed and not lying at an angle. If the cassette is not flat, there may be grid cut-off of the radiation beam, which may give the appearance of a lesion of increased radio-opacity, such as an intra-abdominal mass due to loss of image density.

Direction and centring of the X-ray beam

- Direct the central ray at right-angles to the cassette and in the midline at the level of the iliac crests.
- Exposure is made on arrested expiration.

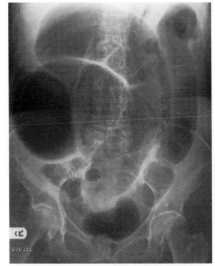

Supine portable radiograph of abdomen showing distal colonic obstruction

Notes

- Radiographs may be taken using a high kVp technique to shorten the exposure time and reduce movement blur, although the increased scatter may degrade the contrast and reduce the ability to see the organ outlines.
- Foam pads may be used to prevent rotation of the patient.

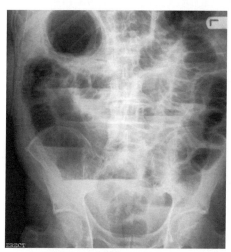

Antero-posterior – erect

The mobile set is positioned to enable horizontal beam radiography necessary for the demonstration of fluid levels.

Position of patient and cassette

- Depending on the patient's medical condition, the patient's bed is adjusted to enable the patient to adopt an erect or semi-erect position. If necessary, a number of pillows or an alternative supporting device are positioned behind the patient to aid stability.
- The patient's thighs are moved out of the beam to ensure that they are not superimposed on the image.
- A 35 × 43-cm grid cassette is placed against the posterior aspect of the patient, with the upper border of the cassette positioned 2 or 3 cm above the xiphisternal joint to ensure that the diaphragm is included on the image to enable demonstration of free air in the peritoneal cavity.

Direction and centring of the X-ray beam

- The horizontal central ray is directed to the centre of the cassette using a 100 cm FFD with care taken to avoid grid cut-off.

Antero-posterior erect radiograph of abdomen showing small bowel obstruction, with gas in the bowel wall (right upper quadrant) indicating impending perforation

Antero-posterior (left lateral decubitus)

This projection, which uses a horizontal central ray, is selected as an alternative to the antero-posterior erect projection when the patient is unable to sit. It is also useful in demonstrating free air in the peritoneal cavity.

Position of patient and cassette

- The patient is turned on to the left side, ideally for 20 minutes, allowing any free air in the abdominal cavity to rise toward the right flank to avoid the problem of differential diagnosis when air is present on the left side of the abdomen within the region of the stomach.
- The grid cassette is supported vertically at right angles to the horizontal central ray, and is positioned against the posterior aspect of the patient to include the right side of the diaphragm.

Direction and centring of the X-ray beam

- The horizontal central ray is directed to the centre of the cassette using a 35 × 43-cm grid cassette.

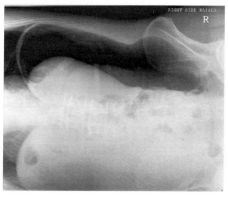

Antero-posterior left lateral decubitus image of the abdomen showing free air in the abdominal cavity

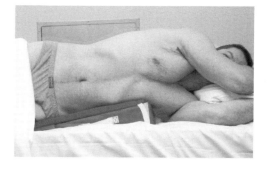

Lateral dorsal decubitus – supine

This projection is selected as an alternative to the antero-posterior projection, with the patient in the left lateral decubitus position, when the patient is too ill to move. It is also used to demonstrate calcification of the abdominal aorta. Abdominal aortic calcification is variable, even in the presence of an aneurysm, and in modern practice it would be more usual to perform ultrasound to assess the size of the aorta and the possibility of abdominal aneurysm. Ultrasound can be done in the emergency room. Computed tomography (CT) scanning offers a greater possibility of demonstrating leak from an aneurysm if the patient is sufficiently stable.

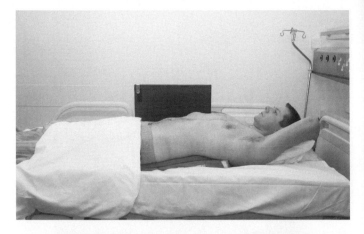

Position of patient and cassette

- The mobile set is positioned so as to enable horizontal beam radiography.
- The patient lies supine and, if possible, is raised off the bed on to a supporting foam pad.
- The arms are extended and supported above the head.
- A grid cassette is supported vertically against the lateral aspect of the abdomen and adjusted parallel to the median sagittal plane.
- The image should include the dome of the diaphragm, the anterior abdominal wall and the vertebral bodies.

Direction and centring of the X-ray beam

- The horizontal central ray is directed to the centre of the cassette.

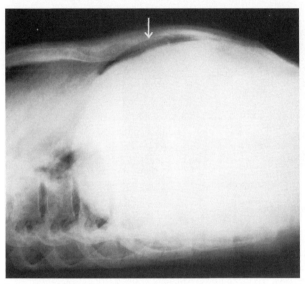

Lateral dorsal decubitus image of the abdomen showing free air in the peritoneal cavity lying adjacent to the anterior abdominal wall

Radiation protection

- A mobile radiation protection barrier should be positioned behind the cassette to confine the primary radiation field.

Note

Free air in the peritoneal cavity can sometimes be demonstrated on a conventional antero-posterior radiograph. In the example opposite, free gas is demonstrated by the presence of a double wall sign. In this image both inside and outside of the bowel wall are seen, as compared with just the lumen side normally, as the result of air both within the lumen of bowel and free in the peritoneal cavity surrounding the section of bowel.

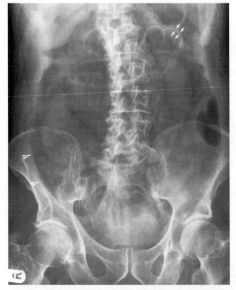

Antero-posterior radiograph of abdomen showing extensive free air in the peritoneal cavity (arrowheads) and double lumen effect demonstrated in left upper abdomen (arrows)

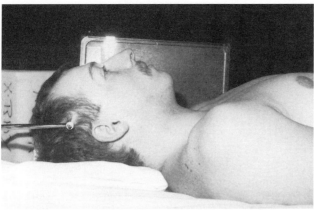

A patient with a spinal fracture dislocation is commonly nursed with skull traction and weights. This is applied by means of a skull calliper secured to the outer table of the parietal regions of the skull. Necessary weights in the early stages of traction may be more than those that are required to maintain realignment of the vertebrae. Traction is continued until there is consolidation.

Lateral projections of the cervical vertebrae, over several weeks, are necessary to assess the effectiveness of the traction and demonstrate the alignment of the vertebrae in relation to the spinal cord. Each radiograph is marked with the weight of the applied traction.

Lateral supine

Position of patient and cassette

- The mobile set is positioned so as to enable horizontal beam radiography.
- With the patient in the supine position, a 24 × 30 or 18 × 24-cm cassette is supported vertically against either shoulder, parallel to the cervical vertebrae and centred at the level of the prominence of the thyroid cartilage.
- The cassette is secured in position using a holder or sandbags.
- The patient's shoulders must be depressed by the supervising doctor gripping the patient's wrists and pulling the arms caudally.

Direction and centring of the X-ray beam

- The horizontal central ray is directed to a point vertically below the prominence of the thyroid cartilage at the level of the mastoid process through the fourth cervical vertebra.

Note

In the radiographs opposite, part of the skull has been included on the film to show where the skull calliper is secured to the parietal regions.

Radiation protection

- A mobile radiation protection barrier should be positioned behind the cassette to confine the primary radiation field.
- The person applying the traction must be medically supervised and wear a radiation protective lead-rubber apron and lead-rubber gloves.

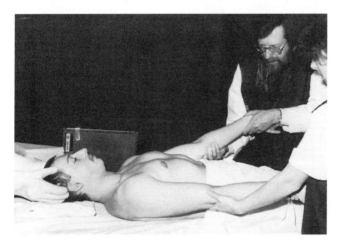

1 day on traction

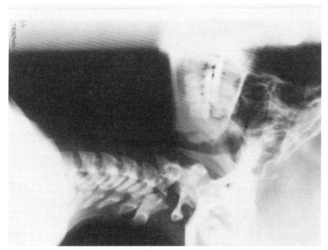

30 days on traction

12 Fractured lower limbs and pelvis

Orthopaedic radiography may be required to be undertaken on the ward immediately following surgery or following the application of traction. For the limbs, two radiographs are taken at right-angles to each other to check on the position and alignment of fractured bones. Examination of the patient will be made difficult if a suspension system is used, which will include weights and a metal pulley rope structure that is connected to the patient's bed. Great care should be exercised not to disturb these appliances, as they may disturb the position of the fractured bones and add to the patient's pain. A heavy patient may tend to sag into the mattress of the bed, which complicates matters when positioning for projections of the upper femur. The patient may be able to lift their bottom off the bed using the overhead hand grip so that a support pad or cassette tunnel device can be introduced under the buttocks.

Antero-posterior

Position of patient and cassette

- The mobile set is positioned carefully relative to any overhead bed supports, with adjustment being made with support of the nursing staff.
- A suitably sized cassette is selected and carefully positioned under the femur or lower leg to include the joint nearest the fracture and as much of the upper or lower limb as possible to enable bone alignment to be assessed.
- The cassette is supported parallel to the femur or lower limb by the use of non-opaque pads.
- For fractures of the neck of femur or pelvis, a cassette tunnel device may be used, which needs only one major disturbance to the patient. Once in position, a cassette may be positioned without any further disruption to the patient. This also serves in aiding the positioning for the lateral projection when the patient is raised, allowing adequate demonstration of the femur.

Direction and centring of the X-ray beam

- Direct the central ray at right-angles to the middle of the cassette with the central ray at right angles to the long axis of the bones in question, in accordance with the techniques previously described in the chapter on the lower limb.

Note

Repeat examinations will be required over a period of time to assess the effectiveness of treatment; therefore, careful positioning and exposure selection are required to ensure that images are comparable.

Radiation protection

- Radiation protection is particularly important, and gonad shields should be used.
- A mobile radiation protection barrier should be positioned behind the cassette to confine the primary radiation field when undertaking lateral projections.

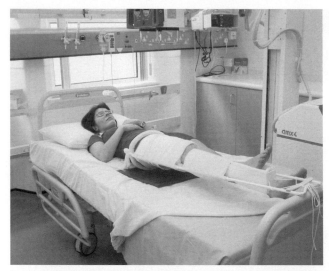

Patient positioned for antero-posterior femur (hip down) following the application of a Thomas's splint

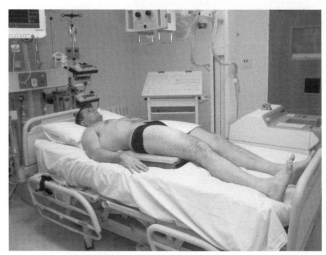

Patient resting on a wooden cassette tunnel device for antero-posterior pelvis

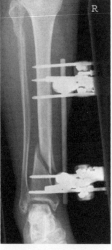

Antero-posterior image of tibia and fibula showing external fixation device

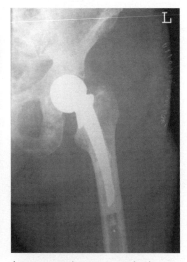

Antero-posterior postoperative image of hip joint following arthroplasty

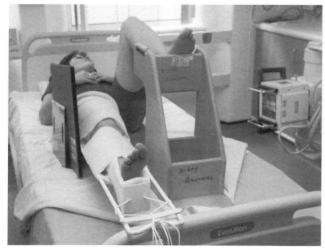

Patient positioned for lateral femur (knee up) following the application of a Thomas's splint

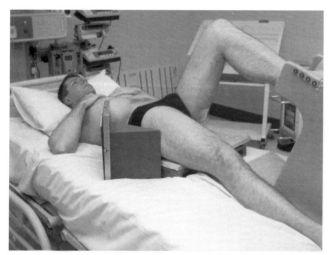

Patient positioned for lateral hip with pelvis raised resting on a cassette tunnel device

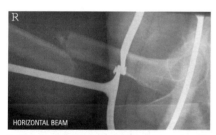

Lateral image of a right fractured femur in a Thomas's splint

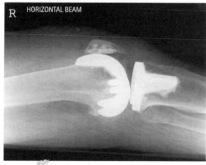

Postoperative lateral image of the knee using a horizontal beam following joint replacement

Position of patient and cassette

- The mobile X-ray equipment is carefully repositioned to enable horizontal beam radiography.
- When the examination is for the distal two-thirds of the femur, the cassette may be positioned vertically against the medial side of the thigh and the horizontal beam directed latero-medially.
- When the proximal part of the shaft or the neck of the femur is being examined, the cassette is positioned vertically against the lateral side of the thigh and the beam is directed medio-laterally, with the opposite leg raised on a suitable support so that the unaffected thigh is in a near-vertical position.
- For the neck of femur, a grid cassette is positioned vertically, with one edge against the waist above the iliac crest on the side being examined and adjusted with its long axis parallel to the neck of femur.
- To demonstrate fractures of the upper femur, it is essential that the patient is raised off the bed on a suitable rigid structure, such as a firm foam pad or a cassette tunnel device.

Direction and centring of the X-ray beam

- For the distal two-thirds of the femur, the horizontal central ray is centred to the middle of the cassette and parallel to a line joining the anterior borders of the femoral condyles.
- To demonstrate the neck of femur, which will include the hip joint, centre midway between the femoral pulse and the palpable prominence of the greater trochanter, with the central ray directed horizontally and at right-angles to the cassette.

Note

When using a grid, it is essential that the cassette remains vertical to avoid grid cut-off.

Arthroplasty postoperative radiography

An antero-posterior projection of the hip is taken within 24 hours of surgery to include the upper third of the femur to demonstrate the prosthesis and the cement restrictor, which is distal to the prosthesis. This may be highlighted by a radio-opaque marker in the form of a ball-bearing, which should appear in all subsequent follow-up images of the hip joint if it has been used.

Loosening of the prosthesis can occur by impaction of the femoral shaft of the prosthesis into the native femur. This is detected most easily by observing a reduction in the distance between the cement restrictor and the tip of the prosthesis. It is therefore most important that the first image includes the cement restrictor.

The nursing management is also determined on confirmation that the hip joint has not dislocated.

Antero-posterior and lateral projections are acquired of the knee joint following knee joint replacement.

12 Fractured femur – paediatric (gallows traction)

This type of traction is used on children from birth to 12 months. Two projections, antero-posterior and lateral, are taken to assess bone alignment and new bone formation. The application of gonad protection and careful collimation of the X-ray beam are essential. Great care should be exercised to avoid disturbing the traction; however, it is still usually possible to maintain traction and rotate the child so that the front of the suspended legs are facing the side of the cot, which can be lowered during exposure to avoid superimposition of the cot's vertical bars.

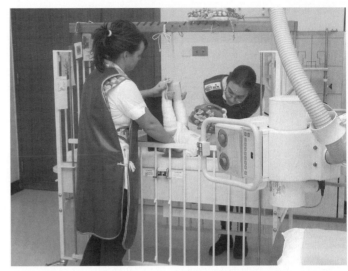

Child in the process of being positioned for antero-posterior femur

Antero-posterior

Position of patient and cassette

- With the child lying supine, with both legs suspended vertically, a cassette is supported against the posterior aspect of the affected leg using foam pads or an L-shaped plastic cassette support device.
- The cassette is positioned to enable full coverage of the femur, including the knee and hip joints.

Direction and centring of the X-ray beam

- Centre to the middle of the anterior aspect of the femur, with the horizontal central ray at right-angles to the cassette.

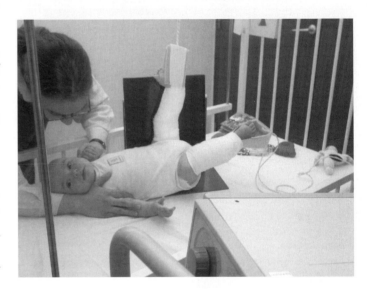

Lateral

Position of patient and cassette

- To avoid superimposition of the unaffected femur, the sound limb is carefully removed from the traction by the medical officer and held in a position outside the radiation beam.
- Alternatively, the traction may be adjusted and the sound limb supported temporarily in a different position.
- The medical officer or health professional must wear a lead-rubber apron and lead-rubber gloves.
- A cassette is supported vertically against the lateral aspect of the affected leg and adjusted parallel to the femur.

Direction and centring of the X-ray beam

- Centre to the middle of the medial aspect of the femur, with the horizontal central ray at right-angles to the cassette.

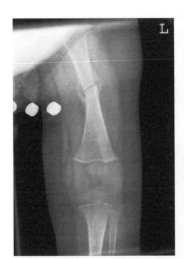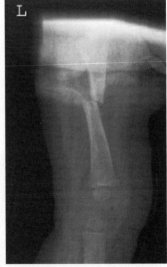

Antero-posterior and lateral images of left femur two weeks post-trauma

Neonates suffering from respiratory distress syndrome are examined soon after birth to demonstrate the lungs, which are immature and unable to perform normal respiration. The baby will be nursed in an incubator and may be attached to a ventilator. The primary beam is directed through the incubator top, with care being taken to avoid any opacity or cut-outs in the incubator top falling within the radiation beam.

Many designs of incubators are available, with many requiring the cassette to be placed within the incubator. However, a number are designed to facilitate positioning of the cassette on a special tray immediately below and outside the incubator housing.

A full account of neonatal radiography is given in Section 14.

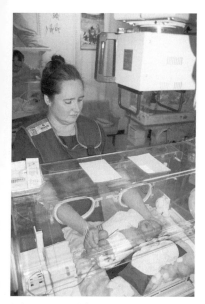

Baby positioned for antero-posterior chest and abdomen

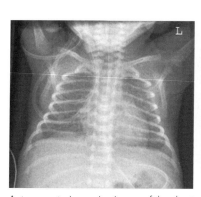

Antero-posterior

- An 18 × 24-cm cassette that is at body temperature is selected. Disposable sheets should be used between the baby and the cassette.

Position of patient and cassette

- The baby is positioned supine on the cassette, with the median sagittal plane adjusted perpendicular to the middle of the cassette, ensuring that the head and chest are straight and the shoulders and hips are level. When using the cassette tray the incubator head end is raised five to ten degrees to avoid a 'lordotic' chest or alternatively a wedge pad is used to raise the shoulders.
- The head may need holding with the chin raised up to avoid the chin obscuring the lung apices, or supported using small covered sandbags. Arms should be on either side, slightly separated from the trunk to avoid being included in the radiation field and to avoid skin crease artefacts, which can mimic pneumothoraces. The arms can be immobilized with Velcro bands and/or sandbags.

Direction and centring of the X-ray beam

- No single centring point is advised.
- Centre the beam to the correct size of the chest.
- The central ray is directed vertically, or angled five to 10 degrees caudally if the baby is completely flat, but if doing so, care should be exercised not to cause the chin to be projected over the apices.
- Constant maximum FFD should be used.

Notes

- Very short exposure times are required for these procedures. A high-frequency generator will give very low mAs and extremely short exposure in the millisecond range.
- Lead-rubber shapes should be placed on the incubator top to protect the gonads and thyroid gland.
- Exposure factor details should be recorded for subsequent imaging, and image comparisons with positioning legends should be recorded on the image.

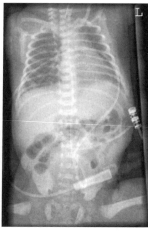

Antero-posterior supine image of the chest in a neonate of 28 weeks gestation

Antero-posterior supine image of the chest and abdomen showing position of an arterial line which has been enhanced using contrast media

Section 13

Theatre Radiography

CONTENTS

INTRODUCTION   368
Liaison   368
Personnel preparation   368
Equipment   368
Darkroom facilities/PACS connectivity   369
Accessory equipment   369
Radiation protection   369
Sterile areas   369

NON-TRAUMA CORRECTIVE
ORTHOPAEDIC SURGERY   370

TRAUMA ORTHOPAEDIC SURGERY   371

DYNAMIC HIP SCREW INSERTION   374
Introduction   374
Imaging procedure   374
Surgical procedure   375

INTERVENTIONAL UROLOGY   376
Introduction   376
Retrograde pyelography   376
Percutaneous nephrolithotomy   377

OPERATIVE CHOLANGIOGRAPHY   378
Imaging procedure   378

HYSTEROSALPINGOGRAPHY   379
Imaging procedure   379

EMERGENCY PERIPHERAL VASCULAR
PROCEDURES   380
Imaging procedure   380

Theatre radiography plays a significant role in the delivery of surgical services. The following settings are typical examples where the radiographer is required:

- non-trauma corrective orthopaedic surgery;
- trauma orthopaedic surgery;
- interventional urology;
- operative cholangiography;
- specialized hysterosalpinography procedures;
- emergency peripheral vascular procedures.

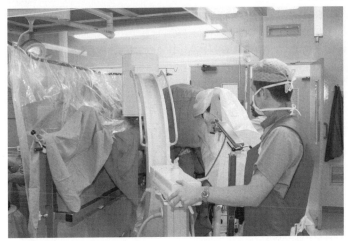

Liaison

- The radiographer must contact the theatre superintendent upon arrival and maintain a close liaison with all persons performing the operation, consequently working as part of the multidisciplinary team.
- The radiographer must be familiar with the layout and protocols associated with the theatre to which they are assigned, demonstrate a working knowledge of the duties of each person in the operating theatre, and ascertain the specific requirements of the surgeon who is operating.

The above photographs are taken during a dynamic hip screw procedure and show the use of a sterile protective barrier as described on page 374

Personnel preparation

- Personal preparation is the first concern of the radiographer before entering an aseptic controlled area.
- The radiographer removes their uniform (and any jewellery), and replaces them with theatre wear. The hair is covered completely with a disposable hat. Theatre shoes or boots are worn, and a facemask is put on. In addition, a film-monitoring badge is pinned to theatre garments.
- Special attention is made to washing the hands using soap, ensuring that the hands are washed before and after each patient. If the skin has an abrasion, this should be covered with a waterproof dressing.

Equipment

- A mobile X-ray unit or mobile image intensifier is selected, depending on the requirement of the radiographic procedure. For example, a mobile X-ray unit may be used for plain-film chest radiography, while a mobile image intensifier may be used for the screening of orthopaedic procedures such as hip pinning.
- Before use, an image intensifier should be assembled and tested ahead of the procedure to ensure that it is functioning effectively prior to patient positioning.

- For the prevention of infection, the unit selected should be cleaned and dried after each patient. Where appropriate, protective plastic coverings can be used to reduce blood contamination during surgical procedures. When blood or other bodily fluids do come into contact with the imaging equipment, an appropriate cleaning solution, as advised by the local infection control officer, should be used.
- Exposure parameters are then adjusted to those required for screening or image recording on film.

Darkroom facilities/PACS connectivity

In many theatre suites, it is customary for X-ray equipment and darkroom processing facilities to be housed within the complex. Processing equipment should be switched on and tested upon arrival. Adequate levels of film processor replenisher solutions should be prepared if required and a supply of cassettes and films made available for use. With modern mobile image intensifiers a PACS DICOM link should be established to facilitate image capture and retrieval of previous images.

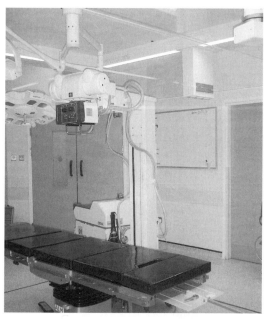

Mobile X-ray set positioned for plain image radiography using a 'Baker's tray' to accommodate a cassette

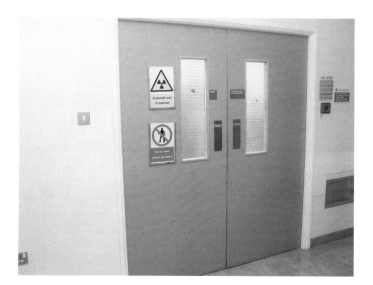

Accessory equipment

- Cassette holders, stationary grids, cassette tunnels and serial changer devices should be cleaned and checked if required.
- An operating theatre table with an adjustable cassette tray should be checked for movement, and the radiographer should be familiar with the function and be able to position cassettes, when requested, with the minimum of fuss.
- Contrast media, if required, should also be supplied to the theatre staff.

Radiation protection

- Radiation protection is the responsibility of the radiographer operating the X-ray equipment. Therefore, the radiographer should ensure that film monitoring badges, lead protective aprons and thyroid shields are worn by all staff wherever possible. Furthermore, as soon as the imaging equipment is switched on, a controlled area exists. Therefore, all doors that have access to the controlled area must display radiation warning signs.
- The inverse square law principle must be applied in the theatre environment. Therefore, staff must be standing at the maximum distance from the source of radiation, and outside the path of the radiation field during exposure.
- The radiation field should be collimated to at least the size of the film or intensifier, and cassette support devices should be used to hold cassettes.
- The radiographer should use the fastest film/screen combination consistent with the examination to reduce radiation dose, or they should aim to maximize the use of dose-saving facilities whilst using an image intensifier.
- Patient identification must be confirmed with either the anaesthetist or an appropriate member of the theatre team before any radiation exposure.
- Records should be kept of patient details, exposure time and radiation dose when screening is employed.
- The radiographer must give clear instructions to staff before exposures are made regarding their role in reducing the risk of accidental exposure.

Sterile areas

The radiographer should avoid the contamination of sterile areas. Ideally, equipment should be positioned before any sterile towels are placed in position, and care should be exercised not to touch sterile areas when positioning cassettes or moving equipment during the operation.

13 Non-trauma corrective orthopaedic surgery

- The radiographer plays a significant role as part of the orthopaedic theatre team, where imaging control is required for an operative procedure.
- Imaging control is required most frequently to aid trauma orthopaedic surgery. However, in a small number of cases it is also required for non-trauma corrective orthopaedic surgery. In both instances, however, the radiographer will be required to work in a theatre environment primarily using a mobile C-arm image intensifier equipped with an image memory device.
- A long list of non-trauma corrective orthopaedic procedures are performed throughout the world. The majority involve the replacement of joints as a result of chronic bone or joint disease, e.g. severe osteoarthritis of the hip can be corrected using the implantation of a prosthetic total hip joint replacement. These procedures, however, no longer require the aid of imaging control due to the advancements of surgical techniques.
- Nevertheless, more complex paediatric operative procedures do require imaging control, namely osteotomies, which are carried out in order to correct defects in bone and joint alignment. Such procedures vary in complexity in terms of corrective surgery and will involve the use of fixation plates. The table opposite lists some examples.

Common corrective orthopaedic operative procedures include:

Pathology	Operative procedure
• Congenital dislocation of the hip/Perthes' disease/hip dysphasia	• Salter pelvic osteotomy
• Persistent femoral anteversion	• Deviation femoral osteotomy
• Varus deformity of the knee	• Proximal tibial osteotomy

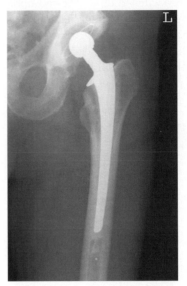

Antero-posterior hip image showing a 'Thompson's' hip prosthesis

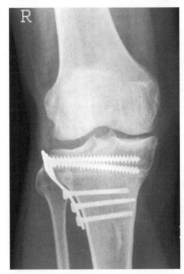

Antero-posterior knee image showing an example of a tibial osteotomy

Common trauma orthopaedic operative procedures include:

Fracture type	Operative procedure
Hip fracture	
Intracapsular	
• Subcapital or transcervical – displaced	• Hemiarthroplasty
• Subcapital or transcervical – undisplaced	• Cannulated hip screws
Extracapsular	
• Intertrochanteric or basal fracture	• Dynamic hip screw (DHS) or gamma nail
• Subtrochanteric fracture	• Dynamic condylar screw (DCS) or gamma nail
Upper and lower extremities	
• Simple fracture of finger/hand/wrist/elbow/foot	• Manipulation under anaesthetic (MUA)
	• Kirschner ('K') wire insertion
• Complicated fracture of ankle/elbow/wrist/forearm	• Open reduction and internal fixation (ORIF) with compression plates and screws
• Comminuted fracture	• External fixation
• Open fracture of tibia or femur with significant soft tissue involvement	• External fixation
	• Unreamed intramedullary nail insertion with proximal and/or distal locking
• Closed fracture of tibia or femur	• Reamed intramedullary nail insertion with proximal and/or distal locking
	• Intramedullary rod
• Fracture of humerus	• Tension band wiring
• Olecranon and patella fracture/displacement following trauma	

- The orthopaedic surgical procedures highlighted previously are necessary to correct defects in paediatric bone and joint alignment. However, the majority of the radiographer's workload in the theatre environment will focus on trauma orthopaedic surgery, assisting the successful reduction of fractures and the implantation of internal or external fixing devices.
- There are various trauma orthopaedic procedures where radiographic imaging is required. The table opposite provides examples of familiar trauma operative procedures in relation to fracture types.
- Image examples and important factors to note during the imaging procedure are provided on p. 372.
- A more extensive explanation of the typical dynamic hip screw (DHS) surgical and imaging procedure can be found on p. 374.

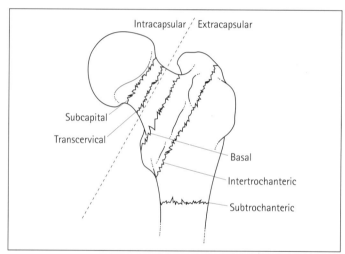

Diagram illustrating types of intracapsular and extracapsular hip fractures

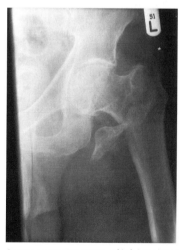

Antero-posterior image of left hip showing extracapsular fracture

The Kirschner wire insertion is performed mostly in corrective simple fracture extremity surgery.

When positioning the image intensifier for this surgical procedure, it is important to ensure that the C-arm is rotated through 180 degrees, therefore placing the affected limb closest to the detector. This reduces magnification and improves image quality.

Open reduction and internal fixations (ORIFs) are performed mostly in complicated fractures where the fracture cannot be held satisfactorily by any other means, e.g. midshaft forearm fractures can be stabilized using compression plates and screws. Again, the image intensifier must be positioned with the affected limb closest to the detector, allowing minimum magnification and distortion of the image yet permitting ease of movement when positioning for both the antero-posterior and lateral images. Imaging control is often required at the end of this procedure as the surgeon can often visualize the fracture site due to the procedure being 'open'.

External fixation and Steinmann pin insertions for traction often require imaging control to visualize the progress of the surgical procedure. Various external fixators are in use, ranging from the Ilizarov (ring fixator) to the AO ((Arbeitsgemeinschaft für Osteosynthesefragen) tubular) system. In either instance, image guidance is often required to demonstrate the true position of the screw or pin during surgical positioning and to aid in the reduction/manipulation of the fracture site when the fixator is in place.

Tension band wirings, like ORIFs, are essentially an open surgical procedure. In these cases, imaging control to assist the surgeon is often kept to a minimum and is upon the surgeon's request.

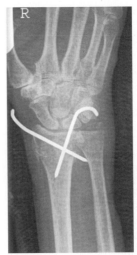

Example of Kirschner wire insertions

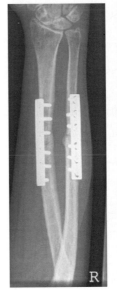
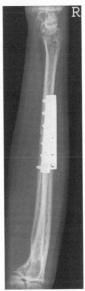

Example of internal plates and screws in forearm following ORIF

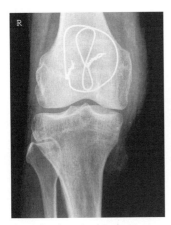
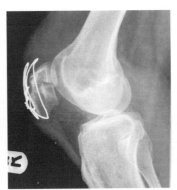

Example of tension band wiring

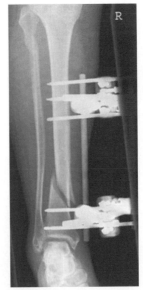
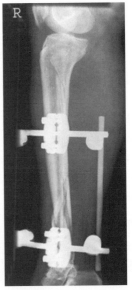

Example of external fixation of tibia and fibula

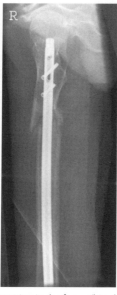

Example of intramedullary nail insertion in the femur (hip down)

Intramedullary nailing requires intermittent imaging control throughout the majority of the surgical procedure, not only to assist the surgeon in visualizing the nail as it passes through the medulla of the long bone but also, more importantly, to assist in the proximal and distal locking of the nail with cortex screws.

During the proximal and/or distal locking of the surgical procedure, the radiographer must aim to image the nail within the medulla of the long bone, demonstrating the circular holes within the nail *en face*, thus allowing the surgeon to insert the cortex screws with ease. Laser guidance facilities are available on some image intensifiers to assist in this procedure.

Cannulated hip screws are used mostly for undisplaced subcapital or transcervical fractures. The imaging procedure for this technique is similar to the DHS procedure, which is discussed in more detail in the following section.

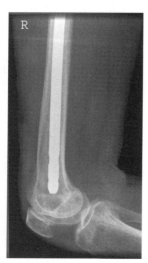

Example of intramedullary nail insertion in the femur (knee up) showing distal locking

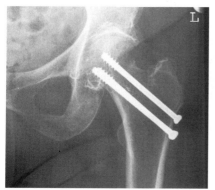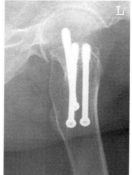

Example of cannulated screws in different patients

13 Dynamic hip screw insertion

Introduction

The procedure described for a DHS insertion is typical of that employed in an orthopaedic theatre. There are, however, a number of variations to be found in the approach of different surgeons, and the radiographer should be aware of the technique employed in their own hospital.

The technique described employs the use of a sterile protective barrier, which separates the image intensifier from the surgeon and the operative field.

During the operative procedure, images of the hip and neck of femur are taken at right-angles at various stages. Care should be taken, therefore, when moving the imaging intensifier into these required imaging positions to ensure that the sterile field is not compromised.

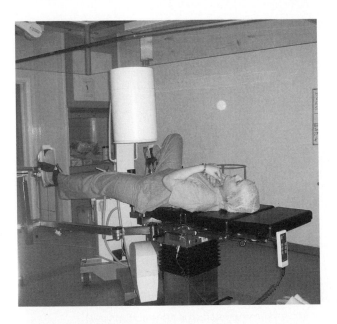

Imaging procedure

A mobile C-arm image intensifier is preferred for this procedure as it provides a real-time image to assist the surgeon in positioning the guide wire and subsequent DHS internal fixator. Ideally, image intensifiers in use should be equipped with a memory device that gives an immediate playback of the image last seen on the television screen. Most modern image intensifiers fulfil this requirement.

Using a system equipped with a memory device helps to reduce the radiation dose to the patient, since the surgeon is able to study an image without further irradiating the patient. This also allows the surgeon to store the last image, so that comparisons can be made of any alterations to the position and direction of the guide wire or DHS. In addition, hard-copy images can be taken at the end of the operation to help demonstrate the completed procedure.

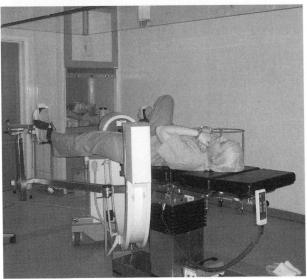

Before the operation commences, the patient, whilst anaesthetized, is transferred to a special orthopaedic operating table with leg supports. The patient is positioned by the orthopaedic surgeon with the unaffected leg raised, flexed and in abduction, and the affected leg extended and in medial rotation. Traction is applied to the affected limb, enabling manipulation and alignment of the fracture site.

At this stage, the mobile image intensifier is positioned to enable screening of the hip in both the postero-anterior and lateral directions. The long axis of the intensifier is positioned between the legs and adjacent to the unaffected limb, enabling the C-arm to be rotated through 90 degrees, parallel to the neck of the femur. Once positioned correctly, the image intensifier is locked into position and checked to ensure that the C-arm rotates freely from the postero-anterior to lateral imaging positions and that the femoral neck is imaged in the middle of the image intensifier face.

As the image intensifier is positioned on the opposite side of the sterile protective barrier, a sterile cover is not required (see page 368). However, a plastic protective cover is placed over the X-ray tube housing to protect the X-ray tube covering in the event of blood spillage from the operative site.

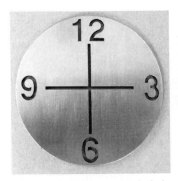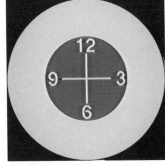

Example of a radio-opaque clock device used for orientation of an image intensifier and an X-ray image of the device

During the surgical/imaging procedure, the radiographer makes appropriate alterations to exposure factors and orientation controls. The use of a radio-opaque clock device is invaluable in determining the correct orientation of the hip joint. A record is made of the total screening time and radiation dose employed during the operation.

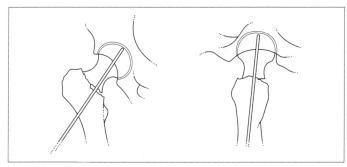

Antero-posterior and lateral hip diagrams showing a reduced fracture

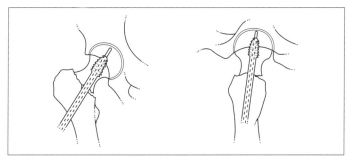

Antero-posterior and lateral hip diagrams showing a guide pin positioned through the centre of the neck of the femur

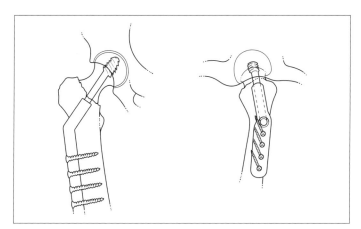

Antero-posterior and lateral hip diagrams showing insertion of a lag screw

Surgical procedure

The diagrams opposite illustrate the typical images that are acquired during an operative procedure using the DHS.

For this procedure, a DHS guide pin and angle guide are first required. The guide pin is positioned through the centre of the neck of femur and an appropriate triple reamer is placed over the guide pin to allow a channel to be reamed for the insertion of a lag screw. When the channel is completed, the lag screw is inserted, with the threaded tip lying approximately 10 mm from the joint surface. A DHS plate is then placed over the distal end of the lag screw assembly and positioned until it is in contact with the lateral cortex of the proximal femur. Cortex screws are then used to secure the DHS plate in position.

Imaging is necessary during the procedure to demonstrate:

- the fracture before it is reduced;
- the fracture reduced, with the angle guide and guide pin during positioning;
- the reaming of a channel before the insertion of the lag screw;
- insertion of the lag screw and DHS plate;
- completed operation, with a DHS inserted to stabilize the fracture site.

As outlined earlier, there are a variety of other operative procedures for the treatment of intertrochanteric and femoral neck fractures. Common to each technique adopted is the placing of guide pins along the femoral neck and into the head of the femur before the insertion of screws or securing plates.

Whist acquisition of images during these operative procedures is a dynamic process, with images acquired at each stage in the postero-anterior and lateral planes, permanent images are acquired at the end of the procedure for completeness. These images are best acquired using the image intensifier memory device, since this reduces radiation dose to the patient and staff. It is important, however, that the hip joint and proximal end of the femur are demonstrated to ensure that the full extent of fixation plates, pins and screws can be seen on these images.

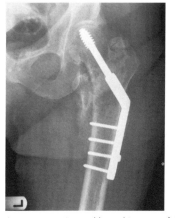
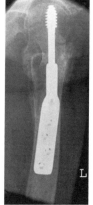

Antero-posterior and lateral images of the hip showing a DHS implant

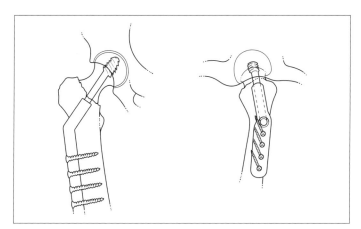

Antero-posterior and lateral hip diagrams showing the completed operation with lag screw and DHS plate secured in position

13 Interventional urology

Introduction

Interventional urology plays an important role in the theatre setting, particularly for those patients who require general anaesthesia. The following procedures are typical examples:

- retrograde pyelography;
- percutaneous nephrolithotomy.

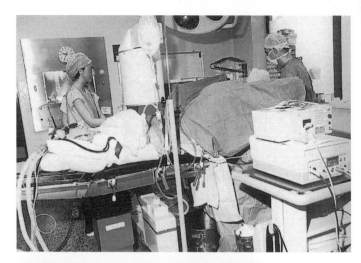

Retrograde pyelography

Retrograde pyelography, also known as ascending pyelography, involves a mechanical filling procedure to demonstrate the renal calyces and pelvis with a suitable organic iodine contrast agent.

A theatre table suitable for cystoscopy, with a radiolucent top, is used. The mobile image intensifier with a C-arm is usually selected to provide real-time images for the surgeon during the operation.

Cystoscopy is first performed to pass a catheter into the ureter and up to the pelvis of the affected kidney. Fluoroscopy may be needed to assist with this.

The patient is positioned supine during the operation.

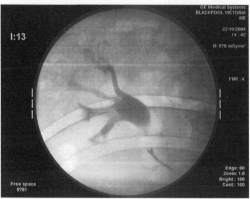

Imaging procedure

- When a mobile image intensifier is employed, the intensifier is positioned on the opposite side of the table to which the surgeon is operating and moved into position over the operation site to adopt a postero-anterior projection of the abdomen. The patient is positioned on the table before the operation to ensure that the intensifier will move into position without being obstructed by the table's main support pillar.
- During fluoroscopy, between 5 and 20 ml of a 150-mg I/ml strength contrast agent is introduced via the ureteric catheter into the affected renal pelvis.
- Permanent images are acquired of the contrast-filled calyces and ureter using the machine's last-image-hold facility or an exposure technique.
- The catheter is withdrawn using fluoroscopy to observe the emptying of the contrast into the bladder.
- Images are acquired as and when required to record any abnormalities.

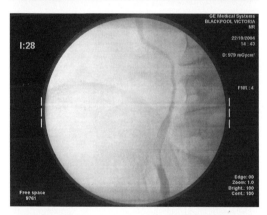

Note

This procedure may be undertaken in the imaging department as part of a two-staged procedure, with the patient having had the cystoscopy in theatre and catheter placement under anaesthetic and imaging subsequently undertaken in the radiology department.

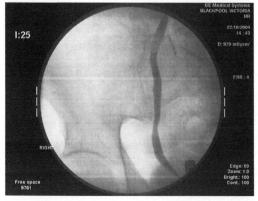

Above images demonstrate a contrast-filled renal collection system and ureter acquired in theatre using a mobile image intensifier and digital image capture device

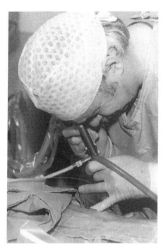

Surgeon with nephroscope and irrigation tubing

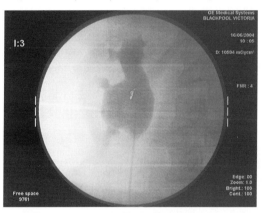

Image showing retrograde filling of kidney

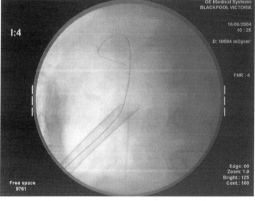

Image showing sheath situated in the renal pelvis

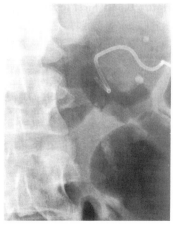

Image showing pigtail catheter left *in situ*

Percutaneous nephrolithotomy

Percutaneous nephrolithotomy (PCNL) is an interventional procedure used to remove renal stones directly via a nephrostomy tract.

A mobile image intensifier with a C-arm and a theatre table for cystoscopy with a radiolucent tabletop are usually selected for this procedure, since this provides a real-time fluoroscopy image of the positioning of catheters and instrumentation and the flow of contrast media through the renal tract.

Small stones less than 1 cm that have proved unsuitable for treatment by lithotripsy are removed by special instruments in conjunction with endoscopy. Larger stones, e.g. stag-horn calculus, require first to be disintegrated by electrohydraulic lithotripsy or ultrasound shock waves.

Imaging procedure

- With the patient supine on the operating table for cystoscopy, a retrograde catheter is placed in the renal pelvis or upper ureter on the affected side. This facilitates contrast medium (150 mg I/ml) and/or methylene blue solution to be injected into the renal pelvis throughout the procedure. The patient is then turned carefully into the prone oblique position, with the affected side uppermost.
- After opacification of the collecting system with contrast and/ or methylene blue solution, the posterior calyx of the lower calyceal group is punctured with an 18-gauge needle cannula. Imaging is performed as necessary during this procedure, with the C-arm vertical and angled obliquely across the long axis of the body to aid localization of the kidney.
- Following removal of the central needle and aspiration of the mixture of urine, contrast and/or methylene blue to ensure accurate position within the collection system, a soft J-wire and then a stiff wire are passed in an antegrade manner into the kidney. The tract is then dilated up to a 30F size (1 cm) using either a series of plastic dilators or a combination of dilators and a dilation balloon. A 1-cm sheath is then placed over the largest dilator or dilated balloon directly into the renal pelvis.
- A nephroscope, with its light source, is passed through the sheath to visualize the collecting system and facilitate the passing of instruments required to disintegrate and remove the calculus. During the procedure, an irrigation system incorporated into the nephroscope will wash clear any calculus fragments from the renal pelvis. Attention should be paid to ensuring that any water spillage from this process does not come into contact with the image intensifier.
- At the end of the procedure, a pigtail catheter is left in the renal pelvis to allow antegrade drainage of the kidney and to perform antegrade contrast studies if required to check for residual stone fragments.
- Careful collimation of the X-ray beam should be employed during this long imaging procedure.
- Permanent images are acquired of the contrast-filled calyces using the machine's last-image-hold facility or an exposure technique.

13 | Operative cholangiography

Cholangiography refers to the demonstration of the hepatic, cystic and bile ducts by direct injection into the biliary tree. The examination may be requested during cholecystectomy to demonstrate the presence of any gallstones within the biliary ducts. The patient will be positioned supine during the operation.

A mobile image intensifier with a C-arm and a theatre table with a radiolucent tabletop are often selected for this procedure as this provides a real-time image for the surgeon to assess the flow of contrast media through the biliary tree.

Alternatively, the examination is performed using a specially adapted theatre table with a radiolucent tabletop, a device commonly known as a 'Baker's tray', and a mobile X-ray machine. A 24 × 30-cm grid cassette with a fast film/screen combination is usually selected. This method does have limitations, since a film has to be processed, thereby adding a delay in the operation. Also, optimum selection of exposure factors is critical.

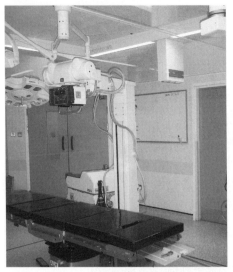

Theatre table with a 'Baker's tray' to accommodate a cassette

Imaging procedure

Mobile image intensifier

When a mobile image intensifier is employed, the intensifier is positioned on the opposite side of the table to which the surgeon is operating and moved into position over the operation site to adopt a postero-anterior projection of the abdomen. It is preferred that the patient is positioned on the table before the operation commences to ensure that the intensifier will move into position without being obstructed by the table's main support pillar.

Under carefully controlled conditions, the surgeon injects 20–30 ml of a water-soluble organic iodine compound (150 mg I/ml), without bubbles, into the biliary tract. The contrast is observed as it flows through the biliary tree into the duodenum.

Images of the contrast-filled biliary tree are acquired using the machine's last-image-hold facility or a single exposure technique.

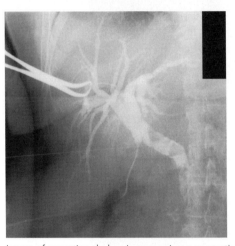

Image of operative cholangiogram using a conventional mobile X-ray set and 'Baker's tray'

Mobile X-ray machine

When a cassette tray (Baker's tray) mechanism is employed, an initial antero-posterior projection of the right upper abdomen may be taken before the operation. The cassette is positioned on the tray mechanism, offset relative to the centre to coincide with the right side of the abdomen. It is then moved to a position, using a long handle, along the table to coincide with the operation field, which should include the biliary tree and the duodenum. A note is made of the correct film position.

When required, antero-posterior projections of the abdomen are taken during and at the termination of the injection of contrast to ensure that any filling defect is constant and that contrast medium is seen flowing freely into the duodenum.

A 24 × 30-cm grid cassette (6 : 1 or 8 : 1 grid ratio) is used with a fast film/screen combination. Exposure is made using a significantly high kilovoltage technique of approximately 85–90 kVp in order to obtain a sufficiently short exposure time and a sharp outline of the biliary tree. In addition, movement blur may be reduced by the anaesthetist stopping the patient's respiration during the exposure.

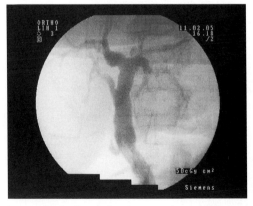

Image of operative cholangiogram using a mobile image intensifier and digital image capture device

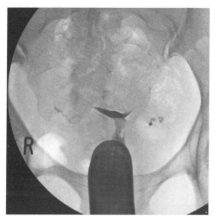

Initial image showing uterine cavity and tubal filling

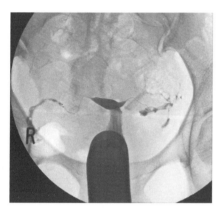

Second image in the series showing tubal spillage

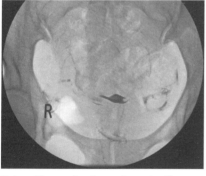

Delayed image showing peritoneal spillage

Hysterosalpingography is commonly carried out in the general X-ray department, and nowadays is increasingly done using ultrasound and appropriate contrast media. However, a small percentage of examinations are carried out under general anaesthetic in theatre using radiographic contrast. (The procedure is described in detail in Whitley *et al.* 1999.)

The examination is requested to demonstrate the patency of the uterine tubes, demonstrating any cause of obstruction or abnormalities of the uterine cavity.

A mobile image intensifier with a C-arm and a theatre table with a radiolucent tabletop are selected for this procedure as this provides a real-time image for the surgeon to assess the flow of contrast media through the uterine cavity via the cervix.

The patient is positioned supine during the operation.

Imaging procedure

- The mobile image intensifier is positioned to adopt a postero-anterior projection of the lower abdomen/pelvic region.
- The patient is positioned on the table before the operation to ensure that the intensifier will move into position without being obstructed by the table's main support pillar.
- The patient is placed in the lithotomy position.
- Using an aseptic procedure, a speculum is introduced to dilate the vagina and a special cervical catheter is introduced through the cervix of the uterus.
- Under carefully controlled conditions, the surgeon injects 10–20 ml of a water-soluble organic iodine compound (300 mg I/ml), without bubbles, into the uterine cavity so that spill into the peritoneal cavity can be seen. This should happen almost immediately with corresponding termination of the injection and withdrawal of the cervix adapter.
- The contrast is soon absorbed in the peritoneal cavity.
- Images of the contrast-filled uterus showing peritoneal spill are acquired using the machine's last-image-hold facility or a single exposure technique.

Note

During exposure, careful collimation of the X-ray beam is employed to reduce the doses to the patient and the surgeon.

13 Emergency peripheral vascular procedures

Emergency angiography is sometimes performed in the theatre environment as part of corrective surgery to vessels following major trauma or bypass grafting to assess the patency of vessels.

A mobile image intensifier with a C-arm and a theatre table with a radiolucent tabletop are usually selected for this procedure. The C-arm will provide the surgeon with a real-time image of the flow of contrast media through the vessels. The procedure is best undertaken with a relatively large image intensifier with a generator capable of rapid image acquisition, subtraction, road-mapping and last-image-hold facilities and with two television monitors, one giving real-time display of imaging and the other showing post-processed images of the vessels in normal or subtracted modes.

The patient is positioned supine during the operation. An arterial catheter will be inserted, usually by Seldinger technique as described in Whitley *et al.* (1999).

Imaging procedure

Mobile image intensifier

When a mobile image intensifier is employed, the intensifier is positioned to adopt a postero-anterior projection of the affected area. The image intensifier face is positioned as close as possible to the skin surface to reduce magnification. For the lower limb, for instance, the patient is positioned on the table before the operation to ensure that the intensifier will move into position without being obstructed by the table's main support pillar. The intensifier should be positioned with its wheels adjusted such that the intensifier can be moved, if necessary, along the length of the limb to follow the flow of contrast.

For subtraction angiography, the image intensifier is positioned over the region of interest, with the region screened to check for collimation of the X-ray beam. With the subtraction technique, selected fluorography is activated, following which up to 20 ml of a contrast agent (300 mg I/ml) is injected into the blood vessel (proximal to the affected site) and images are acquired as directed by the intensifier image acquisition software.

Continuous filling of the blood vessels with contrast agent is observed in the subtracted mode, showing the patency and any pathology of the affected vessel. An image acquisition rate of 1–2 frames/s (fps) is selected and run time is determined visually.

If necessary, a road-map technique may be performed, which facilities the accurate positioning of a catheter/guide wire under fluoroscopic control after first acquiring an image of the area of interest and then superimposing this image on the real-time fluoroscopic image.

Reference

Whitley AS, Alsop CW, Moore AD (1999). Hysterosalpingography. In: *Clark's Special Procedures in Diagnostic Imaging*. London: Butterworth-Heinemann, p. 238.

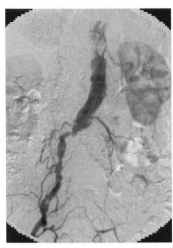

Angiogram of aorta showing complete occlusion of the left common iliac artery

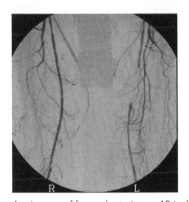

Angiogram of femoral arteries on 12-inch image intensifier, showing short segment occlusion of the left superficial femoral artery

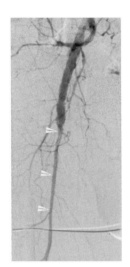

Localized angiogram of right common femoral artery showing flow into the profunda (deep) branch (arrowheads), and occlusion of the superficial femoral artery

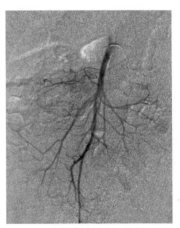

Selective catheterization of the mesenteric circulation looking for a source of intestinal haemorrhage. This examination is normal

CONTENTS

INTRODUCTION	382
General comments	382
Legislation	382
Justification	382
Optimization	382
THE PATIENT	383
Psychological considerations	383
Child development	384
Anatomical differences between children and adults	384
Approach to a paediatric patient	385
Pregnancy	386
Children with physical/learning disabilities	386
The environment: dedicated paediatric areas	386
IMAGING EQUIPMENT	387
IMAGE QUALITY, RADIATION PROTECTION MEASURES AND DOSIMETRY	389
COMMON PAEDIATRIC EXAMINATIONS	390
CHEST – NEONATAL	390
Antero-posterior – supine	390
CHEST – POST-NEONATAL	393
Postero-anterior – erect	394
Antero-posterior – erect	394
Postero-anterior/antero-posterior – erect	395
Antero-posterior – supine	396
Lateral	397
Cincinnati filter device	397
ABDOMEN	398
Antero-posterior	398
Modifications in technique	400
SKULL	402
Fronto-occipital	403

Fronto-occipital – 30 degrees caudad	404
Lateral – supine	405
SINUSES	406
Post-nasal space – lateral supine	406
DENTAL RADIOGRAPHY	407
PELVIS/HIPS	408
Antero-posterior	408
Antero-posterior– erect (weight-bearing)	409
Von Rosen projection	410
Lateral – both hips (frog projection)	410
SPINE – SCOLIOSIS	411
Postero-anterior – standing	412
Lateral	414
SPINE – CERVICAL, THORACIC AND LUMBAR	416
Cervical spine	416
Age under four years	416
LEG LENGTH ASSESSMENT	417
Single exposure method	418
Localized exposure method	419
Digital fluoroscopy method	419
ELBOW	420
Lateral (alternative positioning)	420
Antero-posterior (alternative positioning)	421
BONE AGE	423
FEET – SUPPORTED/WEIGHT-BEARING PROJECTIONS	424
Dorsi-plantar – weight-bearing	424
Lateral – weight bearing	425
SKELETAL SURVEY FOR NON-ACCIDENTAL INJURY	428
SKELETAL SURVEY FOR SYNDROME ASSESSMENT	431

14 Introduction

General comments

Achieving diagnostic quality radiographs whilst minimizing patient dose is the goal of any imaging department, and this is no more important than in paediatrics. Children are special cases, since they have a two to four times higher risk of late manifestations of the detrimental effects of radiation (UNSCEAR Report 2000).

Staff working with children need skill and experience in order to gain their patients' confidence and cooperation. A clear commitment to paediatrics is essential and a dedicated core group of staff responsible for children and for advising others is vital. In this way there can be an understanding of a child's needs, development, psychology and range of pathology.

Dedicated paediatric areas, rooms, equipment and staff all lead to a far higher likelihood of a high-quality examination, at an achievable low dose, without protracted investigation times and without causing undue stress to the child, parent or staff.

Legislation

An environment of quality and safety within diagnostic imaging departments has been progressively promoted and encouraged throughout the European Community over the last few years. The Commission of European Communities has provided support by establishing legal requirements for the radiation protection of the patient and it has been clearly recognized that particular emphasis must be placed on paediatrics. The key to the optimization of paediatric imaging is to produce a radiograph which is of sufficient quality for a radiological diagnosis, at the lowest achievable dose. The need for specific recommendations with regard to objectively defining quality led to the publication of *European Guidelines on Quality Criteria for Diagnostic Radiographic Images in Paediatrics* in 1996. The guidelines contain image quality criteria and entrance surface doses for a standard 5-year-old child, with examples of good technique which would allow these criteria to be met. The criteria given in this chapter are based on the recommendations of the European text but are separated into two categories so that problems due to technique can be differentiated from those arising from varying physical parameters (e.g. kVp, grid).

National Reference Doses are produced and published by the National Radiological Protection Board (NRPB). These are based on rounded 3rd quartile values of a national survey and are reviewed every five years (IPEM Report 2004). In children it is not possible to produce meaningful reference doses without considering their varying size. The NRPB have addressed this by providing normalization factors which can be applied to reference doses for five standard sizes (O, −1, −5, −10 and 15 years) (Hart *et al.* 2000).

The Ionising Radiations (Medical Exposure) Regulations (IRMER) 2000 require the establishment of local diagnostic reference levels derived from local dose audit in addition to National Reference Doses. The Ionising Radiation Regulations emphasize responsibilities for all professionals involved in the use of ionizing radiation and stress the importance of justification, optimization and protection, which should be considered before undertaking a radiographic examination.

Justification

The dose reduction measures achieved by improving radiographic practice are insignificant compared with the doses saved from not performing the examination at all.

Justification is the essential first step in radiation protection, and it is the duty of all radiographers and radiologists to ensure that every investigation performed is the correct examination and is essential in the management of the patient. The Royal College of Radiologists' (RCR 2003) handbook *Making the Best Use of a Department of Clinical Radiology* addresses the need for advice on justification and where at all possible recommendations are evidence based.

The RCR lists a simple series of questions that should always be answered before the investigation is undertaken:

- Is this investigation going to change the patient's management?
- Does the investigation need to be done now?
- Has the investigation been done already?
- Has the appropriate clinical information been given to justify the request?
- Are too many investigations being requested simultaneously?

The guidelines also give advice regarding appropriate imaging pathways in paediatrics.

Referral criteria for 17 common paediatric investigations have also been described by Cook *et al.* (1998). The criteria include not only when investigations should be performed but also, importantly, when investigations should not be performed and when a more senior clinical referral is required. For example, an abdominal radiograph in non-specific abdominal pain is unlikely to demonstrate pathology in the absence of loin pain, haematuria, diarrhoea, a palpable mass, abdominal distension or suspected inflammatory bowel disease; a follow-up chest X-ray (CXR) is not required routinely for follow-up of simple pneumonia in a clinically well child; and some radiographs should not be performed routinely before there has been development of certain normal structures, e.g. sinuses, nasal bones, scaphoids. Where formal referral criteria are not given, reference should be made to the manual of Cook *et al.* (1998) and the RCR (2003) guidelines, which can be adapted to conform with local protocols and requirements.

Optimization

Once it has been decided that an investigation needs performing, choice of the most appropriate technique is essential. In view of the plethora of imaging techniques now available, radiologists and radiographers are best placed to give clinicians advice.

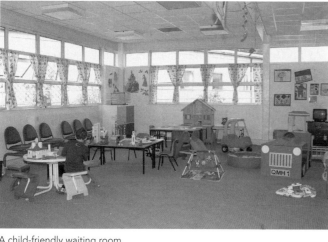

A child-friendly waiting room

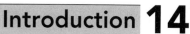

One simple form of immobilization is relatively non-sticky cellotape applied over the fingers

Optimization

However, due to the pressures on most departments, individual advice is not possible for every case, and agreed written guidelines between clinicians and X-ray staff should be compiled. Justification and optimization need good clinico-radiological cooperation.

Examples of optimization include the use of faster image acquisition systems such as screen/film systems for follow-up studies, using a lower kVp/higher mAs to optimize bony definition in non-accidental injury (NAI) CXR examination, and the use of additional lateral coning devices to protect the developing breast in follow-up studies of scoliosis in the adolescent female.

The patient

Psychological considerations

Children are not mini-adults. There are significant differences in the way children of various ages will react in X-ray departments. Young children are sometimes unable to fully comprehend explanations given and can misinterpret well-meaning intentions of staff. Children also do not have a clear perception of time, and to a child staying still for a few minutes can seem like hours. Ill children in particular can become disoriented and have even greater difficulty in cooperating; pain, fear and anxiety can all be exaggerated. Illness can also cause emotional withdrawal, leading to lack of interest and loss of confidence. A sympathetic, kindly approach here is essential.

Parents usually bring their children for investigations, but sometimes another member of the family or a care worker is in attendance and it is important to understand the relationship of the accompanying persons from the beginning.

Parental/carer participation is vital. Regardless of how empathic the staff are, children feel at their most comfortable with their parents and in surroundings that they might consider familiar. Parents can be encouraged to be as supportive as possible and to bring the child's favourite toy, special blanket or books. It is preferable for staff to initially direct all their explanations to the child with the parents listening in. Great care must be taken to talk slowly, clearly and in short, succinct sentences. Children and parents can misunderstand; for complex procedures, they are advised to visit the department beforehand. Written handouts are very helpful so that both the parents and the child can be as aware as possible of the nature of various procedures.

Sometimes parents are extremely distressed. It is essential to be calm and behave in a completely professional manner at all times. Escorting the parents and any disconcerted child to a private area is advisable so that other children and parents do not become upset. Sometimes a more senior member of the department or a radiologist may be needed to discuss any significant problems.

Child development

In the context of diagnostic imaging, childhood can be divided into six main age groups, each of which has different needs and capabilities:

- birth to six months;
- infancy (six months to three years);
- early childhood (three to six years);
- middle childhood (six to 12 years);
- early adolescence (12–15 years);
- late adolescence (15–19 years).

Each age group requires a different level of interaction, tolerance and understanding (Von Waldenburg Hilton and Edwards, 1994).

In the age group birth to six months, it is relatively easy to examine a child, as such children are not yet fearful of strangers. They sleep easily and can usually be quietened by a simple bottle-feed.

At six months to three years, children become increasingly fearful of strangers and cling to their parents. Communication with children of this age may be particularly difficult. Parents will usually have to maintain very close body contact with their child. The use of flashing or musical toys, blowing bubbles, simple rattles or bells may be useful in distracting children of this age. It may also be useful to allow some time for the child and their parents to become familiar with new surroundings before a procedure is undertaken.

At three to six years, communicating is easier but should be limited to simple, child-friendly terminology. Children of this age will often be more cooperative if there is an element of play involved, e.g. describing various pieces of equipment as space ships, seesaw rides, etc. They also have an awareness of modesty, and allowing them to leave on some of their normal clothes can be helpful. Projectors or videos showing exciting changing pictures on walls are also very useful. Children of this age are often extremely physically active and often do not respond well to attempts at physical restraint. If close parental involvement is not helpful, then swaddling young children in cotton blankets or towels can be useful for some examinations.

Children aged six to 12 years are of school age and have a growing capacity to understand what degree of cooperation is required of them and how the results of any tests will be helpful in treating their problems. An awareness of the most fashionable popular toys is very useful. It is also essential that any posters, books, games, etc. in the department are as up-to-date as possible to maintain credibility.

At 12–19 years, children become increasingly embarrassed and aware of their bodies and their development. It is essential at this age that communication and explanation should match their level of maturity. Their right to privacy must be respected at all times. This may include ensuring that there are areas of the department where confidentiality can be maintained, which may involve discussions without the parents being present if the adolescent so desires. If there is a male radiographer, it is advisable that a parent or carer accompanies a female child.

Anatomical differences between children and adults

Not only are children smaller, but their bodies are also different, e.g.:

- Young babies have thin skull vaults and vascular markings are not present before the age of one year.
- The nasal bones are not ossified before three years of age.
- Paranasal sinuses are not normally pneumatized until six years of age.
- The scaphoid bone is not ossified before six years of age.
- The smaller depth of the thorax (antero-posterior diameter) results in less enlargement of the heart, due to magnification, on antero-posterior projections of the chest compared with adults.
- The thymus contributes to the cardio-mediastinal shadow in young children and its variable presentations can mimic pathology.
- Multiple ossification centres at various sites can cause confusion, and reference texts (Keats and Anderson 2001) should always be available. This, in combination with high-quality images, will aid interpretation.
- Children have faster heart and respiratory rates than adults.
- More radiosensitive red bone marrow is more widespread in children and is present in almost all bones of a neonate.

These anatomical differences should be taken into account when optimizing techniques in paediatric radiography, e.g. it is obvious that specific scaphoid views are unnecessary in children under the age of six years.

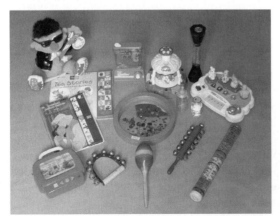

Examples of toys and accessories used to distract the child

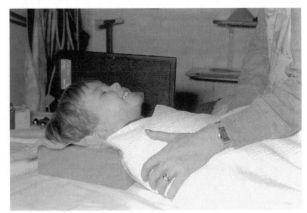

Child swaddled in cotton blanket with head resting on shaped foam pad for lateral skull examination using horizontal beam technique

Approach to a paediatric patient

One should always introduce oneself to a child and parent in a friendly and capable manner. The child's name, age and address should be verified. It is important to speak to the child at their level. A firm but kindly approach is required, and the child should be escorted into the already prepared imaging room. It is preferable for the X-ray tube to be in the correct position. Adjusting its height over the child can be disconcerting. Usually only one parent is asked to accompany the child into the room. This complies with radiation protection guidelines. However, both parents are sometimes required for holding.

A very encouraging, reassuring attitude has to be adopted, and an enormous amount of praise should be given for every single act of cooperation, e.g. 'You are the best child at keeping still we have had all day!' and 'You are so clever!'

Always be honest in answering any questions, as keeping one's credibility is essential in maintaining rapport with children. Allow the child to see the effect of switching on the light beam diaphragm or riding on a chair or table beforehand if necessary.

Rewards of stickers, balloons and bravery certificates are a must. If a child's first experience of an X-ray department is a pleasant one, then any future attendances will be far easier.

Given the right approach and surroundings, most children are cooperative. However, there are some who become physically aggressive and abusive, throwing temper tantrums at every suggestion. In these situations, it is better to get on with the procedure as quickly as possible; a firm approach and a range of simple, well-tried immobilization devices are recommended. Lots of cuddles with the parents/carer afterwards should soon calm the child.

Children attending as outpatients rarely need more preparation than the above for uncomplicated radiology. However, children over four years of age and having abdominal radiographs for suspected calculi/calcification or intravenous urography examination are given oral bowel preparation depending on bowel habits and age.

Children admitted as inpatients need more specific preparation, including liaising with the ward nursing staff and arranging a nurse escort where necessary. Planning of any radiograph should allow for the presence of any intravenous lines, drainage tubes, stomas, etc. It should be ascertained whether the patient will have adequate oxygen supply or intravenous fluid before arranging the examination.

If any patient has a contagious disease, then barrier methods of handling must be instituted. A decision should be made as to whether the patient should be brought to the department or whether the examination should be performed with mobile equipment. In addition, careful timing of the examination in order to avoid close proximity with other vulnerable patients is recommended (e.g. immunocompromised patients, neonates). Plastic aprons, gloves and careful hand-washing are required of all attendants. Masks or eyewear are necessary only if splattering of any body fluids is likely. All items contaminated by body fluids should be disposed of carefully according to local health and safety rules. All equipment that comes into contact with the child should be disinfected with the recommended cleaning agent for that equipment.

As in outpatients, other specific preparation for simple radiographs is rarely required. However, a prone invertogram (see page 401) for assessment of imperforate anus should not be performed in neonates less than 24 hours after birth, so as to allow more distal bowel to be delineated, and should be taken after the patient has been kept in the prone position for 15 minutes. In our experience, sedation has not been required for plain radiography. However, more lengthy procedures, which are beyond the scope of this book, may need sedation. Our preference is to use chloral hydrate (50 mg/kg for scanning procedures). Complex procedures may require a short general anaesthetic. It is essential that all those involved in the sedation of children are well trained and updated in resuscitative techniques.

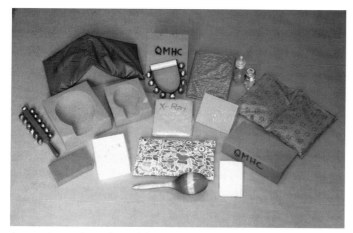

Accessories used to aid immobilization and distraction aids

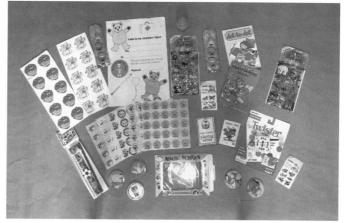

Certificates and rewards

14 The patient

Pregnancy

This can be a difficult issue, but the guidelines of the RCR (2003) state that the possibility of pregnancy should be broached in all female patients who have started menstruating (approximately over the age of 12 years). Discretion is essential, and honest answers are more likely to be given if the child is not with her parents. It is preferable for the child to be taken into the imaging room on her own and then asked tactfully whether she is menstruating and whether she might be pregnant. The choice of a female radiographer or radiologist may be more acceptable. As in adults, the '28-day' rule applies for examinations that directly include the abdomen or pelvis. The 'ten-day' rule applies for fluoroscopic examinations of the abdomen, abdominal computed tomography (CT) and intravenous urograms. A clear explanation of the risk of radiation to any unborn baby is necessary.

It is also important to ensure that all those assisting in restraining a patient are not pregnant.

Children with physical/learning disabilities

It is important to ascertain or make an assessment as to whether a child has a physical or learning disability. It is easy to assume that a physically disabled child also has learning disabilities; however, whatever the degree of disability, all children should be given the opportunity to be spoken to directly and to listen to explanations. The parents or carers of these children are almost always invaluable and completely dedicated to them. They are usually the best people for describing the optimum way to approach physical needs, such as lifting or transferring on to the X-ray table or introducing oral contrast. In some cases, it may be preferable to examine the child in their normal position, e.g. still in the wheelchair.

The environment: dedicated paediatric areas

Waiting area

The reception area is the child's and the parents' first contact with the X-ray department. It is essential that the staff and the environment put the child and parents at their ease as quickly as possible. Working with children requires a child-friendly approach from all individuals involved.

The waiting area should be as well-equipped as possible. It does not have to involve much expense, but toys and games aimed at all age groups should be available. Even more general departments could consider having video/computer games available in the paediatric area, even if this is shared with the paediatric outpatients.

More specialized departments may be able to employ a play therapist. This is particularly useful in gaining children's confidence for more complex procedures. Drawing and colouring activities are often appreciated, and children love donating their own compositions to the department's decor.

Imaging room

The room should already be prepared before the child enters. It is preferable to keep waiting times for examinations to a minimum, as this will significantly reduce anxiety. The room must be immediately appealing, with colourful decor, attractive posters and stickers applied to any equipment that may be disconcerting. Soft toys undergoing mock examinations are also helpful.

A fairly low ambient lighting is preferred, unless fluoroscopy equipment, for example, can be operated in normal daytime lighting. This avoids darkening the room later, which may frighten a child.

As mentioned already, time can appear to pass very slowly for some children. If they can be distracted with music (CD/tape) or moving images (projectors/video), they are far less likely to need physical restraint. Any devices, e.g. syringes, that may upset the child should be kept out of view until they are needed.

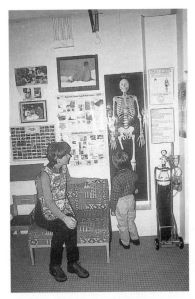

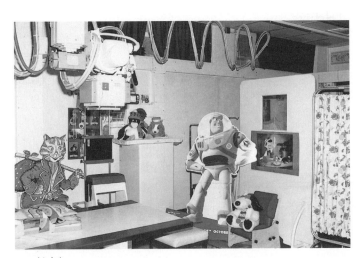

Examples of child-friendly waiting area with poster information (left) and imaging room (right)

X-ray generators

Children have faster heart/respiratory rates and they generally have difficulty in staying still. Very short exposure times are required, and a nearly rectangular voltage waveform and a minimal amount of ripple are desirable. Only 12-pulse or high-frequency multiples can provide this. Similarly, mobile equipment should have converter generators (European Commission 1996).

Timers should also be very accurate. Meticulous quality-control programmes should be in place to ensure that the chosen radiographic voltage matches the effective voltage. Inconsistencies can arise at short exposure settings (European Commission 1996). In order to keep exposure times to a minimum, the cable length between the transformer and the tube should be as short as possible, and all equipment being used for paediatrics should be able to accurately reproduce exposure times of <1 ms.

The radiation emitted takes some time to reach its peak voltage. This is not significant in the longer exposure of adults, but in children long pre-peak times may result in a lower effective voltage. Equipment should be used that has short pre-peak times, or the addition of added filtration should be considered to eliminate any unnecessary low-kVp radiation.

Selection of tube potential

Several publications have recommended selection of a high-kVp technique as a dose-saving measure (European Commission 1996, Warren-Forward and Millar 1995). For example, the EC Guidelines (European Commission 1996) recommend a minimum kVp of 60 kV for neonatal radiographs. Selection of kVp should be as high as possible consistent with desired image quality. This does result in less contrasted radiographs, and a radiological preference for these types of images should be developed.

Focal spot

A focal spot size of 0.6–1.3 mm is acceptable for paediatrics. A change in focal spot size does not affect the dose, but a smaller size improves the image quality at a cost of increased tube loading and possibly longer exposure times.

Additional filtration

Most X-ray tubes have an inherent filtration of 2.5 mm of aluminium. The EC Guidelines (European Commission 1996) recommend the additional use of 0.1 mm of copper or up to 3 mm of additional aluminium, and several authors have demonstrated the dose-saving advantage of additional copper filtration whilst maintaining diagnostic quality (Hansson et al. 1997). Additional filtration further removes the soft part of the radiation spectrum, which is completely absorbed by the patient, uselessly increasing the dose but not contributing to the production of the radiographic image. In our experience, 0.1 mm of additional copper with an initial inherent filtration of 2.5 mm aluminium leads to an entrance dose reduction of 20% with no significant loss of quality in the majority of examinations.

A reduction in image quality has only been noticed in low-kVp techniques of small children's peripheries (e.g. for NAI and on special-care baby units (SCBU)). In order to take this into account, easily removable added filtration may be advisable so that it can be removed when appropriate. In order to avoid confusion of exposure factors, some equipment may be left without added filtration should more than one piece of equipment be available.

It is generally not recommended to have additional filtration on mobile equipment for SCBU, if possible, due to the noticeable reduction in quality (Cook et al. 1998, Wraith et al. 1995).

Anti-scatter grid

An anti-scatter grid is not always required in children. An anti-scatter grid results in an increase in dose of approximately 100%, and its use should always be justified by the need for an increase in image quality. Skull radiographs under one year of age, and pelvis, abdominal and spine radiographs under the age of three years, do not routinely require the use of an anti-scatter grid and can also be avoided in older children of small size. The experience of the radiographer is essential here. If a grid is to be used, then a grid ratio of 8:1 and a line number of 40/cm are recommended. The grid should contain low-attenuation materials such as carbon fibre, and the correct focus-to-film distance (FFD) for a focused grid should be used.

Focus-to-film distance

Increasing the FFD necessitates an increase in exposure factors, but the overall effective dose to the patient is reduced and the blurring due to magnification effect is also reduced. A maximum FFD should be used, a minimum of 100 cm for over-couch tubes, and a minimum of 150 cm for vertical stands in chest and spinal radiography. If designing new departments, consideration should be given to allow for long FFDs (e.g. over 200 cm), which can be particularly useful for erect spinal projections for scoliosis assessment using an air gap technique (Andersen et al. 1982, Jonsson et al. 1995, Kottamasu and Kuhns 1997, McDaniel et al. 1984).

Automatic exposure control

Very few automatic exposure chambers have been made specifically for children, and therefore they are not always able to compensate fully for the wide range of body sizes in children. Usually, use of automatic exposure control (AEC) devices results in higher doses in paediatric practice, and well-tried and structured exposure charts are more likely to produce higher-quality images at lower doses.

Exposure charts are normally based on children's ages, although size is more accurate and this means that radiographic experience and training is vital in selecting appropriate exposure factors.

AEC chambers are also usually built behind the grid. Therefore, an examination using an AEC in these conditions also necessitates using the grid.

Intensifying screen/film systems

High-speed image acquisition systems such as screen/film systems, high-kVp techniques and the deselection of a grid have been found to be the most important methods of reducing dose in radiographic practice.

In our opinion, high-resolution, 200-speed screen/film systems should be limited to peripheries. Most examinations can be performed with rare earth or equivalent screens, i.e. speed classes of 400–600. Many follow-up examinations and radiographs for swallowed foreign bodies can be performed with very fast screen/film systems (700–800).

It should be recognized that various manufacturers do not have the same effective speed of screen/film system for the same numerical description, and the speed of the system can also vary with the kVp. Thus, optimum kVp for the system chosen should be used.

Film processing and viewing conditions

As in adults, the gains obtained in perfecting radiographic practice are lost if simple measures are not taken to ensure that both film processing and lighting conditions for viewing radiographs are not optimized fully.

Film processing should be the subject of daily quality assurance assessment. The brightness of a film viewing box should be 2000–4000 cd/m for radiographs in the density range of 0.5–2.2. A low level of ambient light in the viewing room is essential, as described in the EEC guidelines (European Commission 1996).

Digital radiography

A new digital age is fast replacing conventional techniques in radiography. It has been shown that there are distinct advantages with dose savings of up to 60% when comparing a 1000-speed computed radiography (CR) system with the commonly used 400-speed systems used in most departments (Hufton *et al.* 1998). However, post-processing can mask high-dose techniques, and careful optimization and regulation of digital equipment are essential.

Accessories, including immobilization devices

The hallmark of successful paediatric imaging is by the use of accessories, which in the main are simple and inexpensive. Most important is to have an adequate range to comply with the needs of a wide range of body sizes. The various accessories are described in the following text according to the anatomical area and corresponding radiographic technique.

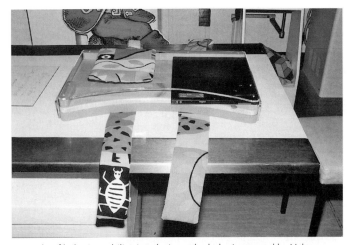

Example of baby immobilization device – the baby is secured by Velcro strapping with the cassette inserted under a Perspex sheet

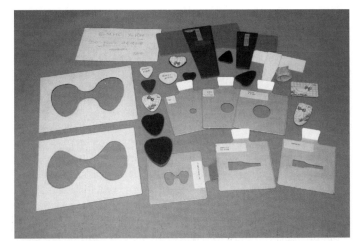

Examples of paediatric gonad and coning devices. The latter can all be placed above the diamentor chamber

Essential image characteristics

The essential image characteristics that should be demonstrated in any of the projections described in this chapter are found by reference to the CEC publication (European Commission 1996). This publication provides guidance on technique, representative exposure factors and corresponding patient doses by age. Visibility of a structure is described in three grades, as follows:

Visualization	Characteristic features are detectable but only just visible
Reproduction	Anatomical details are visible but not defined clearly
Visually sharp reproduction	Anatomical details are defined clearly

Image quality assessment

'Unharmonized, and in many places unoptimized, examination techniques' have been shown to produce a great variation in the absorbed dose to children examined (Almen *et al.* 1996), and many dose surveys have demonstrated wide dose ranges (Kyriou *et al.* 1996, Lowe *et al.* 1999, Ruiz *et al.* 1991).

As described above, image quality criteria for paediatrics have been introduced by the CEC to address this situation (European Commission 1996). These image criteria are an attempt to objectively assess a radiograph and determine diagnostic quality.

However, it is stated clearly in the guidelines that 'under no circumstances should an image which fulfils all clinical requirements but does not meet all image criteria ever be rejected'. This is an important point, as although one should always strive for excellence, the aim is always for a diagnostic image that answers the clinical question. Unnecessarily high quality that results in higher doses should be avoided.

The quality criteria consist of those that depend on correct positioning of the patient and those that depend on the physical parameters that reflect the technical performance of the imaging system.

There is still a subjective element to the criteria. However, several authors have explored the value of the CEC criteria and have found that they allowed a reduction in effective dose by up to 50% without a significant reduction in diagnostic image quality (Cook *et al.* 1998, McParland *et al.* 1996, Mooney and Thomas 1998, Vano *et al.* 1995).

Dose is influenced most by a choice of physical parameters, such as kVp, speed of screen/film system and use of a grid. However, image quality is far more dependent on radiographic technique.

Departments should use all the appropriate dose-saving measures whilst ensuring that high standards of professional training and expertise are maintained. It is recommended that there should be at least one experienced radiographer with additional specialized paediatric training in each department.

Coning devices and gonad protection

Careful coning is an important tool in dose reduction and also improves image quality; primary and scattered radiation are also reduced. All radiographs should show all four diaphragm edges or circular cones, and the coning should be limited strictly to the region of interest. It is important when using additional devices that the light beam diaphragm is coned initially, before inserting the additional device. The latter alone is not sufficient protection if the primary cones are left widely open. Shaped additional coning such as window protection for hips can be used for either male or female patients, being inverted for the latter.

A wide range of gonad protection is required in various sizes and shapes. Gonad protection should be applied even in the erect position. It can be secured in position with sticky tape.

Lead protection on the patient next to the primary beam, if used correctly, is important in reducing exposure to tube-scattered radiation. However, current X-ray equipment allows very precise collimation of the X-ray beam resulting in very little tube scatter. Therefore, in examinations such as erect chest radiographs, it is considered to be more important to ensure good collimation and to produce a diagnostic quality radiograph at the first attempt. If a lead apron or mobile lead screen is used, it should not obscure essential anatomical detail and should not be in the primary beam.

Dose measurement

All radiographic equipment, including mobile and fluoroscopy equipment, should have dose area product (DAP) meters in place. These have been shown to provide a sensitive and simple method of monitoring and recording doses in paediatric radiography (McDonald *et al.* 1996). They need to be of a high specification for children, otherwise the dose readings will not be accurate. Careful monitoring and recording of these DAP meter readings is essential in providing feedback to staff. In due course, a record of accumulative dose in children will become a legal requirement.

Balancing dose and image quality

An attempt should always be made to obtain the best-quality radiograph at the first attempt. Careful preparation is the key. Radiographs should be repeated only at a radiologist's request or if they are undiagnostic. A different approach could be requested, e.g. supine antero-posterior instead of erect CXR. With conventional radiography, copying over exposed images to make them lighter can be performed in some indications without significant loss of quality and should be considered. However, the aim is to obtain radiographs with the correct exposure at the first attempt.

Comparison should be made with available diagnostic reference levels. However, the National Reference Doses (Institute of Physics and Engineering in Medicine 2004) are those above which corrective action should be taken and may be considered high. In addition to the National Reference Doses, therefore, local diagnostic reference levels should be derived from local dose audit.

Lower doses, whilst maintaining diagnostic images, can be achieved with digital radiography in some departments. The aim is to obtain a diagnostic image at the lowest achievable dose.

14 COMMON PAEDIATRIC EXAMINATIONS

A range of common paediatric X-ray examinations are described, which differ in approach and technique to those performed on adults:

- chest – neonatal;
- chest – post-neonatal;
- skull;
- sinuses and post-nasal space (PNS);
- dental;
- abdomen;
- pelvis and hips;
- spine for scoliosis;
- spine;
- leg length assessment;
- elbow;
- bone age, hand and knees;
- feet for talipes assessment;
- skeletal survey for non-accidental injury;
- skeletal survey for syndrome assessment.

Chest – neonatal

Chest radiographs are the most common requests on the SCBU/NNU, with the infant nursed in a special incubator.

All requests should be strictly justified. Image acquisition just before insertion of lines or catheters should be avoided when a post-line insertion film is adequate. Good-quality technique is essential. The range of diagnoses possible in neonatal chest radiography is fairly limited, and differing pathologies can look similar. Correlation with good clinical information is essential. Study of a sequence of films over a period may be necessary for correct interpretation, and therefore accurate recording and reproduction of the most appropriate radiographic exposure are essential for comparisons to be made.

Referral criteria

- respiratory difficulty;
- infection;
- meconium aspiration;
- chronic lung disease;
- pleural effusion/pneumothorax;
- position of catheters/tubes;
- heart murmur/cyanosis;
- oesophageal atresia;
- previous antenatal ultrasound abnormality suspected;
- thoracic cage anomaly;
- as part of a skeletal survey for syndrome/NAI;
- postoperative.

A request for chest and abdomen on one radiograph, with centring to the chest, is sometimes indicated in the following cases:

- localization of tubes or catheters;
- suspected diaphragmatic hernia;
- suspected abdominal pathology causing respiratory difficulty.

Recommended projections

Examination is performed by means of the following projections:

Basic	Antero-posterior – supine
Alternative	Postero-anterior – prone
Supplementary	Lateral

Antero-posterior – supine

An 18 × 24-cm cassette that is at body temperature is selected. Disposable sheets should be used between the baby and the cassette. Modern incubators with cassette trays can be used to avoid disturbance of a very sick baby (see below).

Position of patient and cassette

Sleeping baby

- The baby is positioned supine on the cassette, with the median sagittal plane adjusted perpendicular to the middle of the cassette, ensuring that the head and chest are straight and shoulders and hips are level.
- The head may need a covered sandbag support on either side. A 10-degree foam pad should be placed under the shoulders to avoid a lordotic projection and to lift the chin and prevent it obscuring the lung apices.
- Arms should be on either side, separated slightly from the trunk to avoid being included in the radiation field and to avoid skin crease artefacts, which can mimic pneumothoraces.
- Arms can be immobilized with Velcro bands and/or sandbags.

Baby requiring holding

Positioning is similar to that described for the sleeping baby and can be performed by a single assistant with the following adaptations:

- The arms should be held flexed on either side of the head.
- Arms should not be extended fully, as this can cause lordotic images.
- When needed, legs should be held together and flexed at the knees.

Direction and centring of the X-ray beam

- No single centring point is advised.
- Centre the beam to the midline of the cassette.
- The central ray is directed vertically, or angled five to 10 degrees caudally if the baby is completely flat, to avoid projecting the chin over the lung apices.
- Constant maximum FFD should be used.
- Although some incubators have cassette trays, placing the cassette under the baby is recommended as routine, to avoid magnification and change of exposure factors.

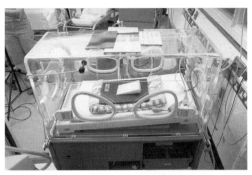

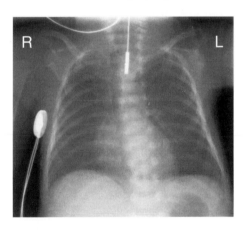

Accessories and position of neonate for antero-posterior chest X-ray taken in an incubator. Note the positioning of the lead coning devices on the top of the incubator and the wedge sponge to avoid a lordotic projection

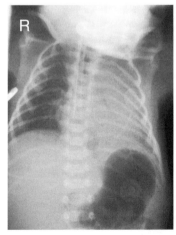

Image of correctly positioned normal neonatal chest radiograph demonstrating high position of pH probe in the upper oesophagus (top) and poorly positioned neonatal antero-posterior chest radiograph (bottom) with chin projected over upper mediastinum, patient rotated to the left with heart obscuring the left thorax and ET tube in the oesophagus

Antero-posterior – supine

Essential image characteristics

- Peak inspiration to include eight to nine posterior ribs (four to five anterior ribs).
- No rotation. Medial ends of the clavicles should overlap the transverse processes of the spine symmetrically, or anterior rib ends should be equidistant from the spine.
- No tilting or lordosis. Medial ends of the clavicles should overlie the lung apices.
- Superior/inferior coning should be from cervical trachea to T12/L1, including the diaphragms.
- Lateral coning should include both shoulders and ribs but not beyond the proximal third of the humeri.
- Reproduction of the vascular pattern in the central two-thirds of the lungs.
- Reproduction of the trachea and major bronchi.
- Visually sharp reproduction of the diaphragm and costophrenic angles.
- Reproduction of the spine and paraspinal structures.
- Visualization of retrocardiac lung and mediastinum.
- Visually sharp reproduction of the skeleton.

Common faults and remedies

- Classically, the port hole of the incubator must not overlie the chest.
- All extraneous tubes and wires should be repositioned away from the chest area.
- Exposure should be made in inspiration. Watching for full distension of the baby's abdomen rather than the chest best assesses this. Expiratory images mimic parenchymal lung disease.
- Arms should not be extended fully above the head, as this will lead to a lordotic position.
- Lordotic images show anterior rib ends pointing upwards, and the lung bases are obscured by the diaphragm.
- The head must be supported to avoid the chin lolling forward and obscuring the upper chest.
- Minimal exposures of less than 0.02 seconds should be used to avoid motion artefact.
- Rotated images should be avoided, as this can cause misinterpretation of mediastinal shift and lung translucency. The separate ossification centres of the sternum, projected over the lungs can also cause confusion.
- As in all radiographs, but particularly in neonatal work, where the name label is large compared with the size of the image, the label should not obscure any of the anatomical detail.
- Taking a radiograph when a baby is crying should be avoided, as this can cause overexpansion of the lungs, which may mimic pathology.
- Overexposure of neonatal chest radiographs results in loss of lung detail.

Antero-posterior – supine (*contd*)

Radiological considerations

- If the baby is intubated, great care must be taken not to dislodge the endotracheal tube. Even small movements of the head can result in significant movement of the tip. This should lie in the lower third of the trachea, approximately between T1 and the carina.
- An umbilical arterial catheter (UAC) follows the umbilical artery down inferiorly to either internal iliac artery and then via the iliacs to the aorta. This catheter is usually finer and more radio-opaque than an umbilical venous catheter (UVC). The former should ideally be placed with its tip in the mid-thoracic aorta between T4 and T9, which avoids the risk of causing thrombosis if the tip is opposite the origins of any of the abdominal vessels. Some UACs can be left with their tips in the lower abdominal aorta if there has been difficulty with advancing them. The UVC passes directly upwards through the ductus venosus in the liver and should lie with its tip in the IVC or right atrium. If lines are only faintly radio-opaque, then 0.5 ml of non-ionic intravenous contrast (iodine 200 mg/ml) can be used for opacification.

Notes

- Minimal handling and the avoidance of heat loss from any incubator are essential. Babies are very vulnerable to infection, and therefore strict hygiene rules and hand-washing are paramount.
- All the cassettes and foam pads inserted into an incubator should be washable.
- Experienced nursing help in immobilization techniques is invaluable.
- All preparation of the X-ray equipment should be performed before placing the X-ray cassette under the baby.

Radiation protection

- Accurate collimation of the X-ray beam using light beam diaphragm with additional lead masking within the primary field balanced on top of incubator.
- It is the radiographer's responsibility to ensure that the holder's hands are not in the direct beam.
- The abdomen should be included on a chest radiograph only if assessment of catheters or relevant pathology is present. In this case, male gonads should be protected.
- All mobile equipment on SCBU should have short-exposure capability to allow kVp selection of over 60 kV as a dose-reduction measure. If this is not possible, then additional filtration can be considered, but this can affect the quality of the image.
- An accurate exposure chart according to infant weight should be available.
- All mobile equipment should have a dose area product meter.

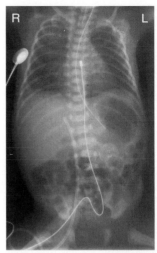

Image of chest and abdominal radiograph post insertion of UAC and UVC

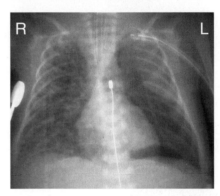

Image of antero-posterior chest in a neonate with pulmonary interstitial emphysema of the right lung and a chest drain draining a left pneumothorax

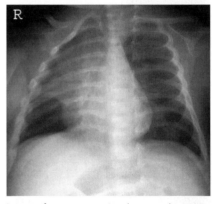

Image of antero-posterior chest poorly positioned due to the neonate being rotated; the normal right lobe of thymus obscures the right upper lobe

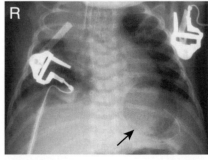

Image antero-posterior chest with shadow of incubator port hole overlying the left diaphragm, ECG clips obscuring right hemithorax and right upper lobe consolidation

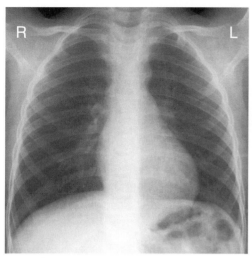

Image of antero-posterior erect normal chest

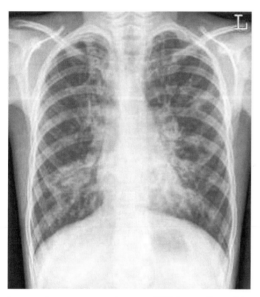

Image of a postero-anterior erect CXR in a patient with cystic fibrosis

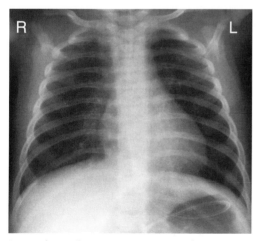

Image of normal antero-posterior supine chest

Recommended projections

Examination is performed by means of the following projections:

Basic	Postero-anterior – erect
Alternative	Antero-posterior – erect
	Antero-posterior – supine
Supplementary	Lateral
	Antero-posterior with Cincinnati filter

There is some controversy as to whether chest radiographs of children beyond the neonatal period should be taken supine or erect and postero-anterior or antero-posterior.

It is recommended that a postero-anterior erect projection should be adopted when a child can stand or when age allows. This results in a lower breast dose. An erect projection also allows better expansion of the lungs and demonstration of pleural effusions and pneumothoraces. However, if this is not possible, then supine projections are taken. For all projections, it is important that the child should be straight, with no rotation.

Specific technique depends on the clinical referral, as follows.

Congenital heart disease

The dimensions of the small paediatric chest are such that the choice of postero-anterior/antero-posterior projection does not have such an influence on the impression of cardiac size, unlike in adults. However, in some cases of known congenital heart disease, it may be advisable to use the same projection for initial follow-up studies (Hochschild and Cremin 1975).

Inhaled foreign body

A high index of suspicion is required.

Use of fluoroscopy or an antero-posterior image of the chest using a Cincinnati filter should be performed where possible to demonstrate the trachea and mediastinum and any mediastinal shift. Otherwise, antero-posterior projections in inspiration and expiration, or, if under two years of age, horizontal beam radiography with the patient in each lateral decubitus position, may be performed to demonstrate air trapping in the obstructed dependent lung. All images should include the pharynx, trachea, major bronchi and lungs and should be as straight as possible to allow assessment of mediastinal shift.

Oesophageal pH probe for reflux study

A postero-anterior/antero-posterior rather than a lateral projection is preferred as it gives a lower dose. It should be coned in laterally to the mediastinum, and the tip of the probe should be at T7/T8. (See image on p. 395.)

Radiation protection

- Very accurate collimation using light beam diaphragm. The four edges of the cones should be visible on the radiograph. The X-ray beam should not be coned to the cassette edges.
- Adequate immobilization essential.
- Postero-anterior projection to reduce breast dose.
- Holder should wear a lead-rubber apron and stand to the side.

Postero-anterior – erect

The key to erect chest radiography is a specifically designed paediatric chest stand. The cassette holder should be in such a position that a parent or carer is able to hold the child easily. A cassette is selected relative to the size of the child.

Position of patient and cassette

- Depending on the child's age, the child is seated or stood facing the cassette, with the chest pressed against it.
- The arms should be raised gently, bringing the elbows forward. The arms should not be extended fully.
- The parent or carer should hold the flexed elbows and head together and pull the arms gently upwards and slightly forward to prevent the child from slumping backwards.

Direction and centring of the X-ray beam

- The horizontal central beam is directed at right-angles to the midline of the cassette at the level of the eighth thoracic vertebra (spinous process of T7).

Antero-posterior – erect

This is done when the postero-anterior projection is not possible.

Position of patient and cassette

- The child is seated with their back against the cassette, which is supported vertically, with the upper edge of the cassette above the lung apices.
- The arms should be raised gently, bringing the elbows forward. The arms should not be extended fully.
- The parent or carer should hold the flexed elbows and head together with their fingers on the forehead, to prevent the child's chin from obscuring the upper chest.
- The holder should pull gently upwards to prevent the child from slumping forward.
- Place a 15-degree foam wedge behind the shoulders to prevent the child from adopting a lordotic position.

Direction and centring of the X-ray beam

- The horizontal central beam is angled five to ten degrees caudally to the middle of the cassette at the level of the eighth thoracic vertebra, approximately at the midpoint of the body of the sternum. This is particularly important in children with hyperinflated chests due to diseases such as bronchiolitis, which predisposes to lordotic projections.
- The radiation field is collimated to the cassette, thus avoiding exposure of the eyes, thyroid and upper abdomen.

Notes

- A comfortable seat, with Velcro straps encased in foam that can be applied over the thighs, is extremely useful.
- Mobile lead shielding (see p. 389).

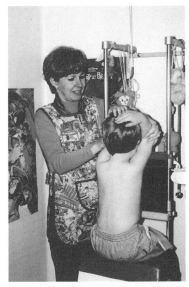

Position of child for postero-anterior erect chest radiograph

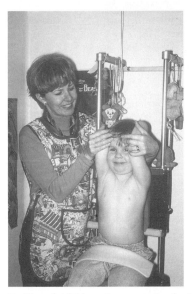

Position of child for antero-posterior chest radiograph

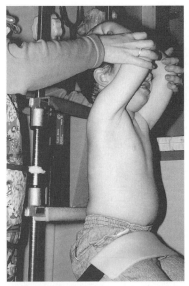

Position of child for antero-posterior chest radiograph seen from the side. Note wedge-shaped sponge to prevent lordotic projection

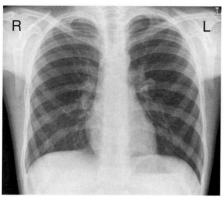

Image of normal postero-anterior erect chest

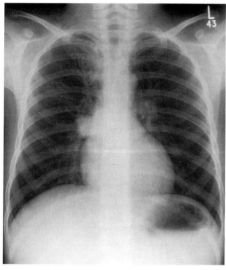

Image of postero-anterior erect chest showing dense right hilum and RUL bronchiectasis in a patient with TB

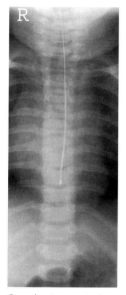

Coned antero-posterior supine chest X-ray to show the position of pH probe which should be at the level of T7/T8

Postero-anterior/ antero-posterior – erect

- Correct interpretation of paediatric chest radiographs requires images taken in maximum inspiration without rotation or tilting. The radiographer should watch the child's chest/ abdominal movements to obtain a maximum inspiration.

Common faults and remedies

- Incorrect density – needs radiographer experience in assessing the size of the child and careful exposure charts.
- Thorax tilted backwards (antero-posterior projection), with clavicles shown high above the lung apices. This lordotic projection results in the lower lobes of the lungs being obscured by the diaphragms. Pneumonia and other lung pathology can be missed. See Position of patient and cassette for how to correct this fault.
- Holder's hands on the shoulders – avoid by following the technique as described.
- Wide cones including arms, skull and abdomen on the radiograph should be avoided.

Essential image characteristics

Antero-posterior/postero-anterior projection:

- Peak inspiration (six anterior ribs (postero-anterior, 5/6 for antero-posterior) and nine posterior ribs above the diaphragm).
- Whole chest from just above the lung apices to include the diaphragms and ribs.
- No rotation (medial ends of clavicles or first ribs should be equidistant from the spine).
- No tilting (clavicles should overlie lung apices). Anterior ribs should point downwards.
- Reproduction of vascular pattern in central two-thirds of the lungs.
- Reproduction of the trachea and proximal bronchi.
- Visually sharp reproduction of the diaphragm and costophrenic angles.
- Reproduction of the spine and paraspinal structures and visualization of the retrocardiac lung and mediastinum.

Radiological considerations

- Chest radiographs are not required routinely for simple chest infections, and follow-up chest images are not required routinely if there has been a good response to treatment, unless the initial chest image showed lobar pneumonia, extensive sublobar pneumonia involving several segments, pneumatocoeles, adenopathy or pleural effusion.
- Follow-up radiographs, where indicated, should not be taken in less than three weeks, as radiological resolution lags behind clinical resolution. Repeat images are required earlier if there is any deterioration. Prompt follow-up chest radiography is required following physiotherapy and antibiotics for areas of collapse.

Antero-posterior – supine

The antero-posterior (supine) projection is performed as an alternative to the erect position when the latter is not possible.

Special attention is required when imaging a baby's chest. With the chest being conical in shape, positioning a baby supine with the back against a cassette results in a lordotic projection, with the clavicles projected above the apices and a large part of the lower lobes superimposed on the abdomen. The heart also appears foreshortened. In a correct projection, the anterior rib ends will be projected inferiorly to the posterior rib ends, and the clavicles will be seen superimposed on the lung apices. This can be accomplished either by leaning the baby forward or by angling the X-ray tube caudally, or both.

The projection is often performed as part of a mobile X-ray examination on children of all ages.

A cassette size is selected depending on the size of the child.

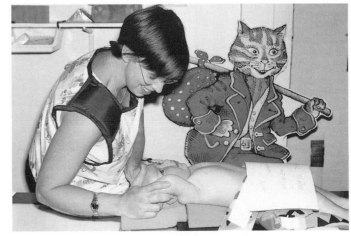

Patient positioned for antero-posterior supine chest

Position of patient and cassette

- The child is positioned supine on the cassette, with the upper edge positioned above the lung apices.
- When examining a baby, a 15-degree foam pad is positioned between the thorax and the cassette (thick end under the upper thorax) to avoid a lordotic projection. A small foam pad is also placed under the child's head for comfort.
- The median sagittal plane is adjusted at right-angles to the middle of the cassette. To avoid rotation, the head, chest and pelvis are straight.
- The child's arms are held, with the elbows flexed, on each side of the head.
- A suitable appliance, e.g. Bucky band or Velcro band, is secured over the baby's abdomen and sandbags are placed next to the thighs to prevent rotation.

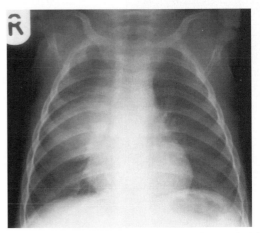

Image of antero-posterior supine chest with large right lobe of thymus

Direction and centring of the X-ray beam

- The vertical central beam is directed at right-angles to the middle of the cassette at the level of T8 (mid-sternum).
- For babies with a very hyperinflated barrel chest (due to bronchiolitis or asthma), the tube is also angled five to 10 degrees caudally to avoid a lordotic projection.

Notes

- Care should be taken not to have the lung apices being obscured by the chin.
- Lead-rubber coverage of the abdomen in immediate proximity to beam is recommended.

Common faults and remedies

- Tilted, with clavicles high above the lung apices. This lordotic projection results in the lower lobes of the lungs being obscured by the diaphragms. Pneumonia and other lung pathology can

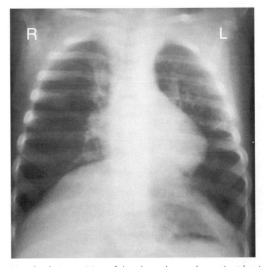

Very lordotic position of the chest due to the patient having marked hyperinflation as a result of bronchiolitis. Clavicles are well above the lung apices. Diaphragms could obscure a basal pneumonia. Note that in the correctly exposed radiograph, the lungs are fully demonstrated with the anterior rib ends inferior to the posterior ends. In the incorrectly positioned radiograph with excessive lordosis of the chest, the rib ends appear to be on the same level or can be above the posterior ribs

be missed. See Position of patient and cassette for how to correct this fault.

Lateral

This supplementary projection is undertaken to locate the position of an inhaled or swallowed foreign body, to evaluate middle lobe pathology or to localize opacities demonstrated on the postero-anterior/antero-posterior projection. A 24 × 30-cm cassette is selected.

Position of patient and cassette

- The patient is turned to bring the side under investigation towards the cassette. The median sagittal plane is adjusted parallel to the cassette.
- The outstretched arms are raised above the head and supported.
- The mid-axillary line is coincident with the middle of the cassette, and the cassette is adjusted to include the apices and the inferior lobes.

Direction and centring of the X-ray beam

- Direct the vertical central ray at right-angles to the middle of the cassette in the mid-axillary line.
- Exposure is made on peak inspiration.

Essential image characteristics

- Peak inspiration (six anterior ribs above the diaphragm).
- Whole chest from C7 to L1.
- Sternum and spine to be included and to be true lateral.
- Visualization of whole trachea and major bronchi.
- Visually sharp reproduction of the whole of both domes of the diaphragm.
- Reproduction of the hilar vessels.
- Reproduction of the sternum and the thoracic spine.

Cincinnati filter device

The use of this filter device is employed in cases of suspected inhaled foreign body when an antero-posterior image of the chest is acquired with the child lying supine.

The Cincinnati filter is composed of 2 mm of aluminium, 0.5 mm of copper and 0.4 mm of tin inserted into the collimator box so that the copper layer is towards the -X-ray tube. Exposures used are in the range of 125–140 kVp and 10–16 mAs, using a cassette and grid system.

On the exposed radiograph, bone detail is effaced to a considerable degree, allowing soft tissue and air interfaces in the mediastinum and adjacent lung to be seen. The trachea and proximal bronchial anatomy are demonstrated well.

A CT scout scanogram can be considered as an alternative.

Careful handling is always advisable in children suspected to have an inhaled foreign body, as dislodgement can result in total airway obstruction.

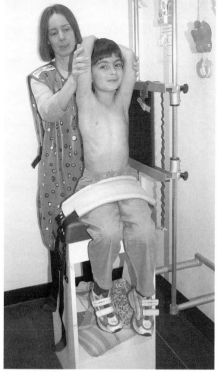

Child position for lateral projection of the chest

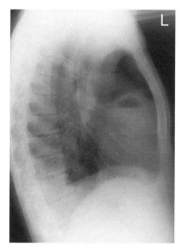

Lateral chest radiograph showing a pulmonary abscess and fluid level

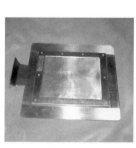

Cincinnati filter device

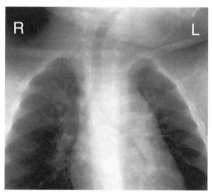

Coned image of antero-posterior chest with Cincinnati filter to show the trachea and proximal bronchi

14 Abdomen

Abdominal radiography of the acute abdomen in children is normally performed in conjunction with abdominal ultrasound. It is not routine in cases of non-specific abdominal pain, as a radiographic abnormality is unlikely to be demonstrated in the absence of any one of the following: loin pain, haematuria, diarrhoea, palpable mass, abdominal distension, or suspected inflammatory bowel disease.

Referral criteria will include suspected intussusception, chronic constipation (suspected Hirschprung's disease), possible swallowed foreign body, and suspected necrotizing enterocolitis. More specific referral criteria of abdominal radiographs are given by Cook *et al.* (1998).

Modification to the standard technique is described on pp. 400–401.

Recommended projections

Examination is performed by means of the following:

Basic	Antero-superior – supine
Alternative	Postero-anterior – prone
Supplementary	Lateral
	Postero-anterior – left lateral decubitus
	Antero-posterior – erect

Antero-posterior

Position of patient and cassette

- The child lies supine on the X-ray table or, in the case of a neonate, in the incubator, with the median sagittal plane of the trunk at right-angles to the middle of the cassette.
- To ensure that the child is not rotated, the anterior superior iliac spines should be equidistant from the cassette.
- The cassette should be large enough to include the symphysis pubis and the diaphragm.

Direction and centring of the X-ray beam

- The vertical central ray is directed to the centre of the cassette.

Notes

- All acute abdominal radiographs should include the diaphragms and lung bases. Lower-lobe pneumonia can often masquerade as acute abdominal pain.
- Radiographs for the renal tract can have more lateral coning, and a fizzy drink may be used to distend the stomach with air, thus displacing residue in the transverse colon and better demonstrating the renal areas.
- Collimation is as for adults, but babies' and infants' abdomens tend to be rounder; therefore, slightly wider lateral cones are required.

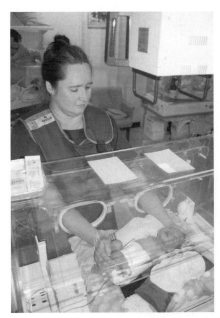

Baby positioned in an incubator for antero-posterior abdomen

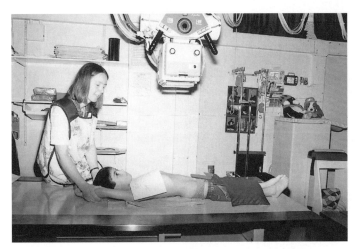

Older child positioned on imaging table for antero-posterior abdomen

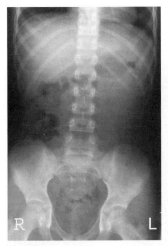

Image of normal antero-posterior abdomen in older child. Note inclusion of diaphragms

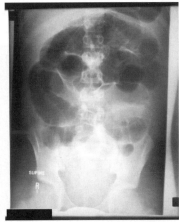

Image of antero-posterior abdomen of an older child with small bowel obstruction. Note use of male gonad protection

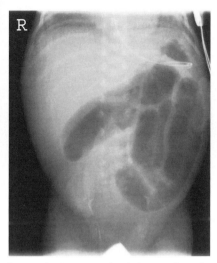

Image of antero-posterior abdomen of a male neonate showing intestinal obstruction due to small bowel atresia

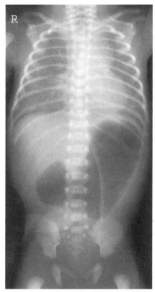

Image of antero-posterior chest and abdomen in a female neonate with duodenal atresia

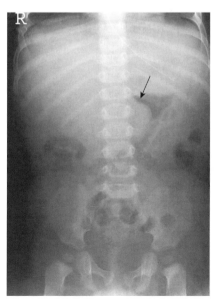

Image of an antero-posterior abdomen of a female infant with an intussusception in the transverse colon (arrow)

Essential image characteristics

Antero-posterior projection for whole abdomen:

- Abdomen to include diaphragm, lateral abdominal walls and ischial tuberosities.
- Pelvis and spine should be straight, with no rotation.
- Reproduction of properitoneal fat lines consistent with age.
- Visualization of kidney and psoas outlines consistent with age and bowel content.
- Visually sharp reproduction of the bones.

Common faults and remedies

- Usually inadequate coning but occasionally too tight coning excludes the diaphragm.
- Male gonads not protected.
- Careful technique is needed to address these problems.

Radiation protection

- Optimization of abdominal radiographs includes using a lower-dose technique, e.g. no grid and a very fast image acquisition system, in the assessment of examinations such as chronic constipation and swallowed foreign body is recommended. Serial images in the latter are not necessary.
- All boys should have testicular protection.
- Radiographs of the renal tract can be more collimated laterally (Cook *et al.* 1998).
- Although it has been demonstrated that a postero-anterior abdominal technique results in a lower dose (Marshall *et al.* 1994), a supine technique with male gonad protection is preferred in children.
- In supine neonates who cannot be moved, a horizontal beam lateral should be taken from the left to reduce the dose to the liver (see below).

Radiological considerations

- Unlike adults, erect images are rarely required or justified.
- Left lateral decubitus images may be required in cases of suspected necrotizing enterocolitis. In this projection, with the patient lying on the left side, free gas will rise, to be located between the lateral margin of the liver and the right abdominal wall.
- Lateral projections may demonstrate Hirschprung's disease or a retroperitoneal tumour in some rare cases.
- Abdominal ultrasound has replaced radiography in many conditions.
- In non-specific abdominal pain, radiographic abnormality is unlikely to be demonstrated in the absence of one of the following: loin pain, haematuria, diarrhoea, palpable mass, abdominal distension or suspected inflammatory bowel disease.

14 Abdomen

Modifications in technique

Constipation

- A very fast film/screen system should be used in chronic cases. A study of colonic transit time may also be requested.
- The patient swallows 30 radio-opaque plastic pellets and an antero-posterior radiograph with the child in the supine position is performed at day 5 following ingestion.
- If pellets are not present on day 5, this is normal.
- If there is a general delay in colonic transit, then the pellets will be distributed throughout the colon.
- If the pellets are grouped in the sigmoid/rectum, then there is poor evacuation.
- A medium-speed screen/film system is used in children under two years of age when Hirschprung's disease is suspected.
- All images should allow adequate assessment of the spine.

Suspected swallowed foreign body

- The initial radiograph should be with a fast-speed screen/film system to include the neck and upper abdomen.
- The radiograph should demonstrate the mandible to iliac crests. Lead protection should be used.
- The most likely sites of hold-up are the neck, mid-oesophagus where the left main bronchus crosses the oesophagus, and at the gastro-oesophageal junction.
- If a foreign body is demonstrated in the neck or chest, a lateral radiograph should be taken to confirm position.
- If history is less than four hours and the foreign body is in the oesophagus, the child should be given a fizzy drink, kept erect and an antero-posterior radiograph repeated in 30 minutes to see whether the foreign body has been dislodged.
- If history is greater than four hours, the patient should be kept nil by mouth and referred for consideration of physical removal.
- If no foreign body is demonstrated, no further radiographs are required unless the patient returns with symptoms of abdominal pain and vomiting. A supine abdominal radiograph should then be performed.
- Parents should always be advised to return if any of these symptoms develop, but pressure to obtain serial radiographs of foreign bodies passing through the abdomen should be resisted strongly, as this involves unnecessary exposure without any added benefit.
- In cases of lead acid or mercury batteries, the radiographs are acquired as described above. However, if the battery is still in the stomach, then it can react with gastric acid. Therefore, the child is normally given metoclopramide and the abdominal radiograph repeated in 24 hours. If the battery is still in the stomach, surgical referral is normally advised.
- Open pins and needles are occasionally swallowed. Surprisingly, most pass unhindered if they are beyond the oesophagus; therefore, the same radiographs are indicated as above.
- If a swallowed foreign body is suspected to be radiolucent, then a contrast study may be indicated.

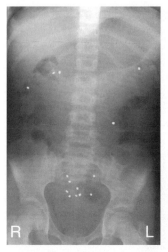

Image of antero-posterior abdomen taken at five days showing delayed transit

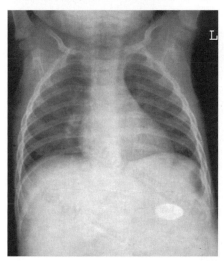

Image of chest and upper abdomen showing coin-shaped foreign body overlying the stomach

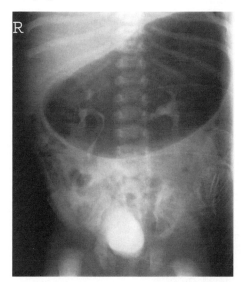

Image of antero-posterior abdomen showing improved visualization of the kidneys in an IVU series following a fizzy drink to cause gaseous distension of the overlying stomach

NB: the use of a metal detector in determining the presence of a metal object in the abdomen may reduce the need for unnecessary irradiation of a child (Arena and Baker 1990, Ryan and Tidey 1994).

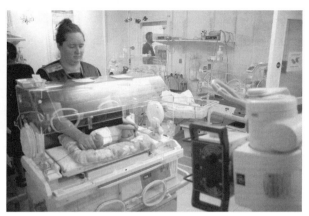

Photograph of neonate in left lateral decubitus position. For minimal handling, dorsal decubitus is an alternative

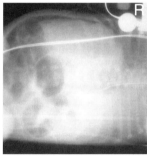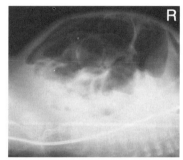

Image of antero-posterior abdomen, left lateral decubitus with free air around the liver and dorsal decubitus with free air anteriorly

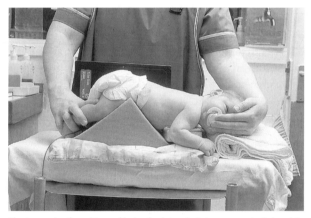

Photograph of position of baby for lateral abdomen ventral decubitus

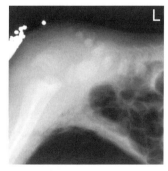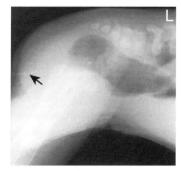

Images of lateral abdomen, ventral decubitus in imperforate anus. Lower limit of air-filled bowel is demonstrated in relation to the pubococcygeal line. Left: high obstruction with lead pellets at anatomical position of anus; right: low obstruction with barium-filled tube tip at level of anus

Modifications in technique

Suspected necrotizing enterocolitis

- An antero-posterior supine abdominal radiograph is obtained, with the legs and arms held in a similar position to that described for the neonatal chest radiograph in a non-sleeping infant (see p. 390).
- The abdomen is normally distended in these cases. Care must be taken not to collimate within the margins of the abdomen.
- If a perforation is suspected, an antero-posterior (left lateral decubitus) projection is selected using a horizontal beam, with the child lying in the lateral position. The right side of the patient is positioned uppermost, as it is easier to demonstrate free air around the liver. The patient should be kept in this position for a few minutes before the radiograph is taken to allow the air to rise.
- If the infant is too ill to be moved, then a lateral (dorsal decubitus) projection is preferred, using a horizontal beam, with the tube directed to the left side of the abdomen to reduce the dose to the liver. This requires less exposure than the antero-posterior projection.
- Lead protection should be used for boys.

Suspected diaphragmatic hernia

A combined antero-posterior chest and abdomen radiograph is recommended.

Imperforate anus (prone invertogram)

A lateral (ventral decubitus) projection is selected using a horizontal beam. This allows intraluminal air to rise and fill the most distal bowel to assess the level of atresia. Radiography should not be performed less than 24 hours after birth.

Position of patient and cassette

- The infant should be placed in the prone position, with the pelvis and buttocks raised on a triangular covered foam pad or rolled-up nappy.
- The infant should be kept in this position for approximately 10–15 minutes.
- The cassette is supported vertically against the lateral aspect of the infant's pelvis, and adjusted parallel to the median sagittal plane.

Direction and centring of the X-ray beam

- The horizontal central ray is directed to the centre of the cassette.

Note

A lead marker is taped to the skin in the anatomical area where the anus would normally be sited. The distance between this and the most distal air-filled bowel can then be measured.

14 Skull

Obtaining diagnostic quality radiographs of the skull in small children is probably one of the most difficult challenges to any radiographer. The technique described for adults is not so straightforward when the patient is a screaming, red-faced, determined toddler accompanied by anxious parents.

Young children may be wrapped in cotton blankets for immobilization. The use of shaped foam pads is strongly recommended.

A feed or use of a pacifier is very beneficial. All clothing, fasteners, hair clips, beads and extra-stiff hair gel need to be removed. The carer accompanying the child, provided the carer is not pregnant, should be encouraged to distract the child with a toy for the exposure.

Children's head sizes are variable and also are of variable density, depending on skeletal maturation and various congenital malformations. Below the age of one year, there are no visible vascular markings, and it is only the range of additional sutures that can cause confusion with fractures. Grids are not used routinely in skull radiography of children under the age of one year, which allows for shorter exposure times and reduced patient dose. If an isocentric skull unit is used, the grid should be removed for children up to the age of one year.

Referral criteria

Referral criteria for skull projections include those specific recommendations by the RCR (2003) on the management of head injury.

Recommended projections

Examination is performed by means of the following:

Basic	• Occipito-frontal
	• Fronto-occipital – 30 degrees caudad
	• Lateral
Alternative	• Fronto-occipital

Modifications of technique are recommended (according to the referral) as follows, in cases of trauma:

Condition	Projections
If not knocked unconscious and specific frontal injury	• Occipito-frontal/ fronto-occipital • Lateral of affected side
If not knocked unconscious and specific occipital injury	• Fronto-occipital – 30 degrees caudad • Lateral of affected side
If knocked unconscious or showing signs of fracture	• Occipito-frontal/ fronto-occipital • Fronto-occipital – 30 degrees caudad • Lateral of affected side

Trauma

- The lateral view should include the first three cervical vertebrae.
- A horizontal beam lateral is usually performed but is not considered essential before the age of six years, as the sphenoid sinus is not pneumatized before this age. After this, air fluid levels might indicate a base of skull fracture. All trauma images should demonstrate adequately the soft tissues.

Craniosynostosis

- For assessment of craniosynostosis, a lateral and under-tilted fronto-occipital, 20 degrees caudad projection will demonstrate all the sutures adequately in most children.
- Tangential views may be required in some cases of a bony lump.

A detailed description of adult skull radiography is given on pp. 238–245 and the techniques described can be readily adopted for older children. The projections described in the following pages are for a one-year-old child and are typical of most departments. The projections are:

- fronto-occipital;
- fronto-occipital – 30 degrees caudad;
- lateral of affected side with horizontal beam.

Radiological considerations

As skull X-rays involve a moderately high dose in terms of plain radiographs, often including a series of radiographs, justification is essential. Good clinico-radiological cooperation, agreed referral criteria and audit are essential in keeping the number of unnecessary radiographs to a minimum (Cook et al. 1998). Some studies suggest that over a third of requests following trauma are unnecessary (Boulis et al. 1978), and many have reported that absence of a fracture does not alter management (Garniak et al. 1986, Lloyd et al. 1997, Masters et al. 1987).

Radiation protection

- Justification, optimization and careful technique are the best ways of conforming to radiation protection guidelines.
- Avoidance of the use of a grid in children under the age of one year is an important dose-saving measure.
- A short exposure time is particularly important in performing skull radiography to avoid movement unsharpness. The maximum exposure time should be less than 40 ms.
- Children's skulls are almost fully grown by the age of seven years; therefore, children over this age need almost as much exposure as an adult.
- The hands of the person holding the child should not be visible on the radiograph.
- Tight collimation with circular cones of variable size is best suited for the shape of the cranium. In this way, unnecessary thyroid radiation can also be avoided in non-trauma cases. The collimation can be inserted above the diamentor chamber (see p. 388).
- Occipito-frontal projections, where possible, will reduce the dose to the eyes (Rosenbaum and Arnold 1978).

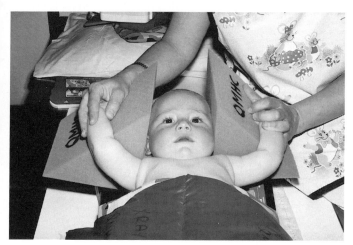

Position of infant for antero-posterior skull with triangular sponges supporting the head on either side

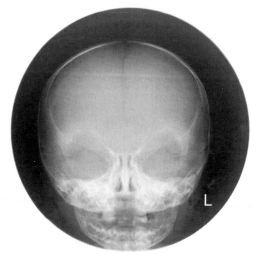

Image of normal fronto-occipital skull radiograph

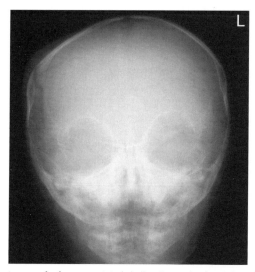

Image of a fronto-occipital skull radiograph of an infant demonstrating a right parietal fracture

Fronto-occipital

A 24 × 30-cm or 18 × 24-cm cassette is selected, depending on the size of the cranium.

Position of patient and cassette

- The child is positioned carefully in the supine position, with the head resting on a pre-formed foam pad positioned on top of the cassette. The head is adjusted to bring the median sagittal plane at right-angles to and in the midline of the cassette. The external auditory meati should be equidistant from the cassette.
- The child is immobilized in this position with the assistance of a carer, who is asked to hold foam pads on either side of the skull during the exposure. The carer usually stands at the head end of the imaging table to undertake this procedure. Occasionally, a second carer is required to assist in keeping the child still.

Direction and centring of the X-ray beam

- The central ray is directed to the nasion at the necessary angle to allow it to pass along the orbito-meatal plane.
- If it is required that the orbits are shown clear of the petrous bone, the central ray should be angled cranially so that it makes an angle of 20 degrees to the orbito-meatal plane and centred to the nasion.

Essential image characteristics

- Whole cranial vault, orbits and petrous bones should be present on the radiograph and should be symmetrical.
- For occipito-frontal 20 degrees, petrous bones should be projected over the lower orbital margins.
- Lambdoid and coronal sutures should be symmetrical.
- Visually sharp reproduction of the outer and inner tables of the cranial vault according to age.
- Reproduction of sinuses and temporal bones consistent with age.
- Visualization of the sutures consistent with age.
- Soft tissues of scalp should be reproduced with a bright light.

Common faults and remedies

- Holder's hands around the face.
- Wide cones.
- Rotated patient with respect to the cassette.
- Whole cervical spine or upper chest unnecessarily on the radiograph.
- Use of a feeding bottle or pacifier often allows the correct position to be maintained.
- Obtaining the child's confidence and following the advice in positioning the patient should avoid these problems.

Fronto-occipital – 30 degrees caudad

Position of patient and cassette

- The child is positioned in a similar way to that described for the fronto-occipital position. However, the chin is depressed so that the orbito-meatal line is at right-angles to the table.
- The carer immobilizes the head using foam pads positioned gently but firmly either side of the head.
- The cassette is positioned longitudinally on the tabletop, with its upper edge at the level of the vertex of the skull.

Direction and centring of the X-ray beam

- The central ray is angled caudally so that it makes an angle of 30 degrees to the orbito-meatal plane.
- To avoid irradiating the eyes, a collimation field is set such that the lower border is coincident with the upper orbital margin and the upper border includes the skull vertex. Laterally, the skin margins should also be included within the field (Denton 1998).
- If the child's chin cannot be sufficiently depressed to bring the orbito-meatal line at right-angles to the table, it will be necessary to angle the central ray more than 30 degrees to the vertical so that it makes the necessary angle of 30 degrees to the orbito-meatal plane.

Essential image characteristics

- The arch of the atlas should be projected through the foramen magnum.
- Lambdoid and coronal sutures should be symmetrical.
- Inner and outer table, soft tissues and sutures as above.

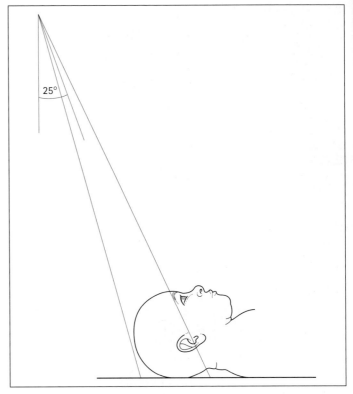

Line diagram demonstrating Denton beam-limiting technique

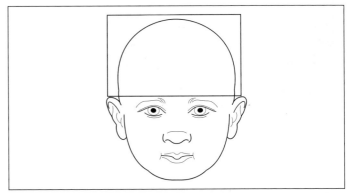

Frontal diagram of skull showing light beam collimation

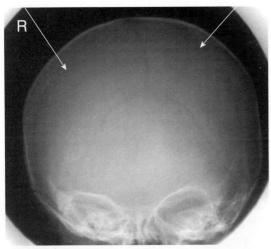

Image of under-tilted fronto-occipital skull radiograph using a 15-degree pad under the skull with a 10-degree caudal tube angle for optimal demonstration of the coronal and lambdoid sutures on a single image

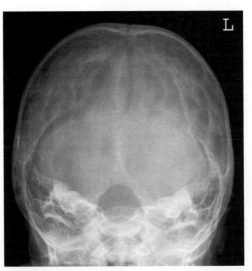

Image of correctly positioned fronto-occipital 25 degrees caudad radiograph of skull as in Denton technique (Denton 1998)

Lateral – supine

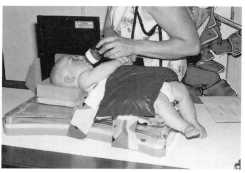

Position of a six-month-old child for lateral skull with horizontal beam technique with patient supine demonstrating immobilization and distraction with a feeding bottle

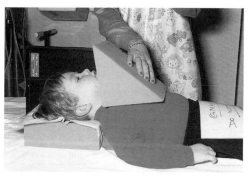

Position of a 3-year-old child positioned for lateral skull, patient supine showing use of foam pad to immobilize the head

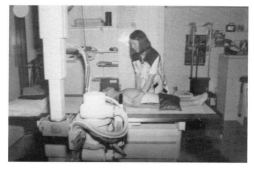

Position of 6-year-old child for lateral skull, patient supine showing position of X-ray tube

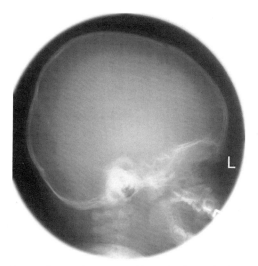

Image of correctly positioned lateral radiograph of a baby's skull

Position of patient and cassette

- With the patient supine on the Bucky table, a pre-formed foam pad is placed under the head so that the occiput is included on the image.
- The patient's head is now adjusted to bring the median sagittal plane of the head at right-angles to the table by ensuring that the external auditory meati are equidistant from the table.
- The head is immobilized with the aid of a carer (see photographs opposite for technique according to age).
- A cassette is supported vertically against the lateral aspect of the head parallel to the median sagittal plane, with its long edge 5 cm above the vertex of the skull.

Direction and centring of the X-ray beam

- The horizontal central ray is directed parallel to the interorbital line so that it is at right-angles to the median plane and the cassette.
- The central ray is centred midway between the glabella and the external occipital protuberance.

Essential image characteristics

- The whole cranial vault and base of the skull should be present and symmetrical.
- The floor of the pituitary fossa should be a single line.
- The floors of the anterior cranial fossa should be superimposed.
- The mandibular condyles should be superimposed.
- The first three cervical vertebrae should be included for trauma and should be lateral.
- Visually sharp reproduction of the outer and inner tables and floor of the sella consistent with age.
- Visually sharp reproduction of the vascular channels and trabecular structure consistent with age.
- Reproduction of the sutures and fontanelles consistent with age.
- Reproduction of the soft tissues and nasal bones, consistent with age.
- Reproduction of sphenoid sinus (not pneumatized below the age of six years).

Maxillary antra are not well pneumatized before the age of three years and the frontal sinuses are not developed before the age of six years. Sinus X-rays are therefore rarely justified in children below this age. An occipito-mental projection of the sinuses is performed erect in a similar way to that described for adults (see p. 263). However, in children the patient's nose and mouth are first placed in contact with the midline of the vertical Bucky and then the head is adjusted to bring the orbito-meatal line at 35 degrees to the horizontal at the centre of the Bucky.

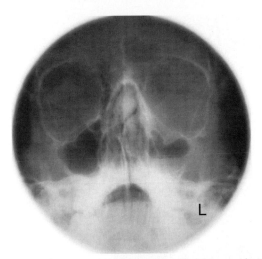

Image of occipito-mental projection of facial bones of a 13-year-old boy demonstrating a blowout fracture of the left inferior orbital margin with fluid levels in the left maxillary antrum and left frontal sinus

Essential image characteristics

- The X-ray beam should be well collimated and should include the frontal sinuses (when developed in children over six years of age) and the bases of the maxillary sinuses and upper maxillary teeth.
- Petrous bones should lie at the base of the antra.
- Orbits, sinuses and petrous bones should be symmetrical.
- Bony detail should have visually sharp reproduction.
- Soft tissues and mucosa of sinuses should be visible.

Post-nasal space – lateral supine

PNS radiography is usually performed on children between four and 10 years of age, with the common problem of mouth breathing due to nasal obstruction. A lateral projection (taken supine) of the PNS is performed to demonstrate enlarged adenoids, hence the PNS must be air-filled to be radiographically visible.

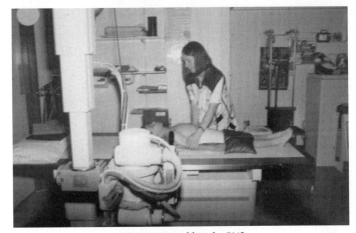

Child positioned for lateral projection of face for PNS

Position of patient and cassette

- The child lies supine on the table, with the lateral aspect of the head in contact with a cassette supported vertically. The head is adjusted to bring the medial sagittal plane parallel to the cassette.
- The jaw is raised slightly so that the angles of the mandible are separated from the bodies of the upper cervical spine.

Direction and centring of the X-ray beam

- The horizontal beam is centred to the ramus of the mandible, and coned to include the maxillary sinuses to the third cervical vertebrae and the posterior pharynx.

Note

The image should be taken with the mouth closed. If the PNS is obliterated, the view should be repeated with the child sniffing.

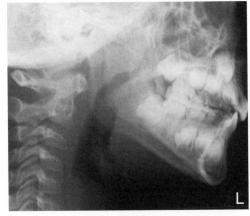

Image of lateral projection of PNS in a 6-year-old child

Essential image characteristics

- The condyles of the mandible should be superimposed.
- Bony detail should have visually sharp reproduction.
- Soft tissue of adenoidal pads should be reproduced.

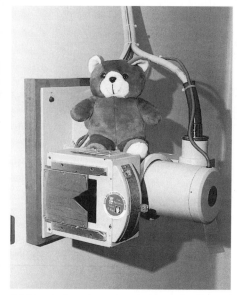

Additional triangular coning device on the X-ray tube assembly for lateral cephalograph

Cephalometric radiography and dental panoramic tomography (DPT) are now the most commonly requested imaging techniques in teenagers due to the increasing requirement for orthodontics. These types of radiographs should not be performed routinely in children under the age of seven years for orthodontic assessment alone. However, paediatric dentists often request DPT on children from three years onward to demonstrate 'state of teeth' before dental treatment. This should be performed only if extensive caries are present. Special attention must be given to justification of exposure and optimization, collimation and avoiding unnecessary repeats.

A detailed description of the radiographic techniques in adults is given in Section 10.

- For lateral cephalometry, in addition to the graduated filter, a triangular coning device is recommended to avoid irradiating the back of the skull and the thyroid.
- The whole skull will need to be demonstrated in cranio-facial deformity.
- CT lateral cephalolometry can also be considered as a low-dose alternative.
- For DPT, additional eye shields are also recommended, where only a fixed aperture is available.

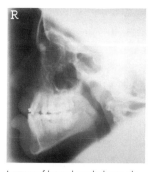

Image of lateral cephalograph of a 9-year-old girl

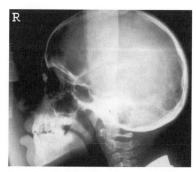

Lateral cephalograph without triangular coning or filter device with unnecessary irradiation of the base of the skull and thyroid

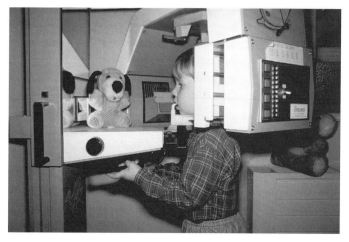

DPT machine with eye shield and child positioned for DPT

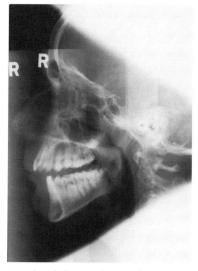

Lateral cephalogram showing fault of teeth not being apposed

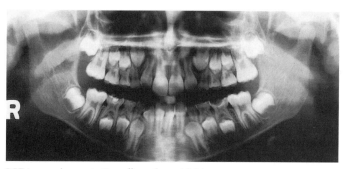

DPT image demonstrating effect of eye shield

Initial pelvic and hip radiography is normally performed in conjunction with ultrasound. Radiation protection measures should be applied strictly. The examination is undertaken using a fast screen/film system, with no grid in children under the age of three years, to ensure that the patient dose is kept to a minimum. The size of the cassette will depend on the age and size of the child.

Radiography may be performed before or during treatment, when a child may present wearing a special splint or plaster-cast.

Referral criteria

- hip pain/limp (irritable hips, Perthes' disease, slipped upper femoral epiphysis, osteomyelitis);
- development dysplasia of the hip (DDH)/congenital dislocated hip (CDH);
- trauma;
- post-surgery;
- part of a skeletal survey for NAI or suspected syndrome.

Recommended projections

The antero-posterior projection is the most commonly requested projection for children of all ages.

Examination is performed by means of the following:

• DDH/CDH	• Antero-posterior – supine • Antero-posterior – erect
• Irritable hips	• Antero-posterior • Lateral – frog view
• Post op for slipped epiphysis	• Antero-posterior – supine • Turned lateral
• Trauma	• Antero-posterior – supine • Lateral – horizontal beam

Antero-posterior

The following describes the technique adopted for a three-month-old baby. A cassette is selected that is large enough to include the pelvis and upper femora.

Position of patient and cassette

- The child lies supine on the X-ray table, on top of the cassette or a specially designed cassette holder, which is placed at the end of the table, with the median sagittal plane of the trunk at right-angles to the middle of the cassette.
- To maintain this position, a sandbag is placed on either side of the baby's trunk, with the child's arms left unrestrained.
- The baby's legs are held straight, with the holder's hands positioned firmly around each leg, the holder's fingers under the baby's calves and the holder's thumbs on the knees.
- If using the cassette holder at the end of the table, the knees should be held together and flexed.

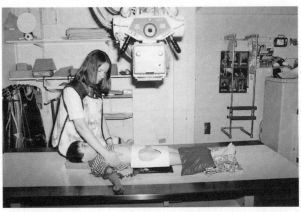

Male child positioned for antero-posterior supine projection of hips with window protection

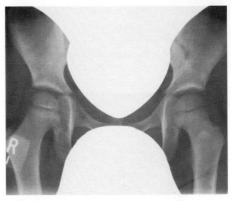

Image of an antero-posterior pelvis showing window gonad protection with additional female protection over the gonads

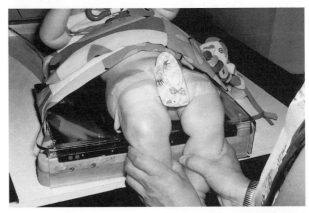

Four-month-old baby boy positioned for hips in an immobilization device with shaped lead protection

- For the older child, positioning is similar to that described for the adult (see p. 148).

Direction and centring of the X-ray beam

- The vertical central ray is directed to the centre of the cassette.

Note

Following surgery, low-dose CT may be used to demonstrate the position of the femoral head in patients treated with the use of a long-term plaster cast.

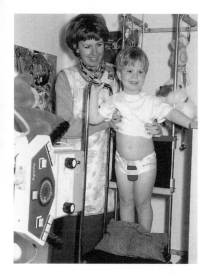

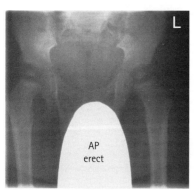

Photograph and image of a male follow-up antero-posterior pelvis erect with gonad protection

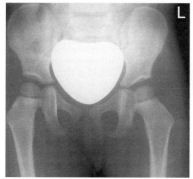

Image of a female antero-posterior pelvis - erect with heart shaped gonad protection

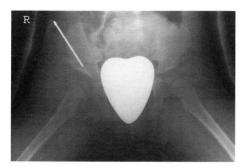

Image of child in plaster cast following right acetabuloplasty

Antero-posterior – erect (weight-bearing)

As soon as a child is able to stand, weight-bearing erect images are frequently requested.

- The child stands with the posterior aspect of the pelvis against a cassette held vertically in the cassette holder.
- The anterior superior iliac spines should be equidistant from the cassette and the median sagittal plane vertical and coincident with the centre of the cassette.
- The ankles should be apart and separated by a small 40-degree foam pad, with the toes straight and pointing forwards.
- The child is supported at the waist whilst standing on a raised platform, with sandbags secured around the feet. Any pelvic tilt is corrected with the use of a small block.

Essential image characteristics

- Whole pelvis, sacrum and subtrochanteric regions of both femora. (Iliac crests can be excluded in specific hip pathology, e.g. Perthes' disease.)
- Symmetrical, with iliac wings and pubic rami of equal length. Femoral necks should not be foreshortened.
- Visualization of sacrum and intervertebral foramina depending on bowel content and presence of female protection. Reproduction of sacro-iliac joints according to age, with reproduction of the femoral necks.
- Reproduction of spongiosa and cortex.
- Visualization of trochanters consistent with age.
- Visualization of soft tissue planes.

Common faults and remedies

- Rotated patient with respect to the cassette needs careful observation of supine patient and holding technique.
- Gonad protection missing, inadequate, too large or slipped over region of interest. Gonad protection is most necessary during hip radiography. A very careful technique is required. A wide range of sizes and types are required. Experience is essential.

Radiation protection

- Gonad protection is not used for the initial examination.
- Subsequent examinations require the use of gonad protection. If erect position is required, then gonad protection can be taped into position. Alternatively, a window-shaped coning device can be inserted beneath the light beam diaphragm.

Radiological considerations

- Hip radiographs are a common request in children, but initial ultrasound examination should always be considered.
- A line drawn from the mid-sacrum through the triradiate cartilage should pass through the medial aspect of the femoral metaphysis to exclude dislocation. Similarly, Shenton's line (along superior obturator foramen and femoral neck) should be uninterrupted.

Von Rosen projection

This supplementary projection was sometimes employed to confirm diagnosis of DDH. The disadvantage of the projection is that it produces a number of false positives and negatives, and it has been largely superseded by hip ultrasound.

The ossification centre of the femoral head tends to be a little eccentric and lateral, particularly following treatment for DDH. This may give the false impression of decentring. The degree of dislocation and decentring is best assessed by drawing a line through the mid-sacrum and triradiate cartilage. This line should pass through the medial aspect of the femoral metaphysis. The use of this line in a straight antero-posterior radiograph of the hips is preferred to the Von Rosen projection.

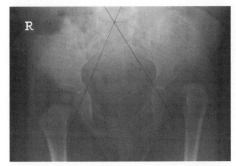

Pelvis of an infant with a line drawn from the mid sacrum through the triradiate cartilage which should cross the medial upper femoral metaphysis showing obvious left dislocation

Lateral – both hips (frog projection)

This projection may be employed to supplement the antero-posterior projection in the investigation of irritable hips.

Position of patient and cassette

- The child lies supine on the X-ray table, on top of the cassette, with the median sagittal plane of the trunk at right-angles to the middle of the cassette.
- To maintain this position when examining a baby, a sandbag is placed either side of the baby's trunk, with the arms left unrestrained.
- The anterior superior iliac spines should be equidistant from the couch top to ensure that the pelvis is not rotated.
- The hips and knees are flexed.
- The limbs are then rotated laterally through approximately 60 degrees, with the knees separated and the plantar aspects of the feet placed in contact with each other.
- A child may be supported in this position with non-opaque pads.
- The cassette is centred at the level of the femoral pulse and must include both hips.

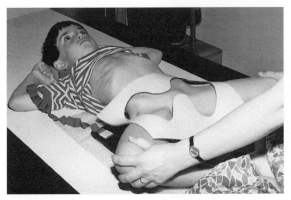

Child positioned for frog projection of hips with window protection

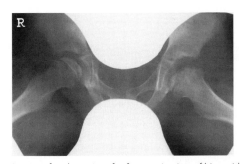

Image of male patient for frog projection of hips with window protection demonstrating bilateral Perthes' disease

Direction and centring of the X-ray beam

- The vertical central ray is directed in the midline at the level of the femoral pulse.

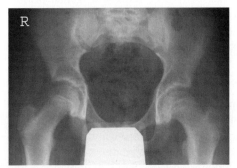

Image of antero-posterior hips with SUFE on left

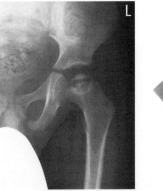
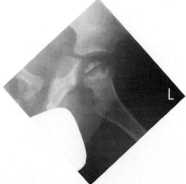

Image of antero-posterior and turned lateral of left hip showing left femoral head Perthes' disease. Note: gonadal protection for all follow-up images

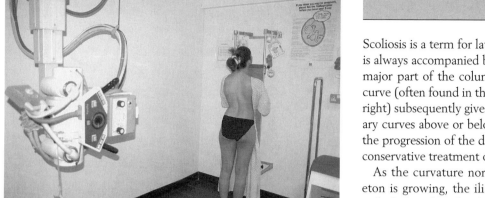

Photograph of patient positioned for postero-anterior projection spine

Scoliosis is a term for lateral curvature of the vertebral column. It is always accompanied by rotation of the involved vertebrae. The major part of the column is usually involved, since the primary curve (often found in the thoracic spine with the convexity to the right) subsequently gives rise to one or two compensatory secondary curves above or below it. Radiography is performed to assess the progression of the disease and to measure the effectiveness of conservative treatment or when surgical treatment is considered.

As the curvature normally will progress only while the skeleton is growing, the iliac crests on postero-anterior images are included so that the degree of maturity can be estimated from the degree of apophyseal fusion. Alternatively, the non-dominant hand can be radiographed for bone age.

The majority of patients encountered will be children or adolescents, most commonly suffering from idiopathic scoliosis. Images will be taken at regular intervals as progression of the disease is monitored. Given the relatively high radiation doses associated with this examination, and the heightened radiosensitivity of children, radiation protection considerations are paramount (see below).

Referral criteria

The referral criteria for all types of pathology where a whole spine, rather than a segmental spine, examination is indicated are as follows:

- idiopathic/congenital/paralytic and post-infective scoliosis;
- spina bifida;
- suspected syndrome;
- severe injury;
- metastatic disease;
- metabolic disorder.

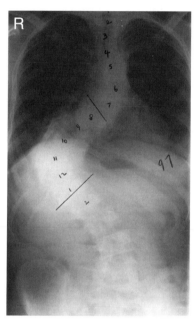

Postero-anterior erect spine showing example of initial image at presentation taken with a grid and limited collimation to include the thorax and abdomen. Cob angles demonstrated to measure the degree of lateral curvature

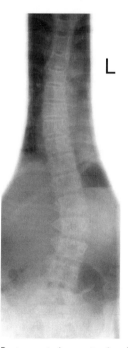

Postero-anterior erect spine showing example of follow-up study taken without a grid, with faster screen/film speed and tailored collimation to restrict the X-ray beam to the spine and avoid the developing breast

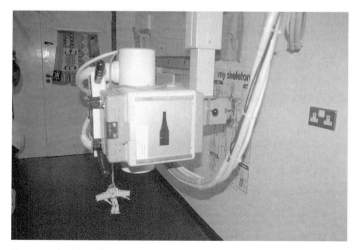

Photograph of lateral coning device used for follow-up studies

411

14 | Spine – scoliosis

The projections required will vary considerably, depending on the stage of the disease, the age of the patient, treatment and the preferences of the orthopaedic surgeon. Close liaison between the radiology and orthopaedic departments is of paramount importance.

Image acquisition may be undertaken using conventional or digital radiography. Conventional radiography is described, and the reader is directed to the manufacturers' literature for details relating to digital acquisition and measurement procedures.

- A standing postero-anterior image is often all that is required.
- A lateral projection may be performed at the time of the initial investigation.
- Images may be required with the patient wearing a brace and repeated with the brace removed in order to monitor its effectiveness.
- Additional frontal images with the patient supine and recumbent, bending to each side may be requested to assess the degree of passive correction and determine the extent of any planned fusion.
- Postoperative radiographs of the chest are required to assess lung expansion and spinal radiographs to ensure integrity of the spinal instrumentation.

Postero-anterior – standing

A 35 × 43-cm cassette with a 400-speed film/screen system is selected and positioned in a chest stand or erect Bucky. A grid is used for the initial examination.

For examination of taller children, when it is not possible to include the whole spine on a 35 × 43-cm cassette, a specialized long cassette (typically 30 × 90 cm or 35 × 105 cm) loaded with ungraduated screens is used and held erect in a special upright holder mounted on a wall.

Position of patient and cassette

- The patient stands with the anterior aspect of the trunk in contact with the vertical Bucky or grid cassette.
- The lower edge of the cassette is placed 1.5 cm below the iliac crests, with the chin resting on the top of the cassette to include from C7 to S1.
- The median sagittal plane should be at right-angles to the cassette and should coincide with the vertical centre line of the Bucky.
- The patient's arms should be by their sides, although it may be necessary to raise the arms of smaller children to assist in stretching the vertebral column.
- If the patient is standing, shoes should be removed and the feet placed slightly apart in the anatomical position to ensure that the patient is bearing weight equally on both legs.
- Occasionally, a wooden block (height previously determined) is positioned under one foot to correct for pelvic tilt.
- A line joining the highest point of the iliac crests should be horizontal if possible.

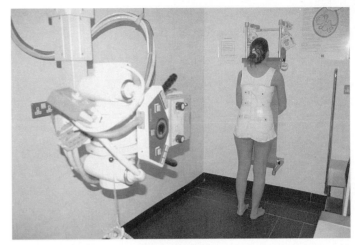

Photograph of patient in a brace positioned postero-anterior projection of the spine

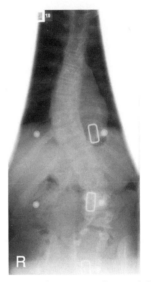

Image of a patient with spina bifida in a brace postero-anterior projection of the spine without a grid

- The middle of the cassette should be positioned just above the thoracolumbar junction (T11/Tl2 region).

Radiation protection

- The most effective protection for the breasts is to undertake the examination in the postero-anterior position.
- Follow-up examination does not require the same quality for definition as the initial examination.
  - The grid can be dispensed with, unless the patient is particularly large.
  - A fast screen/film system (700–800-speed) can be used. This can result in a dose reduction of 80% compared with the initial radiograph. The iliac crests do not need to be included for every radiograph.
  - Developing breast tissue in adolescent females is highly radiosensitive; unnecessary irradiation of the breasts should be avoided where possible and breast shields considered.
  - A pre-shaped filter device can be attached to the light-beam diaphragm (LBD) when undertaking conventional film radiography, to protect the developing breasts, ribs and gonads.

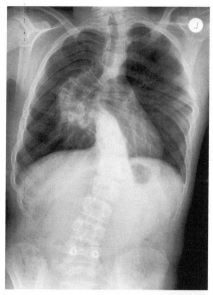

Image of postero-anterior spine erect without cones

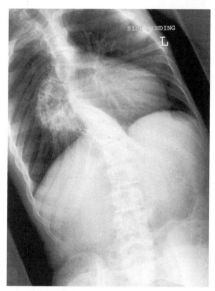

Image of postero-anterior spine erect – patient bending to the right

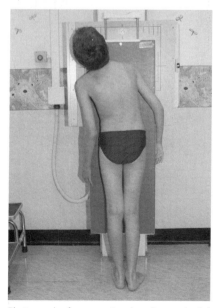

Photograph of erect patient bending to the left

Postero-anterior – standing

Direction and centring of the X-ray beam

- A horizontal central ray is employed, and the beam is collimated and centred to include the whole spinal column.
- The lower collimation border is positioned just below the level of the anterior superior iliac spines, thus ensuring inclusion of the first sacral segment. The upper border should be at the level of the spinous process of C7.
- An increased FFD is used to ensure the correct cassette coverage (180–200 cm).

Notes

- For follow-up radiographs, a preshaped filter device of appropriate size is attached to the LBD to protect the developing breasts, ribs and gonads.
- If there is clinical suspicion of a structural abnormality then the cervical spine, ribs and hips may need to be included on the initial radiograph.
- It is important that the medial aspects of the iliac crests are not excluded to enable assessment of the spinal maturity from epiphysis growth.

Common faults and remedies

- It is important to ensure consistency in technique so that valid comparisons can be made. Note the technique and exposure factors employed and keep these with the patient's records for future reference. This will also help to reduce unnecessary repeats.

Essential image characteristics

- The first image should demonstrate the spine to include above and below the curvature, ribs and iliac crests (latter if aged 10–18 years in girls and 13–20 years in boys). For an idiopathic scoliosis, lower cervical spine to sacrum is adequate.
- If a structural abnormality is demonstrated, an antero-posterior cervical spine and additional coned views may be required.
- The image should give good reproduction of the vertebral bodies and pedicles, visualization of the posterior facet joints and reproduction of spinous processes and transverse processes consistent with age. Clear visualization of the endplates is required, essential for measuring the Cobb angle.
- Follow-up images should be coned to the spinal curvature and iliac crests as above.

Lateral

A 35 × 43-cm cassette with a 400-speed film/screen system is selected and positioned in a chest stand or erect Bucky. A grid is used for the initial examination.

Position of patient and cassette

- The patient stands with their bare feet slightly apart, with the side of the convexity of the primary curve against the vertical Bucky.
- Care is taken to ensure that the patient does not lean towards the cassette.
- The lower edge of the cassette is placed 1.5 cm below the iliac crests.
- The mid-axillary line is centred to the cassette. The coronal plane should be at right-angles to the cassette.
- The latter may be assessed by palpating the anterior iliac spines and rotating the patient so that a line joining the two sides is at right-angles to the cassette.
- Similarly, a line joining the lateral end of the clavicles should be at right-angles to the cassette.
- The arms are folded over the head.

Direction and centring of the X-ray beam

- A horizontal central ray is employed, and the beam is collimated and centred to the cassette to include the whole spinal column.
- The lower collimation border is positioned at the level of the anterior superior iliac spines, thus ensuring inclusion of the first sacral segment.
- The upper border should be at the level of the spinous process of C7.
- An increased FFD is used to ensure the correct, whole anatomical area is covered (180–200 cm).

Notes

- Care should be taken to ensure that the beam is well collimated to exclude the breast tissues, especially in follow-up radiographs.
- Additional views, fluoroscopy, CT or MRI may be required to reveal the complete extent of the 3-dimensional nature of some severe deformities.

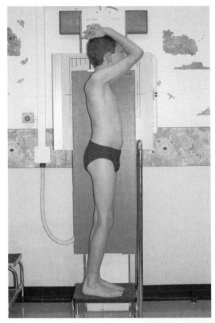

Patient positioned for lateral projection of the spine

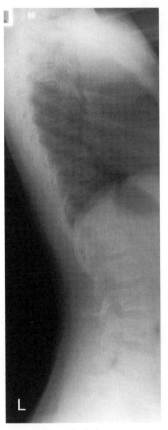

Image of lateral whole spine using grid and cones collimated to the spine

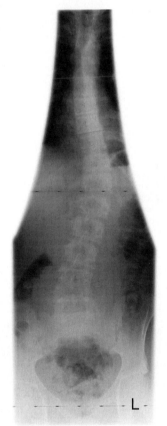

Image of postero-anterior whole spine scoliosis and uncorrected pelvic tilt using a long cassette

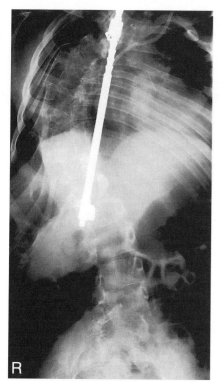

Postero-anterior erect image showing Harrington rod

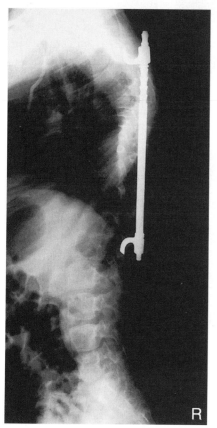

Lateral erect image showing Harrington rod

Radiological considerations

- The most common referral for scoliosis is now idiopathic scoliosis. Affected children are otherwise completely normal, with a normal life expectancy. Multiple radiographs for monitoring are required, and therefore dose-saving measures are important.

- Scoliosis is described as being of early onset (before five years) and late onset. Those who develop large curves early have a higher risk of developing cardiovascular complications.

- Secondary spinal scoliosis is now less common in most centres. The main causes being: congenital (including hemivertebrae), neuromuscular disorders and neurofibromatosis. Tuberculosis is uncommon and polio is now rare. However, it is still extremely important to exclude underlying disease and MRI or scintigraphy is advised in all patients with atypical 'idiopathic' scoliosis or painful scoliosis (the latter typically being due to an osteoid osteoma). MRI should also be considered preoperatively to exclude lesions such as syringomyelia.

- When a secondary scoliosis is suspected due to abnormalities seen on the first thoraco-lumbar spine image, coned views, cervical spine and pelvic radiographs can be considered for additional assessment.

- The lateral curvature of an idiopathic scoliosis is usually convex to the right giving a right-sided hump and is accompanied by rotation of the vertebrae on a vertical axis. This thrusts the ribs backwards in the thoracic area and increases the ugliness of the deformity. The rotary component makes the disease more complex than a cosmetic deformity and rotation of the thorax can lead to compression of the heart and lungs, whereas lumbar curves can predispose to later degenerative changes.

- The goal of therapy is to keep the primary curve less than 40 degrees at the end of growth; small curves of less than 15 degrees are usually not treated. Curves of 20–40 degrees are managed in a body brace, and curves of more than 40 degrees usually have spinal fusion (e.g. a metal Harrington rod). Follow-up images of patients with a Harrington rod will need to show any breakage of the rods or surrounding Luque wiring.

- An assessment of skeletal age is required so that appropriate treatment can be planned. The development of the iliac apophyses (Risser's sign) correlates well with skeletal maturity, as determined by assessing bone age at the hand and wrist (Dhar *et al.* 1993). The iliac apophyses first appear laterally and anteriorly on the crest of the ilium. Growth develops posteriorly and medially, followed by fusion to the iliac crests. Increasing ossification correlates with decreased progression.

14 Spine – cervical, thoracic and lumbar

This section addresses modifications in technique for the cervical spine for those patients aged four years and under. Readers are referred to Section 6 for guidance in the technique for the adult spine.

Referral criteria for the spine as a whole are slightly different and include:

- low back pain (any back pain is abnormal in a child);
- scoliosis (the whole spine should be performed as described for whole spine);
- lower motor neuron signs in legs/neuropathic bladder;
- congenital anomaly of spine or lower limbs;
- suspected infection (isotope bone scan/MRI may also be indicated);
- tethered cord (lumbar region) suspected because of skin changes (ultrasound is normally selected first, up to six to eight months of age);
- trauma (however, this is not routine, since spine fractures are uncommon in children but indicated when significant injury).

Cervical spine

The technique is as in adults, but it is a difficult area to image in children and needs to be modified according to age. The odontoid peg is not ossified before age 3 years and peg projections are not routinely indicated in trauma below the age of 10 years.

Lateral projections require the patient to be as straight as possible to allow optimal evaluation, particularly in cases of trauma. Consideration should be given to the wider retropharyngeal space, particularly seen on expiratory images where the trachea can bow anteriorly and pseudo-subluxation of C2/C3 is a normal variant due to movement as a result of slightly flatter facet joints at this age. The growth plate between the peg and body of C2 needs to be recognized and not confused with a fracture.

Age under four years

For the **antero-posterior projection**, an 18 × 24-cm cassette (no grid) is placed longitudinally on the table. The child is positioned supine, with the shoulders lying in a 15-degree foam pad to lift the chin. The head rests in the hollow of a skull pad to maintain a straight position.

To aid positioning and immobilization, a Bucky band may be secured over the trunk. The carer is asked to stand by the side of the table and to hold the child's arms gently by the side of the child's body.

For the **lateral projection**, the child is maintained in the same position as for the antero-posterior projection, with a horizontal beam used to acquire the image. In trauma, the carer is asked to pull the arms downwards, to move the shoulders for the C7/T1 junction. A pacifier or drink may be employed to distract an infant.

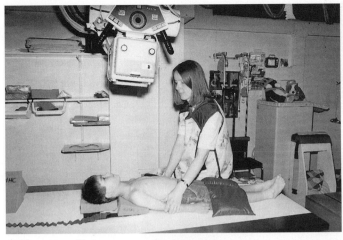

Child positioned for antero-posterior cervical spine

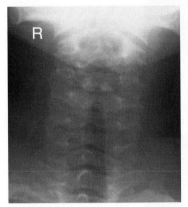

Image showing antero-posterior cervical spine

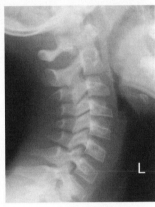

Image of lateral cervical spine in an older child

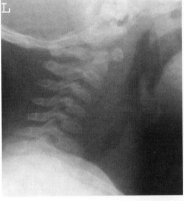
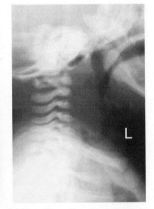

Images of lateral cervical spine in younger children. Note the physiological tracheal bowing during crying and physiological subluxation. Note: Images are best taken when child is as quiet as possible

Notes

- An FFD of 100 cm may be employed to reduce the dose, as the object-to-film distance of the spine is much reduced compared with the adult distance.
- For the investigation of lumbar spondylolisthesis in the older child, both right and left postero-anterior oblique projections may be requested.

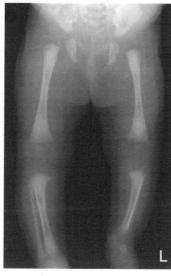

Image of antero-posterior both limbs in a neonate with a short left leg due to hypoplastic tibia, fibula and foot

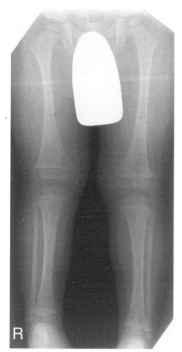

Image of antero-posterior both limbs in a male child with short right femur and gonad protection

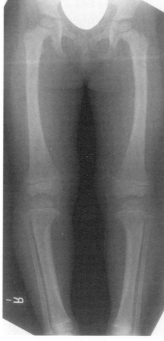

Erect both lower limbs with female gonad protection

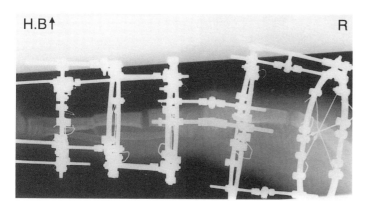

Image of lower leg in Ilizarov frame

Leg length assessment is undertaken to assess discrepancy in leg length that has been confirmed to be real rather than as a result of pelvic tilt due to scoliosis.

Assessment can be undertaken by means of the following:

- Single exposure of both limbs on a large cassette using a large FFD.
- Localized exposures of the hips, knees and ankles on a single cassette employing radio-opaque graduated rulers.
- Digital acquisition and reconstruction techniques using a remote-controlled digital fluoroscopy table/C-arm imaging system, or a single exposure technique using a CR system.
- CT scanogram of both legs.

Conventional methods are described here, with the digital fluoroscopy scanning method outlined briefly. The reader is directed to the manufacturers' instruction manuals for more detailed instruction of the digital acquisition and CT scanogram methods.

Radiological considerations

- Differences in limb length can occur as a result of a variety of congenital conditions or as a result of infection or trauma to the growth plates. Successful surgical correction depends on accurate radiographic measurement of the limbs.
- There are two main methods for equalizing limb length. The first is to fuse the growth plates at one end of a long bone. Alternatively, one can increase the length of the shorter limb by performing a transverse osteotomy and using a device and frame outside the limb to separate the cut ends to allow healing. External fixators or the Ilizarov (Ilizarov 1988) device can be used. The Ilizarov device results in less movement at the osteotomy sites; therefore, fewer postoperative radiographs are required compared with lengthening using external fixators.

Essential image characteristics

The following characteristics are essential:

- Pelvis, knees and ankles should be straight.
- Density of the pelvis, knees and ankles should be appropriate for radiological assessment.
- Reproduction of hip, knee and subtalar joints with careful collimation.
- Reproduction of spongiosa and cortex.
- Visualization of soft tissue planes.
- When a ruler technique is employed, the ruler(s) should be straight and visible on the image at each of the joints.

Radiation protection

- Children undergoing such procedures need multiple radiographs, and it is important to always use gonad protection on all follow-up images.

Single exposure method

Assessment by single exposure may be undertaken using a long cassette (35 × 105 cm) fitted with graduated screens and preferably loaded with a single film (triple-fold film) and a large FFD (typically 180–200 cm). The fastest end of the screens is placed under the hips and the slowest under the ankle joints. The cassette is mounted vertically in a special holder to facilitate radiography in the erect position or alternatively is placed on the floor with the child examined in the supine position.

With this technique, the divergent beam will magnify the limbs. However, the inaccuracy of the measurement of the difference in length due to magnification will probably be less than 5%, i.e. an inaccuracy of less than 2.5 mm when the difference in actual length is 50 mm. This degree of inaccuracy may be considered surgically insignificant.

Alternatively, when examining a baby or small child, especially when they cannot stand and may be uncooperative, a smaller cassette is selected to match the length of the limbs. If possible, the child is examined on the imaging table provided a large enough FFD can be obtained.

Position of patient and cassette

- The patient stands with the posterior aspect of the legs against the long cassette and ideally with the arms folded across the thorax.
- The anterior superior iliac spines should be equidistant from the cassette and the medial sagittal plane should be vertical and coincident with the central longitudinal axis of the cassette.
- The legs should be, as far as possible, in a similar relationship to the pelvis, with the feet separated so that the distance between the ankle joints is similar to the distance between the hip joints, with the patella of each knee facing forwards.
- Foam pads and sandbags are used to stabilize the legs and ensure that they are straight.
- If necessary, a block is positioned below the shortened leg to ensure that there is no pelvic tilt and that the limbs are aligned adequately.

Direction and centring of the X-ray beam

- The horizontal central ray is directed towards a point midway between the knee joints.
- The X-ray beam is collimated to include both lower limbs from hip joints to ankle joints.

Common faults and remedies

- Reduce magnification by placing body parts as close as possible to the cassette and increasing the FFD to the maximum distance (180–200 cm).

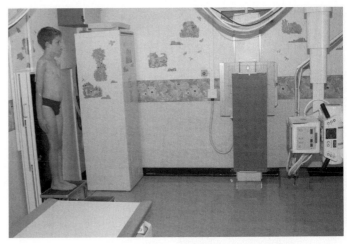

Photograph of a tube positioned for erect leg length single exposure technique

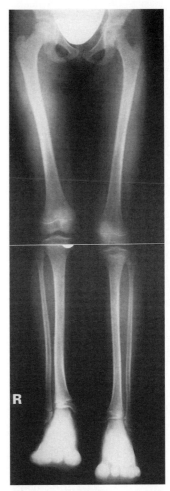

Image of both legs taken erect with wooden block under right foot to correct pelvic tilt

Notes

- For CR acquisition, three 35 × 43-cm cassettes, with slight overlap, are held in an adjustable vertical cassette holder.
- For leg alignment studies, the legs from hips to ankles should be included and any clinical defect should not be corrected.

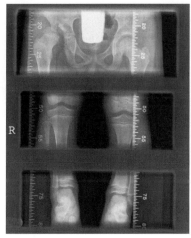

Image of leg length using localized exposure technique

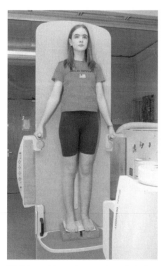

Child positioned erect for digital exposure technique

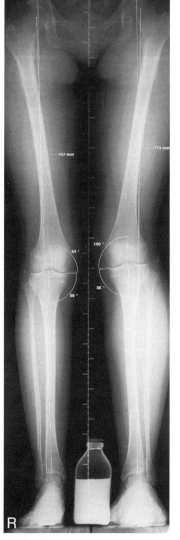

Image of leg lengths using digital fluoroscopy method

Localized exposure method

- Assessment is made using three separate exposures, using a 35 × 43-cm cassette placed length-wise in the Bucky tray. The procedure is undertaken with the use of two 100-cm plastic rulers, each with an opaque scale at 1-cm intervals, which produces an image on the radiograph, which is necessary for drawing lines on the radiograph and obtaining the required measurements.
- The rulers are placed longitudinally on the X-ray table top in such a way that they are parallel to each other with their scales corresponding and separated approximately 20 cm apart so that they will be visible on the radiograph. The rulers are secured in position by Velcro.
- The patient lies between the rulers with the hips, knees and ankles adopting the antero-posterior position, with the legs straight and the hips positioned at the top end of the rulers' scales.
- Three separate exposures are made, with the X-ray beam collimated and centred midway between the hip joints, knee joints and ankle joints, starting first at the hips so that their image is recorded on the top third of the radiograph. The process is repeated so that the knees occupy the middle third and the ankles the lower third of the radiograph.
- Inaccuracy of the measurement due to using the technique is insignificant since the central ray is perpendicular to the cassette at the appropriate level of each joint.
- The exposure is adjusted accordingly at each of the joints to ensure that the density and contrast at each joint are similar. The dose may be reduced accordingly by removing the grid from the Bucky mechanism.

Digital fluoroscopy method

This method employs the use of a remote-controlled digital fluoroscopy unit and specialist software to enable reconstruction and measurement of distances and angles.

During this process, images are acquired in stages of the lower limbs, as the image intensifier and X-ray tube are moved in a vertical direction from hips to ankles at a constant speed so that the images overlap slightly with each other.

A special ruler located in a central position is also imaged during this process to enable reconstruction and calibration. The overlapped images are then reconstructed into one overview image, using reconstruction software, after which calibration of distances is performed. The operator having defined measurement settings, landmarks are applied to the image and measurements taken. This procedure has negligible magnification error and a minimal parallax effect.

The patient is positioned with both legs as straight as possible. Lead pennies are placed under the weight-bearing part of the patient's heels, and a wooden block may be placed under the shorter limb. To improve image quality, X-ray compensating filters are positioned between the legs and adjacent to the ankles. Right and left anatomical markers are attached to the tabletop so that they do not overlap with the patient's bone.

The elbow can be one of the most difficult examinations to interpret in children, and excellent technique is required.

The most common injury in children is a fracture of the lower end of the humerus, just above the condyles (supracondylar fracture). Not only is the injury very painful, but also careless handling of the limb can aggravate the injury, causing further damage to the adjacent nerves and blood vessels.

The arm should not be extended forcibly, and rotation of the limb should be avoided.

Radiography is often also undertaken with the elbow flexed in plaster or in a sling. Any supporting sling should not be removed.

As with the adult, radiography is undertaken using antero-posterior and lateral projections, with an additional antero-posterior oblique used to detect a fracture of the radial head. However, children are sometimes reluctant to extend their elbow for the antero-posterior projection. Modification of the basic technique is necessary, with images acquired with the child erect or supine, so that the child may be able to extend the arm more easily.

It is important that both antero-posterior and lateral images are acquired with all three joints in the same plane in order to demonstrate any displacement of the humerus.

Lateral (alternative positioning)

Child supine/prone

- When examining a baby, it is preferable to lay the patient prone on a soft pillow or pad, as shown opposite.
- The unaffected arm is placed by the side of the trunk, with the head turned towards the affected side and the affected elbow flexed and gently raised on to the cassette.
- The carer immobilizes the patient by holding the wrist on the affected side, with the other hand placed firmly across the patient's back.
- It may be necessary to angle the X-ray tube to direct the central ray perpendicular to the shaft of the humerus, centring on the lateral epicondyle.
- If the child is cooperative, they may be seated on the holder's lap, with the elbow flexed and placed on a cassette.

Child standing

- This projection should be undertaken such that any supporting sling is not removed.
- A cassette is supported vertically in a cassette holder.
- The child is stood sideways, with the elbow flexed and the lateral aspect of the injured elbow in contact with the cassette. The arm is gently extended backwards from the shoulder. The child is then rotated forwards until the elbow is clear of the rib cage but still in contact with the cassette, with the line joining the epicondyles of the humerus at right-angles to the cassette.
- The horizontal central ray is directed to the medial epicondyle and the beam collimated to the elbow.

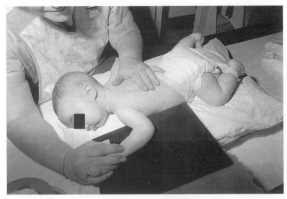
Baby positioned for lateral projection in prone position

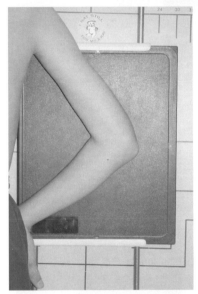
Child positioned erect for lateral projection

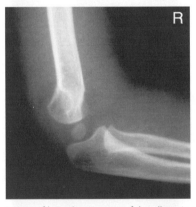
Image of lateral projection of the elbow in a young infant demonstrating a supracondylar fracture (capitellum is posterior to the anterior humeral line)

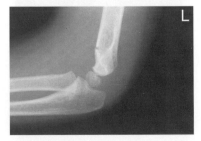
Lateral image of a supracondylar fracture in an older child

Antero-posterior (alternative positioning)

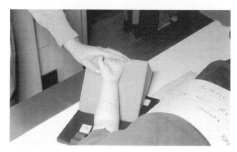

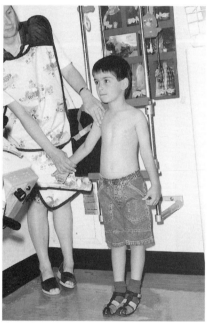

Child positioned supine for antero-posterior projection: (top) elbow extended, (bottom) elbow flexed

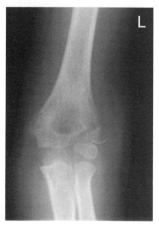

Child positioned erect for antero-posterior projection

Child supine

- The patient lies supine on the imaging couch or patient trolley with the shoulder and hip of the unaffected side raised to bring the side being examined into contact with the cassette.
- The arm is slightly abducted and extended or, if not possible, slightly flexed with forearm supported on a foam pad. Medial and lateral epicondyles should be equidistant from the cassette.
- Specific oblique views of the radial head can also be performed if there is significant clinical suspicion.
- The vertical central ray is directed midway between the epicondyles.

Child standing

- For the antero-posterior projection, a cassette is supported vertically in a cassette holder.
- The patient can either stand or sit with their back to the cassette. The arm is abducted slightly, and the trunk is rotated until the posterior aspect of the upper arm is in contact with the cassette, with the epicondyles of the humerus equidistant from the cassette.
- If the elbow is flexed fully, the central ray is directed at right-angles to the humerus to pass through the forearm to a point midway between the epicondyles.
- If there is less flexion at the elbow, it should be possible to direct the horizontal central ray to the midpoint between the epicondyles, without the X-ray beam having to pass through the forearm.

Radiation protection

- Patients must sit lateral to the X-ray table and not with their legs under the table.
- Avoid the holder's hands in the X-ray beam.
- All holders must wear a lead apron.
- Accurate coning of the LBD is essential.

Image of antero-posterior projection of the elbow demonstrating lateral condylar fracture

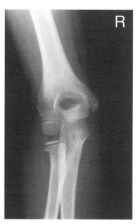

Image of antero-posterior elbow demonstrating a Salter–Harris II fracture of radial neck

Common faults and remedies

- Suboptimal view of the humerus and radial head due to the child being unable to extend the elbow and radiograph being taken with point of elbow balanced on the cassette. See above for how to avoid this.
- If the child is unable to extend the elbow, or if the elbow is flexed in a plaster cast, initially the humerus should be placed parallel to the cassette to best demonstrate a supracondylar fracture. If in acute trauma no fracture is evident on this radiograph, then a repeat image is acquired with the forearm parallel to the cassette to demonstrate the proximal radius and ulna.
- Forearm pronated instead of correct supination.
- Rotated joint. The joints of the shoulder, elbow and wrist should be in the same plane to obtain best positioning.

Essential image characteristics

Antero-posterior projection of elbow:

- Distal end of humerus should be straight, with no rotation or foreshortening.
- Radius and ulna should be parallel and aligned with the humerus, allowing for the carrying angle.
- Radial head should not overlap the capitellum.
- Coning should include distal thirds of the humerus and proximal thirds of the radius and ulna.
- Cortex and trabecular structures should be visually sharp.
- Reproduction of muscle/fat planes.

Lateral projection of elbow:

- Humerus should be in true lateral position, with superimposition of the condyles.
- Humerus should be at right-angles to the radius and ulna.
- Coning should include distal third of humerus and proximal thirds of radius and ulna.
- Soft tissue detail should include the coronoid and olecranon fat pads if displaced.
- Cortex and trabecular structures should be visually sharp.
- Reproduction of muscle/fat planes.

Radiological considerations

- A good knowledge of ossification centres around the elbow is required, with suitable texts (e.g. Keats and Anderson 2001) being available to avoid the necessity for comparison views.
- The radio-capitellar line should pass through the radius and mid-capitellum on both projections.
- The anterior humeral line should pass through the anterior third of the capitellum on the lateral projection.
- The ossification centres appear in order of the pneumonic CRITOE (capitellum, radius, internal epicondyle, trochlea, olecranon and external epicondyle).

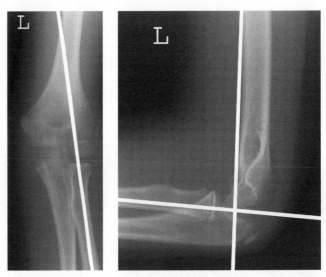

Antero-posterior and lateral radiographs of the elbow showing ossification centres, anterior humeral line and radio-capitellar line

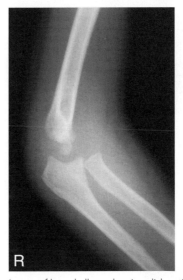

Image of lateral elbow showing dislocation of the radial head and olecranon fracture

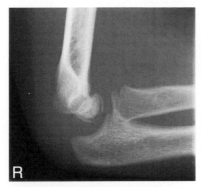

Image of lateral elbow showing Salter – Harris III fracture of the capitellum

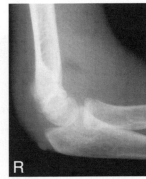

Image of lateral elbow showing joint effusion

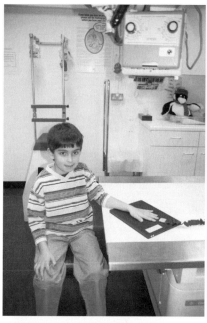

Child positioned for dorsi-palmar projection of a non-dominant hand

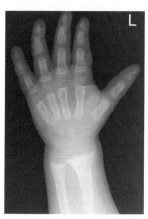

Image of a postero-anterior hand in an 18-month-old child with cystinosis and rickets who has delayed bone age of 6 months (G&P)

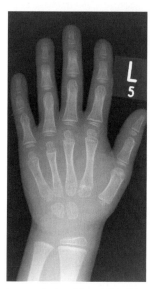

Image of a hand in a child of 6 years and 10 months with growth hormone deficiency and a dissociated bone age. The phalangeal bone age is 5 years and the carpal bone age is 2 years (G&P)

Recommended projections

There are two main methods of bone age assessment: atlas matching by Greulich and Pyle (Greulich and Pyle 1959) and the point scoring system by Tanner and Whitehouse (Tanner *et al.* 1983). Slightly different results are produced and the same method should be used for serial measurements.

The non-dominant hand should be selected.

The protocol requires a dorsi-palmar projection of the whole hand, including all digits and the wrist joint.

The fingers should be straight, with the metaphyses in profile.

Radiography of the dorsi-palmar projection of the hand is described on p. 40.

The determination of osseous maturation is based on the number, size and appearance of the ossification centres and on the width of the growth plate or the degree of fusion present.

Radiological considerations

Girls are more advanced than boys, and separate standards are available. Nineteen of 20 children are within two standard deviations (SDs) from the mean of their chronological age. The SDs vary with age, and any assessment of bone age should include the degree of deviation from the mean and value of one SD at that age.

If there are no ossification centres visible in the carpus, then an antero-posterior of the knee can be taken to demonstrate the presence of the distal femoral and proximal tibial ossification centres, which appear at 36 and 37 weeks, respectively.

Children with retarded or advanced bone ages may be short or tall for their age. Children with advanced bone age may undergo premature fusion of the epiphyses and be short in adult life. A predicted adult height can be obtained from standard tables, which require an assessment of current height and bone age.

Bone age is normally required in patients suspected of having an underlying endocrine abnormality and is commonly requested in patients with precocious puberty. A bone age is also performed in patients with suspected significant nutritional deficiency, chronic disease and possible underlying syndrome. Occasionally, the diagnosis of a syndrome can be inferred from the hand radiograph, e.g. Turner's syndrome, with such patients having short fourth and fifth metacarpals.

14 Feet – supported/ weight-bearing projections

Radiographic examination of the feet, with the child standing weight-bearing, is undertaken in the assessment of:

- talipes (congenital foot deformity present at birth);
- painful flat foot.

Recommended projections

Examination of the affected foot is undertaken for both babies and toddlers using the following projections:

Basic	Dorsi-plantar (antero-posterior) – weight-bearing
	Lateral – weight-bearing
Supplementary	Lateral – with forced dorsiflexion
	Dorsi-plantar oblique

Dorsi-plantar – weight-bearing

A cassette is selected that is large enough to include the foot.

Position of patient and cassette

Babies

- The baby is supported supine on the X-ray table, and the knee of the affected side is flexed so that the foot rests on the cassette.
- The foot is adjusted so that the tibia is perpendicular to the cassette.
- Both feet may be examined together, with the knees held together.
- Pressure should be applied to the bent knee to simulate weight-bearing.

Toddlers

- The toddler is seated in a special seat, with both feet resting on the cassette in a similar way as that described above. Or, if the child is old enough, they adopt a standing position.
- Downward pressure is applied to both knees.
- No attempt should be made to correct alignment of forefeet.

Direction and centring of the X-ray beam

- The vertical central ray is directed midway between the malleoli and at right-angles to an imaginary line joining the malleoli.
- The central ray may be angled five to 10 degrees cephalic to avoid the tibiae overlapping the hind feet.

Essential image characteristics

- The alignment of the talus and calcaneus of the hind foot should be clearly visible, with no overlapping by the shins.
- Visualization of the bones of the feet consistent with age.
- Visualization of the soft tissue planes.
- Reproduction of the spongiosa and cortex.

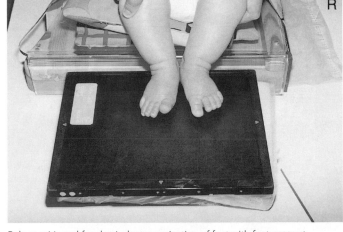

Baby positioned for dorsi-plantar projection of feet with feet support

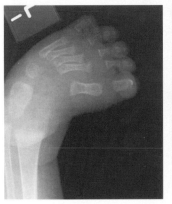 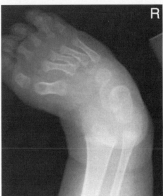

Image of dorsi-plantar feet in a baby with talipes equinovarus. Note calcaneus and talus are parallel and superimposed

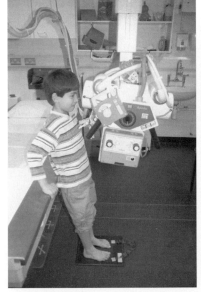 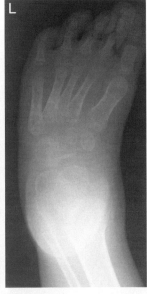

Left: older child positioned for weight-bearing, dorsi-plantar projection of feet. Note the slight posterior lean to avoid the long bones overlying and obscuring the hind feet. Right: image of 4-year-old boy's foot with corrected CTEV and residual varus of the forefoot

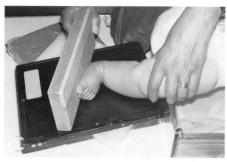

Baby positioned for lateral projection of foot with pressure applied by a wood block support in order to try and correct any equinus deformity of the ankle

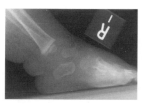 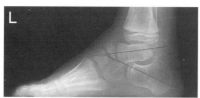

Image of lateral foot in neonate and older child with talipes equinovarus demonstrating talus and calcaneus parallel in former and dorsal dislocation of navicular in the corrected foot of the latter

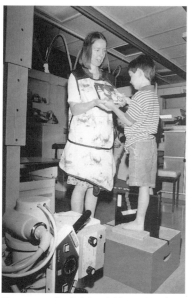

Photototograph of older child standing for a lateral projection of the foot

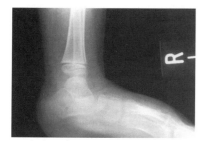

Image of lateral foot of a child hind foot valgus and almost vertical talus in a patient with cerebral palsy

Lateral – weight bearing

A cassette is selected that is large enough to include the foot.

Position of patient and cassette

Babies

- With the baby supine on the imaging couch, the affected leg is preferably internally rotated so that the inner border of the foot is placed against the cassette with the ankle (not fore-foot) in the true lateral position. Alternatively, the leg is externally rotated, with the lateral aspect of the foot against the cassette.
- A wooden block support is positioned beneath the sole of the foot, with dorsiflexion pressure applied during exposure to demonstrate the reducibility of any equinus deformity at the ankle.

Toddlers

- The child can be examined standing, with a cassette placed in a groove against the inner foot.
- To stop the foot from being inverted, the leg should not be externally rotated.
- Forced dorsi-/plantarflexion views may also be required.

Direction and centring of the X-ray beam

- The central ray is directed to the lateral/medial malleolus at right-angles to the axis of the tibia. For toddlers, the beam is directed horizontally.

Essential image characteristics

- The alignment of the talus and calcaneus in the true lateral position should be clearly visible.
- The sole of the foot should be flat against the block, with no elevation of the heel.
- See dorsi-plantar projection characteristics, above.

Common faults and remedies

- For the dorsi-plantar projection, the shins often obscure the hind feet. Angle the beam 10 degrees cephalad to overcome this problem.
- The density of the image (dorsi-plantar) is correctly appropriate for forefeet but does not demonstrate the hind-foot, which is more important. A wedge can be used to avoid over-penetration of the forefeet.
- For the lateral projection, care should be taken to avoid oblique projection of the foot as this could simulate a valgus/varus position.

14 Feet – supported/weight-bearing projections

Radiological considerations

Foot radiographs should allow correct assessment of the alignment of the bones of the hindfoot, midfoot and forefoot. Various terminology is used to describe their position.

The term **talipes** originates in an old description of a patient walking on his ankle (talus) rather than the foot (pes). The terms **calcaneus** and **equinus** refer to the position of the foot in relation to the ankle. The former indicates dorsiflexion with elevation of the anterior end of the calcaneum and equinus indicates plantarflexion of the calcaneum like a horse's foot

Hindfoot varus

Hindfoot varus means that an axial reference line through the calcaneum is deviated towards the midline of the body. The degree of varus angulation is determined by measurement of the talo-calcaneal angle on an antero-posterior projection, which will be decreased leading to parallelism and overlapping of the talus and the calcaneus. The long axis of the talus (midtalar line) passes lateral to the base of the first metatarsal and the talus and calcaneus are also parallel on the lateral view.

Hindfoot valgus

Hindfoot valgus means that an axial reference line though the calcaneum is deviated away from the midline of the body. The talo-calcaneal angle on an antero-posterior projection of the foot will be increased and similarly on the lateral projection, leading to a more vertical talus.

The talo-calcaneal angles vary with age and should be compared with recognized tables (Keats and Sistrom, 2001). However, it is to be noted that calculated angles are not always abnormal in abnormal feet.

Lateral radiographs allow assessment of the plantar arch. Increased height of the arch (**cavum arch**) is associated with valgus/varus foot deformities. A flattened arch (**pes planus**) may be due to a flexible flat foot, tarsal coalition or other congenital conditions.

Congenital talipes equinovarus (CTEV or club foot) is the most common abnormality. This consists of hindfoot equinus, hindfoot varus and forefoot varus. It occurs in 1–4/1000 live births, males being more commonly affected, it is usually idiopathic and there is a slight genetic preponderance.

Congenital talipes calcaneus is a common neonatal condition which normally corrects spontaneously but those with valgus of the calcaneum may have underlying hip dislocation.

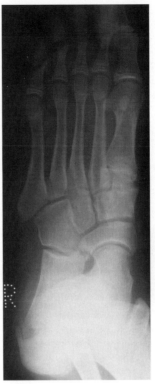

Dorsi-plantar oblique image of a right foot demonstrating calcaneo-navicular coalition

Congenital vertical talus produces a more severe valgus deformity. Eighty percent are associated with syndromes or CNS disorders. The vertical talus and equinus of the calcaneum produce a convex plantar arch (rocker bottom foot).

Metatarsus adductus, which should be distinguished from CTEV, has a normal hindfoot with adduction of the forefoot and most correct with passive reduction.

Tarsal coalition

If a tarsal coalition is suspected because of a painful flat foot, evidence of talar beaking should be sought on the lateral image, which may be due to talo-calcaneal fusion, for which CT is required for confirmation. A dorsi-plantar oblique (45 degrees) projection of the foot is necessary for the demonstration of a calcaneo-navicular coalition. Both forms of coalition can be fibrous/osseous.

Note

Foot deformities need careful positioning, and analysis of the derangement and care must be taken to produce high-quality radiographs. Radiographs should be performed weight-bearing or with stressed dorsiflexion in order to appreciate the true alignment and to determine the degree of unreducable equinus in patients with CTEV.

Examples of various foot derangements are shown overleaf.

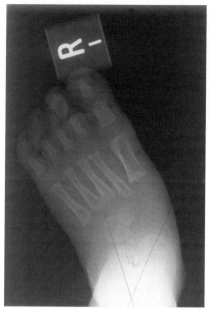

Neonate - right dorsi-plantar calcaneovalgus right foot

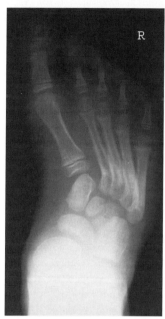

Older child - dorsi-plantar with skew-foot

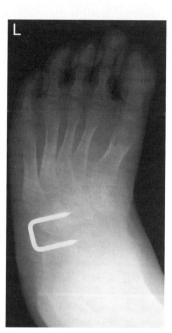

Dorsi-plantar left foot on older child with CTEV following cuboid osteotomy and calcaneo-cuboid stapling

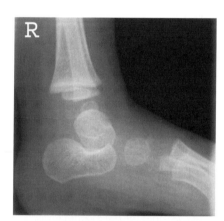

Neonate – lateral foot with calcaneovalgus and vertical talus

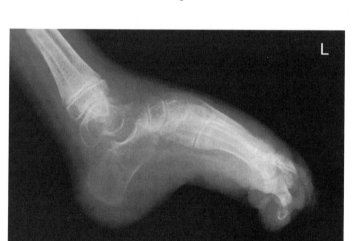

Recumbant image of lateral foot demonstrating pes cavus in a patient with cerebral palsy

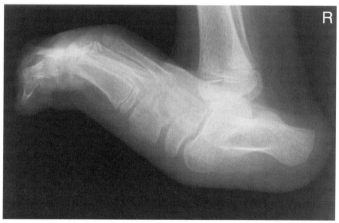

Recumbant lateral foot showing severe planus valgus and a vertical talus in a patient with a meningomyelocele

14 Skeletal survey for non-accidental injury

A skeletal survey is the main radiological investigation for NAI. It comprises a series of images taken to assess the whole skeleton.

Evidence of NAI to children is an all too common occurrence in any department dealing routinely with children. It can result in serious long-term emotional and physical injuries. The latter include serious neurological deficits, mental retardation and in, the worst cases, death of the child.

Certain skeletal injuries in this condition are highly suspicious. Posterior rib fractures (Kleinman and Schlesinger 1997) and metaphyseal fractures are almost pathognomonic of NAI. Carefully evaluated, well-collimated, high-detail, skeletal radiographs are vital in all cases of suspected infant abuse (Carty 1997, Kleinman and Marks 1992, Nimkin and Kleinman 1997, Nimkin et al. 1997).

Rationale for projections

A skeletal survey is needed to demonstrate pathology, but it is equally important in dating skeletal injuries, as accurate evaluation and dating of these injuries will be vital in providing legal argument (Kleinman et al. 1989). This may require further views of certain specific areas, and this has to be tailored to the appearances of the initial injuries and to the clinical history given (Kleinman et al. 1996).

Post-mortem skeletal studies may also be required in some cases and can provide useful additional information (Thomsen et al. 1997).

It is rarely, if ever, necessary for a skeletal survey to be performed by junior staff outside normal hours (see radiological considerations).

Referral criteria

The referral criteria that would justify a skeletal survey are as follows:

Criteria	Examples
Clinical suspicion	• Skin lesions • Retinal haemorrhage • Torn frenulum under the age of 3 years
Incidental detection of suspicious fractures on radiographs taken for other reasons	• Skull fractures > 6 mm wide • Fractures that do not correspond with the history given • Fractures that are older than the history given • More than one fracture of differing age • Metaphyseal fractures • Posterior or anterior rib fractures • Long bone fractures <1 year • Abnormal periosteal reactions

Occult bony injury is rare over three years of age, and most NAI surveys are performed on infants under two years of age. They are also indicated in siblings under two years of age when the index case is proven NAI.

Projections

The projections advised below are suggested by the RCR (British Society of Paediatric Radiologists, BSPR). Fifty per cent of rib fractures are occult, compared with 20% of limb fractures, and as they are diagnostically important, oblique rib projections are justified. Oblique views of the hands are preferred as they are more likely to show buckle and subtle cortical fractures (Nimkin et al. 1997).

The advised projections are as follows:

- antero-posterior chest (chest to show all ribs, clavicles and shoulders);
- abdomen (to include pelvis);
- antero-posterior right and left femur (to include hip and knee joints and upper two-thirds of tibia and fibula);
- antero-posterior right and left ankle (to include distal third of tibia and fibula);
- antero-posterior right and left humerus;
- antero-posterior right and left forearm;
- lateral cervical, thoracic and lumbar spines;
- antero-posterior skull, lateral skull (and Towne's if occipital fracture suspected);
- oblique ribs (may be delayed by up to 10 days);
- anterior oblique of both hands;
- antero-posterior both feet;
- coned/lateral views of fractures or abnormalities.

The practice of imaging the entire body on one radiograph 'babygram' should never be performed. This is a totally inadequate and uninterpretable examination. Two healthcare personnel should always be present in the room for the examination, e.g. radiographer and nurse. Both should sign the radiograph and request form, and the timing of the examination should be recorded accurately. This is important for legal documentation. In the case of digital imaging and electronic request forms, a signed record should be made in the patient's notes.

Current recommendations are that a CT of the head should routinely be performed under one year of age and with a very low threshold for those under two years of age, to exclude associated subdural collections.

Radiological considerations

A high index of suspicion is required. However, a skeletal survey should be requested only following discussion between the consultant paediatrician and consultant radiologist, as the radiation dose from an inappropriate skeletal survey should be avoided and is just as much a reason for litigation as failure to identify fractures. It requires radiologist involvement to ensure diagnostic quality, to allow additional projections of any injury to be taken, and to suggest the timing of any repeat studies. The outcome, whether positive or negative, may have huge implications (for the family especially). Good clinico-radiological cooperation at the highest level is vital, supported by the highest standard of radiography.

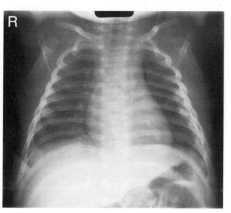

Antero-posterior chest showing bilateral anterior rib fractures

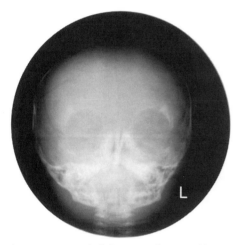

Antero-posterior skull showing right parietal fracture

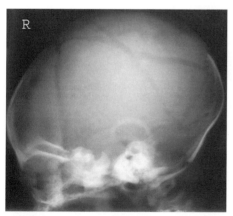

Image of lateral skull showing biparietal fractures

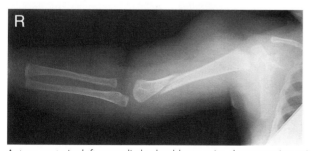

Antero-posterior left upper limb, shoulder to wrist, demonstrating spiral fracture of the humerus

Radiation protection

Well-collimated, carefully positioned images provide not only a far higher quality but also a lower radiation dose. Higher-kVp techniques with additional filtration are usually recommended as dose-saving measures in paediatrics. However, in an NAI survey, low kVp/high mAs should be employed for best demonstration of bony detail and soft tissues. It may be advised to avoid additional filtration (inherent of approximately 2.5 mm aluminium) because it will have the most detrimental effect on image quality when low-kVp techniques are used.

Radiographic technique

Well-tried and tested restraining methods are most important in performing skeletal surveys to ensure high quality.

A patient, careful, non-judgemental approach is essential, and full explanation should have been given to the parents by the requesting clinician. Patient positioning and X-ray beam centring has already been described for the individual examinations, but there are some differences in technique, which are outlined below.

Chest/abdomen

- Shoulders and all ribs should be included on the image.
- A minimum of 400-speed class film/screen system is used to reduce movement unsharpness.
- The tube potential should be between 60 and 70 kVp to ensure optimum bony detail.

Spine (cervical, thoracic and lumbar)

- A minimum of 400-speed class film/screen system is used to reduce movement unsharpness.
- A single lateral image is acquired without the use of a grid in children under three years of age.
- Tube potential up to 70 kVp.

Skull

- The antero-posterior and lateral images are acquired without the use of a grid if the child is under one year of age.
- The lateral image is acquired using a lateral horizontal beam.
- Tube potential up to 70 kVp.

Upper and lower limbs

- A 200-speed class film/screen system and 45–60-kVp range is used to provide optimum soft tissue and bony detail.
- Separate images of the humerus and radius and ulna are normally acquired after 18 months of age.
- Separate images of the femur and tibia and fibula are acquired. The image of the femur should include the knee joint.
- May need adhesive tape ruler/strapping for restraint (see p. 430).

Common faults and remedies

- Views of epiphyses and metaphyses in profile are needed to show the classical metaphyseal fractures as corner fractures. The actual fracture occurs right across the metaphysis. If the radiographic beam is divergent or the metaphyses are tilted, then the fracture appears as a bucket-handle fracture, but this can easily be missed or thought to be due to a normal variation in the appearance of the ossification of the metaphyses. Correct interpretation needs precise technique.

- An attempt to radiograph the whole leg together should be avoided. Immobilization can be provided only at the feet, and excessive plantarflexion whilst holding can result in tilted metaphyses and the heels obscuring the ankle joints.

Essential image characteristics

- These are as described for the individual anatomical areas. Extremely good-quality radiographs are essential, with excellent bone and soft tissue detail.

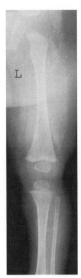
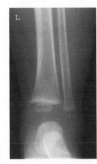

Image of antero-posterior left ankle with the ankle straight and the beam straight allowing an 'end-on' appearance of the metaphysis

Radiograph of left femur and upper two-thirds of tibia and fibula and ankle separately imaged

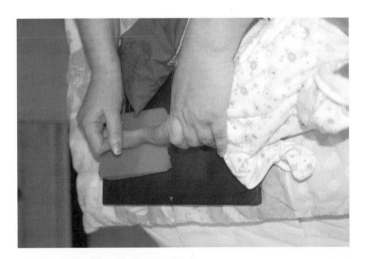

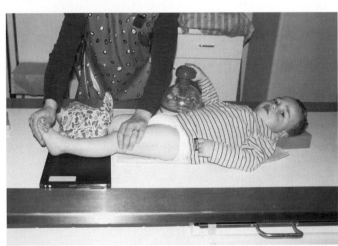

Holding of patient in optimal position for demonstration of left lower limb

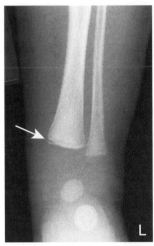

Image of left ankle of a neonate with a corner tibial fracture

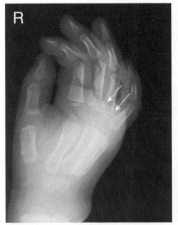
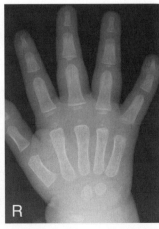

Image of oblique position of right hand. Note fractures of the third and fourth proximal phalanges not seen on the dorsi-palmar projection of the same patient (left)

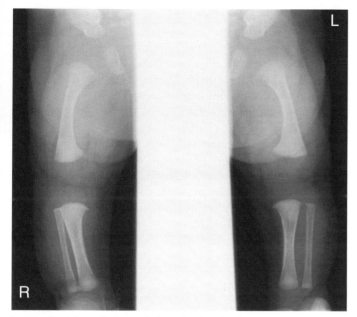

Image of both lower limbs in a baby with achondroplasia

A similar technique can be used for syndrome assessment.

The radiographs performed will depend on the suspected syndrome or clinically visible abnormalities. However, a syndrome skeletal survey will normally include:

- antero-posterior skull;
- lateral skull;
- postero-anterior/antero-posterior chest;
- antero-posterior whole spine;
- lateral whole spine;
- pelvis;
- antero-posterior both whole legs, separately or together on one image depending on ease of handling;
- postero-anterior of non-dominant hand for bone age.

Notes

- Additional radiographs of the upper limbs, hand and feet can be performed if there is clinical deformity.
- Lateral projections may be required for bowed limbs.

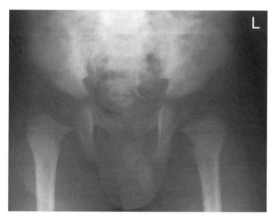

Image of antero-posterior hips in a patient with a vitamin D-resistant rickets

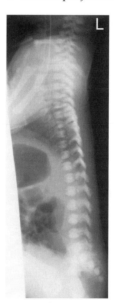

Image of lateral spine in a child with Jeune's asphyxiating thoracic dystrophy with very short ribs

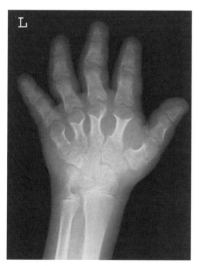

Image of a postero-anterior hand in a child with acrodysostosis

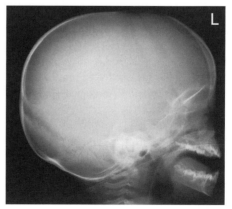

Image of a lateral skull radiograph demonstrating a J-shaped sella

14 Acknowledgements

We would like to thank Mrs Wendy Appleby and Mrs Jane Radford for their much-valued support in the typing and layout of the text. We would also like to thank Mr M Fitzgerald, Mr J Kyriou and Mrs A Pettet (Radiological Protection Centre, St George's Hospital, London) and Dr S M Pablot and Dr Mary Warren (Queen Mary's Hospital for Children, Epsom and St Helier University NHS Trust, Carshalton, Surrey) for their respected and extremely useful comments, encouragement and honest opinion. Also Mr Robert Wade and the Medical Illustration Department at Queen Mary's Hospital for Children for their much appreciated attention given to providing most of the illustrations.

We are also very grateful to the Medical Engineering Research Unit (MERU) at QMHC for their assistance and skills in producing the immobilization device with Perspex top and wooden cassette holder, the chest stand with seat and the various shaped coning devices and filters described in the text. They have all been designed by Kaye Shah and the staff of QMHC.

Further acknowledgements

We would also like to express our sincere thanks to Stewart Whitley and all the members of staff of Blackpool Victoria Hospital and Alder Hey Hospital, Liverpool, for the contributions on the Denton skull radiography technique and alternative techniques for the leg lengthening.

References

Almen A, Loof M, Mattsson S (1996). Examination technique, image quality, and patient dose in paediatric radiology. A survey including 19 Swedish hospitals. *Acta Radiol* **37**(3 Part 1): 337–42.

Andersen PE Jr, Andersen PE, van der Kooy P (1982). Dose reduction in radiography of the spine in scoliosis. *Acta Radiol* **23**:251–3.

Arena L, Baker SR (1990). Use of a metal detector to identify ingested metallic foreign bodies. *Am J Roentgenol* **155**:803–4.

Boulis ZF, Dick R, Barnes NR (1978). Head injuries in children – aetiology, symptoms, physical findings and x ray wastage. *Br J Radiol* **51**:851–4.

Carty H (1997). Non-accidental injury: a review of the radiology. *Eur Radiol* **7**:1365–76.

Cook JV, Shah K, Pablot S, Kyriou J, Pettet A, Fitzgerald M. (1998). *Guidelines on Best Practice in the X Ray Imaging of Children*. London: Queen Mary's Hospital for Children, Epsom and St Helier University NHS Trust and Radiological Protection Centre, St George's Hospital.

Denton BK (1998). Improving plain radiography of the skull: the half-axial projection re-described. *Synergy* August, pp. 9–11.

Dhar S, Dangerfield PH, Dorgan JC, Klenerman L (1993). Correlation between bone age and Risser's sign in adolescent idiopathic scoliosis. *Spine* **18**:14–19.

European Commission (1996). *European Guidelines on Quality Criteria for Diagnostic Radiographic Images in Paediatrics*. Luxembourg: Office for Official Publications of the European Communities. (Available from HMSO Books, London.)

Garniak A, Feivel M, Hertz M, Tadmor R (1986). Skull X-rays in head trauma: are they still necessary? A review of 1000 cases. *Eur J Radiol* **6**:89–91.

Greulich WW, Pyle SI (1959). *Radiographic Atlas of Skeletal Development of the Hand and Wrist*. Stanford, CA: Stanford University Press.

Hansson B, Finnbogason T, Schuwert P, Persliden J (1997). Added copper filtration in digital paediatric double-contrast colon examinations: effects on radiation dose and image quality. *Eur Radiol* **7**:1117–22.

Hart D, Wall BF, Shrimpton PC, Bungay DR, Dance DR (2000). *Reference Doses and Patient Size in Paediatric Radiology*. Chilton: National Radiological Protection Board.

Hilton SvW, Edwards DK (1994). *Practical Paediatric Radiology*. Philadelphia: W.B. Saunders.

Hochschild TJ, Cremin BJ (1975). Technique in infant chest radiography. *Radiography* Jan **41**(481):21–5.

Hufton AP, Doyle SM, Carty HM (1998). Digital radiography in paediatrics: radiation dose considerations and magnitude of possible dose reduction. *Br J Radiol* **71**:186–99.

Ilizarov GA (1988) The principles of the Ilizarov method. *Bull Hospital Joint Dis Orthop Inst* Spring **48**(1):1–11.

Institute of Physics and Engineering in Medicine (2004). IPEM Report 88 *Guidance on the Establishment of Diagnostic Reference Levels for Medical X ray Examination*. York: IPEM.

Jonsson A, Jonsson K, Eklund K, Holje G, Pettersson H (1995). Computed radiography in scoliosis. Diagnostic information and radiation dose. *Acta Radiol* **26**:429–33.

Keats TE, Anderson MW (2001). *Atlas of Normal Roentgen Variants that May Simulate Disease* 7th edn. St Louis, MO: Mosby.

Keats TE, Sistrom C (2001). *Atlas of Radiologic Measurement* 7th edn. St Louis, MO: Mosby.

Kleinman PK, Marks SC (1992). Vertebral body fractures in child abuse. Radiologic-histopathological correlates. *Invest Radiol* **27**:715–22.

Kleinman PK, Schlesinger AE (1997). Mechanical factors associated with posterior rib fractures: laboratory and case studies. *Pediatr Radiol* **27**:87–91.

Kleinman PK, Blackbourne BD, Marks SC, Karellas A, Belanger PL (1989). Radiologic contributions to the investigation and prosecution of cases of fatal infant abuse. *N Engl J Med* **320**:507–11.

Kleinman PK, Nimkin K, Spevak MR, Rayder SM, Madansky DL, Shelton YA, Patterson MM (1996). Follow-up skeletal surveys in suspected child abuse. *Am J Roentgenol* **167**:893–6.

Kottamasu SR, Kuhns LR (1997). Musculoskeletal computed radiography in children: scatter reduction and improvement in bony trabecular sharpness using air gap placement of the imaging plate. *Pediatr Radiol* **27**:119–23.

Kyriou JC, Fitzgerald M, Pettet A, Cook JV, Pablot SM (1996). A comparison of doses and techniques between specialist and non-specialist centres in the diagnostic X-ray imaging of children. *Br J Radiol* **69**:437–50.

Lloyd DA, Carty H, Patterson M, Butcher CK, Roe D (1997). Predictive value of skull radiography for intracranial injury in children with blunt head injury. *Lancet* **349**:821–4.

Lowe A, Finch A, Boniface D, Chaudhuri R, Shekhdar J (1999). Diagnostic image quality of mobile neonatal chest x-rays and the radiation exposure incurred. *Br J Radiol* **72**:55–61.

Marshall NW, Faulkner K, Busch HP, March DM, Pfenning H (1994). A comparison of radiation dose in examination of the abdomen using different radiological imaging techniques. *Br J Radiol* **67**:478–84.

Masters SJ, McClean PM, Arcarese JS *et al.* (1987). Skull X-ray examinations after head trauma. Recommendations by a multi disciplinary panel and validation study. *N Engl J Med* **316**:84–91.

McDaniel DL, Cohen G, Wagner LK, Robinson LH (1984). Relative dose efficiencies of antiscatter grids and air gaps in paediatric radiography. *Med Phys* **11**:508–12.

McDonald S, Martin CJ, Darragh CL, Graham DT (1996). Dose-area product measurements in paediatric radiography. *Br J Radiol* **69**:318–25.

McParland BJ, Gorka W, Lee R, Lewall DB, Omojola MF (1996). Radiology in the neonatal intensive care unit: dose reduction and image quality. *Br J Radiol* **69**:929–37.

Mooney R, Thomas PS (1998). Dose reduction in a paediatric x-ray department following optimization of radiographic technique. *Br J Radiol* **71**:852–60.

Nimkin K, Kleinman PK (1997). Imaging of child abuse. *Pediatr Clin North Am* **44**:615–35.

Nimkin K, Spevak MR, Kleinman PK (1997). Fractures of the hands and feet in child abuse: imaging and pathologic features. *Radiology* **203**:233–6.

Rosenbaum AE, Arnold BA (1978). Postero-anterior radiography: a method for reduction of eye dose. *Radiology* **129**:812.

Royal College of Radiologists (2003). *Making the Best Use of a Department of Clinical Radiology*, 5th edn. London: Royal College of Radiologists.

Ryan J, Tidey B (1994). Metal detectors to detect aluminium. *Br Med J* **309**:131.

Ruiz MJ, Gonzalez L, Vano E, Martinez A (1991). Measurement of radiation doses in the most frequent simple examinations in paediatric radiology and its dependence on patient age. *Br J Radiol* **64**:929–33.

Thomsen TK, Elle B, Thomsen JL (1997). Post mortem examination in infants: evidence of child abuse? *Forensic Sci Int* **90**:223–30.

Tanner JM, Whitehouse RH, Cameron N, Marshall WA, Healy MJR, Goldstein H (1983). *Assessment of Skeletal Maturity and Prediction of Height* 2nd edn. London: Academic Press.

United Nations Scientific Committee on the Effects of Atomic Radiation (2000). *Unscear Report: Sources and Effects of Ionizing Radiation* Vol. II. Vienna: United Nations Scientific Committee on the Effects of Atomic Radiation.

Vano E, Oliete S, Gonzalez L, Guibelalde E, Velasco A, Fernandez JM (1995). Image quality and dose in lumbar spine examinations: results of a 5 year quality control programme following the European quality criteria trial. *Br J Radiol* **68**:1332–5.

Warren-Forward HM, Millar JS (1995). Optimization of radiographic technique for chest radiography. *Br J Radiol* **68**:1221–9.

Wraith CM, Martin CJ, Stockdale EJ, McDonald S, Farquhar B (1995). An investigation into techniques for reducing doses from neo-natal radiographic examinations. *Br J Radiol* **68**:1074–82.

Section 15

Mammography

CONTENTS

INTRODUCTION	436
Recommended projections	436
Positioning terminology	437
Female breast anatomy	438
X-ray equipment features	439
General features	439
Image acquisition	440
Exposure factors	440
Film identification	440
Imaging parameters	440
Diagnostic requirements	440
Criteria for good imaging performance	440
Example of good radiographic technique	441
Processing	441
Radiation protection	442
Quality assurance	442
Overview of the UK Breast Screening Service	443
RADIOLOGICAL CONSIDERATIONS	444
General comments	444
Lesion characteristics	445
Lesion diagnosis	446
Therapy-related changes	446
Other techniques	447
45-DEGREE MEDIO-LATERAL OBLIQUE (MLO) BASIC – LUNDGREN'S OBLIQUE	448
CRANIO-CAUDAL – BASIC	450
EXTENDED CRANIO-CAUDAL – LATERALLY ROTATED	452
EXTENDED CRANIO-CAUDAL – MEDIALLY ROTATED	453
EXTENDED CRANIO-CAUDAL PROJECTION	454
LATERAL PROJECTIONS	455
Medio-lateral	455
Latero-medial	456
AXILLARY TAIL	457
LOCALIZED COMPRESSION/PADDLE PROJECTIONS	458
MAGNIFIED PROJECTIONS	459
Full-field magnified projections	459
Paddle-magnified projections	459
STEREOTACTIC NEEDLE PROCEDURES	460
Technique	461
Stereotactic preoperative marker localization	461
BREAST IMPLANTS	462
CORE BIOPSY AND SPECIMEN TISSUE RADIOGRAPHY	463
Core biopsy	463
Breast tissue radiography	463

Mammography is the radiographic examination of the breast tissue (soft tissue radiography). To visualize normal structures and pathology within the breast, it is essential that sharpness, contrast and resolution are maximized. This optimizes, in the image, the relatively small differences in the absorption characteristics of the structures comprising the breast. A low kVp value, typically 28 kVp, is used. Radiation dose must be minimized due to the radio-sensitivity of breast tissue.

Mammography is carried out on both symptomatic women with a known history or suspected abnormality of the breast and as a screening procedure in well, asymptomatic woman. Consistency of radiographic technique and image quality is essential, particularly in screening mammography, where comparison with former films is often essential. Whilst other techniques such as magnetic resonance imaging (MRI) and ultrasound have a role in breast imaging, mammography is undertaken to image the breast most commonly and is hence considered in detail in this chapter.

Recommended projections

Examination is performed by means of the following projections:

Basic projections	• 45-degree medio-lateral oblique (Lundgren) • Craniocaudal
Supplementary projections	• Extended cranio-caudal laterally rotated • Extended cranio-caudal medially rotated • Extended cranio-caudal • Medio-lateral • Latero-medial • Axillary tail • Localized compression/paddle • Magnified (full-field/paddle) projections

The two basic projections are done both for asymptomatic and for symptomatic women. Supplementary projections may be used if these projections fail to demonstrate a clinically detected lesion, or to demonstrate a lesion more clearly.

Author's note regarding projections

All projections are described on breasts of an average size, with the woman standing, unless otherwise stated. The projections can, however, be achieved with the woman seated, even in a wheelchair. The word 'woman' is used to describe those undergoing the examination as not all attendees for mammography will be patients. It is acknowledged that mammography is also performed on men, albeit rarely.

The exception to the use of the word 'woman' is in the heading 'Position of patient and cassette', which is retained for consistency with the rest of the book.

The heading 'Direction and centring of the X-ray beam' has been omitted from all descriptions of the projections. The linked nature of the tube and image-recording mechanism make the direction and centring of the X-ray beam implicit in the description of the position of the patient and cassette.

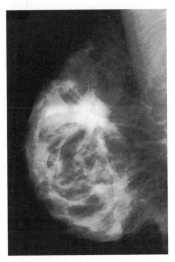

Image showing lesion with spiculated edges

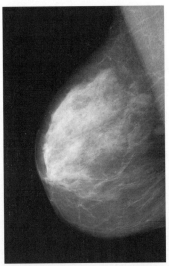

Image showing good differentiation between adjacent soft tissues

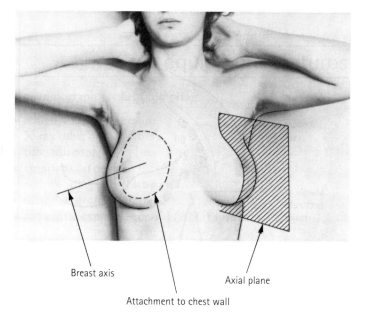

Breast axis

Attachment to chest wall

Axial plane

Positioning terminology

Despite the great individual variation in the external form of the breast, the approximately circular attachment to the chest wall is constant. Vertically the attachment extends from the second to the sixth rib, and at the level of the fourth costal cartilage it extends transversely from the side of the sternum to the mid-axillary line.

A line drawn from the centre of the circle to the nipple can be termed the **breast axis**. Two planes of importance in radiographic positioning pass through the breast axis. The **axial plane** divides the breast into inner and outer portions; the **transverse plane** lies at right-angles to the vertical axial plane, intersecting it along the breast axis. The breast is thus divided into quadrants, termed upper outer, lower outer, lower inner and upper inner, respectively. In the normal erect resting position, the axial plane makes an angle of 20–30 degrees with the sagittal plane of the body, and the transverse plane makes an angle of 30–50 degrees with the horizontal.

A prolongation into the axilla of the supero-lateral portion of the breast along the lower border of pectoralis major is called the **axillary tail**. The **retromammary space** lies behind the glandular tissue and should be visible (at least in part) on a correctly positioned mammogram. Microscopically, the breast consists of 15–20 **lobes**, supported by a **stroma** of fibrous tissue, which contains a variable quantity of fat. Each lobe has a main duct, opening in the nipple. Deeply, the ducts branch within the breast to drain **lobules**. Each lobule consists of a cluster of small **ductules**, into which the glandular **epithelium** cells pass their secretions. Lobules are demonstrated radiographically as fine, nodular opacities, individually measuring 12 mm in diameter but usually superimposed to give a more or less homogeneous opacity.

With progressive **involution**, the lobules successively shrink and become invisible. Involution commences in the subcutaneous and retromammary regions, then progresses sequentially through the lower inner quadrant, the upper inner and lower outer quadrants, and finally the upper outer quadrant.

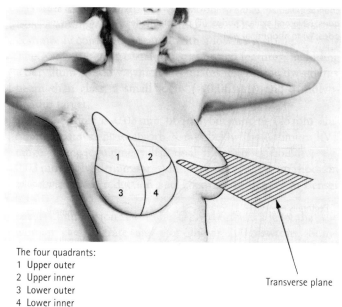

The four quadrants:
1 Upper outer
2 Upper inner
3 Lower outer
4 Lower inner

Transverse plane

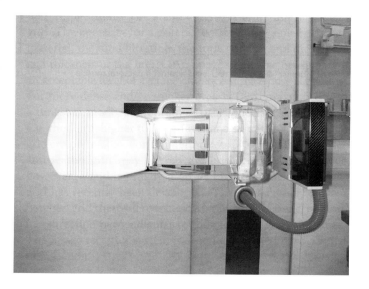

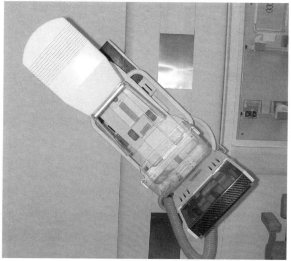

Radiation protection

Absorbed doses are high in mammography due to the low kVp necessary to maximize the small differences in attenuation between tissues in the breast. A considerable proportion of the X-ray spectrum will, at the kVp used, not contribute to image formation but will increase breast dose. The breast is one of the most radio-sensitive tissues in the body. Careful technique is essential to avoid the need for repeat projections. Gonad protection, e.g. a lead-rubber apron, should be used, particularly in young women and in projections where the primary beam is directed towards the gonads, e.g. the cranio-caudal projection. Selection of the X-ray tube target material and the filtration used is important in dose reduction. The aim is to produce optimum image contrast but minimum dose. With careful choice of target material and filtration, the majority of the radiation that would contribute only to dose, and not to image formation, can be removed. This is done by using the characteristic radiation of a target material as close to that ideally required, giving an image of good contrast with low dose. This radiation is then filtered using a material whose absorption spectrum has a K-edge positioned such that it will filter out as much of the unwanted radiation as possible whilst leaving as much of the image-forming radiation as possible.

In practice, the target material required by the EC standards is molybdenum. This must be incorporated into specially dedicated equipment. The molybdenum target produces a very narrow band of low-energy radiation, particularly when used with a 0.03-mm molybdenum filter. This gives high-contrast films but means a relatively high radiation dose to the woman. In some units, it is possible to change the molybdenum filter to a 0.5-mm aluminium equivalent filter. The beam then simulates that produced by a tungsten target. A tungsten target with a 3-mm aluminium filter gives a narrow beam spectrum but at higher energy levels than from a molybdenum target. Contrast is reduced but radiation dose is lower than with a molybdenum target. Another advantage is that penetration of dense breasts is better. Other filtration material, e.g. rhodium, is available in some equipment for dense breasts.

It must be appreciated that the choice of anode material, total filtration, tube voltage and the use of a moving grid required to produce optimal image quality at an acceptable level of average entrance skin dose (7 mGy for a standard-sized woman, 4.5 cm compressed breast, with anti-scatter grid – EC standards) will depend substantially on the density and thickness of the breast examined. For denser and/or thicker breasts (>6 cm compressed), a tungsten anode, aluminium or other special filtration, higher tube voltages and an anti-scatter grid may be preferable; for thinner breasts (<4 cm), the use of an anti-scatter grid may not be necessary.

The compression device, a Perspex plate, which can be positioned manually but is more commonly motor-driven, has a role in radiation protection as it reduces dose because exposure factors are reduced. Additionally, it maintains close object-to-film contact, thus reducing geometric unsharpness and reducing movement unsharpness. It improves contrast by reducing the production of scattered radiation, flattens out tissues resulting in a film of even density that will demonstrate both anterior and posterior parts of the breast, and spreads out intra-mammary structures, allowing them to be visualized more easily.

Quality assurance

This is the application of techniques to ensure that a system or individual is performing at an optimal level. Quality control contributes to quality assurance by ensuring that pieces of equipment, e.g. the processor, are performing at optimal levels.

The Forrest Report 1986 recognized the importance of quality assurance in mammography, where the accuracy of diagnosis is very dependent on the image quality. Furthermore, consistency of standards was recognized to be essential, as subsequent screening examinations would use images from previous screening rounds for comparative purposes during mammography reporting. The Forrest Report 1986 recommended that a report regarding quality assurance should be commissioned. This resulted in the Pritchard Report 1987, which stated that 'the adoption of quality assurance system was crucial to the success of the introduction of breast screening in the UK'. The report gave guidelines on the establishment of a quality assurance system. Clearly, the performance of the service as a whole is dependent on all its integral parts, and no quality assurance initiative should be seen in isolation, even though the performance of each part of the system is measured against a specific stated objective. Parameters that were identified in the Pritchard Report 1987 for assessment were: equipment specification and performance, film/screen combination and cassettes, film processing, image quality, dose to the woman examined, and personnel performance.

The Pritchard Report provided detailed guidance on outcome objectives and standards, process objectives, quality assurance manuals, management of quality assurance, equipment procurement, testing and maintenance, training and performance of staff.

The guidance provided by the Pritchard Report 1987 on each parameter to be monitored was detailed. For example, it required radiographic performance to be monitored, such that 97% of examinations performed had to be diagnostic and less than 3% of women should need a repeat examination due to technical reasons.

Subsequent to this, the UK Mammography Trainers Group, with the support of the College of Radiographers (CoR), devised a way of evaluating radiographer performance via evaluation of the quality of the medio-lateral oblique mammograms. This method is used both for the accreditation of radiographers through the CoR's Certificate of Competence in Mammography and for long-term performance monitoring. Postgraduate courses incorporating this

Certificate of Competence are now available at several universities. In order to address the Pritchard Report and ensure that all women, irrespective of location, are assured of a high standard of service, a centrally monitored, formally organized quality assurance (QA) exists within the NHS Breast Screening Programme in the UK. In essence, at national level there is a specialist coordinating committee, consisting of all regional QA radiographers and regional representatives for each associated profession, e.g. physicists. Meetings are held in association with the relevant professional bodies, and they identify objectives and set standards. This committee reviews performance of the whole programme and the input of their professional elements down to regional level. At regional level, there is a regional QA manager, who chairs a committee consisting of a member of each of the professions that form the multidisciplinary breast-screening team. This committee institutes QA procedures and monitors regional performance. It considers details of performance down to unit level. This committee organizes multidisciplinary visits to units to discuss quality on an informal basis. Within each unit, a QA manager exists, commonly a radiographer whose role is to institute internal QA procedures and to ensure participation in external QA. Considering QA issues in the unit itself requires great tact, particularly with respect to assessment of the performance of individuals.

The NHS Breast Screening Programme publishes a series of booklets explaining the QA procedures pertinent to each profession. The QA programme has been so successful that similar measures have been extended into the Cervical Cytology Programme. EC standards were issued recently giving guidelines for QA in mammography and have been referred to above.

Overview of the UK Breast Screening Service

Breast cancer is the commonest form of cancer in the UK, affecting one in 12 women. As the incidence of and mortality from breast cancer in the UK were the highest in the world, in 1985 the government commissioned a report to consider how this serious problem could be addressed. The Forrest Report 1986 recommended that all females between the age of 50 and 64 years should be screened three-yearly. This led to the setting-up of the Breast Screening Service nationally. Screening mammography was advocated as the preferred method to promote early detection of breast cancer. As the cause of breast cancer was unknown, attempts at its prevention seemed futile. However, it had been recognized for some years that if cancers were detected at a time when they were too small to be clinically detected and early treatment initiated, then prognosis improved.

Forrest predicted that, with screening, mortality could be reduced by 30%. The age group of 50–64 years was selected because in younger women the disease was less prevalent, and if it occurred it was thought to be more malignant and spread more rapidly. Younger breasts also contain more glandular tissue, making visualization of suspicious areas, e.g. micro-calcifications, more difficult. Previous trials had, however, shown screening of women over 50 years of age to be efficacious.

The screening interval was set at three years as a balance between letting as few as possible interval cancers escape detection and the cost, dose, etc. associated with more frequent screening. The working party in the Forrest Report acknowledged that the screening interval should be subject to amendment when the optimum screening interval was established.

Asymptomatic women attending for screening mammography initially had only the medio-lateral oblique projection of each breast taken. Many centres, however, also performed the cranio-caudal projection. Both a cranio-caudal and a medio-lateral oblique projection of both breasts at the prevalent screen became mandatory from the summer of 1995, to increase accuracy of breast cancer detection. At incident screening, normally only a medio-lateral oblique projection of both breasts is undertaken.

Forrest's other conclusions were that each screening service should have access to a skilled multidisciplinary team of radiographers, radiologists, clinicians, pathologists, breast-care nurses and surgeons. Each basic screening unit should serve a population of 41 500 women, and the requirement for units throughout England and Wales would be 120 centres.

The multidisciplinary team should take referrals from one to three basic screening units. The need for rigorous quality control to maintain the highest service standards was acknowledged.

Women with negative mammographic examinations were to be recalled in three years. In women where further projections were necessary as a result of a positive or equivocal result, the women would be asked to attend the assessment centre for additional projections, e.g. repeat mammography, magnified or paddle projections, ultrasound and/or FNA. This was to establish whether a lesion seen on initial mammography existed and, if so, whether it was benign or malignant. If it was established in this process that no significant abnormality existed, then the woman would be returned to the three-yearly screening recall. Her treatment otherwise would depend on the nature of the abnormality and the policy of the medical team in charge.

Screening is also available on demand to women over 65 years of age, and routine screening is being extended to age 70 years.

15 Radiological considerations

General comments

Similar considerations apply to most projections in mammography and they will therefore be considered here in one section. Mammographic changes of disease are often very subtle so that fastidious attention to technique is necessary at all stages of the process from image acquisition, through processing to interpretation.

Small artefacts, slight unsharpness of any cause, and any defect of technique may lead to serious errors of omission or interpretation.

Movement unsharpness may result from discomfort due to compression of the breast and should be assessed when checking the films. The major role of mammography is detection of malignant disease, which may occur in any area of breast tissue, so that full coverage of the breast is essential.

Images are viewed back to back, so that the corresponding projections are facing away from each other. Correct and clear marking of the side and projection make reading much easier, and the name details should always be clearly visible.

Emulsion pick-off artefact is usually obvious as such, but large amounts may mask micro-calcifications. Talc or aluminium in deodorants may produce small densities in the axilla that may be mistaken for, or mask, micro-calcifications. (Density in this context means area of dense breast tissue, which will produce a lighter area on the film.) Skin lesions may be visible as small, often well-demarcated masses and could therefore be mistaken for breast disease, so it is helpful for the radiographer to mark the position of any such abnormalities. The senile seborrhoeic wart is one common such lesion, though this may have a characteristic appearance. Skin folds produce dark lines, the cause of which is usually obvious, but they may be confusing, especially if subtle, and are to be avoided.

Composite or summation shadows are artefacts due to superimposition of two or more normal structures, or areas of glandular tissue, which produce an appearance simulating pathology. These can often be resolved by the use of further projections, in particular the spot compression view. Magnification projections are more useful for assessment of genuine lesions by giving more detail of the surface of a mass or more detailed images of calcifications.

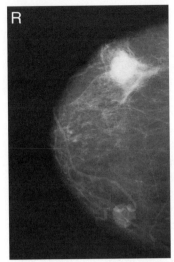

Seborrhoeic wart in inner part of breast (lower part of image). Compare with the appearance of a carcinoma in the outer part of the breast (upper half of image)

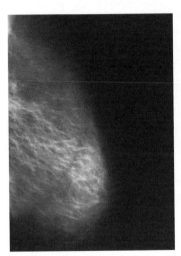

Skin fold appears as low density line across breast

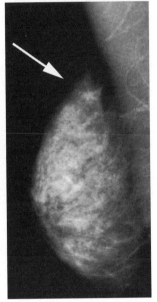

Composite artefact right axillary tail (confirmed by compression view and ultrasound)

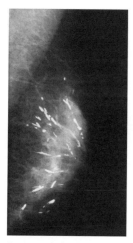

Large ill-defined mass in elderly patient, highly suspicious of carcinoma

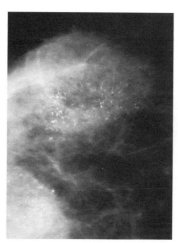

Benign calcification ductal calcifications

Malignant irregular unilateral micro-calcification typical of malignancy

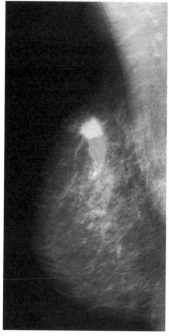

Spiculated mass typical of carcinoma, with added diagnostic feature of micro-calcification

Lesion characteristics

Four main types of lesion are visible mammographically, namely masses, calcifications, architectural distortion and density, each of which is assessed according to a variety of features:

Masses

Masses are assessed by shape, margin and density. The shape may be round, oval, irregular or lobulated, and the margin (or surface) may be smooth, obscured (by surrounding tissue), indistinct or spiculated. Any of these may be hyper-, iso- or hypodense. Benign lesions tend to be round or oval and well-defined, whereas malignancies tend to be irregular in shape and outline and are often hyperdense. A low-density lesion suggests fat and is usually benign, e.g. oil cyst, lipoma, galactocoele. Lymph nodes often have a distinct appearance due to the fatty centre or hilum.

Calcifications

Calcifications vary in size, shape, number, grouping and orientation. There are many typically benign forms of calcification, such as dermal, vascular and popcorn calcifications. Milk of calcium is amorphous calcification in microcysts and has a characteristic teacup shape on the oblique projection. Many types of rod- and ring-like calcifications are also benign. Malignant calcifications are often grouped, linear or branching and irregular in size, shape and separation. New calcifications are suspicious, e.g. those appearing since the prevalent screening round, although new benign calcifications do appear. A significant number of calcifications are indeterminate, requiring further assessment.

Architectural distortion

Architectural distortion is a feature of many carcinomas. It also occurs with benign conditions, such as sclerosing adenosis, radial scar and fat necrosis. In most of these cases, it can be proven benign only by histology. Surgical scarring causes linear distortion, which may be remarkably subtle with modern surgical technique; if gross, it will mask early features of recurrent disease.

Focal increased density

Focal increased density may be a sign of malignancy, but it has low specificity unless combined with other features. Breast density may be asymmetrical, reflecting previous surgical resection of the less dense breast or more rapid involution of the less dense breast as part of normal ageing. Benign disease may also cause asymmetric increased density, but focal density is regarded with suspicion.

Other features

Other features may be present, such as skin thickening, skin retraction, nipple retraction and trabecular thickening. These are assessed with the main features outlined above and in light of the clinical picture.

Lesion diagnosis

Some lesions are obviously benign or malignant. For example, a dense, spiculated mass with surrounding distortion, skin thickening and clustered, irregular micro-calcifications in a 70-year-old is almost certainly malignant, whereas a smooth, oval, well-defined isodense mass with popcorn calcification in a 35-year-old is most likely to be a fibroadenoma.

Typical lymph nodes have a fatty centre and hilum, oil cysts are well-defined and of fatty density, and duct ectasia may produce typical coarse ductal rod- or tube-like calcifications.

Many abnormalities, however, do not show diagnostic features and require further assessment by ultrasound and/or biopsy. Simple cysts are very common and appear as round, well-defined masses or clusters of masses, but there are no mammographic signs that are absolutely diagnostic of a cyst, so ultrasound or aspiration is usually required for diagnosis.

Some lesions are notoriously difficult to diagnose and closely mimic malignancy. One such is radial scar, which produces a spiculated area, often with an apparent small central mass. These are surgically removed, as even core biopsy does not exclude fibrosis next to a scar. Fat necrosis may produce all the features of malignancy and even at histology can be difficult to diagnose.

Therapy-related changes

Surgical scarring varies from a subtle isodense line at the site of earlier operation to a large, irregular, dense, spiculated area with marked surrounding distortion and skin change. In the latter case, detection of recurrent disease is more difficult and comparison with previous films is very helpful. For this reason, early follow-up films after wide local excision are often performed.

Radiotherapy produces an increased density of the breast, with diffuse trabecular thickening and often visible skin changes. Similar changes in a patient with carcinoma who has not had radiotherapy suggest lymphangitis of the breast.

Breast implants are very dense and obscure much tissue normally, but use of the Eklund technique allows adequate assessment in most cases. If this is not successful or cannot be achieved, then ultrasound and MRI are useful alternatives, depending on the clinical problem.

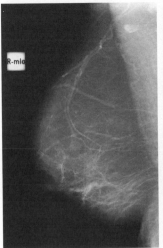 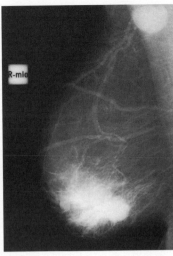

Axillary lymph nodes on mammogram. Left image shows normal node with a fatty centre. Right image shows same node later replaced by tumour

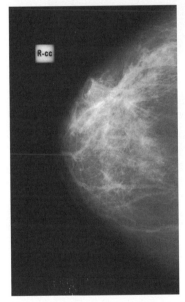

Mammogram appearance consistent with radial scar

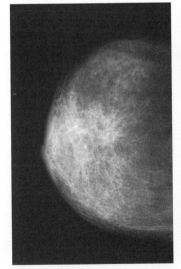 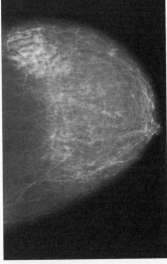

Left image shows surgical scar and radiotherapy changes in the right breast. Right image shows normal left breast for comparison

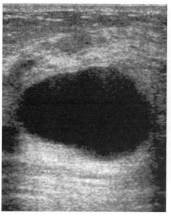

Ultrasound of breast cyst

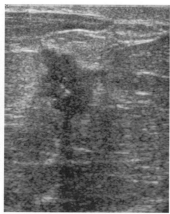

Ultrasound showing typical appearance of carcinoma

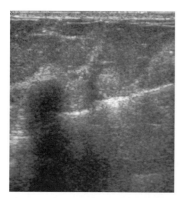

Ultrasound image showing biopsy needle in position

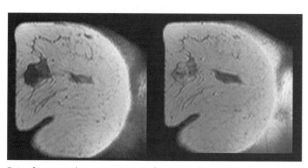

Pair of images showing cancer before and after gadolinium enhancement

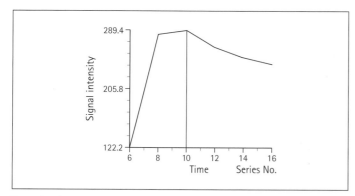

Typical malignant time intensity curve drawn from 5 pixels of previous image set

Other techniques

Mammography may be supplemented by a variety of alternative imaging techniques, and in some cases these are used instead. These modalities are covered more exhaustively in Chapter 11 of *Clark's Special Procedures in Diagnostic Imaging* (Whitley *et al.* (1999). London: Butterworth-Heinemann).

Ultrasound

Ultrasound is the most widely used and readily available alternative imaging technique. It is the best test for determining whether a lesion is a cyst. Other fluid-containing diseases may also be detected, such as abscesses and duct ectasia. Intracystic tumours are rare but are seen better on ultrasound (often as an incidental finding) than on mammography. Ultrasound gives different tissue information from that obtained by X-ray (e.g. homogeneity of tissue, acoustic shadowing), making this a useful supplementary tool. It also allows assessment of fixation of surrounding tissue and vascularity. It may be used, therefore, to assess mammographically indeterminate masses or to guide core biopsy.

In younger patients, where the density of breast makes mammography less sensitive and where suspicion is lower, ultrasound has an important role in diagnosis and avoidance of radiation exposure.

Being a real-time technique, ultrasound is simpler and faster and will be the guidance method of choice for most interventional techniques, assuming that the lesion is visible.

Magnetic resonance imaging

MRI is expensive, relatively time-consuming and not available widely. Some patients cannot tolerate it due to claustrophobia. In addition to showing the morphological features demonstrated by other modalities, a graph of signal against time after administration of intravenous gadolinium-based contrast agent allows quantification of the rate of tissue enhancement and gives a sensitive method of differentiating fibrosis (scarring) from recurrent tumour. Core biopsy is often preferred as it is quicker and more specific. MRI may be used to assess multiple lesions, implants and tissue around implants. It may be useful in some young patients who have a strong family history and will require many years of screening, or for screening of young patients after mediastinal radiotherapy for Hodgkin's lymphoma.

Nuclear medicine

Nuclear medicine is currently not a major modality in breast imaging. Scintimammography using technetium sestamibi will detect carcinoma with sensitivity and specificity equal to MRI in some series, but the expertise is not widely available. In most centres, core biopsy is more often used for assessment of indeterminate lesions.

Radionuclide imaging will have an increasing role to play as sentinel node biopsy replaces axillary dissection as the standard investigation for lymph nodes in the axilla. This will reduce the morbidity of breast surgery.

15 45-degree medio-lateral oblique (MLO) basic – Lundgren's oblique

This projection demonstrates the greatest amount of breast tissue of any single projection. It was recommended by the Forrest Report 1986 as the single projection mandatory for screening mammography. In 1995, that advice was superseded and this projection, now done in conjunction with the cranio-caudal projection, is the routine examination of the breast. EC standards state that in a complete breast examination, there must be visually sharp reproduction of the whole glandular breast and visually sharp reproduction of the cutaneous and subcutaneous tissue, and the nipple should be parallel to the film.

Position of patient and cassette

- The mammographic equipment is routinely angled at 45 degrees from the vertical. However, the precise angulation required will depend on the woman, e.g. for a very thin woman, the breast-support table will be almost vertical.
- The anatomical marker is oriented vertically to prevent confusion of the image with those produced by other mammographic projections.
- The woman faces the equipment, with the breast about to be examined closer to the breast-support table. She has her feet apart for stability, in preparation for the leaning she will have to do later to achieve the correct position.
- The woman's arm is placed on the top of the table, with the elbow flexed and dropped behind it. The table height is adjusted so that the lower border of the breast is 2–3 cm above the edge of the film.

- The radiographer places his or her hand against the rib cage and brings the breast forwards, with his or her thumb on the medial aspect of the breast. The breast is gently extended upwards and outwards to ensure it contacts the breast-support table. This is aided by leaning the woman forward.
- With the breast still supported manually, the shoulder on the side under examination is lifted and extended with the other hand to ensure inclusion of the axilla, the axillary tail and as much as possible of the breast tissue.
- The hand that is supporting the breast maintains an upward and outward lift on it, whilst the other hand is gently removing any skin folds, especially between the lateral aspect of the breast and the film support behind it.
- The compression plate is applied to fit into the angle between the humeral head and the chest wall. Great care must be taken not to hurt the woman, commonly in her ribs or sternum. Initially slightly pushing away the opposite side of the body, until the compression plate touches the breast, and then rotating it inwards again helps overcome this.
- When the compression is almost complete, the breast is checked for skin folds and the radiographer's hand is removed. Premature removal will cause the breast to droop.
- The nipple must be in profile and about a third of the way up the film. To ensure that the entire breast back to the chest wall margin is included, the infra-mammary skin fold should be included if possible. Compression is adequate if, when the breast is squeezed gently, it feels firm.

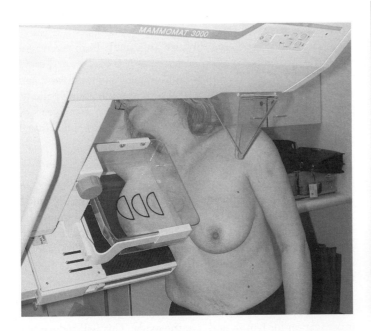

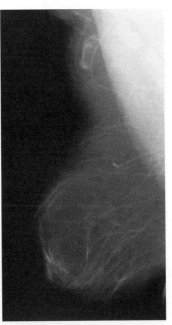

Radiograph of 45-degree medio-lateral oblique

Essential image characteristics

- The axilla, axillary tail, glandular tissue, pectoral muscle and infra-mammary fold should be demonstrated.
- The pectoral muscle should be demonstrated to nipple level.
- When both medio-lateral oblique projections are viewed together 'mirror image', they should be symmetrical, matching at the level of the pectoral muscle as a deep 'V' and at the inferior border of the breasts.

Common faults and remedies

- The breast may be positioned incorrectly. If the axillary area is not well demonstrated, then the breast-support table was too low and the axillary area and infra-mammary nodes will not be visualized. This can be rectified by ensuring, when positioning, that the nipple is a third of the way up the film.
- If the pectoral muscle is not well demonstrated, then this is due to the woman not leaning in towards the equipment, thus allowing the breast to relax, and not extending the arm and shoulder up and over the breast-support table adequately. The woman must be encouraged to lean in to the equipment and to stretch her arm and shoulder over the breast-support table to ensure inclusion of the pectoral muscle.
- There are several causes for all the breast tissue not being included on the film. If, in the initial positioning, the radiographer's hand was not placed against the woman's rib cage to ensure that the whole breast was present to be stretched across the breast-support table, then this must be rectified. If the woman was standing back from the breast-support table, then she must be encouraged to stand further forward.

- If it is the inferior aspect of the breast that is visualized inadequately, then this is because the woman was standing in a position where her feet and hips were not aligned with the rest of her body as it faced the equipment.
- If the lower border of the breast is cut off the film, then the film height was incorrect or the breast was released by the radiographer before adequate compression was applied to hold it in place.
- If the nipple is not in profile and there is no reason for this, e.g. inverted nipple, surgery, etc., then the woman's body was not parallel with the film support. If the woman stands too far forward, the nipple will rotate under the breast tissue. If she stands too far back, the nipple will lie above the midline and not all of the breast tissue will be demonstrated.
- An under-penetrated image with poor definition commonly results from inadequate compression. If compression was applied, then the usual cause is that the top edge of the compression plate was too near the humeral head, resulting in minimal compression being applied to the breast. This can be avoided by checking the breast tissue by gentle squeezing to ensure that it feels firm.
- If the exposure is incorrect, then this is usually due to incorrect centring of the glandular tissue over the automatic exposure chamber.
- Skin folds show as opaque linear shadows, which can obscure detail. Folds in the skin must be smoothed out while the breast is still supported manually, so that the movement does not alter the position of the breast. (See image below.)

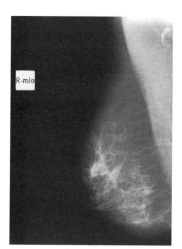
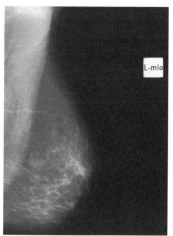

Two medio-lateral radiographs (right and left) presented for viewing

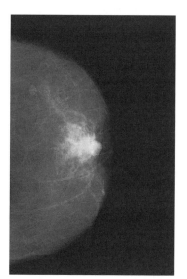
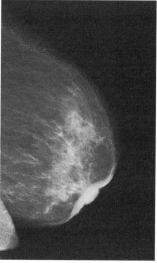

Left image shows cc view with nipple not in profile. Right image shows oblique view with nipple in profile for comparison. Note extensive radiotherapy changes make nipple more obvious

15 Cranio-caudal – basic

This projection demonstrates the majority of the breast, excluding the superior posterior portion, the axillary tail and the extreme medial portion (which contains less glandular tissue than the lateral portion).

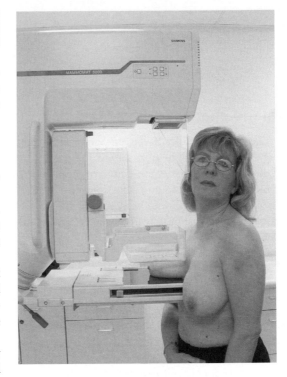

Position of patient and cassette

- The mammography equipment is positioned with the X-ray beam axis pointing vertically downwards.
- The woman faces the machine, with her arms by her sides. She is standing and is rotated 15–20 degrees to bring the side under examination close to the horizontal breast-support table. The table is at the level of the infra-mammary crease.
- The radiographer stands on the side of the woman that is not being examined and lifts the breast up in the palm of the hand to form a right-angle with the body. It is rested on the breast-support table and the radiographer's hand is slipped out. The nipple should be in the midline of the breast and in profile.
- Film markers are placed on the axillary side of the film (by international convention) close to the woman's axilla and well away from the breast tissue.
- The woman's head is turned away from the side under examination, and the shoulder on the side under examination is dropped to promote coverage of the lateral posterior portion of the breast, to bring the outer quadrant of the breast in contact with the breast-support table, and to relax the pectoral muscle.
- The breast is then lifted up and rotated medially five to 10 degrees so that the nipple is just medial to the midline of the film. The position of the breast is checked to ensure that the nipple is still in profile.
- The breast is smoothed by the radiographer's hand to remove any skin folds and is also stretched carefully across the film support.
- As the hand is removed, the breast is compressed firmly to a level that the woman can tolerate (EC standards). This should result in an equal thickness of tissue anteriorly and posteriorly. A remote-controlled foot compression device allows this to be achieved more easily, as the radiographer then has both hands free.
- Care must be taken when the compression is applied to ensure that exposure is immediate. Compression must be released as soon as the exposure ends.

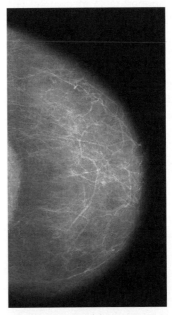

Normal cranio-caudal projection

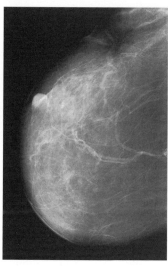

Radiograph demonstrating nipple not in profile, in this case due to surgical distortion

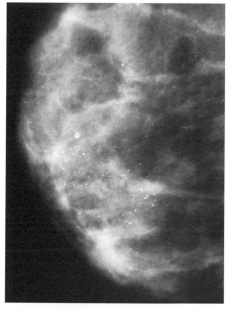

Radiograph showing two types of benign calcification

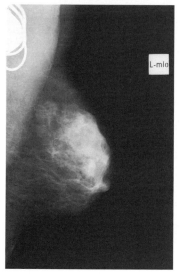

Radiograph of patient with pacemaker *in situ*

Essential image characteristics

- No overlying structures should be seen.
- The pectoral muscle will be seen in 30–40% of patients.
- The nipple should be in profile and shown medial to the mid-line of the film.
- The medial portion of the breast should be included on the film.
- There should be no folds in the breast tissue.

Common faults and remedies

- Overlying structures, such as the clavicle, the mandible or large earrings, may be seen. This can be prevented by taking care when positioning, using a deep compression plate, canting the head away from the tube, and removing earrings, respectively.
- The nipple may not be in profile. This is due most commonly to the cassette/image receptor holder being at the wrong height. If the support is too low, then the nipple will be tilted below the majority of the breast tissue; if it is too high, then the nipple will lie above the majority of the breast tissue.
- The nipple may also not be in profile if the skin on the underside of the breast is caught at the edge of the cassette/image receptor holder. The breast must be lifted and the underside of the breast pulled forward. If there is loose skin on the superior surface of the breast, then the nipple may not be positioned in profile. In such a case, the nipple position must be controlled by applying tension to the skin surface but not the underlying tissue as the compression is applied.
- If the nipple is not in profile in a woman with a fixed nipple, then no improvement can be made without the loss of visualization of breast tissue. Hence, either a clear view of the retro-areolar area is needed on the medio-lateral oblique projection or a supplementary projection of this area is essential.
- If the breast is positioned incorrectly, then areas of breast tissue will be lost from the image. If the medial portion of the breast is not on the film, then the breast has been over-rotated. If the breast was rotated inadequately medially, then the lateral aspect of the breast will be lost.
- Folds in the breast tissue result if the breast is not smoothed out before compression is completed. As folds can obscure detail, e.g. micro-calcifications, great care must be taken to ensure that they do not occur.
- Under-penetrated images, which lack detail, are generally a result of inadequate compression. This can be overcome by checking the breast manually for firmness before exposure.
- Incorrect exposure when using an automatic exposure device is usually because the glandular portion of the breast was not positioned accurately over the ionization chamber.

The routine cranio-caudal projection will not show many abnormalities in the upper quadrant of the breast, which will be demonstrated on the medio-lateral oblique projection.

As all lesions must be demonstrated on two projections, this extended cranio-caudal projection is useful for demonstrating the outer quadrant, axillary tail and axilla.

Position of patient and cassette

- The woman faces the equipment and the side under examination is rotated about 45 degrees to the equipment.
- The breast is elevated in the radiographer's hand to form a right-angle with the body and to position the nipple in profile. The breast-support table is raised to contact the inferior part of the breast closest to the chest wall.
- The hand is removed gently, leaving the breast with the nipple area on the extreme medial edge of the breast-support table.
- The woman's arm is placed on the side of the breast-support table holding the equipment.
- The radiographer stands behind the woman and lifts up the breast, extending it as far as possible to show as much breast tissue as possible.
- The woman leans back about 45 degrees if possible, depressing her shoulder to enable the outer quadrant and axilla to contact the breast-support table.
- The woman's arm is extended. She holds on to the equipment with her other hand for stability and to maintain her position.
- Whilst the breast is held in position on the breast-support table, the woman is asked to lean towards the equipment and is gently pushed in. If she cannot lean as far back as 45 degrees, then a satisfactory projection of the upper outer quadrant will still be possible provided that she is rotated adequately.

- The nipple must be kept in profile. Not all of the medial aspect of the breast will be demonstrated.
- The breast is supported manually while the compression is initiated. The hand is removed forwards but not until the compression is almost complete, so that the breast does not move.
- The compression plate fits into the angle between the humeral head and the rib cage.

Essential image characteristics

- The breast must be positioned so that the axillary tail is present on the film, with as much of the breast tissue as possible shown.

Common faults and remedies

- If the breast image shows insufficient axillary tail and axilla, then the nipple was not at the far medial edge of the film support before the woman leant back.
- If the nipple was not in profile, then the woman did not lean in enough to allow the medial part of the breast to be rotated inwards.
- If compression is inadequate, then the breast was not checked for firmness and the compression may have been too close to the humeral head.
- If the exposure is incorrect, then this is usually due to incorrect centring of the glandular tissue over the automatic exposure chamber.
- Folds in the breast tissue result if the breast is not smoothed out before compression is completed. As they can obscure detail, e.g. micro-calcifications, great care must be taken to ensure that they do not occur.

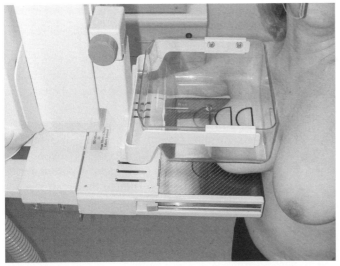

Radiograph of laterally extended cc view demonstrates axillary nodes

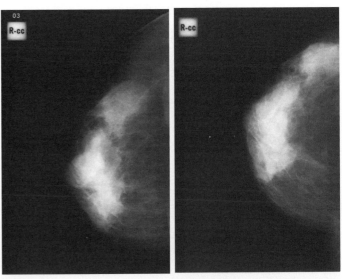

Radiograph pair showing benefit of laterally extended cc view in completing coverage of the axillary tail

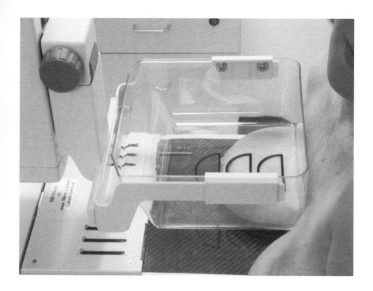

This is useful for demonstrating lesions in the medial portion of the breast.

Position of patient and cassette

- The woman faces the equipment. Her sternum is about 8 cm from the medial edge of the breast-support table.
- Both breasts are lifted on to the breast-support table, which is lowered for this purpose. It is then raised to the correct height, enabling the nipple on the side under examination to be in profile.
- The woman is pushed gently towards the equipment.
- The breast to be demonstrated is stretched in and rotated to enable the medial posterior area to be visualized. The breast is held while the initial compression is applied. Then the radiographer's hand is removed so the final compression can be achieved.

Essential image characteristics

- The maximum inclusion of the medio-posterior part of the breast is demonstrated.

Common faults and remedies

- If the inner quadrant is not fully visible, then the woman needs to be encouraged to move further forward into the equipment and the medial part of the breast needs rotating more.
- If the nipple is not in profile, then the breast-support table was not at the correct height or the breast was not lifted and stretched enough.
- If compression is inadequate, then the film will be under-exposed. The breast was not checked for firmness.
- If the exposure is incorrect and the film is under-penetrated, then this is usually due to incorrect centring of the glandular tissue over the automatic exposure chamber.
- Folds in the breast tissue result if the breast is not smoothed out before compression is completed. As they can obscure detail, e.g. micro-calcifications, great care must be taken to ensure that they do not occur.

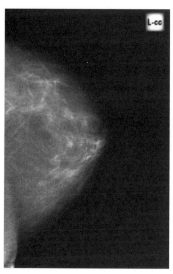

Radiograph of extended cranio-caudal – medially rotated projection

15 Extended cranio-caudal projection

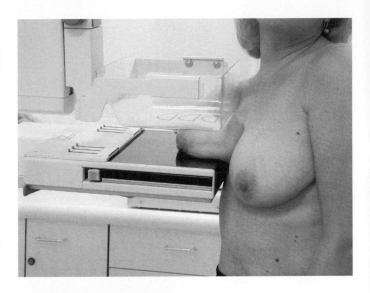

This projection is of value if a lesion was seen high in the axillary tail on the medio-lateral oblique but was not shown on the cranio-caudal projection. It demonstrates the axillary tail and the upper midline portion of the breast tissue.

Position of patient and cassette

- The breast-support table is horizontal and positioned slightly below the infra-mammary angle.
- The woman stands close to the equipment, with her breast aligned slightly to the medial side of the midline of the breast-support table. Her feet and hips point towards the table.
- The breast is lifted gently and placed on the table. The woman is then encouraged to lean 10–15 degrees laterally, extending her arm away from the side of her body. The woman should not rotate her body so that her thorax is positioned obliquely, but she must remain squarely facing the equipment.
- Compression is applied, the exposure made, and compression released immediately.

Essential image characteristics

- The nipple should be in profile.
- The anterior edge of the pectoral muscle lateral to the midline of the breast should be visualized.

Common faults and remedies

- This is a difficult position to achieve and maintain. It is essential that the woman's body remains square to the equipment and that she does not turn obliquely. Compression, exposure and release must be done expeditiously due to the awkward nature of this position.
- Folds in the breast tissue result if the breast is not smoothed out before compression is completed. As they can obscure detail, e.g. micro-calcifications, great care must be taken to ensure that they do not occur.
- Under-penetrated images, which lack detail, are generally a result of inadequate compression. This can be overcome by checking the breast manually for firmness before exposure.
- Incorrect exposure when using an automatic exposure device is usually because the glandular portion of the breast was not positioned accurately over the ionization chamber.

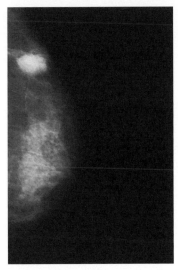

Radiograph of extended cranio-caudal projection showing a laterally placed mass

Lateral projections are valuable in localizing areas of abnormality, e.g. micro-calcification, and in the clarification of suspicious lesions.

Lateral images are taken at 90 degrees to the cranio-caudal projection and show the relationship of lesions to the nipple.

Both medio-lateral and latero-medial projections can be taken. The medio-lateral is more common, because although the axillary area is not shown, more of the breast overall is visualized.

Medio-lateral

Position of patient and cassette

- The equipment is positioned with the tube and breast-support table vertical.
- The woman faces the equipment, with the breast-support table at the lateral side of the breast. The woman places her arm behind the breast-support table and holds the equipment for stability. She leans in from the waist to ensure that the breast tissue closest to the chest wall will be visualized.
- The equipment is adjusted to the height at which the inferior portion of the breast will be included.
- The radiographer's hand is placed against the side of the rib cage and slid forward to support the breast, the palm of the hand on the lateral aspect and the thumb on the medial aspect.
- The woman is pushed in gently and the breast extended outwards and upwards against the breast-support table, ensuring that the nipple remains in profile.
- The shoulder of the opposite side is pushed back so that the compression plate can be brought into contact with the breast under examination. Firm support of the breast is necessary at this time so that the breast tissue at the chest wall margin is not pulled away.
- Compression is applied gently. When the plate contacts the breast at the chest wall, the other shoulder is brought

forward again to ensure that the woman is in a position for a true lateral projection.
- The breast position is maintained manually, with the radiographer using his or her other hand to remove any skin folds between the breast-support table and the lateral aspect of the breast.
- The hand is removed, ensuring that the position is maintained as final compression is applied.

Essential image characteristics

- The breast, including its inferior border, should be demonstrated adequately.
- There should be the same depth of tissue as in the cranio-caudal projection.

Common faults and remedies

- If all the breast tissue is not seen, then the radiographer's hand was not taken back to the rib cage and the breast not slid forward sufficiently across the breast-support table.
- If the nipple was not in profile, then the woman was standing too far in front of the breast-support table if the nipple lies behind the majority of the breast tissue, and too far behind if the nipple is lying in front of the majority of the breast tissue.
- If compression is inadequate, then the film will be under-exposed. The breast was not checked for firmness.
- If the exposure is incorrect and the film under-penetrated, then this is usually due to incorrect centring of the glandular tissue over the automatic exposure chamber.
- Folds in the breast tissue result if the breast is not smoothed out before compression is completed. As they can obscure detail, e.g. micro-calcifications, great care must be taken to ensure that they do not occur.
- If the nipple of the other breast is demonstrated, then the other breast may need to be held back.

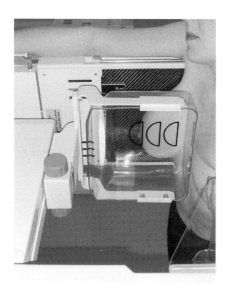

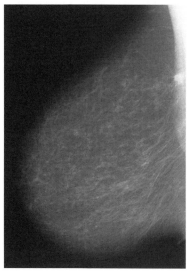

Radiograph of medio-lateral projection showing small tumour close to the chest wall

Latero-medial

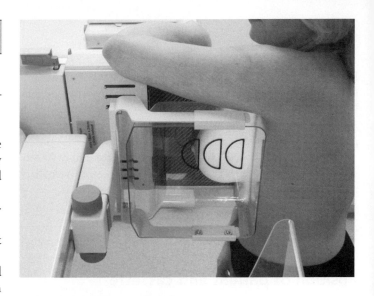

Position of patient and cassette

- The breast-support table is placed against the sternum. The arm on the side being examined is lifted up to clear the X-ray tube and is rested on the equipment. The body is rotated inwards slightly to contact the breast-support table.
- The equipment height is altered in order that the lower border of the breast is included.
- The breast is gently guided across and upwards, ensuring that the nipple is in profile.
- Compression is applied while the radiographer's hand supports the breast. The hand is removed as final compression is achieved.
- This projection is taken for demonstration of medially situated lesions.

Essential image characteristics

- The breast is demonstrated fully, including its inferior border.
- The same depth of breast tissue should be visualized as on the cranio-caudal projection.

Common faults and remedies

- If not all of the breast is demonstrated, then the woman's body was not pushed in adequately.
- If the nipple was not in profile, then the arm was pulled over too much, thus rotating the body into an oblique position and causing the nipple to lie under the majority of the breast tissue.
- Folds in the breast tissue result if the breast is not smoothed out before compression is completed. As they can obscure detail, e.g. micro-calcifications, great care must be taken to ensure that they do not occur.
- Under-penetrated images, which lack detail, are generally a result of inadequate compression. This can be overcome by manually checking the breast for firmness before exposure.
- Incorrect exposure when using an automatic exposure device is usually because the glandular portion of the breast was not positioned accurately over the ionization chamber.

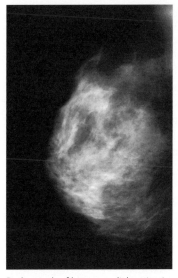

Radiograph of latero-medial projection

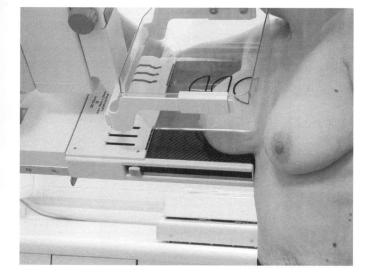

This projection is valuable in women where lymph gland involvement of a breast carcinoma is suspected or there is accessory breast tissue, as it demonstrates tissue high into the axilla.

Position of patient and cassette

- The woman faces the equipment. Her feet are turned at an angle of approximately 15 degrees towards the midline. Her arm on the side under examination is raised and her hand placed on her head. She must remain close to the equipment.
- The equipment is at 45 degrees to the horizontal and level with the suprasternal notch and the humeral head when her arm is raised.
- The woman is leant forwards towards the machine so that the corner of the table is deep in the axilla.
- The radiographer should take hold of the woman's arm on the side under examination, from behind the breast-support table, and pull her arm and thus her humeral head firmly across the top of the breast-support table, ensuring that the corner of the film is deep in the axilla. The arm is rested on top of the table and the woman encouraged to lean against the cassette/image receptor holder.
- The breast is held forward by the radiographer, to ensure even thickness of the breast and to improve the compression of the axillary region.
- Compression is applied, the exposure made and compression released.

Essential image characteristics

- The axillary region must be demonstrated.

Common faults and remedies

- Inadequate compression can occur, visualized as an underpenetrated image with poor definition. This is often due to the humeral head or the clavicle being caught by the compression plate.
- Folds in the breast tissue result if the breast is not smoothed out before compression is completed. As they can obscure detail, e.g. micro-calcifications, great care must be taken to ensure that they do not occur.
- Incorrect exposure when using an automatic exposure device may result from the glandular portion of the breast being positioned inaccurately over the ionization chamber.

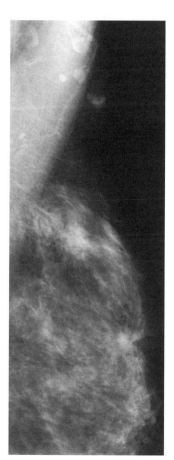

Radiograph demonstrating axillary tail projection

15 Localized compression/paddle projections

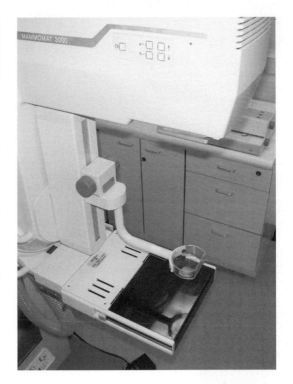

Localized compression/paddle projections can provide extra information in a suspicious area, e.g. by demonstrating whether the borders of a lesion are defined clearly or indistinctly.

The paddle projections required are usually selected by the radiologist, with the aim of repeating those projections that initially demonstrated the possible lesion.

A small compression paddle is needed, but the projections are done with a full-field diaphragm to allow landmarks to be identified.

For accurate localization of the region of interest, the original mammogram must be examined. It is essential that the radiographer measures and records the depth of the lesion from the nipple back towards the chest wall, the distance of the lesion from the nipple (above, below, medial or lateral), and the distance from the skin surface to the lesion.

Position of the patient and cassette

- The woman is positioned as for the original projection.
- The recorded coordinates are used to move the woman until the affected breast tissue lies over the automatic exposure control and the paddle is centred over it. Allowances have to be made for the fact that the coordinates recorded were from a fully compressed breast.
- The compression is applied sufficiently to hold the breast in place.
- The coordinates are then rechecked. Provided that the region of interest is centred under the paddle, the centring point is marked on the skin surface and compression applied fully.
- If the area of interest was not under the paddle on checking, then the woman's position is adjusted, before proceeding as above.
- The compression used should be firmer than usual. It is essential that the woman understands the purpose and necessity for this, to ensure her cooperation.

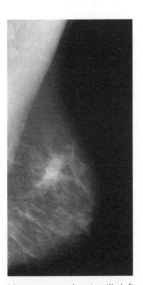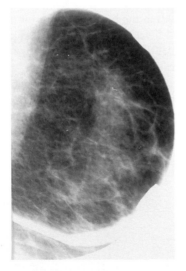

Mammogram showing ill-defined region, and repeat mammogram using paddle to show the effect of compression

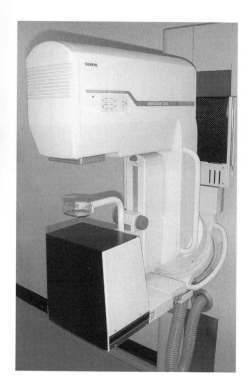

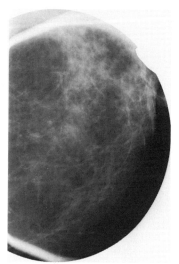

Radiograph of paddle-magnified projection

Projections of the breast using a magnification technique, using either a localized or full-field technique, are sometimes employed to give enhanced visualization of the breast architecture and detail, thus promoting better diagnosis.

- Magnification is used most commonly to examine areas of calcification.
- Magnified projections are done in the cranio-caudal and medio-lateral projections.
- A fine focus of $0.1\,mm^2$ is essential, and a magnification factor of two is commonly used.
- A specially designed platform or tower fits on to the breast-support table to allow this projection to be undertaken. Magnification factors are typically 1.5, 1.8 or 2.0.
- No grid is used.
- Small and large paddles may be utilized for magnified projections and a full-field diaphragm.
- The advantage of using a small paddle is that compression can be applied firmly to the area of interest. However, if the suspicious area, e.g. calcification, is extensive, then a larger paddle is needed to allow visualization of the entire area on the film.

Full-field magnified projections

- The woman is placed in the position for the lateral and cranio-caudal projections in turn.
- It is important to realize that the field will cover only the half of the breast under examination and that in large breasts some measuring may be needed.

Paddle-magnified projections

- As with standard paddle projections, the recording of the coordinates of the lesion from the original images and the positioning technique, as described above, is essential in order to accurately centre the lesion under the paddle.
- In magnified projections, the use of a fine focus will lengthen the exposure time greatly, and the projections should be taken on arrested respiration.

15 Stereotactic needle procedures

Due to improvements in the technical quality of mammography and the introduction of screening mammography, an increasing number of clinically impalpable breast lesions are being detected. These, like palpable lesions, require further radiological investigation to establish a diagnosis. Commonly, further mammographic projections and ultrasound examinations are undertaken to confirm the presence of the suspected abnormality and to assess its clinical importance. Any impalpable lesion that cannot be stated definitively to be benign after such procedures must have a tissue diagnosis. This is achieved by:

- image-guided FNA cytology; and/or
- image-guided core biopsy wherever possible.

Open surgical biopsy is thus avoided. Whilst FNA or core biopsy can be done freehand in palpable lesions, impalpable lesions produce unique problems.

Ultrasound-guided biopsy is preferable for impalpable lesions, since it is quick to perform, very accurate, and associated with minimal discomfort and morbidity to the woman. It is the guidance technique of choice for biopsy if the lesion is visualized clearly on ultrasound. X-ray-guided FNA, however, is essential if there is any doubt that what is seen on ultrasound is the same lesion as visualized on the mammograms, and when the lesion is not shown on ultrasound. The most accurate way of performing X-ray-guided FNA is using stereotactic equipment. Accuracy is clearly essential to ensure that the relevant area is sampled, as the definitive treatment, ranging from non-excision of a benign lesion to mastectomy in a malignant lesion, is based on the outcome of the cytological/histological sample. Two main types of stereotactic equipment exist: a purpose-built table where the woman lies prone, and an accessory that can be fitted to conventional mammographic equipment. The latter is described, since it is more common.

Any woman undergoing this procedure will be anxious, and a good rapport between the woman and the radiographer is essential. A thorough explanation of the procedure before it commences and at each step along the way is important as this will relax and reassure the woman.

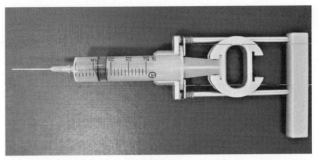

Example of FNA needles in specialized needle holder

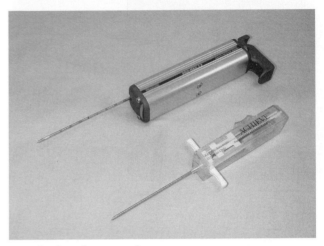

Example of core biopsy needles

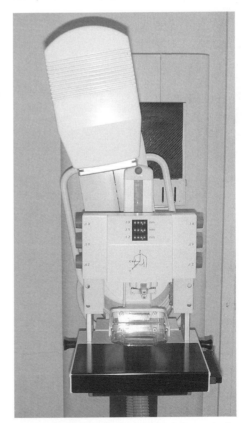

Stereotactic device which is attached electronically to the mammography unit, with stereo image pair in position

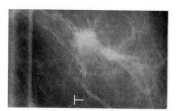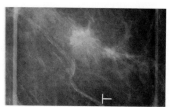

Example of stereo imaging pair showing a localized lesion

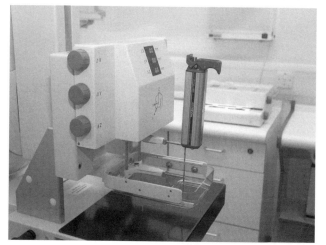

Mammogram unit with needle biopsy 'gun' in position

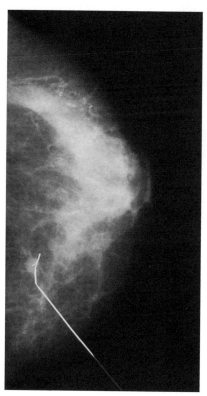

Mammogram showing lesion and marker wire *in situ*

Technique

The way the breast is to be positioned for the localization to be done is agreed with the radiologist. The woman is seated and positioned, and the compression plate, with its integral window, is applied. An outline of the compression plate window is drawn on to the woman's skin so that any breast movement during the procedure is evident. The tube movements necessary to produce the stereo images are performed (typically the tube is swung 20 degrees to each side of the midline). The radiographs are processed as quickly as possible and the images checked with a radiologist, ensuring that the lesion is shown clearly and that it is not too close to the edge of the compression plate window. The coordinates of the lesion will be calculated by the equipment from the stereo images. A local anaesthetic injection to the skin over the biopsy area is given. The needle holder is positioned correctly, and the radiologist places the needle in the breast. A check film is essential after the first needle has been placed to confirm that the needle is located correctly. Aspiration is then performed. The procedure may be repeated with several needles, and multiple passes may be undertaken with each needle, if necessary.

Modern equipment has a digital system for biopsy and spot imaging. The film processing is replaced with digital image acquisition and reconstruction, which can be done very swiftly and accurately. Core biopsy is performed in a similar way typically using a 14G wide-core biopsy needle.

Stereotactic preoperative marker localization

This procedure is very similar to that described for stereotactic FNA or core biopsy. Whilst stereotactic equipment is not essential, it does increase the accuracy. The marker wire that is used instead of the fine needle or the biopsy gun will depend on the preferences of the surgeon performing the biopsy or excision. The purpose of this localization is for a marker wire to be placed accurately in the breast lesion so that the surgeon can perform a diagnostic biopsy of the lesion. It is essential that the marker wire tip lies within the lesion so accurate assessment of the depth of the abnormality in the compressed breast is made. The position of the wire in relation to the abnormality in the breast must therefore be checked mammographically after marker insertion.

15 Breast implants

As breast implants are radio-opaque, visualization of breast tissue is often not possible. This is especially so if the implant forms a large proportion of the breast. Women with breast implants and who attend for mammography need to be made aware of the limited nature of any mammographic examination performed on them. Breast awareness in these women is vital, and its value to them should be stressed. The radiologist in charge will have a policy regarding the mammography of these women, many of whom are still keen to be examined even though they recognize the limitations of this. Many radiologists prefer to undertake breast ultrasound or MRI in breasts substantially augmented with prosthetic material.

Women with implants may be embarrassed about them and/ or worried that mammography will cause them to rupture. Thus, establishing a rapport with the woman is vital.

Women with breast implants may be imaged using standard projections, tangential projections or the Eklund technique.

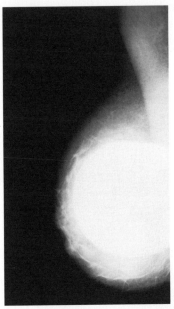

Mammogram showing appearance of a breast implant

Imaging procedure

- Using the standard technique, the cranio-caudal projection is undertaken first.
- The breast is positioned routinely, but compression is applied only to a point at which the breast will be held in position.
- A manual exposure must be set, as the AEC would not terminate the exposure due to the radio-opacity of the breast.
- The resultant mammogram is evaluated particularly with respect to exposure factors, and repeated if necessary.
- The medio-lateral oblique projection is then taken, with an increase of exposure factors of about one-third of those for the cranio-caudal projection.

Notes

- Tangential projections should be undertaken in any woman with breast implants and who is undergoing mammography due to a localized breast lump.
- The Eklund technique is suitable for women in whom there is a large volume of breast tissue relative to the prosthesis. The implant is displaced to the back of the breast so that only the breast tissue is compressed and imaged.

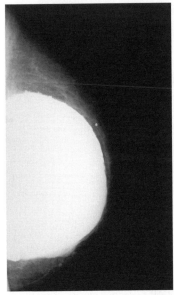

Mammogram showing appearance of a breast implant with surface irregularity due to ageing of the implant

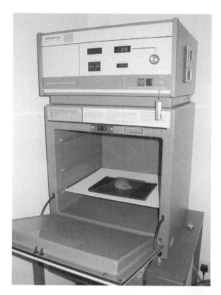

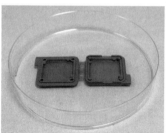

Core biopsy container

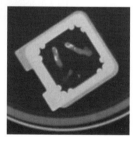

Specimen radiograph taken using special container

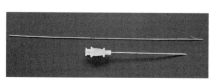

Example of hookwire and insertion needle used for wire localization procedures

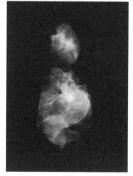

Radiograph showing wire localization specimen

Core biopsy and specimen tissue radiography 15

Core biopsy

Both core biopsy and specimen breast radiography, involving a magnification technique, play an important role in the diagnosis, management and treatment of breast cancer.

Breast tissue cores, which are obtained in the manner described on p. 461, are examined radiographically to determine the presence of a breast lesion that may contain or be solely composed of calcifications.

Procedure

Following core biopsy, the excised tissue cores are laid out on a fibre-free sheet or in a dedicated specimen holder kept moist with isotonic saline to prevent desiccation. Radiography may be performed on the mammography table using the magnification facility or in a specimen radiography cabinet.

Radiographic technique using specimen cabinet

The tissue cores on the fibre-free sheet are placed on top of an 18 × 24-cm cassette containing a single emulsion film. The tissue is exposed using an exposure of 26 kVp and 3 mAs.

Once adequate radiographs have been obtained, the tissue cores must be transferred to a fixative, usually formalin, and transported to the laboratory immediately for processing for subsequent histology.

Breast tissue radiography

Prior to surgical excision of a breast abnormality, a wire is inserted in the centre of the lesion using the stereotactic preoperative marker localization technique, as described on p. 461.

Following excision of the breast abnormality, the breast tissue specimen is sent for radiographic examination while the patient is still under anaesthetic to ensure that there is a minimum 1 cm clear margin of normal breast tissue surrounding the lesion.

The radiographic procedure is performed while the patient is still under anaesthetic; thus, the procedure is carried out as quickly and as efficiently as possible.

Procedure

The procedure may be performed on the mammography table using the magnification facility or in a specimen radiography cabinet and using an 18 × 24-cm cassette containing a single emulsion film.

Two projections of the specimen are obtained, each image at right-angles to the other.

The specimen is first positioned on one half of the film, with the other half masked with lead rubber, and an exposure is made with careful collimation of the beam. The specimen is then positioned on the other half of the film and turned through 90 degrees.

Section 16

Miscellaneous

CONTENTS

TRAUMA RADIOGRAPHY	466	
Assessment of the patient's condition	466	
Planning the examination	466	
Adaptation of technique	467	
Patient's condition	468	
Equipment and imaging considerations	468	
Advanced Trauma and Life Support (ATLS)	471	
FOREIGN BODIES	472	
Introduction	472	
Percutaneous foreign bodies	473	
Ingested foreign bodies	474	
Inhaled foreign bodies	475	
Inserted foreign bodies	476	
Transocular foreign bodies	477	
TOMOGRAPHY	479	
Introduction	479	
Principles	480	
Types of tomographic movement	482	
Image quality	485	
Radiation protection	485	
Procedure	486	
Exposure time and exposure angle	486	
Applications	486	
Kidneys	487	
Antero-posterior	487	
Larynx – antero-posterior	488	
Trachea – antero-posterior	488	
MACRORADIOGRAPHY	489
Principles	489
Applications	491
SKELETAL SURVEY	492
Introduction	492
Recommended projections	493
SOFT TISSUE	494
Introduction	494
Exposure technique	494
FORENSIC RADIOGRAPHY	496
Introduction	496
Classification of forensic radiography	496
Anatomical terminology	496
Legal issues	497
Equipment and accessories	497
Local radiation rules	497
De-briefing	497
Dental radiography	498
Recommended dental projections	498
General radiography	499
Still born (15–40 weeks)	500
Antero-posterior 'babygram'	500
Lateral 'babygram'	501
Still born (15–40 weeks): skull projections	502
Lateral	502
Skeletal survey – out of hours	503
Further reading	504

16 Trauma radiography

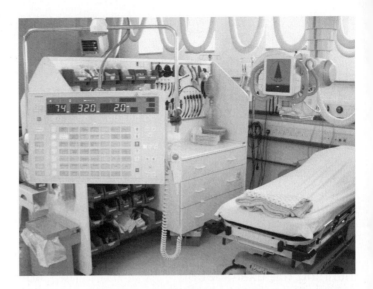

Radiographers are aware that image quality is often compromised when examining a patient who has suffered acute trauma as their mobility and ability to cooperate is often reduced greatly. It is ironic that these patients, who require the highest-quality diagnostic images to detect the serious injuries associated with trauma, often will have a set of images that are of reduced quality as a result of their inability to cooperate.

Plain radiography of trauma, whether undertaken in the emergency room or within the imaging department, should therefore be considered as an imaging speciality in its own right. Radiographers undertaking these examinations need to have specialist knowledge that will help them to be aware of all the factors that reduce image quality and how to minimize their effects. It is beyond the scope of this section to give a detailed account of all the relevant imaging factors relevant to trauma radiography. However, it is possible to provide a series of points that all radiographers should be mindful of when undertaking any radiography of the acutely injured patient.

Assessment of the patient's condition

A vital first step in the examination is to scrutinize the imaging request and assess the patient's condition. An assessment of the mechanism of injury and a discussion with the patient (if possible) relating to their condition and capabilities will enable the radiographer to properly plan the examination for the maximum diagnostic outcome.

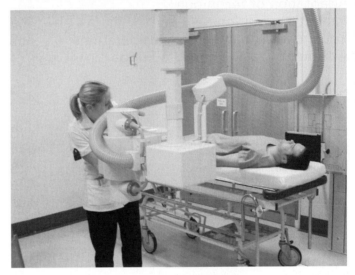

Planning the examination

When the radiographer is presented with a patient requiring multiple examinations, it is important to spend some time planning the whole examination so that it can be conducted efficiently, using the most appropriate equipment for the task.

Consider a patient who requires examinations of the whole spine, chest and pelvis. It would be more efficient if all the lateral radiographs were performed before all the antero-posterior radiographs. This avoids wasting time in moving the tube back and forth between exposures.

When examining patients on stretchers, it is also worth considering the side of any lateral examinations as the trolley enters the X-ray room. By doing this, the appropriate side of the body can be positioned against the vertical Bucky at this stage, rather than disrupting the examination halfway through by moving the trolley around.

Good communication with the accident and emergency (A&E) department staff is also of vital importance at the planning stage of any procedure. This will provide the radiographer with valuable information about the patient's condition and ability to cooperate. In addition, if the procedure is being undertaken as a mobile examination, then good communication is vital to ensure that the radiographer takes the correct equipment to the emergency room and correctly times their arrival in the department.

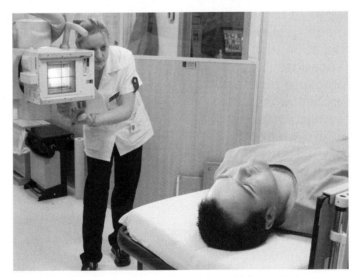

When undertaking trauma examinations involving multiple examinations, it will save time if all the examinations in one plane (e.g. laterals) are undertaken before others

Adaptation of technique

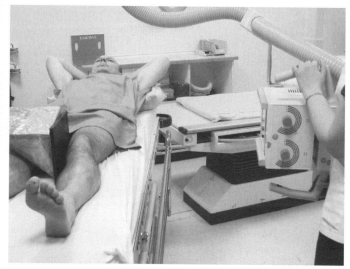

Horizontal beam lateral for knee examination

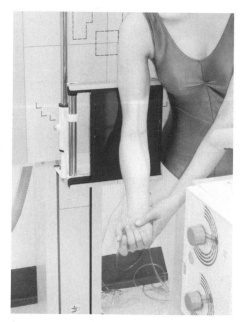

Antero-posterior elbow standing for supracondylar fracture

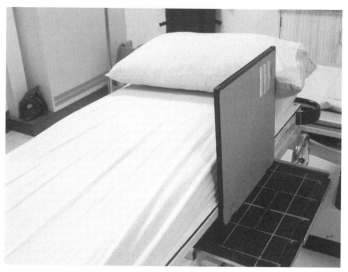

Accident and Emergency trolley with 30 × 40-cm cassette for lateral C spine

Much of the skill of a trauma radiographer stems from an ability to be able to produce radiographs of diagnostic quality when the patient is unable to cooperate to such an extent that the standard positioning cannot be undertaken.

It is beyond the scope of this section to give a full account of all the common adaptations that are used in trauma radiography. What has been provided is a series of general points and principles that radiographers should consider when presented with a difficult trauma case.

Horizontal beam laterals

This is an extremely useful adaptation that is used when the patient cannot move into the standard lateral position with a vertical central ray. In the example shown opposite, the use of a horizontal beam is actually advantageous to diagnosis. A lipo-haemarthrosis, which is a soft tissue indicator of injury within the knee joint, would not be visible if a standard lateral projection was performed.

Standing up/sitting

Patients may find it difficult to attain the standard positioning when the radiographs are undertaken in the usual seated or supine position. In such cases, asking the patient to stand up (if the condition will allow) may be beneficial. One good example of a situation where this is useful is in the case of a suspected supracondylar fracture of the elbow. The patient may not be able to extend the elbow to attain a good antero-posterior position whilst seated, but they may be able to do this if imaged erect.

Consider the pathology

The radiographer will constantly strive to produce standard projections that meet strict positioning criteria, but it is easy to forget to consider the pathology in question. This could lead to an important diagnosis being overlooked. An example of where this might happen is in a long bone when a joint examination is requested. The radiographer may not include an area of pathology in a long bone near to a joint if the radiation field is restricted to the joint region.

Be flexible

Radiographers should not become accustomed to doing things in a particular manner, otherwise they will become inflexible and unable to deal with unusual situations. Consider the cassette size used for lateral cervical spine radiography. In most cases, an 18 × 24-cm cassette would be used, but it is often difficult to support this cassette in a vertical position, especially in the resuscitation room. In such a situation, a 30 × 40-cm cassette resting on the trolley cassette tray may prove to be a useful alternative (see photograph opposite).

16 Trauma radiography

Patient's condition

It is important to closely supervise trauma patients at all times, as their condition can easily deteriorate. Patients who initially appear quite cooperative may suddenly become unstable and be in danger unless an appropriate intervention is made.

As discussed above, the patient's ability to cooperate will have a strong bearing on the quality of the final images. For the most part, there is nothing that can be done when a patient cannot cooperate, other than to adapt the imaging technique accordingly. There are some situations, however, when the radiographer may have some control over the patient's ability to cooperate. Some of these are outlined below.

- The intoxicated patient: in the absence of serious trauma, if possible delay the examination until the patient is sober enough to cooperate fully. This is particularly important for regions of the body where injuries can be difficult to diagnose. The quality of facial-bone radiographs obtained using a skull unit are far superior to those taken with the patient supine on a trolley. It would be unwise or even dangerous to attempt a facial-bone examination using a skull unit on a patient who is heavily intoxicated.
- Delaying the examination may also be considered when the patient's ability to cooperate is restricted severely by immobilization devices or clothing. Once other injuries have been excluded, these devices may be removed and the patient may be more able to cooperate.

Equipment and imaging considerations

Several X-ray equipment manufacturers offer a range of dedicated systems for trauma radiography. These are certainly useful in terms of time-saving and image quality when undertaking multiple procedures. It is possible, however, to obtain images that are equally as good as those taken using dedicated systems using a general X-ray room equipped with a ceiling-suspended tube, a vertical Bucky, a floating-top table with Bucky, and appropriate emergency equipment. A skull unit, although not essential, will increase the quality of skull and facial-bone images. One of the most desirable features of a room used for trauma radiography is space. If the radiographer has a generous space allocation, then this will give them greater flexibility when adaptations in technique are required.

Other more specific considerations are considered individually.

Immobilization devices

Any room used for trauma radiography should have a generous supply of radio-lucent foam pads and sandbags for supporting patients or cassettes. Specialist devices, such as the leg support used for lateral hip radiography, are often invaluable.

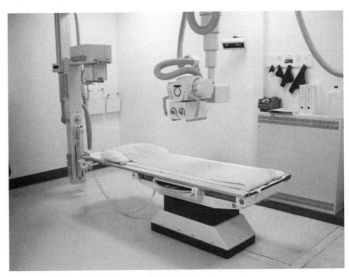
A typical room suitable for trauma imaging

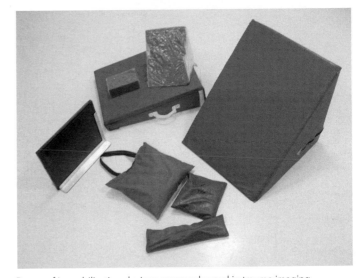
Range of immobilization devices commonly used in trauma imaging

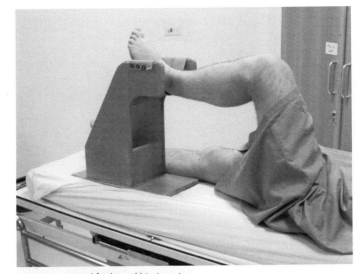
Leg support used for lateral hip imaging

468

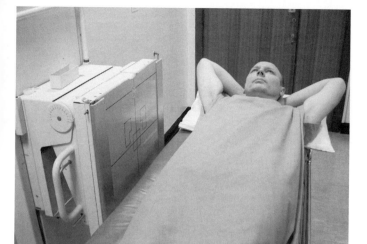

Increase in object-to-film distance leading to greater geometric unsharpness

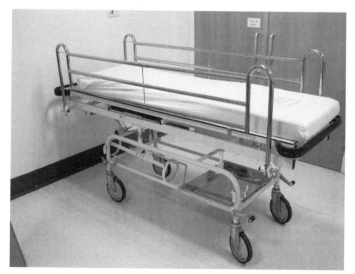

Increased focus-to-film distance to reduce geometric unsharpness

Example of a trolley well suited for Accident and Emergency imaging

Equipment and imaging considerations

Grids

Adaptations in technique will often result in the use of stationary grids for trauma radiography. These should be used only as a last resort due to the poor efficiency of such grids in terms of scatter attenuation compared with that of a Bucky with a moving grid mechanism. The grid lattice pattern from the stationary grid, and the relatively low grid ratio, contribute to a lower image quality when stationary grids are used. The type of grid is also important. If a focused grid is employed, then the radiographer must ensure that the correct focus-to-film distance (FFD) for the type of grid is used, otherwise a 'cut-off' artefact will result.

Object-to-film distance

In many cases, an increase in object-to-film distance (OFD) will result from the modifications in technique required in trauma radiography. A good example is the horizontal beam lateral radiograph of the thoracic or lumbar spine. If the patient is lying in the middle of the trolley, then the spine will often be positioned at some distance from the cassette. This results in an increase in magnification and geometric unsharpness. The problem is easily remedied by increasing the focus-to-object distance (FOD) (within the focus range of the grid) to compensate. Remember that if this strategy is employed, and no automatic exposure device is used, then the radiographer must increase the exposure factors.

Collimation

Many trauma radiographic examinations are prone to high levels of scattered radiation that degrade overall image quality. A good example of such an examination would be the horizontal beam lateral lumbar spine, as described above. The extra tissue from the abdominal viscera lying either side of the spine increases the amount of tissue irradiated compared with a standard lateral, and there is a corresponding increase in scatter production. In such cases, close attention to collimation is important, as this will serve to vastly decrease the scatter produced and will significantly improve image quality.

Type of trolley

There are many different types of trolley available for use in A&E work, some of which are far more suitable for plain film imaging than others. It is strongly recommended that radiographers maintain close links with A&E staff so they can involve themselves with the purchase of new trolleys. A period of evaluation when any potential new trolley is tested in practice is essential as part of the procurement process. Some relevant considerations with respect to trolley design are highlighted on the next page.

Equipment and imaging considerations (*contd*)

Cassette holder

The trolley must have either a moveable tray underneath the patient to accommodate cassettes and grids or a wide platform that runs the length and width of the trolley. The latter may offer greater flexibility if the patient is not central to the trolley. Alternatively, separate cassette holders are available or can be made to suit a particular purpose.

Access to cassettes

Whichever method is used to support the cassette underneath the trolley, it is important that the radiographer can easily gain access and view the cassette wherever it is positioned relative to the patient. This is vital for accurate alignment of the cassette to the beam before exposure.

Object-to-film distance

The distance between the trolley top and the cassette holder underneath should be as small possible but still allowing reasonable access for the positioning of cassettes. If this distance increases, then geometric unsharpness will also increase, thus reducing image quality.

Uniform trolley top

The trolley top should be completely radio-lucent (no metal bars or hinges) and designed in such a way that there is a minimum of joins in the material that the trolley top is constructed of. These may cause artefacts on any images taken using the cassette holder underneath the patient.

Vertical cassette holders

Some trolleys come equipped with vertical cassette holders, which are useful, but not vital, for performing horizontal beam lateral examinations.

Image artefacts

Artefacts from clothing or immobilization devices applied by ambulance staff are an ongoing difficulty for radiographers to deal with. Necklaces or earrings under rigid neck collars cause many problems, as the radiographer may not be aware of their presence until an image is obtained. Again, the establishment and maintenance of good communication links between professional groups will allow communication of such problems and raise awareness of the difficulties that arise as a consequence.

Teamwork

When imaging trauma patients, the efficiency and effectiveness of a radiology department will spring from good teamwork. This applies between professional groups as well as within the radiology department. Close links between radiology and the A&E

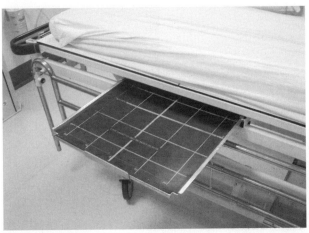

Example of a trolley cassette holder well suited for Accident and Emergency imaging

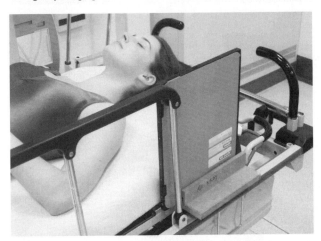

Trolley cassette holder used for horizontal beam imaging

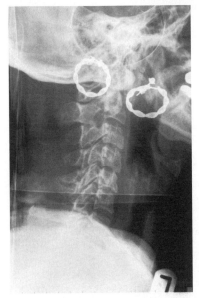

Example of artefact obscuring a spinal fracture

department will help each group to understand their respective difficulties and will help to overcome problems and maximize efficiency. When imaging a patient who has suffered multiple trauma, a team of two – one radiographer positioning the patient and the other processing the images – will serve to maximize efficiency.

Exposure factors

Trauma radiography often requires adaptations in exposure factors due to the non-standard imaging conditions encountered. Some considerations that the radiographer should be aware of are listed below:

Reducing exposure time

If movement unsharpness is likely, then the exposure time can be reduced in a variety of ways:

- Increase the kVp and reduce the mAs.
- If possible, increase the tube mA and reduce the exposure time.
- Increase the tube loading to 100%. Most generators are routinely operated at a loading of less than this.
- Consider using a faster imaging system and thus reducing exposure time.
- Use of a broad focal spot will allow a shorter exposure time.

Enhance contrast

Consider altering the kVp to manipulate the image contrast. A low kVp will be useful for demonstrating foreign bodies such as glass or for highlighting a subtle fracture. A high kVp may be useful for reducing large differences in subject contrast – differing regions within spine being a good example.

Exposure latitude

Systems that offer wide exposure latitude are particularly useful, as they are more able to cope with the variations in conditions encountered in the trauma setting. The digital systems are particularly useful in this respect.

Automatic exposure devices

These are advantageous for trauma imaging, particularly those located in the erect Bucky, which are used for horizontal beam spinal imaging. Care should always be taken to ensure that the tube is centred correctly to the Bucky at all times, otherwise the device will not give the correct exposure. It is easy to decentre the tube from the Bucky whilst making fine alterations to the final centring point.

Correct labelling of images

Given the many modifications in technique often employed in trauma radiography, it is important that the final image is labelled correctly (e.g. supine, erect, horizontal beam, etc.) so an accurate diagnosis can be made.

Advanced Trauma and Life Support (ATLS)

This is a comprehensive protocol introduced by the American College of Surgeons to ensure that any patient suffering major trauma is given adequate emergency care, even remote from a major trauma centre, thus allowing patients to arrive at a centre of excellence in the best possible condition. The ATLS workbook specifies minimum standards of care to all body systems from a variety of viewpoints, including specifications for radiographic examination. It is also being widely adopted outside the USA.

According to protocol, the initial radiographic assessment of the severely injured patient includes: lateral cervical spine, chest X-ray (CXR) and pelvis. N.B. skull X-ray is not included.

These are performed immediately as part of the initial assessment and before full clinical examination. Following full clinical evaluation, further projections or projections of other areas may be requested. At some point (determined by the clinical priorities), full projections of the cervical spine should be obtained.

The definition of 'full projections' will be determined by local protocols, but is usually three projections (antero-posterior, lateral, peg), with the addition of trauma oblique projections in some centres. If adequate basic projections are not obtained, then the use of computed tomography (CT) may become necessary, again as determined by local guidelines. CT is not a quick examination in the unconscious, ventilated patient, and it can be a high-dose examination. It should not be viewed as an easy alternative to good plain-film radiography.

ATLS also calls for flexion projections of the cervical spine under supervision of an experienced doctor, prior to full 'clearance' of the spine in patients who are alert and neurologically normal but suffering neck pain. **Flexion of the spine in an injured patient should be undertaken only under medical supervision.**

As 7–10% of patients with cervical spine fracture have an associated fracture of the thoracic or lumbar spine, projections of these areas may also be indicated.

Significant injury to the thoracic and lumbar spine can occur without local tenderness or pain, especially in the presence of a painful lesion elsewhere. It may therefore be appropriate to perform full spine projections in patients with major trauma and other painful lesions, as well as those with depressed level of consciousness and those with cervical spine injury.

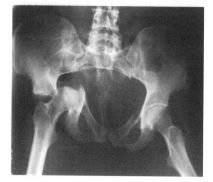
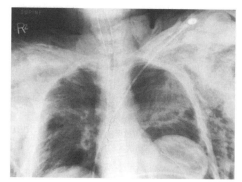

ATLS series of trauma images showing a fracture dislocation of C5/C6, unstable pelvic fractures and a chest image showing pneumothorax and surgical emphysema

16 Foreign bodies

Introduction

Many different objects may enter body tissues and cavities under a variety of circumstances. The main methods of entry are:

- percutaneous
- ingestion
- inhalation
- insertion
- transocular.

If the foreign body is non-metallic and a similar sample of the object is available, then the sample may be placed in a few centimetres depth of water in a non-opaque container and radiographed to establish its radio-opacity. The method adopted to demonstrate the presence and position of a foreign body is governed by its size and degree of opacity and its location. Unless it is radio-opaque or in a position where it can be coated with opaque material to render it visible – as, for instance, in the alimentary tract – then the foreign body cannot be shown on a radiograph. Partially opaque foreign bodies, such as wood, some types of glass and other low-density materials, may sometimes be shown by suitable adjustment of the kVp.

Although the spatial resolution of computed radiography (CR) and direct digital radiography (DR) may be inferior to conventional imaging, the electronic post-processing capabilities of these systems more than compensate. The ability to adjust the image using image magnification, edge enhancement and windowing tools make the presence of a foreign body more easily visualized. Additionally, the contrast resolution of CR and DR is greater than that of conventional imaging, making it possible to visualize foreign bodies previously not seen on radiographs (e.g. splinters of wood).

Removal of bulky dressings from soft tissue lacerations is recommended, especially when using CR and DR, as these artefacts become more obvious on the image and can obscure radio-opaque foreign bodies such as glass fragments. Matted blood in the hair can also prevent glass splinters in the scalp from being seen.

Ultrasound is useful in the localization of non-opaque subcutaneous foreign bodies and the genital system.

CT or magnetic resonance imaging (MRI) may be used when it is necessary to demonstrate the relationship of a foreign body to internal organs.

Notes

- MRI must not be undertaken if there is any possibility that the foreign body is composed of ferromagnetic material.
- Before commencing any examination, it is important to ensure that no confusing opacities are present on the clothing, skin or hair on the tabletop, Bucky, cassette or intensifying screens, or on the Perspex of the light-beam diaphragm.

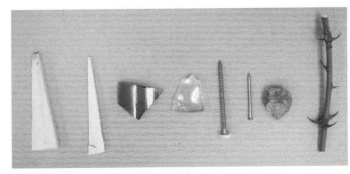

Photograph of samples of wood, glass and metal objects

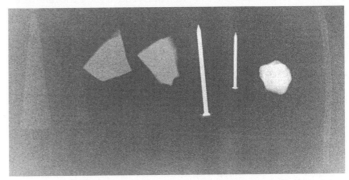

Radiograph of the objects seen above X-rayed through a wax block – note the thin sliver of wood and thorn wood is barely visible

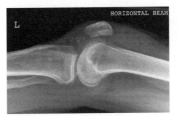 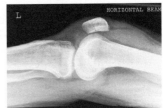

Images of a left knee acquired using a computed radiography system: left, windowed for normal viewing; right, windowed for soft tissues (here demonstrating more clearly a joint effusion in the suprapatellar bursa)

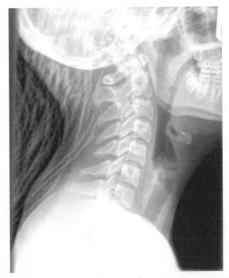

Lateral neck image showing the effect of braided hair with streak-looking structures superimposed over the soft tissue neck region

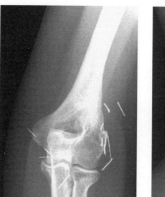
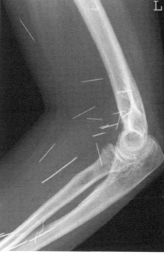

Antero-posterior and lateral images of a right elbow demonstrating multiple needle insertions

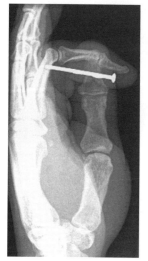
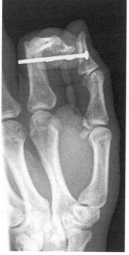

Dorsiplantar and lateral images of the thumb showing embedded nail in the distal soft tissues

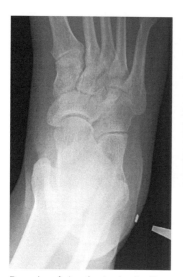
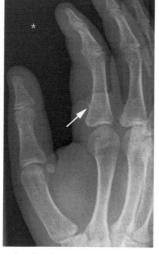

Examples of glass foreign bodies illustrating that the density on the image will vary depending on the thickness and lead content of the glass

Percutaneous foreign bodies

These are commonly metal, glass or splinters of wood associated with industrial, road or domestic accidents and self-harm injuries.

Generally, two projections at right-angles to each other are required, without movement of the patient between exposures, particularly when examining the limbs. The projections will normally be antero-posterior or postero-anterior and a lateral of the area in question, as described in the appropriate chapters.

A radio-opaque marker should be placed adjacent to the site of entry of the foreign body. The skin surface and a large area surrounding the site of entry should be included on the images, since foreign bodies may migrate, e.g. along muscle sheaths, and high-velocity foreign bodies may penetrate some distance through the tissues.

Compression must not be applied to the area under examination.

Oblique projections may be required to demonstrate the relationship of the foreign body to adjacent bone. A tangential (profile) projection may be required to demonstrate the depth of the foreign body and is particularly useful in examination of the skull, face, and thoracic and abdominal walls. Sometimes a single tangential projection may be all that is required to show a superficial foreign body in the scalp or soft tissues in the face.

The exposure technique should demonstrate both bone and soft tissue to facilitate identification of partially opaque foreign bodies and to demonstrate any gas in the tissues associated with the entry of the foreign body.

The most usual exposure techniques for conventional radiography are:

- kVp sufficiently high to demonstrate bone and soft tissue on a single exposure;
- use of two film/screen combinations of different speeds or a film/screen combination and non-screen film to demonstrate bony detail on one film and soft tissue on the other film with one exposure.

The use of digital image acquisition offers significant advantages in the localization of foreign bodies. CR and DR both allow soft tissue and bone to be visualized from one exposure using post-processing. The use of features such as edge enhancement and windowing enable much better demonstration of foreign bodies that have radio-opacity similar to that of the surrounding tissue.

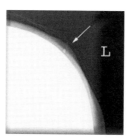

Tangential (profile) projection of the scalp showing glass embedded in the soft tissues

16 Foreign bodies

Ingested foreign bodies

A variety of objects, such as coins, beads, needles, dentures and fish bones, may be swallowed accidentally, or occasionally intentionally, particularly by young children. A technique used to smuggle drugs through customs involves packing the substance into condoms, which are subsequently swallowed.

The patient should be asked to undress completely and wear a hospital gown for the examination. The approximate time of swallowing the object and the site of any localized discomfort should be ascertained and noted on the request card, along with the time of the examination. However, any discomfort may be due to abrasion caused by the passage of the foreign body. It is important to gain the patient's cooperation, especially in young children, since a partially opaque object may be missed if there is any movement during the exposure. The patient should practise arresting respiration before commencement of the examination.

If the patient is a young child, then the examination is usually restricted to a single antero-posterior projection to include the chest, neck and mid- to upper abdomen. The lower abdomen is usually excluded, to reduce the dose to the gonads, as the examination is usually performed to confirm the presence of a foreign body lodged in the stomach unable to pass through the pylorus. Care must be taken to ensure that the exposure selected is sufficient to adequately penetrate the abdomen as well as to visualize the chest.

The examination of older children and adults may require a lateral projection of the neck to demonstrate the pharynx and upper oesophagus, a right anterior oblique projection of the thorax to demonstrate the oesophagus, and an antero-posterior abdomen projection to demonstrate the remainder of the alimentary tract, exposed in that order. Each image should, preferably, be inspected before the next is exposed, and the examination terminated upon discovery of the foreign body, to avoid unnecessary irradiation of the patient. The cassette used should be large enough to ensure overlapping areas on adjacent images.

Non-opaque foreign bodies may be outlined with a small amount of barium sulphate. A few cases require a barium-swallow examination. If no foreign body is demonstrated within the alimentary tract, and particularly if there is doubt as to whether the foreign body has been ingested or inhaled, then a postero-anterior projection of the chest will be required to exclude an opaque foreign body in the respiratory tract or segmental collapse of the lung, which may indicate the presence of a non-opaque foreign body in the appropriate segmental bronchus. All projections should preferably be exposed in the erect position. A fast film/screen combination and short exposure time should be employed.

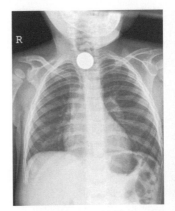
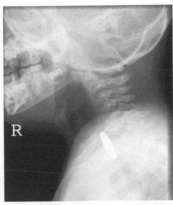

Antero-posterior and lateral images showing a coin lodged in the upper oesophagus of a child

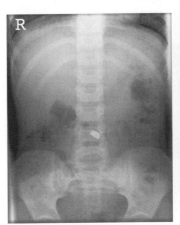

Watch battery in transit in the alimentary tract

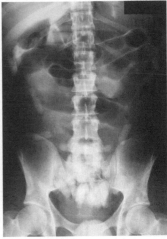

Antero-posterior abdomen image showing multiple condoms filled with drugs lodged in the lower abdomen causing small bowel obstruction

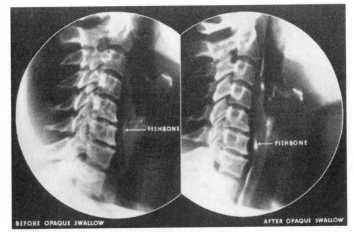

Use of barium sulphate to outline fish bone lodged in the upper oesophagus

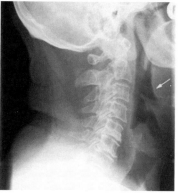

Lateral soft tissue image of the neck showing a fish bone lodged in the larynx

Inhaled foreign bodies

Foreign bodies may be inhaled. Infants and young children habitually put objects into their mouths, and these may be inhaled. Teeth may be inhaled after a blow to the mouth or during dental surgery. Such foreign bodies may lodge in the larynx, trachea or bronchi.

The adult patient should be asked to undress completely to the waist and to wear a hospital gown for the examination. A postero-anterior projection of the chest, including as much as possible of the neck on the image, and a lateral chest projection will be required initially. Alternatively, an antero-posterior chest image is acquired when examining children. A lateral projection of the neck, including the nasopharynx, may also be required. In the case of a non-opaque inhaled foreign body, postero-anterior projections of the chest in both inspiration and expiration will be required to demonstrate air trapping due to airway obstruction. This may manifest itself as reduced lung attenuation on expiration and/or mediastinal shift. The kVp must be sufficiently high to demonstrate a foreign body that might otherwise be obscured by the mediastinum. A fast imaging system (film/screen combination) and short exposure time should be employed.

Cross-sectional imaging such as CT and MRI are additional techniques that may provide useful information. NB: MRI is contraindicated in cases of suspected ferrous materials, since the examination may result in movement of the foreign body.

Bronchoscopy may be used to demonstrate the position of a foreign body, since the foreign body may be removed during this procedure.

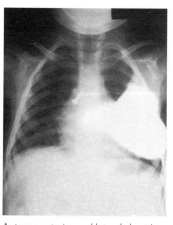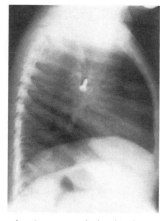

Antero-posterior and lateral chest images showing a screw lodged in the right main bronchus

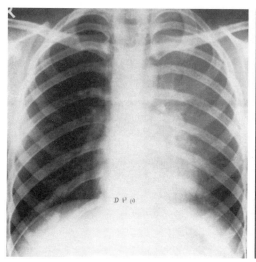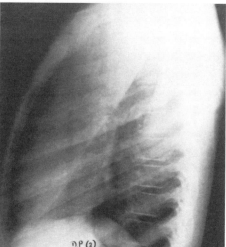

Postero-anterior and lateral chest images demonstrating a tooth in left superior lobar bronchus and atelectasis in the left lung

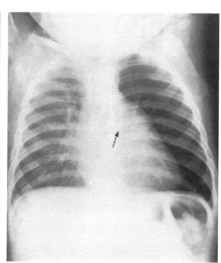

Antero-posterior chest image showing a foreign body in the left main bronchus with obstructive emphysema

16 Foreign bodies

Inserted foreign bodies

Foreign bodies are sometimes inserted into any of the body orifices. Infants and young children, for example, may insert objects into the nasal passages or an external auditory meatus. In these cases, radiography is required only occasionally, since most of these objects can be located and removed without recourse to radiography.

When radiography is requested, two projections of the area concerned at right-angles to each other will be required.

Swabs may be left in the body following surgery. Such swabs contain a radio-opaque filament consisting of polyvinylchloride (PVC) impregnated with barium sulphate for radiographic localization.

Ultrasound should be the initial modality selected for the detection of an intrauterine contraceptive device. It is also very effective in the detection of soft tissue foreign bodies with the advantage of incurring no radiation burden where it is available.

There have been incidents where objects such as vibrators have become lodged in the rectum. In these cases, a single antero-posterior projection of the pelvis may be required.

Patients who are prone to self-harm may insert a variety of objects into their body cavities and under the skin.

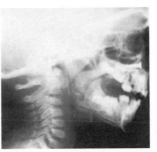 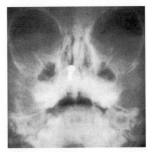

Lateral and postero-anterior facial images showing a screw in the right nasal cavity

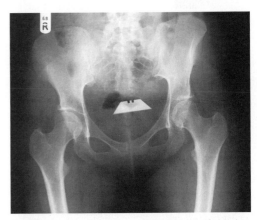

Antero-posterior pelvis showing a Stanley knife blade inserted in the vagina

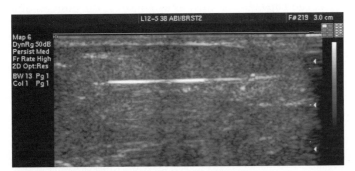

Ultrasound image of a needle in the superficial soft tissue

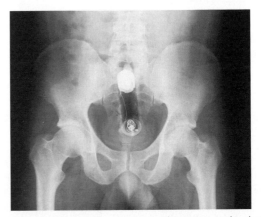

Antero-posterior pelvis showing a vibrator inserted in the rectum

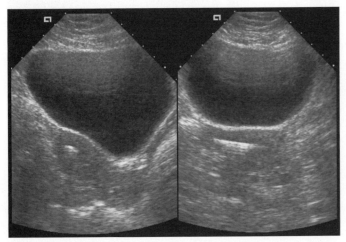

Ultrasound image of an intrauterine contraceptive device

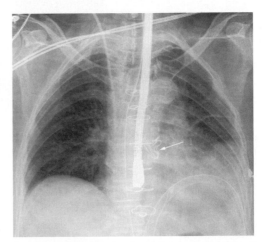

Portable antero-posterior chest taken in theatre to locate missing swab

Transocular foreign bodies

Foreign bodies that enter the orbital cavity are commonly small fragments of metal, brick, stone or glass associated with industrial, road or domestic accidents.

Plain film imaging is the first modality for investigation of a suspected radio-opaque foreign body in the orbit. For further investigation, or assessment of a non-opaque foreign body, CT scanning can be very useful. CT will give information about damage to the delicate bones of the medial and superior orbital

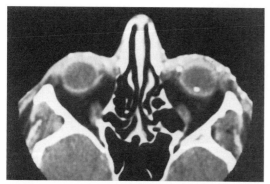

CT image showing multiple foreign bodies

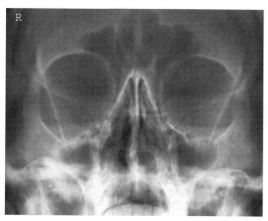

Modified occipito-mental image taken to detect the presence of a radio-opaque foreign body (normal)

margins, and evidence of any damage suffered by the brain if the orbital roof has been breached. Ultrasound is useful for detecting superficial foreign bodies and soft tissue damage but is less useful in the orbit in detecting very small foreign bodies. Access to ocular ultrasound expertise is less likely to be immediately available, and there is the extra hazard of introducing coupling gel into a possibly deep wound.

Radiographic localization may be carried out in two stages:

- To confirm the presence of an intra-orbital radio-opaque foreign body.
- To determine whether the foreign body is intra- or extra-ocular.

Images showing fine detail are essential. A small focal spot (e.g. 0.3 mm^2), immobilization with a head band and a high-definition film/screen combination is recommended. Metal fragments down to $0.1 \times 0.1 \times 0.1$ mm in size may be detected by conventional radiography.

Intensifying screens must be scrupulously clean and free of any blemishes producing artefacts that could be confused with foreign bodies. A cassette with perfectly clean screens may be set aside especially for these examinations.

Confirmation of a radio-opaque foreign body

A modified occipito-mental projection with the orbito-meatal base line(OMBL) at 30 degrees to the cassette is undertaken, with the patient either prone or erect. Whichever technique is adopted, the head must be immobilized. The technique is described in detail on page 269. Ideally, a dedicated skull unit is selected as this will provide the maximum degree of resolution required for the visualization of a small foreign body.

The chin is raised so the OMBL is at 30 degrees to either the vertical or horizontal beam. This position projects the petrous ridges to just below the inferior, anterior orbital margin with the walls of the orbit lying parallel to the cassette. Using a vertical or horizontal beam, the central ray is directed to the interpupillary line. The beam is either collimated to include both orbits or just the orbit under examination, depending on the departmental protocol.

Notes

- If it is suspected that a foreign body is obscured by the skull then a soft tissue lateral image may be necessary.
- It may be necessary to repeat the examination if the artefact is suspected to be from a possible dirty screen.
- If a radio-opaque foreign body is identified in the orbit, before proceeding with any further localization images it may be advisable to wait until the patient has been seen by the ophthalmologist who may decide to remove the foreign body or request CT or ultrasound in preference to radiography localization.

16 Foreign bodies

Transocular foreign bodies (*contd*)

Localization of intra-orbital foreign body

The method described determines the position of the foreign body relative to the centre of the eye and whether it is intra- or extra-ocular. It should be ascertained that the patient is able to maintain ocular fixation, i.e. keep the eyes fixed on some given mark, since the exposures are required with the patient looking in different directions.

The examination is preferably carried out using a skull unit. The following projections are required:

- Occipito-mental (modified) (see p. 269) with the centring adjusted to the middle of the interpupillary line. Two exposures are made, one with the eyes level and looking forward and the other with the eye under examination adducted (turned towards the nose).
- Lateral (see p. 267), with the centring adjusted to the outer canthus of the eye. Three exposures are made, one with the eyes level and looking forward, one with the eyes raised and one with the eyes lowered.

In each case, the patient should look steadily at some predetermined mark or small object during the exposure. A tracing is made from the lateral projections showing the three shadows of the foreign body. Straight lines are drawn to join them. The lines are then bisected at right angles midway between the shadows. The point of intersection of the bisectors indicates the centre of the eyeball if the intersection is slightly anterior to the zygomatic border of the orbit. In this case the foreign body is in the eyeball.

If the intersection is remote from the zygomatic border it will indicate that the foreign body is in the surrounding tissue or muscles.

A second tracing from the occipito-mental projections enables lateral movement of the foreign body to be plotted and shows its antero-posterior position relative to the centre of the pupil.

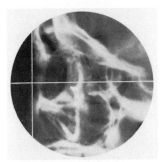
Lateral orbits with eyes level

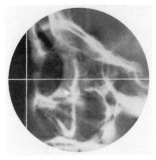
Lateral orbits with eyes raised

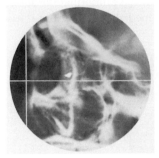
Lateral orbits with eyes lowered

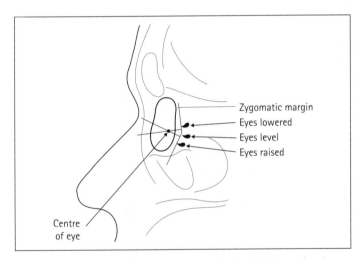
Tracing from lateral projections shows that the foreign body lies within the eye

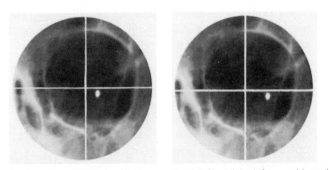
Occipito-mental images with the eyes level (left) and the left eye adducted (right)

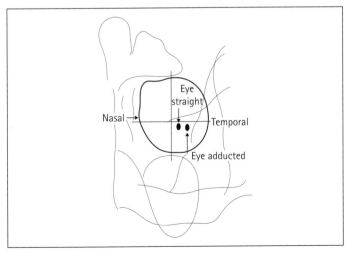
Tracing from occipito-mental projections shows that the foreign body lies posterior to the centre of the eye

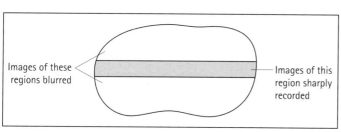

Images of these regions blurred

Images of this region sharply recorded

Diagram illustrating tomography theory

Introduction

A conventional radiograph is a two-dimensional image formed by the superimposition of images from successive layers of the body in the path of the X-ray beam. The image of a structure in one layer of the body is observed with the superimposition on it of images of structures in layers above and below it.

Before the introduction and widespread use of CT, a technique known as (conventional) tomography was employed. This used conventional X-ray equipment, with tomographic attachments, or a dedicated tomographic unit to record images of structures or layers within the patient while images of structures outside the selected layer were made unsharp. There are several methods of achieving this, all of which involve some form of movement of the patient or equipment during the exposure, but in every case the general principle is the same. Throughout the exposure, movement occurs, causing images from the unwanted layers to move relative to the image receptor and therefore to be unsharp; images from the selected layer are kept stationary relative to the film and are recorded in focus. Tomography involves the synchronized movement of the X-ray tube and the cassette while the patient remains stationary. If there is movement only of the patient during the exposure, this is called autotomography.

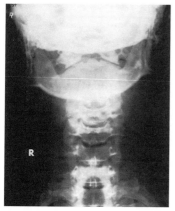

Antero-posterior conventional image of cervical spine with superimposed mandible on the upper vertebrae

Autotomography

In this technique, the part to be visualized remains stationary during the exposure while overlying structures produce unsharp images due to some form of patient movement. The part to be visualized should be immobilized. A long exposure time is used to allow sufficient movement and therefore blurring of unwanted images.

The two most common applications of autotomography are as follows: an antero-posterior projection of the cervical spine, where the patient opens and closes the mouth during the exposure so that the mandible is not recorded as a sharp image obscuring cervical vertebrae; and a lateral projection of the thoracic vertebrae, where the patient continues gentle respiration during the exposure so that images of the ribs and lungs are unsharp, allowing better visualization of the vertebrae.

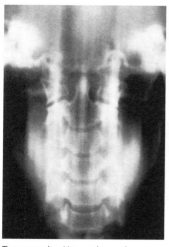

Tomograph – X-ray tube and cassette move during exposure

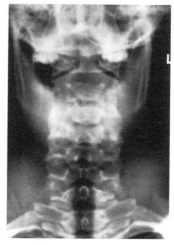

Autotomograph – mandible moving during exposure

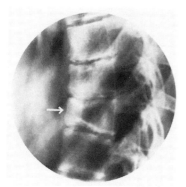

Autotomograph – gentle respiration during long exposure

16 Tomography

Principles

As stated previously, a tomographic image can be produced by relative movement between the patient, the image-recording device and the X-ray tube. In practice, this is normally achieved by the patient remaining stationary while the X-ray tube and the cassette move.

As the X-ray tube and cassette move relative to the patient, the projected images of structures at different levels of the body will move with different velocities. The nearer the structure is to the X-ray tube or cassette, the faster its image will move. The tube is linked to the cassette tray such that the cassette moves at the same velocity as images of structures only at the level of the pivot; therefore, only these images are recorded on the same part of the image receptor throughout the movement. Images of structures at or in all other layers move at a different velocity from that of the cassette and are not recorded on the same part of the image receptor throughout the movement and are therefore blurred.

It is therefore possible to record the outlines of structures more sharply on only one layer of the body free from obscuring images from other layers.

It is an important requirement that throughout the movement there is no change in the magnification of images on the object plane, since this would produce image unsharpness. To ensure constant magnification, the following relationship must be maintained throughout the movement:

$$\frac{\text{Focus-to-film distance}}{\text{Focus-to-pivot distance}} = \text{a constant}$$

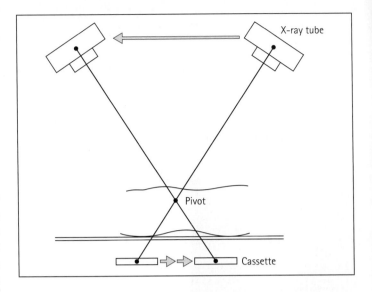

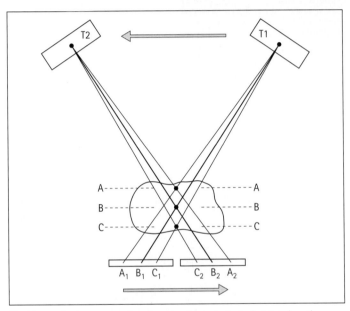

The X-ray tube is connected to the cassette and pivoted at B. When the X-ray tube moves from T1 to T2 during the exposure; images of layer B move at the same velocity as the image receptor and are recorded on the same part of the image receptor throughout the exposure and the image is sharp; images of layer A move faster than the image receptor and are therefore blurred; images of layer C move slower than the image receptor and are therefore blurred

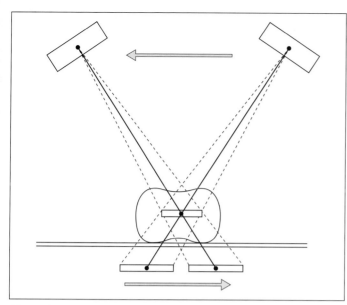

Object plane parallel to the image receptor

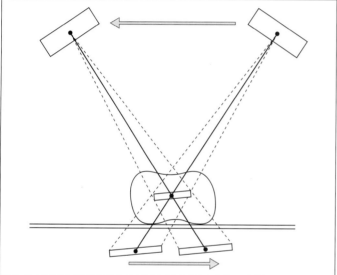

Inclined plane tomography

Principles

The layer recorded sharply is called the object plane and it is parallel to the image receptor.

Normally, the image receptor lies parallel to the tabletop and therefore the object plane is parallel to the tabletop at the level of the pivot. If the image receptor lies at an angle to the tabletop, during the movement the layer visualized will be at the same angle. This is called inclined-plane tomography.

Depth of layer

The height of the pivot table above the tabletop is variable so that any level in the patient can be selected for tomography. Either the pivot can be raised or lowered above the tabletop to the required level in the patient (variable pivot), or the pivot is in a fixed position and the tabletop can be raised or lowered to bring the required level to the level of the pivot (fixed pivot).

The height of the pivot above the tabletop is indicated on a scale. If the upper attachment of the connecting rod is at the level of the focal spot and the lower attachment is at the level of the cassette, then the layer recorded sharply is the layer at the level of the pivot that is parallel to the cassette. If the cassette is situated above or below the lower attachment of the connecting rod, then a layer above or below the pivot level will be recorded sharply.

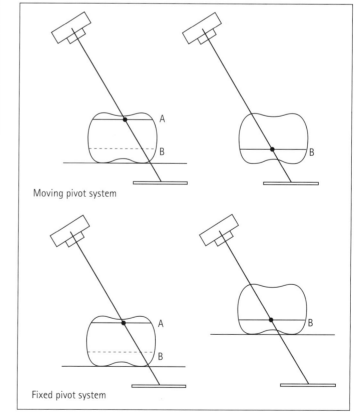

Moving pivot system

Fixed pivot system

16 Tomography

Types of tomographic movement

Before the use of CT, when (conventional) tomography was used more widely, a variety of tube/film movements were employed to produce more effective blurring of unwanted structures, e.g. (in order of increasing complexity):

- linear
- circular
- elliptical
- spiral
- figure-of-eight (Lissajous figure)
- hypocycloidal.

Dedicated tomographic units were required for all movements other than linear. Since the use of conventional tomography is now limited mainly to imaging the renal tract, linear movement produces adequate blurring and we will only consider this movement in our discussions.

Features of linear movement

This is the simplest form of tomographic movement. The X-ray tube and image receptor move in lines parallel to the tabletop. The FFD changes throughout the movement, being least at the midpoint of the movement. Line-to-line movement is often confined to one direction only, which is along the long axis of the table, but some equipment will allow the linear movement to be in any direction parallel to the tabletop. There are different designs:

- **Arc-to-line:** the X-ray tube moves in an arc above the table while the image receptor moves below the table in a line parallel to the tabletop. This is typical of the majority of units. Throughout the movement, there is a change in the ratio of the focus-to-film/focus-to-pivot distance, resulting in a continual change in the magnification of images in the object layer. This results in some unsharpness, but if the change in magnification is kept to a small value then the image can be accepted by the observer as sharp.
- **Arc-to-arc:** the X-ray tube and the image receptor move in arcs, the centre of rotation being the pivot. Throughout the movement, the image receptor remains parallel to the tabletop and the FFD is constant.

NB: linear movements have the disadvantage that they produce 'linear streaks'. These are pseudo-shadows caused by structures just outside the layer, which are incompletely blurred out and appear as indistinct linear images superimposed on the sharp image of the selected layer.

Exposure angle

The exposure angle is the angle through which the tube moves during the exposure. It is inversely related to the thickness of layer visualized on the image. For linear tomography, there is usually a choice of exposure angle ranging from about two to 40 degrees.

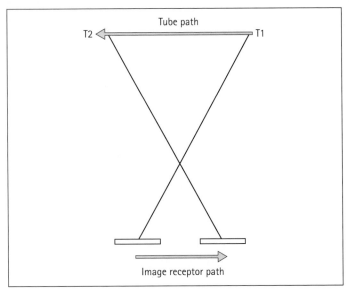

Line-to-line

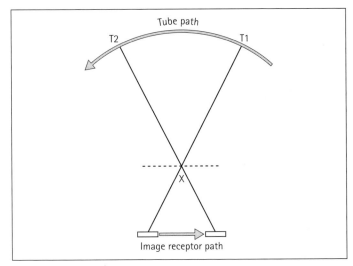

Arc-to-line

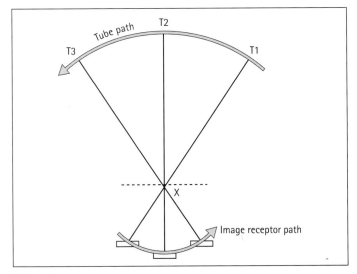

Arc-to-arc

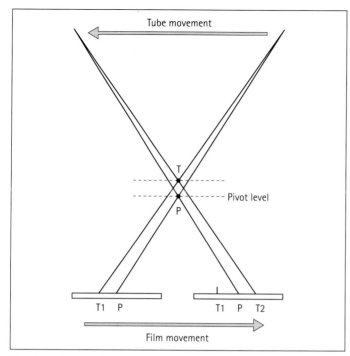

The above diagram demonstrates that during tube movement, the image of P (at the level of the pivot) is recorded on the same part of the film and is a sharp image. T is on a plane higher than the pivot and its image moves on the film from T1 to T2, but if this distance is not greater than about 0.6 mm it is still accepted as a sharp image. Therefore, the thickness of the layer extends up to T. There is a similar thickness of the layer below the pivot

Types of tomographic movement

Thickness of layer

Only images of structures at the level of the pivot and parallel to the film are recorded on the same part of the film throughout the movement. This layer is infinitely thin. Images of structures outside this object plane move relative to the image receptor, but if this movement is small (less than about 0.6 mm), they will be recognizable images. Therefore, the visualized layer has some thickness. The amount of relative movement of the image and therefore the thickness of the layer depends on the exposure angle, i.e. the angle through which the X-ray tube moves during the exposure. The greater the exposure angle, the thinner the layer. The layer has no well-defined boundary as there is a progressive deterioration in the sharpness of images of structures with increasing distance from the object plane.

Layer thickness also depends on the distance of the structure above or below the pivot. Images of structures above the pivot are more blurred than those below the pivot, and thus the layer is thinner above the pivot than below it. The practical significance of this is that structures close to the object plane can be 'blurred out' more easily if they are on the tube side of the patient (see the diagram opposite).

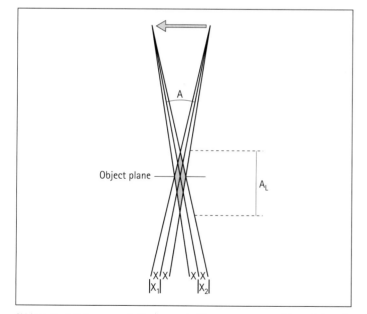

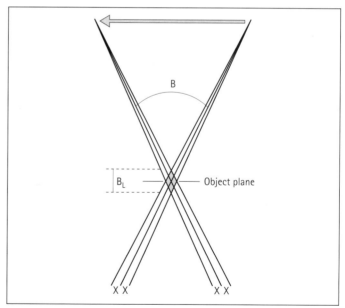

2X (e.g. $X_1 + X_2$) represents the amount of image movement (about 0.6 mm) on the film which the observer can still accept as being a sharp image. Therefore images of objects within the layer A_L are seen as sharp images for exposure angle A and within the layer B_L for exposure angle B. The larger the exposure angle, the thinner the layer

Types of tomographic movement (*contd*)

The graph shows how the thickness of the layer varies with exposure angle. At larger angles there is little change in layer thickness with change in exposure angle, whereas at small angles a small change in the exposure angle causes a large change in layer thickness.

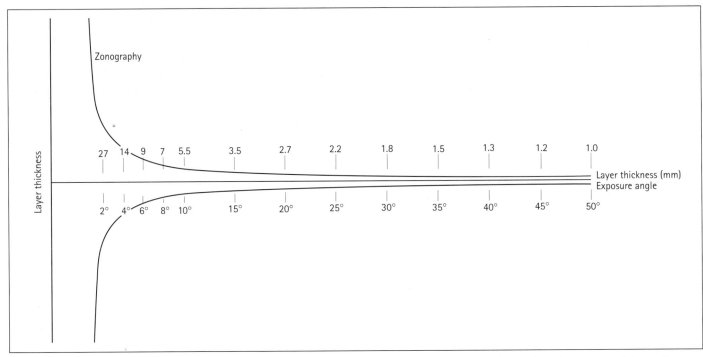

Although layer thickness can be calculated on the basis of the acceptable image blur, the thickness is also dependent on the radio-opacity and shape of structures lying outside the calculated layer. Opaque structures and those lying along the line of the X-ray tube movement are more difficult to 'blur out' and both these factors increase the apparent thickness of the layer

Zonography

This is the term applied to small-angle tomography giving relatively thick layers. There is no fixed exposure angle below which tomography is classified as zonography, but the term is generally reserved for exposure angles of 10 degrees or less.

Thickness of cut and spacing of layers

For zonography, where the layer can be, for example, greater than 2 cm thick, layers at 2-cm intervals can be used. In practice, it is normal to use 10-degree exposure angles and 1-cm intervals. With wide-angle tomography, spacing of layers should be closer, to ensure that the layers overlap.

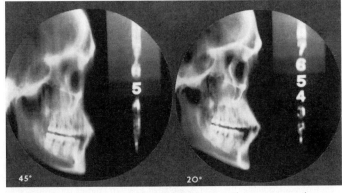

Tomographs illustrating change of layer thickness with exposure angle

Magnification in tomography

As with all projected images, there is some magnification of a tomographic image. The magnification (M) is given by:

$$M = \frac{FFD}{\text{Focus-to-pivot distance}}$$

Generally, the quality of a tomography image, in terms of its sharpness and contrast, is not as good as that of a standard radiographic image.

Contrast

Because only a thin layer of the body is being recorded, inherent contrast is low, the problem being greater with the larger exposure angles that produce very thin layers. If the region is made up predominantly of soft tissue, then the layer might have to be at least 1 cm thick for contrast to be acceptable.

To improve contrast, particular attention should be paid to the control of scattered radiation by collimating the X-ray beam to the smallest possible field. A further method of improving contrast is to select the lowest kVp that will still give effective penetration.

Sharpness

As with a standard radiographic image, unsharpness can be due to patient movement (Um), focal spot size (Ug) and intensifying screens (Us). In addition, the tomographic movement can introduce a source of image unsharpness (Ut).

Particular attention should therefore be paid to the choice of focal spot sizes, immobilization and intensifying screens to reduce unsharpness to a minimum.

Exposure time and exposure angle

The exposure time and control of mA are undertaken automatically once the exposure angle has been selected. Automatic exposure control varies the mA continually during the exposure to ensure consistent film density.

Localization of the depth of the layer(s) required

The approximate depth may be known from past experience or from records kept of similar examinations. If not, then the depth of the layer can be estimated by studying antero-posterior and lateral radiographs.

Clearly, pivot heights will vary from patient to patient. They will also depend on whether a foam mattress is used and, if so, its thickness.

Radiation protection

The usual steps are taken to reduce the radiation dose to the patient, but there are some additional measures that are particularly applicable to tomography:

- The position and depth of the lesion should be localized accurately, preferably before the examination but if not then in the early stages of tomography.
- Whenever possible, the patient is positioned so that the structure of interest is parallel to the film, thus reducing the number of layers required.
- In skull tomography, position the patient prone wherever possible to reduce the radiation dose to the lens.
- The smallest field size compatible with a diagnosis is essential not only for radiation protection but also to improve radiographic contrast.
- The radiographer must follow an organized procedure for all stages of the examination to avoid the necessity of repeating exposure due to a careless omission.

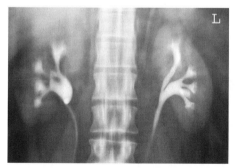

Thick layer (zonogram) required to give contrast in soft tissue region

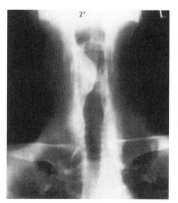
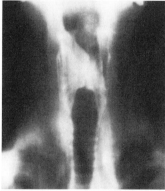

Thirty degrees linear. Contrast can be obtained in a thin layer containing air, bone and soft tissue

16 Tomography

Procedure

The following procedure should be used as a guide in preparing and undertaking tomography:

- Having read and understood the request card, previous images should be studied for the localization of the position, extent and depth of the region to be visualized.
- The exposure angle to be used is selected with reference to the thickness of the zone containing the lesion and the shape of structures to be blurred out.
- An explanation of the examination is given to the patient. The patient is then positioned and immobilized on the table.
- The vertical central ray is directed to the centre of the region and the X-ray beam is well collimated.
- The pivot height is set and the exposure angle is selected.
- The cassette carrying the appropriate radio-opaque legends is placed in position.
- The X-ray tube is moved to the starting position for the movement.
- The patient is given final instructions before the exposure is made.
- On viewing the tomography image, if it is satisfactory in terms of positioning, exposure, contrast and localization, any further required levels are taken.
- The pivot height is changed by a distance that depends on the thickness of the layers being recorded.

Exposure time and exposure angle

The exposure time selected should be greater than the time taken for the X-ray tube to complete the entire movement. This ensures that the exposure angle is symmetrical and that the anticipated angle, and hence layer thickness, is obtained. The choice of complex movements that require an exposure time of several seconds may be restricted if patient movement is a problem.

The use of variable-speed equipment allows for a choice of exposure time and mA for a given mAs.

In some examinations, not all of the exposure angle contributes equally to image formation. In such cases, the exposure can be controlled to take place during part of the movement. For example, in linear antero-posterior tomography of the larynx (caudal → cranial), the exposure can take place only during the first part of tube movement.

Applications

The widespread availability of CT has resulted in a corresponding decrease in the use of conventional tomography. The main use conventional tomography is in intravenous urography examinations to reduce the effects of superimposed bowel gas. It may still be used for other structures where access to CT is limited or not possible.

Two further applications – larynx and trachea – are included as examples.

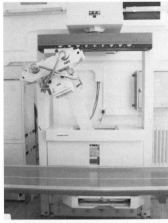

X-ray tube positioned in start position for linear tomography using a dedicated tomography unit

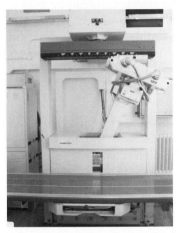

X-ray tube seen in stop position after linear tomography

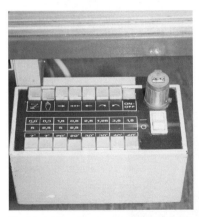

Pivot height and exposure angle adjustment control

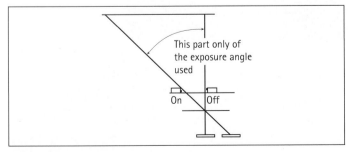

Diagram illustrating asymmetrical exposure angle technique

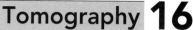
Kidneys

In this situation, tomography is often used as a simple, cheap and relatively effective method of imaging the renal tract free of overlying structures. Since the structures that are required to be visualized are relatively thick (antero-posterior measurement), zonography, or narrow-angle tomography, is used to produce a large layer thickness.

Tomography is used during intravenous urography either at 10–20 minutes after injection, to diffuse the shadows of gas that overlie the calyces preventing their clear visualization, or immediately on completion of the injection to show the nephrogram stage. This latter method – nephrotomography – was used to differentiate between kidney cysts and tumour and between intra- and extra-renal masses, but has been actively superseded by ultrasound and CT.

Notes

Although a narrow angle, e.g. 10 degrees, can produce a large layer thickness (approximately 5 cm) and may enable the whole of the outline of the kidneys to be shown on one exposure it will not efficiently 'blur out' overlying bowel shadows in the bowel.

To 'blur' gas shadows a 20-degree, 30-degree or even a 40-degree angle may have to be used.

Antero-posterior

Position of patient and cassette

- The patient is supine on the table, with the median sagittal plane of the body at right-angles to and in the midline of the table.

Direction and centring of the X-ray beam

- The vertical central ray is centred in the midline, midway between the suprasternal notch and the symphysis pubis.

Pivot height

- 8–11 cm.

Note – if a mattress is used, then allowance for its thickness must be made when selecting the pivot height.

Tomographic movement

- Linear 10 degrees – zonography.
- Linear 30 degrees – to blur out overlying bowel gas.

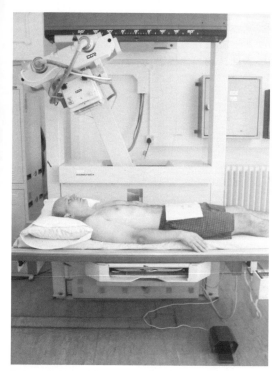

Patient positioned for tomography of the renal areas – note that during IVU abdominal compression is usually in place

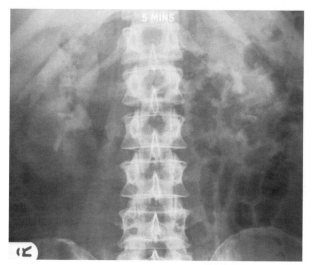

Five-minute post-contrast image with bowel gas obscuring the renal areas

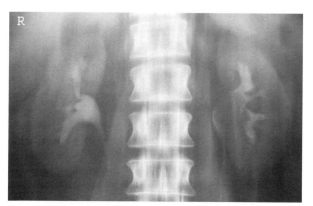

Tomography image showing the renal areas free from gas shadows and a mass in the left renal pelvic region

Larynx – antero-posterior

Position of patient and cassette

- The patient lies supine on the table, with the median sagittal plane of the trunk and head at right-angles to and in the mid-line of the table.
- The patient is located on the table so that a vertical central ray would pass 1 cm inferior to the eminence of the thyroid cartilage.

Pivot height

- From 0.5 cm deep to the skin surface to 4 cm deep to the skin surface.

Tomographic movement

- Linear longitudinal 20 degrees. With the X-ray tube moving in a caudal to cranial direction, the first half of a 40-degree movement can be used to avoid superimposing the images of the mandible and facial bones on to those of the larynx.
- Because the region is one of inherently high contrast, a high kVp (≥90 kVp) can be used; this reduces the amount of linear streaking recorded.
- Tomography may be taken during quiet breathing and also while the patient is phonating 'ee' to demonstrate an abnormal movement of the vocal cord due to a lesion.

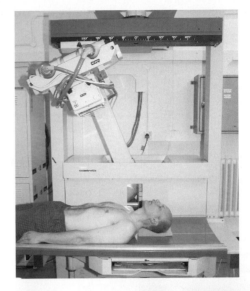

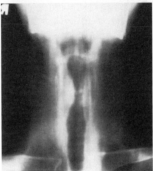
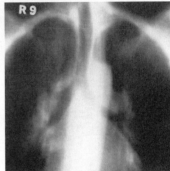

Larynx   Trachea and bifurcation

Trachea – antero-posterior

The trachea passes downwards and slightly backwards from its commencement at the lower border of the cricoid cartilage to its bifurcation just below the level of the sternal angle. With the patient supine, the trachea makes an angle of about 20 degrees with the table, its upper end being further from the table than its lower end. To bring the trachea and the image receptor parallel either the lower trunk is raised on pillows or, if there is sufficient clearance between the cassette tray and the undersurface of the table, the cassette can be inclined about 20 degrees in the cassette tray by raising the edge of the cassette which is under the neck.

Position of patient

The patient lies supine on the table with the median sagittal plane of the trunk and head at right angles to, and in the midline of, the table. The lower trunk is raised as described above, which is essential if the patient has a marked lordosis. The patient is located on the table so that the vertical central ray would pass along the median sagittal plane midway between the cricoid cartilage and the sternal angle.

Pivot height

- 4–5 cm deep to the sternal notch.

Tomographic movement

- Linear transverse 10 degrees; may be followed by large angle movements if thinner layers are required.

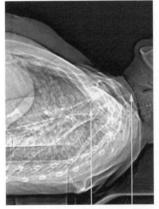

Computed tomography scout image showing the angle of the trachea

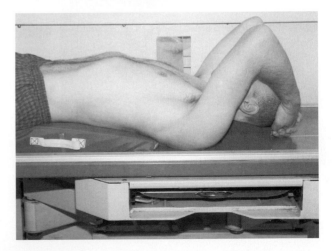

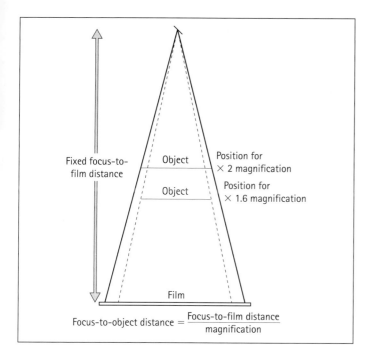

Fixed focus-to-film distance

Object — Position for × 2 magnification

Object — Position for × 1.6 magnification

Film

$$\text{Focus-to-object distance} = \frac{\text{Focus-to-film distance}}{\text{magnification}}$$

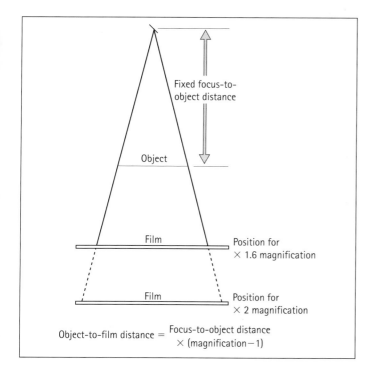

Fixed focus-to-object distance

Object

Film — Position for × 1.6 magnification

Film — Position for × 2 magnification

$$\text{Object-to-film distance} = \text{Focus-to-object distance} \times (\text{magnification} - 1)$$

Principles

In some cases, it is helpful to the person making a diagnosis if the radiographic image can be enlarged, allowing smaller detail to become more obvious. Where digital image recording is used, this magnification can be obtained electronically. Using conventional film/screen technology, an alternative method of producing a magnified image is at the time of exposure, by increasing the object-to-recording medium distance; in this case, the X-rays diverging from a point source will produce a directly magnified image.

The magnification (M) can be calculated from:

$$M = \frac{\text{image size}}{\text{object size}} = \frac{\text{FFD}}{\text{FOD}}$$

$$M = \frac{\text{FFD}}{\text{FOD}}$$

The FOD (or OFD) is taken from the mid-level of the part or lesion.

Fixed focus-to-film distance

For a fixed FFD, magnification is increased by bringing the object nearer to the X-ray tube focus. The FOD for a given magnification is calculated from:

$$\text{FOD} = \frac{\text{FFD}}{\text{magnification}}$$

For example, with a fixed FFD of 100 cm, and if a magnification factor of one to six is required, then the FOD will be:

$$\text{FOD} = \frac{\text{FFD}}{\text{M}} = \frac{100}{1.6} = 62.5 \text{ cm}$$

Fixed focus-to-object distance

So that the skin dose to the patient can be limited, the FOD is kept fixed at, say, 90 or 100 cm, and the required magnification is obtained by moving the film away from the object. The required OFD for a given magnification is than calculated from:

$$\text{OFD} = \text{FOD} (\text{M} - 1).$$

For example, if a magnification factor of one to six, is required at an FOD of 100 cm, then the required OFD will be:

$$\text{OFD} = 100(1.6 - 1) = 60 \text{ cm}.$$

Similarly, for a magnification factor of two at the same FOD, the required OFD will be:

$$\text{OFD} = 100(2 - 1) = 100 \text{ cm}.$$

Some equipment, e.g. the Orbix, has the facility for moving the cassette away from the object along a scale calibrated in magnification factors.

Principles (*contd*)

The technique of producing an image by direct magnification is called macroradiography. It has the advantage that although movement and geometrical unsharpness are increased compared with a technique using minimum OFD, there is no increase in photographic unsharpness. However, it must be remembered that such a magnified image will always be less sharp than one taken with the same focal spot with a minimum OFD.

A magnified image of acceptable sharpness will be produced only if movement unsharpness and geometrical unsharpness are kept to a minimum.

Movement unsharpness

Direct magnification by increased OFD can be carried out only if there is complete immobilization of the patient, because any movement of the patient, be it due to lack of immobilization or involuntary movement, will be magnified on the radiograph due to the increased OFD. The technique, therefore, lends itself to producing magnified images of bony structures or structures contained within bone, e.g. the lacrimal ducts. For macroradiography, immobilization devices should be used, e.g. supports, binders, sandbags and pads, and the instructions should be given to the patient to remain still.

Geometrical unsharpness

Geometrical unsharpness occurs because the source of X-rays is not a point source and any distance between the object and film will cause an image penumbra in addition to magnifying the image. Thus, for a given focal spot size, there is a limit to the magnification of the image beyond which the geometrical unsharpness is so great that significant detail is lost. The smaller the focal spot size, the greater the possible magnification of the image while still retaining acceptable image quality.

The relationship between image magnification (M) and focal spot size (f) with the corresponding geometrical unsharpness (Ug) is given by:

$$Ug = f(M - 1).$$

For example, if geometrical unsharpness is to be limited to 0.3 mm, then the maximum obtainable with the corresponding focal spot size is as follows:

Focal spot size (mm)	Maximum magnification
0.1	4.0
0.2	2.5
0.3	2.0
0.6	1.5
1.0	1.3

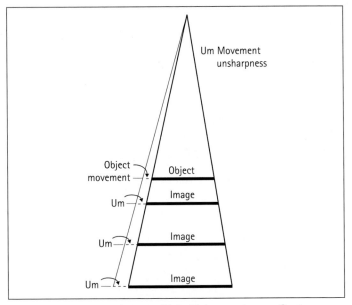

Increasing movement unsharpness (Um) with increase in magnification

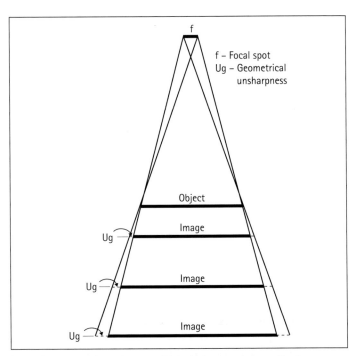

Increasing geometric unsharpness (Ug) with increase in magnification

Principles

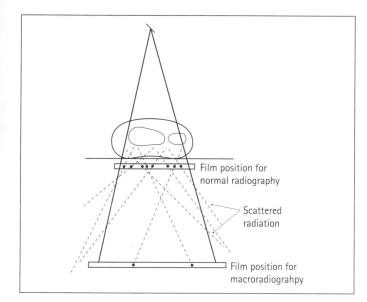

Film position for normal radiography

Scattered radiation

Film position for macroradiograhpy

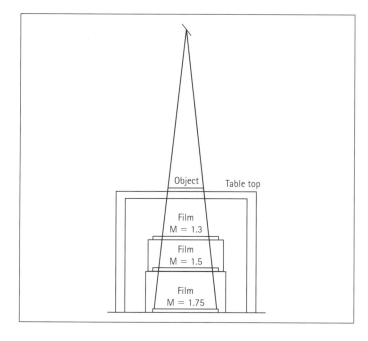

Object — Table top

Film M = 1.3

Film M = 1.5

Film M = 1.75

Scattered radiation

With macroradiography, there is usually an increase in FFD that requires a corresponding increase in mAs. Because an ultra-fine focus must be used, the permissible mA values will be reduced and hence a longer than normal exposure time is required. Immobilization is, therefore, essential. To reduce the mAs, and therefore the exposure time required, a secondary radiation grid may not used. It is possible to dispense with the grid because the amount of scatter reaching the film is reduced due to the air gap between the patient and the cassette. Scattered radiation leaving the patient diverges through the intervening gap and although it would have been incident on a cassette in contact with the patient, some of it is now scattered outside the area of the film.

Additionally, the smallest possible field is used in order to reduce the amount of scatter produced originally.

Cassette support

A method of supporting the cassette a known distance from the patient is required. An isocentric skull unit is ideal for this purpose, as the distance of the cassette holder from the body part under examination, and hence the magnification, can be varied precisely.

Applications

Because of the increased radiation dose in macroradiography and the increasing use of CR and DDR, the use of macroradiography is limited mainly to radiography of the skull in dacrocystography (see Chapter 10 in Whitley *et al.* (1999), p.380).

Macroradiography can also be used for imaging the carpal bones in cases of suspected fracture of scaphoid.

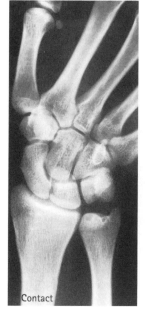

Contact

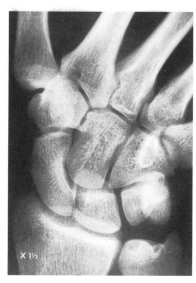

× 1½

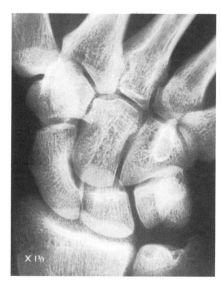

× 1⅔

16 Skeletal survey

Introduction

The commonest application of radiographic survey of the skeletal system is in suspected cases of non-accidental injury in children, when it is necessary to demonstrate the presence, multiplicity and age of any bone injury. The technique and imaging protocols required are described in detail in Chapter 14 (see p. 428).

In adults, multiple trauma, often from moving vehicle accidents, accounts for most situations where a skeletal survey is used. Reference has been made on page 471 to the Advanced Trauma Life Support (ATLS) imaging survey.

Another situation in which a skeletal survey may be useful in adults is the diagnosis and assessment of a patient with suspected myeloma, a malignant disease of the blood plasma cells. The diagnosis is usually made by detection of an abnormal immunoglobulin in the blood, but plain film radiographs are used in equivocal cases to confirm a diagnosis and to assist in monitoring the disease. Myeloma is unusual in that bony deposits of tumour do not usually elicit an osteoblastic reaction, and for this reason a radionuclide bone scan will often be negative.

Before the advent of modern radionuclide imaging, plain-film radiographic skeletal surveys were used as a primary means of diagnosing and assessing bony involvement in various pathological conditions, especially metastatic disease and some metabolic disorders.

Plain film radiography is now reserved for problem-solving when radionuclide scans require clarification, for example to determine whether a 'hot spot' is due to metastasis, degenerative disease, or some other condition such as Paget's disease. Modern biochemical tests have removed the need for skeletal surveys in the management of most metabolic and endocrine disorders, although radiography may be used to assess complications such as development of 'Brown tumours' in hyperparathyroidism or in detection of pathological fractures.

Since the development of disease-modifying drug regimens, serial radiography is increasingly used to monitor the progress and response to treatment of inflammatory arthropathies, particularly rheumatoid arthritis. This will normally be limited to the small joints of the hands and feet, but other areas may be imaged as clinically appropriate.

MRI offers the ability to image the soft tissues in addition to skeletal structures. For this reason, as well as its superior sensitivity and its ability to detect problems at multiple levels, it has largely replaced other imaging modalities in the assessment of suspected spinal cord compression.

Whenever a skeletal survey is considered, the projections should be adapted to the clinical information required and local protocols. Guidance from the clinician and/or radiologist in charge is important in determining the correct projections.

Indication	Projection
Myeloma and metabolic disease (adjust according to clinical picture and local protocol)	Lateral skull Postero-anterior chest Lateral lumbar spine Pelvis (to include upper femora) Antero-posterior left humerus Antero-posterior right humerus
Rheumatoid arthritis (projections to consider; rarely will all be required, others may be requested)	Postero-anterior chest Antero-posterior and lateral thoraco-lumbar spine Antero-posterior pelvis Sacro-iliac joints Cervical spine (flexion and extension) Dorsi-palmar, both hands (to include wrists) Antero-posterior both knees, Dorsi-plantar, both feet

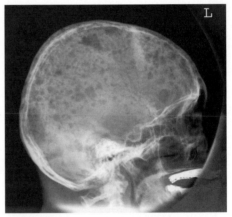

Lateral radiograph of skull showing multiple lytic deposits typical of myeloma

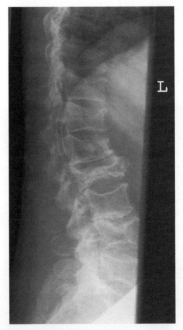

Lateral radiograph of lumbar spine showing multiple areas of vertebral collapse, of varying age, due to myeloma. Excessive collimation has partially obscured the lower two lumbar vertebrae

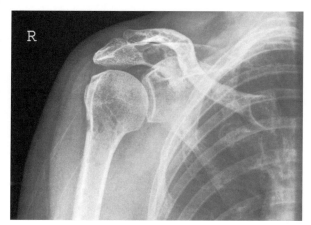

Antero-posterior radiograph of shoulder showing multiple lytic deposits of myeloma in the humerus, scapula, clavicle and ribs

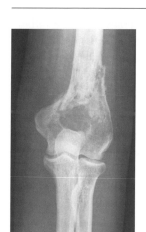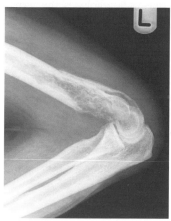

Antero-posterior and lateral radiographs of the elbow in a patient with myeloma, showing multiple tumour deposits and a pathological supracondylar fracture of the humerus

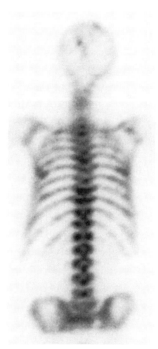

Radionuclide bone scan showing diffusely increased skeletal uptake and absent renal uptake (superscan) in a patient with metastases from carcinoma of the prostate

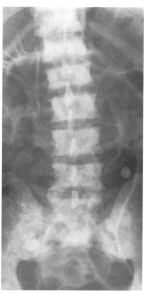

Antero-posterior radiograph of the lumbar spine in a patient with diffuse sclerotic metastases from carcinoma of the prostate

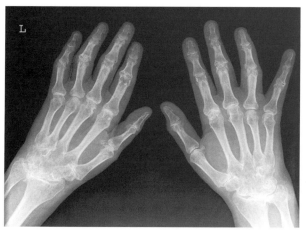

Dorsi-palmar radiograph of both hands and wrists in a patient with seronegative arthritis

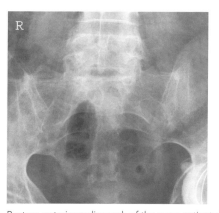

Postero-anterior radiograph of the same patient shown left, demonstrating fusion of the sacro-iliac joints sometimes seen in this condition

16 Soft tissue

Introduction

Soft-tissue radiography is the term generally used for radiography of muscle, skin, and subcutaneous and glandular tissues without the use of contrast media. There is normally only a small differential attenuation between adjacent structures, which results in lower subject contrast. Fat, however has a lower density than other soft tissue and the attenuation coefficient results in a higher optical density on the radiograph. The fat shadow may, therefore, delineate adjacent soft tissue structures and is normally demonstrated in subcutaneous tissue, between faciae, muscles and tendons. In order to successfully demonstrate soft tissues, specifically when using conventional film/screen technology, special attention must be given to:

- **radiographic contrast:** use of appropriate exposure technique, and reduction of scattered radiation;
- **image sharpness:** immobilization, small focal spot, film or film/screen combination chosen according to exposure technique;
- **avoidance of artefacts:** non-screen technique or scrupulously cleaned screens, avoidance of dressings, and avoidance of folds in the skin or in the patient's gown.

Skin tumours such as subcutaneous cysts and warts may cause confusing opacities and should be noted on the X-ray request card along with any other unusual features that may mislead the radiologist.

Exposure technique

Several different exposure techniques may be used. They may be divided broadly into two categories: those employing a normal kVp for the area being examined and those employing a non-standard kVp.

Normal kVp

This category may be divided into three subcategories:

- Use of a normal technique for the part being examined when air shadows or fat pads may delineate abnormalities in adjacent soft tissue structures, e.g.:
  - effusion in a synovial cavity causing a filling defect in a fat pad adjacent to a joint;
  - enlarged adenoids causing a filling defect in the air contained in the nasopharynx.
- Use of two or more films or film/screen combinations to demonstrate both bony detail and soft tissue with one exposure, e.g.:
  - facial bones, nasal bones and soft tissues of the face;
  - calcification of tendons and bony detail of the shoulder joint.

- Use of a wedge filter, where the thicker part of the wedge attenuates the beam over the soft tissues, e.g.:
  - cephalography to demonstrate bony detail of the skull and facial bones along with the soft-tissue outline of the face on one film;
  - to see the soft tissue of the toes when exposing the whole foot.

Non-standard kVp

This category of exposure technique may also be divided into three subcategories: subnormal kVp, low kVp and high kVp.

Subnormal kVp

This term is used when the kVp employed in less than 45 kVp, which is the lowest useful kVp available on many X-ray units. Modified or special equipment is required that has an X-ray tube with reduced added and inherent filtration along with a small focal spot size. The use of such kVp increases differential attenuation of adjacent soft tissues and thus increases subject contrast. Radiographic contrast may be increased further by the use of a film or film/screen combination with a high average gradient, i.e. more than three. An example of the use of this technique is found in mammography.

Low kVp

This term is used when the kVp employed is 15–20 kVp less than normal for a similar projection of the area being examined. Bony detail is not demonstrated in this case. Examples of the use of this technique are calcifications in limbs, e.g. calcification of arteries or tendons, parasitic calcifications and superficial tumours, normally demonstrated in a profile projection of the area.

High kVp

This term is used when the kVp employed is 20 kVp or more than that normally used for a similar projection of the same area. The use of such kVp reduces the differential attenuation of soft tissues, decreasing subject contrast, and thus allowing a greater range of tissues to be demonstrated. An example of this is the greater visualization of the bowel wall in double contrast barium enema examinations. When used with CR, edge enhancement (enhancement of the boundaries of different tissues) offsets the reduced contrast.

Note

Digital imaging technology facilitates the application of 'windowing' the acquired image to visualize soft tissue areas even when normal kVps are employed.

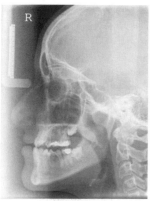

Example of a lateral cephalogram showing both skull bone and facial soft tissues on the one image

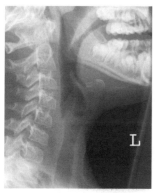

Lateral soft tissue image of the neck

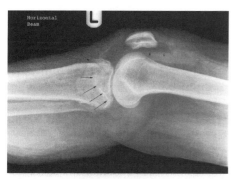

Horizontal beam lateral knee CR image windowed to show soft tissues showing depressed fracture of tibial plateau (arrows) and lipohaemarthrosis (arrowheads)

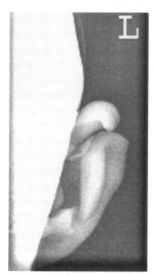
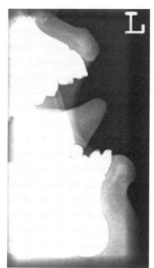

Image of traumatized ear   Soft tissue image of tongue

Exposure technique

Choice of projection

To demonstrate soft-tissue lesions, the most suitable projections are those that will project the area under examination away from the adjacent bone. Normally the projections described in the appropriate chapters of this book will be used, but occasionally a profile projection will be required of the area under examination.

Lesions demonstrated by air

Soft-tissue lesions may be demonstrated by air in body cavities, e.g. enlarged adenoids encroach on the posterior nasopharyngeal air space demonstrated on a lateral projection of the neck. After adenoidectomy, there is no longer soft-tissue encroachment on the air space. A normal exposure technique for the part being examined is used in these cases.

Air in the soft tissue is known as surgical emphysema and may be caused by trauma, especially rib fracture or perforation of an abdominal viscous such as the rectum. A large area must be included on the radiograph; therefore, a high kVp should be used.

Lesions demonstrated by fat

Fat has a lower attenuation coefficient than other soft tissue and shows as a higher optical density on the radiograph. Effusion in a synovial cavity may cause a filling effect in a fat pad adjacent to a joint. Blood-lipid fluid levels may also be demonstrated when a horizontal central ray technique is used. It is, therefore, essential that the kVp used to demonstrate joints is sufficient to demonstrate both bone and soft-tissue structures.

Lipoma is a benign, well-defined fatty tumour that is more transradiant than adjacent tissues and therefore appears as a darker area on the radiograph. A normal exposure is used.

Calcifications in soft tissue

Calcifications in limbs, e.g. calcifications of arteries, tendons and ligaments, and parasitic calcifications, are usually best demonstrated by using a low kVp exposure technique. Calcifications in the trunk are demonstrated using a normal exposure technique.

Bone and adjacent soft tissues

In conditions such as rheumatoid arthritis, gout, myositis ossificans and osteomyelitis, there may be soft-tissue swelling and calcification. It is, therefore, essential that the kVp is sufficient to demonstrate both bone and soft-tissue structures.

Introduction

Forensic medicine is defined as the use of medical knowledge, especially pathology, to the purposes of the law, as in determining the cause of death.

Forensic radiography is the use of radiographic knowledge to aid in the implication of forensic medicine. The word 'forensic' comes from the Latin *'forensic'*, meaning 'to the forum'. The forum was the basis of Roman law and was a place of public discussion and debate pertinent to the law.

Forensic anthropology is the application of the science of physical anthropology to the legal process.

Whilst radiography is necessary when dealing with individual victims, it is also used on a greater scale when associated with major tragedies such as train crashes and air disasters.

Imaging is also required in the identification of individuals whose remains may be badly decomposed or only skeletal. Such identification may be associated with war victims or civil atrocities with victims found in mass graves.

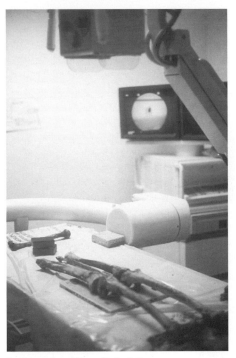

Radiography of lower limb skeleton

Classification of forensic radiography

Radiography of a cadaver is undertaken for several different medical purposes:

- fetal and neonatal;
- identification;
- cause of death.

All of these investigations are usually requested under the direction of the coroner, and the attending pathologist will request specific areas to be examined radiographically.

Post-mortem imaging may also be requested to identify any previous disease processes or trauma that the deceased has suffered and that may or may not have contributed to their death.

Another area of forensic radiography in either the live or deceased patient is in the assessment of non-accidental injury (NAI), usually in paediatric patients but also now in elderly patients.

For elderly abuse queries, the areas to be imaged will be identified by the pathologist. For paediatric abuse queries, the protocol authorized within the place of work must be used for either live or deceased patients.

The foremost pitfalls in the radiological diagnosis of abuse are suboptimal radiological imaging, radiographic underexposure or overexposure, and malposition.

A protocol will specify the projections required and also the high technical image quality needed to identify the fine changes and disruption of normal bone patterns.

Other specific areas to be imaged may also be requested by the pathologist to ascertain the maximum amount of information from the X-ray examination.

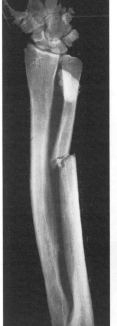
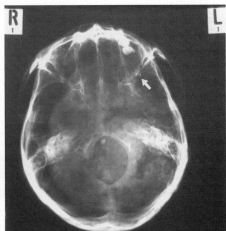

Fractured ulna   Skull base projection

Anatomical terminology

There are few clinical words and terms that are used purely in this scenario. Anatomy references are generic, regardless of whether the patient is alive or post mortem.

Legal issues

The College of Radiographers stated in 1999: 'Forensic radiography refers to the application of medical knowledge in the collection of evidence to be used in a court of law.'

To ensure parity for all forensic examinations, certain guidelines and methods of recording evidence are necessary:

- All radiographs taken must be signed by the radiographer.
- Date and identification (ID) must be photographed on to the image.
- Number of images and all projections taken must be formally noted and signed by the radiographer and a witness.
- No copies of the original images.

Equipment and accessories

The X-ray equipment required for forensic radiography is variable and dependent on what is available and whether the imaging is to take place off site. It may include:

- mobile X-ray machine;
- dental radiographic equipment;
- fluoroscopy equipment;
- digital radiographic equipment;
- CT (on-site or mobile) equipment;
- MRI (on-site or mobile) equipment;
- film-processing facilities with darkroom.

If standard mobile X-ray machines are to be used, then cassettes, grids, film and processing equipment will also be required.

Cassette size and intensifying screen type are dependent on the area being examined.

Electricity and water supplies will also be required if working off site.

Using fluoroscopy or any other digital method of imaging also gives the option of digital storage of the images produced.

Accessories required include:

- protective clothing, including gown/suit, gloves and mask;
- plastic bags to protect cassettes;
- cleaning materials;
- pads and sandbags;
- radio-opaque markers;
- stationery.

Local radiation rules

If forensic radiography is undertaken on site, i.e. on Trust property, then departmental local radiation rules with regard to radiation protection for all radiographic examinations must be adhered to.

Separate local rules will need to be drawn up when working in an emergency mortuary situation. These must include the identification of:

- the radiation protection supervisor (RPS);
- the radiation protection advisor (RPA).

The RPA is the radiographer's employer's (i.e. the Trust's) RPA.

- The definition of a 'controlled area' must be stated, including marking boundaries and erecting warning signs.
- The controlled area must be of at least a 2-m radius from the X-ray tube (vertical beam).
- All personnel within this area must wear protective equipment.
- Monitoring devices must be placed at the boundary of the controlled area.
- For horizontal-beam radiography, where possible the primary beam must be directed towards a primary shield and the controlled area extended to 6 m from the X-ray tube.

De-briefing

This process of assessing the effects of the trauma of undertaking forensic radiography in any situation is essential for the welfare and support of the professionals involved. The radiographers must be made aware of the signs and symptoms of stress, and strategies identified to help them cope with it.

A support mechanism must be provided for these professional volunteers and access to specialist support must be made available.

A de-briefing session after a major incident is standard procedure in the police force, and any radiographers involved in these incidents participate in these sessions.

Forensic radiography should be undertaken by *volunteer radiographers* whenever possible.

16 Forensic radiography

Dental radiography

The primary technique used in the identification of a cadaver is the comparison of dental records. This examination can be used regardless of the stage of decomposition or the post-mortem state of the cadaver.

An odontologist will examine the cadaver's dentition to record a plan. In addition to this visual and clinical assessment by the specialist, dental X-rays may also be requested.

The images produced can be evidential proof of cadaver identification when matched to previous dental records. Radiographic detail of the following will aid the odontologist in the final identification of a cadaver:

- fillings and dental intervention;
- root morphology;
- unerupted teeth;
- dental patterns;
- previous dental surgery.

Recommended dental projections

The odontologist may request several standard radiographic dental and facial projections. The primary projections taken to produce maximum information are:

- lower standard occlusals;
- upper standard occlusals;
- intra-oral radiographs;
- mandibular projections.

The radiographic technique for these projections can be found in the appropriate dental/facial sections of this book (see Section 10).

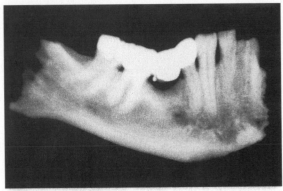

Radiograph of a fragment of mandible recovered from a plane crash. A gold bridge is shown with melting of gold solder due to the heat of the fire following the crash

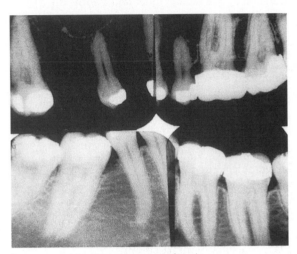

Post-mortem bitewing radiographs of teeth

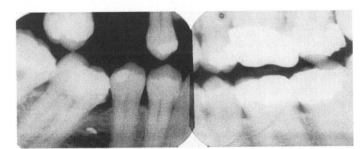

Ante-mortem bitewing radiographs of teeth matching the post-mortem radiographs seen above

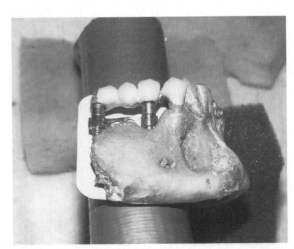

Imaging a section of the mandible

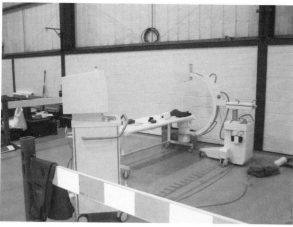

Distant mortuary set up with a mobile image intensifier system

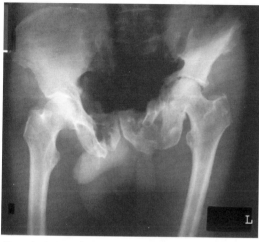

Air crash victim with severe pelvic trauma

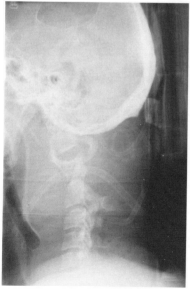

Motorcyclist with extensive neck trauma – note air in the oesophagus

Adaptation of technique

Several changes to normal radiographic technique for both dental and general radiography undertaken will be required.

The majority of forensic radiography is carried out distant from the imaging department and using mobile radiographic equipment. Forensic radiography will usually be undertaken in a mortuary, either permanent or temporary.

The physical state of the cadaver will determine the number of projections that will be taken and the techniques that can be used.

The cadaver may be contained (e.g. in a body bag); whilst this is advantageous with regard to health and safety and cross-infection, it does limit any changes to be made in positioning of the cadaver for X-ray examination.

Care must be taken to ensure that no sharp or dangerous objects are present in the body or body bag. The radiographer needs to be aware of these potential dangers of injury to himself/herself and others.

Thus, no protocol can be formalized for forensic imaging, as the examination is dependent on many variables.

Adaptations will be required to all standard radiographic techniques for each examination being undertaken.

Imaging may be undertaken using a selection of cassettes containing film/screens systems in order to provide full coverage of the body. Alternatively, imaging may be undertaken using a mobile C-arm fluoroscopic system enabling full screening of the body to identify specific abnormalities. Such equipment will incorporate an imaging recording system in order to record and catalogue forensic features.

When using such equipment to image a body bag, it is important that a scanning technique is adopted that allows for overlapping of areas of the body to ensure that no area of the body and body bag are left un-imaged. The C-arm should be moved in a set pattern. The use of floor markings will aid the radiographer to ensure overlapping of the image intensifier field.

When necessary, two plain-film projections at right-angles are taken of a specific area. This may be required to provide further information on the nature and extent of a sustained injury.

Images may also be required of sections of the body that have been removed by the pathologist for more detailed forensic examination.

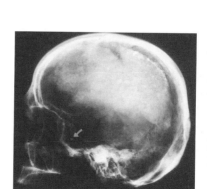

Lateral skull showing a bullet trace

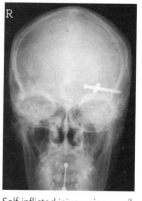

Self-inflicted injury using a nail gun at point blank range

16 Forensic radiography

Still born (15–40 weeks)

General comments

- A full skeletal survey is undertaken, at the request of the coroner for the pathologist.
- Identification is by referral card and is cross-checked with the identification bands on the limbs of the fetus.
- The technique normally employed is that of whole-body 'babygram' with both antero-posterior and lateral projections acquired.
- Dependent upon the gestational age of the fetus, additional fronto-occipital and lateral skull images are taken.
- Images are acquired using a 400-speed film/screen system in a standard cassette or using a CR/DDR system.
- Images are shown to a specialist radiologist.
- Further images may be requested dependent upon any abnormalities that are identified at the time of imaging.

Imaging technique

- As the health and safety of the staff is imperative, the procedure is easier if two radiographers perform the examination. This will reduce the risk of cross-injection and provide added personal protection.
- The X-ray room is prepared. The imaging cassette is covered in a polythene sheet, taking care that it remains smooth to exclude any crease artefacts being recorded on the image.

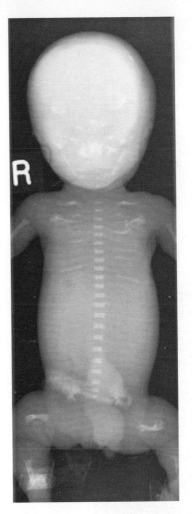

Antero-posterior 'babygram'

- The fetus is placed on the covered cassette in the supine position.
- The limbs are positioned antero-posterior where possible. It may be necessary to support these in place by using plastic strips taped down over the limbs or covered sandbags.
- The X-ray tube is centred and collimated to include all the relevant anatomy. (Specific techniques are detailed in Section 14.)
- Lead markers are placed into the collimated area.
- Exposure factors should be selected consistent with the size of the fetus.

Note

Normally, X-ray rooms used for this purpose have a detailed exposure chart (e.g. 25-week fetus: 56 kV, 1.4 mAs.)

Identification

The imaging cassette is marked immediately following exposure, ensuring that the correct information and orientation are on the image, including date and identification number.

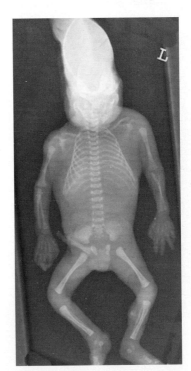

Examples of antero-posterior whole-body images of fetuses

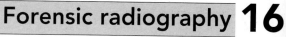

Lateral 'babygram'

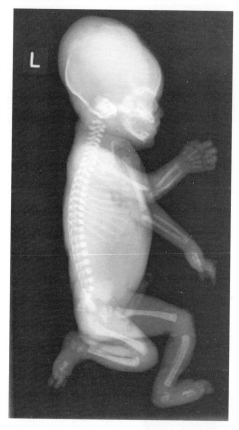

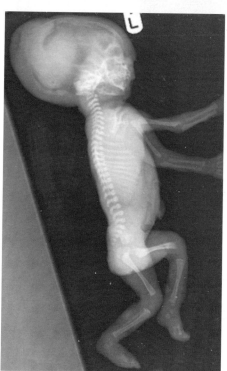

Examples of lateral whole-body images of fetuses

- The fetus is placed on the covered cassette in the lateral position. The cassette size is dependent upon the size of the fetus.
- The limbs are positioned lateral where possible. It may be necessary to support these in place by using plastic strips taped down over the limbs/covered sandbags or soft roll.
- The X-ray tube is centred and collimated to include all the relevant anatomy. (Specific techniques are detailed in Section 14.)
- Lead markers are placed into the collimated area. It may be necessary to mark individual limbs to ensure correct identification.
- Exposure factors should be selected consistent with the size of the fetus.

Note

Normally, X-ray rooms used for this purpose have a detailed exposure chart (e.g. 25-week fetus: 56 kV, 1.4 mAs.)

Identification

The imaging cassette is marked immediately following exposure, ensuring that the correct information is on the image, including the date and patient identification number.

16 Forensic radiography

Still born (15–40 weeks): skull projections

Fronto-occipital

- The fetus is placed on the covered 18 × 24-cm cassette/ imaging plate in the supine position.
- The skull is normally flexed forward at presentation, but a covered 15-degree wedge may be placed under the shoulders to bring the orbito-meatal lie at right-angles to the cassette.
- Soft roll or covered pads are used to immobilize the skull and prevent rotation.
- The remainder of the technique is as described in Section 14.

Note

Normally, X-ray rooms used for this purpose have a detailed exposure chart (e.g. 25-week fetus: 56 kV, 1.4 mAs.)

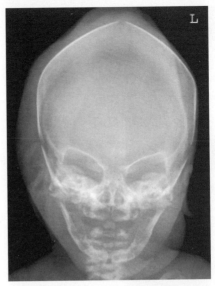

Fronto-occipital skull image of a fetus

Lateral

- The fetus is turned into the lateral position, with the head resting on the covered 18 × 24-cm cassette/imaging plate.
- A soft roll or covered pad may be placed under the face to bring it parallel with the table and cassette.
- The remainder of the technique is as described in Section 14.

Note

Normally, X-ray rooms used for this purpose have a detailed exposure chart (e.g. 25-week fetus: 56 kV, 1.4 mAs.). An alternative technique is to use a horizontal beam lateral. This may be required, dependent upon the presentation of the fetus.

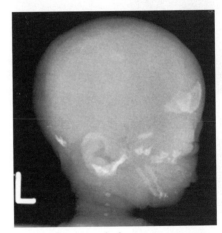

Lateral skull image of a fetus

Identification

The imaging cassette is marked immediately following exposure, ensuring that the correct orientation and information are on the image, including the date and patient ID number.

Post-procedure

- The X-ray equipment and room are cleaned according to hospital protocol.
- The referral card and images (where appropriate) are presented to the radiologist for report.

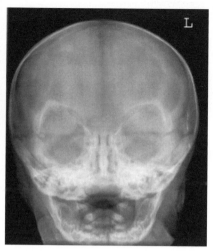

Antero-posterior skull on a 1-year-old child

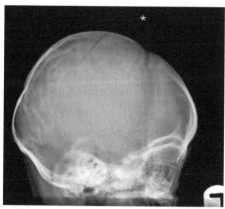

Lateral skull on the same child (above) showing a fracture in the parietal region

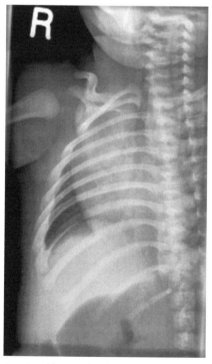

Anterior oblique right ribs

Skeletal survey – out of hours

Skeletal survey protocols for cot death and other such fatalities, as well as non-accidental injury investigations in children, are discussed in detail in Section 14 (see pp. 428–431). However, in the 'out of hours' situation, a protocol should be adopted similar to the one described below, which will assist as a reminder and guide for all those involved in undertaking this task. It is often the case that such requests are made out so infrequently that such a protocol will be helpful in determining the roles and responsibilities of every member of the team. Included on the page are some images for the standard radiography series.

Example protocol

- The accident and emergency (A&E) sister/mortuary technician to liaise with the on-call radiographer.
- All surveys should be performed in the X-ray department.
- A record is made of the names of all staff involved in the imaging procedure and attendant during the procedure.
- A decision is made on the time to perform the survey. (Note that this should be during normal working hours where possible.)
- The lead paediatric radiologist must be informed when the survey is to be performed on a child.
- The on-call radiologist must be informed when the procedure is to be performed on an adult.
- The entire examination must be witnessed. This may be the sister from A&E, a police officer or a coroner officer.
- Witnesses must be present throughout the procedure and must not leave the subject unattended at any time.
- The subject must be identified correctly, and all images must be labelled correctly with name and date. Side-markers should be present on all projections at the time of the examination.
- At the end of the procedure, hard copies of the images with a radiologist report should be handed over to the coroner's officer.
- In extreme circumstances, i.e. when the coroner requests to move the body before a radiologist arrives, it is important to ensure that the referral card is given to the appropriate radiologist for them to issue a report later, as follows:

Compiled by: ....

Name of authorizer: ....

Date of protocol: ....

Review date: ....

16 Further reading

Merten DF, Carpenter BLM (1990). Radiologic imaging of inflicted injury in the child abuse syndrome. *Pediatric Clinics of North America*, 37, 815–37.

College of Radiographers (1999). *Guidance for the Provision of Forensic Radiography Services*. London, College of Radiographers.

Whitley AS, Alsop CW, Moore AD (1999). *Clarke's Special Procedures in Diagnostic Imaging*. London, Butterworth Heinemann, p. 380.

Index

abdominopelvic cavity 331–50, 398–401
  image parameters 335
  imaging protocols 334
  paediatric radiography 337, 398–401
    in survey for non-accidental injury 429
  planes and regions 332–3
  projections 334
  radiological considerations 326–7
  referral criteria for radiography 334
  ward radiography 353, 358–60
abdominothoracic radiography, neonatal 390
abduction 6
  arm in, coracoid process demonstration 103
  hand in, scaphoid imaging with 50
  hip in 147
abscess
  hepatic and subphrenic 343
  pulmonary 397
absorption unsharpness 19, 20, 32
acetabuloplasty 409
acetabulum 155
  anterior oblique (Judet's) projection 151, 155
  fracture 142, 155
achondroplasia 431
acoustic (auditory) meatus, external 230
acrodysostosis 431
acromioclavicular joints 94
adduction 6
adolescents (incl. teenagers) 384
  pregnancy 386
Advanced Trauma and Life Support (ATLS) 471
  spinal radiography 471
    cervical 170, 471
    whole spine/full projections 181, 471
air, free see gas
air cells, mastoid 252
air-gap technique 201
airways
  foreign body see foreign bodies
  lower see lungs
  upper 194–7
alimentary tract, foreign bodies see foreign bodies, swallowed
ambient lighting 16
anatomy
  child–adult differences 384
  terminology 2
    breast 438
    forensic radiography 496
    skull 230
    tooth surface 284
aneurysm, abdominal aortic see aortic aneurysm
angiography, emergency 380
angle board 317
ankle (talocrural) joint 106, 114–17
  movements/positions 107
  in skeletal survey for non-accidental injury 430
anterior oblique projection 8
  biliary system 348
  cervical vertebrae 176
  elbow 62–3

hand 42
heart/aorta 219
hip joint/acetabulum 151, 155
occlusal radiography
  mandible 312
  maxilla 311
scaphoid 51
skull 235, 254
anterior patient aspect 2
antero-posterior oblique projection
  knee joint 134
  sacro-iliac joint 161
  sternum 226–7
  tibiofibular joint (proximal) 125
antero-posterior projection 7, 10, 11
  abdominopelvic cavity 338–42, 358–9
    biliary system 348
    children 398–401
    diaphragm 343, 344, 398
    liver 343
    urinary tract (incl. kidney) 339, 345–6, 347, 487
    ward radiography 358–9
  ankle joint 114–15, 116
    in stress 117
  babygram (stillborn) 500
  cervical spine
    auto-tomography 173, 479
    C1/C2 170–2
    C3/C7 172–3
    child 416
  coccyx 192
  elbow, child 421–2
  femur
    child 364
    shaft 136
    ward radiography 362, 364
  forearm 59
  hips 148–50
    both 145, 148–9
    children 408–9, 410, 431
    one 144, 150, 371
    prostheses/implants 370, 375
  humerus
    neck 74
    shaft 71, 72
    supracondylar 70
  knee joint 126
    in corrective surgery 370
    in stress 129
  leg length assessment 417
  lumbar vertebrae 182–3
  lumbosacral junction 189
  lungs 205, 208–10
    neonatal 365
    post-neonatal children 394–5
  pelvis 143, 145, 148–9, 158
    children 408–9, 410
    ward radiography 362
  ribs
    cervical 225
    lower 222
    upper 225

sacro-iliac joints 160
sacrum 190
shoulder
  calcified tendons 92–3
  clavicle 96
  coracoid process 103
  glenohumeral joint 85–6
  outlet projection 83
  post-manipulation 87
  in recurrent dislocation 88–90
  scapula 101
  survey image 81
thoracic spine 179–80
thorax
  lungs see subheading above
  neonates 390–2
  pharynx/larynx 194, 488
  post-neonatal children 394–6
  ribs see subheading above
  tomography 488
  trachea/thoracic inlet 196, 488
  on ward 354–7, 355, 365
thumb 48
tibia and fibula 124
anthropological baseline 230, 255
anthropological plane 230, 255
anus, imperforate 384, 401
aorta 214–19
  anatomy 214, 215
aortic aneurysm, abdominal 334, 337
  ward radiography 358
apophyseal joint see facet joint
apophysis
  calcaneal 118
  iliac, development 415
arc-to-arc tomographic movement 482
arc-to-line tomographic movement 482
arm see upper limb
artefacts
  abdominopelvic radiography 335
  chest X-ray 205, 217
  mammography 444
  soft tissue radiography 494
  trauma radiography 470
arthritis
  glenohumeral 78
  skeletal survey 491, 492
  see also osteoarthritis
arthroplasty, total (prosthesis), hip joint 148, 362, 363, 370
articulare 327
ascites 336
asphyxiating thoracic dystrophy 431
asthenic abdomen 333
atlanto-axial joint 171
  subluxation 169
atria 214
auditory meatus, external 230
auricular plane 230, 255
automatic exposure control
  abdominopelvic radiography 338
  breast radiography 440, 451
  digital imaging 24

automatic exposure control (*contd*)
  paediatric radiography 387
  trauma radiography 471
auto-tomography 479
  cervical vertebrae 173, 479
  thoracic vertebrae 181, 479
axial (transverse) plane 3
  abdominopelvic cavity, upper and lower 332
  breast 437
  calcaneum 119
  carpal tunnel 54
  cervical vertebrae (upper) 174
  elbow 64–5
    ulnar groove 67
  humerus
    bicipital groove 73
    neck 74
  shoulder 81
  toes 113
axillary lymph nodes 438, 446
axillary tail 437, 457
  artefact 444
azygos lobe 204

babygram 500, 500–1
  see also infants; neonates
Baker's tray, operative cholangiography 378
ball catcher's position 44
Bankhart lesion 88
barium swallow, foreign bodies 474
batteries, swallowed 400, 474
beam-alignment instruments in dental
      radiography 288
  bitewing radiography 292, 294
  paralleling technique 300, 301
beam angulation 7, 10–11
  oblique projection using 9
  in periapical radiography, bisecting angle
      technique 296, 297, 298
  skull 234
    half-axial fronto-occipital 30 degrees caudad
        projection 243, 244
    lateral projection 235
    occipito-frontal projections 240, 241
    problems and warnings 235
  see also specific tissues and their projections
beam collimation *see* collimation
beam dimensions, dental radiography 285
Bennett's fracture 49
bicipital groove 73
biliary system incl. ducts, radiography
      (=cholangiography) 348
  operative 378
bimolar projection 317
biopsy, breast 460–1, 463
  image-guided 447, 460–1
bisecting angle technique 291, 295–8
bit depth 25
bite block 302, 303, 304
bitewing radiography 280, 292–4
  film holding ± beam-holding instruments 288
  forensics 498
  image geometry 294
    optimization 291
bitewing tab 292, 293
bladder 347
  calculi 336, 345, 347
  in retrograde pyelography 376
blood flow mechanics in supine chest X-ray 209

body bag imaging 499
body build 333
Bohler's angle 118
bone
  age assessment 423
  soft tissues adjacent to, demonstration
      495
bone subtraction, dual energy digital imaging of
      lungs 201
bowel (intestine) 334
  dilatation 340
  haemorrhage 380
  obstruction 336, 339, 341
    children 398, 399
    by foreign body 474
    ward radiography 358, 359
  perforation 337
    impending 359
  see also constipation
boxer's fracture 42, 45
breast 435–63
  anatomy 438
  biopsy *see* biopsy
  cancer *see* cancer
  compression (for mammography) *see*
      compression
  developing, avoiding exposure 411, 412
  guidance for interventions 447, 460–1
  implants 446, 462
  radiography *see* mammography
  specimen tissue radiography 463
  UK screening service 443
bronchi 204
  foreign body 475
bronchiectasis, children 395
bronchiolitis 396
buccal tooth surface 284
bullet trace, skull 499
burst fracture, cervical spine 171

cadaver *see* post-mortem imaging
calcaneonavicular coalition 426
calcaneovalgus 427
calcaneus 106, 118–19
  in talipes equinovarus 424, 425, 426
calcification 495
  breast 444, 445
    benign 445, 451
    malignant 445
  heart valve 217
  pericardial 218
  shoulder tendons 91–3
calculi
  salivary 309, 313
  urinary tract 336, 345, 347
    kidney *see* kidney
cancer (malignancy incl. carcinoma)
  breast 445, 446
    UK screening service 443
    ultrasound/MRI/scintigraphy 447
  radiation-related risk 34
canines 281
  in bisecting angle technique 298
  in paralleling technique 301, 302
  unerupted maxillary, vertex occlusal
      radiograph 307
canthus, outer 230
capacitor discharge units 353
capitellum (of humerus), fracture 422

cardiomegaly (heart enlargement) 219
  artefactual 217
cardiothoracic ratio (CTR) 208, 209, 215
carpal bones, recommended projections 38
  see also specific bones
carpal tunnel 54
carpus *see* carpal bones; wrist
cartilages, laryngeal 181, 195
cassette, access in trauma radiography to 470
cassette holder, trauma radiography 470
catheter
  superior vena cava 357
  umbilical artery or vein 392
cathode ray tube 26
cementum 281
central venous pressure line 357
cephalometry 280, 325–8
  paediatric 407
  panoramic machines and 321, 325
  soft tissues in 495
cervical ribs 225
cervical spine/vertebrae (and neck) 164, 168–78
  in Advanced Trauma and Life Support
      170, 471
  auto-tomography 173, 479
  forensic radiography 499
  fracture 171, 181, 471
    and dislocation 361
  levels/landmarks 166, 167
  paediatric 416
    in survey for non-accidental injury 429
  ward radiography 361
cervicothoracic junction 178
charge-coupled device (CCD) 23
  dental radiography 287, 288
chest *see* thorax
chevron square system 282
children 381–433
  abdominopelvic radiography *see*
      abdominopelvic cavity
  bone age 423
  chest *see* thorax
  dental radiography 407
    film mounting and holding in intra-oral
        radiography 289
    film positioning in occlusal radiography 310
    lateral oblique 315
  elbow 420–2
  femoral fracture 364
  foreign bodies
    nasal passages 476
    swallowed 400, 474
  general aspects 382–9
    choice of imaging methods 382–3
    common examinations 390
    environment 386
    justification 382
    legislation 382
    patient considerations 384–6
    radiation risks and protection 34, 382, 389
  hip *see* hip joint
  humerus *see* humerus
  non-accidental injury 496
    post-mortem radiography 428, 503
    skeletal survey 428–30, 492, 503
  paranasal sinuses 406
  radiation risks and protection (in general) 34,
      382, 389
  see also specific tissues/anatomic regions

skull radiography *see* skull
spine *see* vertebral column
see also adolescents; infants and toddlers; neonates
chin position in dental panoramic radiography 323
cholangiography *see* biliary system
Cincinnati filter device 397
clavicle 75, 95–8
CMOS (complementary metal oxide semiconductor)-based sensors in dental radiography 287, 288
coccyx 164, 192
   palpation 166
collapsed lobe (lung) 213
collateral ligaments, ankle, tear 115
Colles' fracture 58
collimation 35
   chest X-ray 205
   dental radiography 285
      panoramic radiography 325
   facial bones 262
   skull radiography
      cephalometry 326
      children 402, 404
   trauma radiography 469
colon
   intussusception 399
   obstruction, ward radiography 358
communication with children 384, 385
complementary metal oxide semiconductor (CMOS)-based sensors, dental radiography 287, 288
compression
   breast (for mammography) 439
      in various projections 448–58
   image 26
   spinal cord 492
computed radiography (CR) 22
   technology 23
   uses 22
      dental radiography 287
      foreign body 472, 477
      leg alignment 139
      paediatrics 388
computed tomography
   head/skull
      cephalometry 407
      in non-accidental injury 428
      skull base 246
   hip joint/acetabulum 155
   intestinal obstruction 336
   shoulder 78
   spine
      cervical 171
      trauma patient 471
   thorax, bony reconstruction 220
computer monitor *see* monitor
condoms, drugs swallowed in 474
congenital disease
   abdomen/bowel 401
   foot deformities 426
   heart 393
   hip (developmental dysplasia) 410
coning devices, children 389
consolidation 354
   neonates 392
constipation 337
   child 400

contrast 13–17, 32
   bitewing radiography 294
   kilovoltage and 14, 29
   lumbar vertebrae 184
   lungs 200, 201
   radiographic *see* radiographic contrast
   shoulder radiography 78
   soft tissue radiography 494
   thoracic vertebrae 179
   tomography 485
   trauma radiography 471
contrast media 14
coracoid process 79, 103
core biopsy 463
   image-guided 460, 461
coronal (frontal) plane 3
   skull 3, 230
coronal sutures 404
cranio-caudal projection, breast 450–4
craniosynostosis 402
cranium *see* skull
cricoid cartilage 181
cross-infection control *see* infection
crown of teeth 281
cyst
   breast 446, 447
   hydatid (liver) 343
   mandibular 309
   pericardial 217, 218
cystic fibrosis 393
cystinosis 423
cystoscopy and cystography preceding retrograde pyelography 376

darkroom, theatre radiography 369
death, radiography after *see* post-mortem imaging
de-briefing, forensic radiography 497
decubitus positions (lying down) 4
   dorsal *see* supine position
   lateral *see* lateral decubitus position
   lateral dorsal *see* lateral dorsal decubitus
   lungs 198
   ventral *see* prone position
degenerative change, knees 132
dens (odontoid peg) 171
density 12, 13
   breast (focal-increased) 445
   contrast and 14–16
   image *see* image
   patient/physical 12
   photographic/optical 12, 13
dental radiography 278–329
   children *see* children
   extra-oral *see* extra-oral radiography
   film
      in bitewing radiography 292, 293, 294
      in dental panoramic radiography, faults and their correction 324
      direct film 286
      mounting and identification 289
      occlusal radiography 310
      in paralleling technique 300
      processing 290, 321
      sizes 286, 292
      third molar images 304, 305
   forensic applications 498
   image reception and acquisition 286–8, 318–23

infection control 290
   intra-oral *see* intra-oral radiography
   radiation protection 290
   uses 280
   X-ray equipment features 285
dentine 281
Denton beam-limiting technique 404
detectors (digital imaging) 23, 24, 26
development (film) *see* processing
developmental dysplasia of hip 410
diaphragm 343
   children 398
   respiratory movements 344
DICOM (Digital Imaging and Communications in Medicine) 25
digit(s) *see* fingers; thumb; toes
digital imaging (DR) 22–7
   advantages 22
   direct *see* direct digital imaging
   image capture/acquisition *see* image
   image optimization 24
   image processing 26
   image quality, factors affecting 23–4
   image size and bit depth 25
   networking 25–6
   technology 23
   uses 22
      dental radiography 287, 288
      leg alignment 139
      leg length assessment 419
      lungs 200, 201
      urinary tract radiography 388
Digital Imaging and Communications in Medicine 25
digital recording in cephalometric analysis 327
direct digital imaging (DDR), uses 22
   foreign body 472
dislocations
   carpus/wrist 58
      lunate 53, 58
   elbow 68
   facet 173
   hip 142, 149
      congenital (=developmental dysplasia) 410
   interphalangeal joint (distal) 47
   radius
      distal 60
      head, child 422
   shoulder 79, 82, 86
      post-manipulation 87
      recurrent 88–90
   ulna (distal) 60
   see also fracture dislocation
distal tooth surface 284
distortion, image 17
dorsal aspect of patient 2
dorsal decubitus position *see* supine position
dorsal surface of foot 107
dorsiflexion (ankle joint) 107
   insufficient 114
dorsi-palmar oblique projection 41
dorsi-palmar projection 40
   child 423
dorsi-plantar erect projection 111
dorsi-plantar oblique projection
   foot 108
      child 426
   subtalar joint 120
   toes 112

dorsi-plantar projection
  foot 108
    child 424, 425, 426, 427
  toes 112
dose
  image quality vs, paediatrics 389
  quantities 33
    dental panoramic radiography,
      reduction 321
    paediatric radiography 382, 389
    reference levels, National Radiological
      Protection Board 33
    paediatric radiography 382
drains, chest
  insertion 357
  neonates 392
drugs swallowed in condoms 474
dual energy digital imaging (±subtraction),
    lungs 201
duodenal atresia 399
dynamic hip screws 368, 374–5

echinococcosis (hydatid disease), liver 343
effusions (joint)
  elbow 68
  knee 130
    suprapatellar bursa 128
effusions (pleural fluid) see pleural fluid
Eklund technique 462
elbow 61–9
  children 420–2
elderly
  abuse 496
  dental radiography, intra-oral film mounting
    and holding 289
emergency peripheral vascular procedures 380
emphysema, pulmonary interstitial 392
employers' responsibilities, radiation
    exposure 34
enamel 281
endodontics
  image acquisition 288
  paralleling technique 300
endotracheal tube 357
  children 392
enterocolitis, necrotizing 399, 401
environment, paediatric radiography 386
epicondyles, humeral avulsion 68
equinovarus deformity 424, 425, 426
equinus deformity, ankle 425
equipment
  dental radiography 285
  facial bone/sinuses 262
  forensic radiography 497
  mammography 439
  paediatric radiography 388
  skull 233
  theatre radiography 368
    cholangiography 378
    dynamic hip screw insertion 374
  trauma radiography 468–70
  ward radiography 353
  erect position (standing) 4, 5, 10
    abdominopelvic cavity 340–1
      on ward 359
    cervical spine 168–9, 176
    elbow, child 420, 421
    foot 111
    lungs 198, 206–8

children 393, 394–5
  ward radiography 354
pelvis/hip 157, 158
  child 409
scoliotic spine 411, 412–13, 415
shoulder
  clavicle 95
  glenohumeral joint 85
  scapula 101
  survey image 81
skull 239, 246
  facial bones in lateral projection 267
trauma patient 467
ethmoid sinuses 260, 275
  demonstration 277
European Commission, image quality standards
    in cephalometry 326
eversion of foot 107
expiration (images acquired on)
  diaphragm movement 344
  lungs 199, 206
  ribs 222
exposure, radiation 28–31
  automatic control see automatic exposure
    control
  detectors (digital imaging) 23, 24, 26
  factors/parameters influencing 30–1
    choice of 31
    dental panoramic radiography and 321
    lung radiographs and 202, 205
    mammography and 440
    soft tissue radiography and 494
    tomography and 482, 486
    trauma radiography and 471
  film 16, 24
  legislation see legal issues
  patient 33–5
    protection see protection
    risk of exposure 34
extension 6
  cervical spine 175
  lumbar spine 186
external fixation see fixation
external rotation see lateral rotation
extra-oral dental radiography 279, 318–23
  image receptors 286
extremities see limbs; lower limb; upper limb
eye, foreign body in/around 269, 477–8
eye shields, children 407

fabella 130
facet (apophyseal/zygapophyseal) joints
  C3/C7, dislocations 173
  lumbosacral 187, 189
facial bones 263–74
  equipment 262
  fracture(s) 243, 245, 260, 268, 270
    children 406
  patient preparation and immobilization 262
  radiographic anatomy for positioning 260–1
  recommended projections 262
  skull units and, and intoxicated trauma
    patients 468
  see also hemifacial hypoplasia
fallopian tubes 379
fat
  breast 438
  in soft tissue radiography, lesions
    demonstrated by 495

fat pads, elbow 68
Fédération Dentaire International notation 282,
    283
feet see foot
femoral artery occlusion 380
femur 148–54
  distal fracture 128
  intramedullary nailing 373
  proximal/upper end (incl. head and neck)
    144, 148–54
    fracture 142, 147, 149, 151, 152, 362, 363,
      375
    Perthes' disease 409, 410
    trabecular patterns 145
  shaft 106
    fracture 136
  short right 417
  in skeletal survey for non-accidental injury
    430
  ward radiography (fractures) 362–4
    children 364
ferromagnetic objects see metal (incl.
    ferromagnetic) objects
fetus
  avoiding irradiation see pregnancy
  stillborn 500–2
fibula 124
  external fixation 362, 372
  fracture see fracture
  hypoplasia 417
  in skeletal survey for non-accidental injury
    430
fill factor 23
film 21
  chest X-ray 203
  density (photographic/optical density) 12, 13
  dental radiography see dental radiography
  fog 16
  mammography, identification 440
  paediatric radiography 388
  processing see processing
  tomography, movement 482–4
  see also exposure; focus-to-film distance
film holder, dental radiography 285, 288
  bitewing radiography 292, 294
  periapical radiography
    bisecting angle technique 295
    paralleling technique 300, 301, 302
    third molar images 304, 305
film-to-object distance see object-to-film
    distance
filtration and filters
  dental radiography 285
    cephalometry 325
  mammography 439
  paediatric radiography 387
    inhaled foreign body 397
  soft tissue radiography 494
fine needle aspiration cytology 460–1
fingers
  holding film for periapical radiography 295
  radiography 38, 46–7
    immobilization in child 383
  see also thumb
fixation
  external 372
    lower leg 362, 372
  internal 372
flail chest 220

flat panel detector 23
flexion 6
  ankle joint 107
  cervical spine 175
    in Advanced Trauma and Life Support 471
  elbow
    full flexion 64
    partial flexion 62–3
  knee joint 107, 127, 131
    insufficient 133
  lumbar spine 186
fluid collections
  abdominopelvic cavity 336
    ward radiography 358
  chest, ward radiography 355
  see also effusions
fluoroscopy/fluorography 21
  leg length assessment, digital method 419
  thorax 220
focal-increased breast density 445
focal spot, paediatric radiography 387
focus-to-film distance (FFD) 17, 29–30
  cephalometry 325
  chest
    lungs 202, 354
    on ward 354
  macroradiography 489
  paediatric radiography 387
  unsharpness and 20
focus-to-object distance (OFD), macroradiography 489
focus-to-skin distance (FSD), dental radiography 285, 300
fogging 16
foot/feet 106, 108–11, 424–7
  child 424–7
    hypoplasia 417
  position/movement terminology 107
foramen magnum 243, 244, 245
forearm 59–60
  internal fixation 372
foreign bodies 334, 472–9
  abdominopelvic cavity 334
    ward radiography 358
  foot 110
  inhaled (airway) 194, 195, 475
    children 393, 397
  inserted 476
  oral 310
  orbit 269, 477
  percutaneous 473
  swallowed/ingested 334, 474
    children 400, 474
  thenar eminence 48, 49
forensic radiography 496–503
  anatomic terminology 496
  applications 496–503
  classification 496
  de-briefing 497
  equipment 497
  legal issues 497
Forrest Report 442, 443
fracture(s) 371–4
  acetabulum 142, 155
  calcaneal 118, 119
  femur see femur
  fibula 116
    and tibia 125

fixation see fixation
hand
  fingers/phalanges see phalangeal fractures
  metacarpal 40, 42, 45, 49
hip 148, 371, 373
humerus
  children 69, 420, 422, 429
  condylar/proximal to condyles 69, 421
  neck 74
  shaft 72, 75
  supracondylar see supracondylar humeral fractures
hyoid bone 195
intercondylar notch 128
ischium 149
malleolus 115
metatarsal (fifth) 115
non-accidental injury (child) 428
olecranon process see olecranon process
patella 128, 130
pelvis 142, 155, 362
pubis/pubic bone 148, 149
radius 60
  distal 58
  head/neck 68, 421
ribs 220
  child, non-accidental 429
  lower 224
  upper 97
  ward radiography 354
sacrum 149, 191
shoulder 82, 86
  clavicle 95, 96, 97
  scapula 102
skull
  facial bones see facial bones
  nasal bones 270
  parietal bone see parietal fracture
  skull base 230, 238
spine
  cervical see cervical spine
  children 416
  lumbar 181, 185, 471
  thoracic 181, 471
sternum 213, 220, 228
surgery 371–4
tibia 128, 130, 135, 362, 372
  and fibula 125
toes 47
tooth, fragments in lip 310
ulna 60, 496
  distal 55
wrist 53
fracture dislocation
  cervical spine 361
  Lisfranc 109
Frankfort plane 327
frog (legs) position 154
  children 410
frontal plane see coronal plane
frontal sinuses 260, 275
  demonstration 277
fronto-occipital projections 234, 242–4
  children 403–4
  stillborn fetus 502
  temporal bones 250–1
fronto-orbital projection 242
full-field magnified projections of breast 459

gadolinium-enhanced MRI, breast cancer 447
Galeazzi fracture 60
gallbladder 348
gallows traction 364
Garden screws, femur 150
gas/air, free (in body cavities)
  in abdominopelvic cavity 337, 342
    children 401
    tomography and blurring of gas shadows 487
    ward radiography 358, 359, 360
  in soft tissue radiography, lesions demonstrated by 495
gastric outlet obstruction 336
gastrocnemius, sesamoid bone in tendon of medial head of 130
gastrointestinal tract, foreign bodies see foreign bodies, swallowed
gastro-oesophageal reflux, oesophageal pH probe in children 391, 393, 395
genetic harm, radiation 34
geometrical unsharpness 18, 20, 43
  macroradiography 490
glabella 230
glenohumeral joint 85–6
  arthritis 78
  trauma 79
glioma, optic nerve 248
glomus jugulare tumour 248
gnathion 327
gonad protection 34, 35
  abdominopelvic radiography 339
    children 398, 399
    urinary tract imaging 345
  children (in general) 389
  femoral shaft radiography 137
  hip/pelvis/upper femur radiography 146, 149, 154
    children 408, 409, 410
    ward radiography 362
  knee joint radiography 131, 132
  leg length assessment, child 417
gonion 327
grids 23
  lung radiography 201
  mammography 439
  secondary/scattered radiation 31
    lung radiography 201
    macroradiography 491
    paediatric radiography 387
  skull radiography, children 402
  trauma radiography 469
growth hormone deficiency, bone age in hand 423
gynaecology 379

haemorrhage
  chest trauma 354
  intestinal 380
half-axial fronto-occipital 30 degrees caudad projection see Townes projection
hallux, lateral projection 113
hallux valgus 111
hand 38, 40–6
  abducted, scaphoid imaging with 50
  child
    in acrodysostosis 431
    bone age assessment 423
    in skeletal survey for non-accidental injury 430

hand 38, 40–6 (*contd*)
  radiographic anatomy 41
  see also finger; thumb
Harrington Rod 415
head *see* facial bones; paranasal sinuses; skull
heart 214–19, 354–7
  anatomy 214, 215
  configuration, assessment 210
  congenital disease 393
  failure, mimicking signs 209
  size
    artefact 217
    assessment 207, 208, 209, 215
    enlargement *see* cardiomegaly
  valves *see* valves
  ward radiography 354–7
  see also thorax
hemifacial hypoplasia 320
hepatic abnormalities 343
high-kilovoltage technique
  lungs 201, 206
  soft tissue radiography 494
hilar regions of lung 204
Hill–Sachs lesion 88, 89
hip joint 142, 148–55
  anatomy and image appearances 144, 145–6
  children 142, 408–10
    in vitamin D-resistant rickets 431
  fracture 148, 371, 373
  prosthesis 148, 362, 363, 370
  in trauma, radiographic lines in assessment of
    integrity 145
hip screws
  cannulated 373
  dynamic 368, 374–5
horizontal beam radiograph
  abdominopelvic cavity 341
    diaphragm 343
  ankle 116
  femoral shaft 137
  knee 128
  lumbar spine 185
  skull 238
  trauma patient 467
hospital information systems 25
humerus 38
  adult fractures *see* fractures
  bicipital groove 73
  child 69
    fractures 69, 420, 422, 429
  epicondyles, avulsion 68
  neck/head 38, 74–6, 88–9
  shaft 72–3
  in shoulder radiography 78, 86
    in recurrent dislocations 88–9
hydatid cyst 343
hydropneumothorax 355
hyoid fracture 195
hypersthenic abdomen 333
hyposthenic abdomen 333
hysterosalpingography 379

iliac artery occlusion 380
iliac bone (ilium) 156, 158
  apophyses, development 415
  spines and crests as lumbosacral landmarks
    166
ilio-ischial line 145
ilio-pubic line 145

ilium *see* iliac bone
Ilizarov device 417
image 12–21
  acquisition/reception/capture (conventional
    radiography) 16
    dental radiography 286–8, 318–23
    lungs 200
    mammography 440
    scattered radiation reaching 16
  acquisition/reception/capture (digital
    radiography) 22
    leg alignment 139
    lungs 200
    workstations 25
  analysis/interpretation
    cranial radiography 230
    leg alignment in digital radiography 139
  artefacts *see* artefacts
  contrast *see* contrast
  density 12, 13, 28
    in bitewing radiography 294
    in digital imaging 13
  digital *see* digital imaging
  display 21
    see also monitor
  distortion 17
  formation 12
  geometry in intra-oral radiography,
    optimization 291
  magnification *see* magnification
  projection *see* projection
  quality/essential characteristics
    abdominopelvic radiography 335
    dental radiography 294, 301
    factors influencing 32
    mammography 440–1, 442–3
    paediatric radiography 389
    skull radiography 236, 326
    tomography 484–5
  sharpness and resolution *see* sharpness
image intensifier, mobile
  in theatre 368
    angiography 380
    cholangiography 378
    dynamic hip screw insertion 374
  on ward 356
imaging methods for children 382–3
imaging room, children 386
immobilization 18, 19
  abdominopelvic radiography 340, 345
  children 388
    finger taping 383
    pelvis/hip radiography 408
    skull radiography 403, 404, 405
    spine 416
  head 236, 262, 403, 405
  trauma patient 468
impingement syndromes, shoulder 78
implants (incl. prostheses)
  breast 446, 462
  heart valve 217
  hip joint 148, 362, 363, 370
  pacemaker 216, 217, 218, 451
incisal surface of tooth 284
incisors 281
  in bisecting angle technique 298
  in C1/C2 radiography 170, 171
  in paralleling technique 301, 302
inclined plane tomography 481

incubators, babies in 365
  abdominal radiography 398
  chest radiography 391
index finger, lateral projection 46
infants and toddlers (6 months–3 years) 384
  femoral fracture 364
  foot radiography 424, 425
  spinal radiography 416
  see also neonates
infection
  chest, children 395
  control
    children with contagious disease 385
    dental radiography 290
    theatre radiography 368
    ward radiography 353
infero-superior projection
  facial bones 268
  humeral neck 76
  patella/knee joint 131
    prone position 133
  shoulder 82
    calcified tendons 93
    clavicle 97–8
    recurrent dislocation 90
infradentale 327
infraorbital line 230
infraorbital margin/point 230
infraorbital plane, isocentric skull technique
  256
infraspinatus and its tendon 91
inion 230
injury *see* trauma *and various types of injury*
innominate bones 145
inspiration (images acquired on)
  diaphragm movement 344
  lungs 199, 205
  ribs 222
  sub-maximal 205
intensifier, image *see* image
intensifying screens 19, 21, 30
  chest X-ray 203
  facial bones 262
  paediatric radiography 388
intercondylar notch 135
  fracture 128
internal fixation 372
internal rotation *see* medial rotation
interorbital line 230
interphalangeal joint, distal, dislocation 47
interpupillary line 230
interstitial emphysema, pulmonary 392
intertuberous sulcus 73
intestine *see* bowel
intoxicated trauma patient 468
intramedullary nailing 373
intra-oral radiography 279, 292–317
  film 289
    mounting and identification 289
    size 286, 292
    image geometry, optimization 291
    image receptors 286
intrauterine contraceptive device, ultrasound
  476
intravenous urography 486, 487
inversion (foot) 107
  ankle injury due to 115
  stress, AP projection of ankle with 117
involution, breast 437

Ionising Radiations (Medical Exposure)
    Regulations (2000) 34
    paediatric radiography 382
IRMER *see* Ionising Radiations (Medical
    Exposure) Regulations
ischium, fracture 149
isocentric skull technique 255–7
isocentric skull unit 233

jaw *see* mandible; maxilla; moving jaw
    technique
Jefferson fracture 171
Jeune's syndrome 431
joint movements *see* movement
Judet's projection 151, 155
    reverse 155
jug-handle projection 268
jugular foramina 248–9

kidney (renal imaging) 334
    calculi 336, 345
        removal 377
    children 400
    retrograde pylography 376
    tomography 487
    trauma 337, 339
kilovoltage 28
    contrast and 14, 29
    lung imaging 201, 206
    paediatric radiography 387
    soft tissue radiography 494
Kirschner wire 372
knee joint 106, 126–35
    lipohaemoarthrosis 128, 130, 495
    movements/positions 107
    theatre radiography 470
kyphotic patients, skull radiography 244

labial tooth surface 284
lambdoid sutures 404
laryngocele 194
larynx 194–5, 488
    cartilages 181, 195
    foreign body 475
    tomography 488
laser printers 26
lateral aspect of patient 2, 107
lateral decubitus position 4, 10, 11
    abdominopelvic cavity 342
        children 399, 401
        on ward 359
    heart/lungs on ward 355
lateral dorsal decubitus position, abdominopelvic
        cavity 342–3
    on ward 360
lateral oblique projection 9
    glenohumeral joint 86
    hip/femoral head and neck 153
    humeral neck 76
    jaws 314–17
    skull 252
    subtalar joint 120, 123
    tibiofibular joint (proximal) 125
lateral occlusal projection of maxilla 310
lateral projection 7, 10, 11
    babygram (stillborn) 501
    breast 455–6
    cervical spine 168–70
        children 416

in flexion and extension 175
    on ward 361
cervicothoracic junction 178
coccyx 192
foot 110–11
    child 425–7
hip/femoral neck 144, 152
    both hips *see* frog position
    dynamic screw 375
    modified technique 153
humerus
    neck/head 75–6, 88
    shaft 71, 72
    supracondylar 69
lower limb
    ankle joint 115, 116, 117
    calcaneum 118
    children 364
    femoral shaft 137, 364
    foot *see subheading above*
    hallux 113
    knee joint 127, 128
    tibia and fibula 124
    toes 113
lumbar spine 183–6
lumbosacral junction 188
pelvis 143, 157
sacrum 191
scoliotic spine 414–15
shoulder
    outlet 84
    scapula 102
    sternoclavicular joint 100
skull/head 234, 238, 257, 431
    with angulation 235
    cephalometry 326, 407, 495
    facial bones 267, 406
    intra-orbital foreign body 478
    mandible 271
    nasal bones 270
    paranasal sinuses 278
    stillborn fetus 502
    temporomandibular joint 274
thoracic spine 180–1
    auto-tomography 181, 479
thorax
    children 397
    heart/aorta 218, 355
    lungs 211, 213, 355, 397
    pharynx/larynx 195
    sternum 228
    trachea/thoracic inlet 196
    on ward 355
trauma patient 467
upper limb
    children 420, 422
    elbow 61, 420, 422
    fingers 46–7
    forearm 60
    hand 45
    humerus *see subheading above*
    radial head 66
    scaphoid 53
    thumb 48
    wrist 55, 56–7
urinary tract 346
lateral rotation (external rotation)
    arm, shoulder tendon calcification
        92

breast, for extended cranio-caudal view
        452
    lower limb in 107
        hip/pelvis radiography with 147
lateral supine position, post-nasal space in
        children 406
lateromedial projection
    ankle joint 116
    breast 456
Lauenstein's projection 144, 151
law *see* legal issues
leg *see* lower limb
legal issues (incl. legislation and regulations)
    forensic examination 497
    on medical exposure 34
        paediatric radiography 382
lighting, ambient 16
limbs/extremities
    calcifications in soft tissue 495
    position, terminology describing 6–7, 107
    surgery 371–3
    see also lower limb; upper limb
lingual tooth surface 284
lip, tooth fragment 310
lipohaemoarthrosis, knee joint 128, 130, 495
lipoma 495
Lisfranc fracture dislocation 109
little finger, lateral radiograph 46
liver 343
lobes
    breast 437
    lung
        anatomy 204
        collapse 213
        tumour 211, 212
localized projections
    breast 458
    leg length assessment 419
    thoracic spine 181
look-up table 26
lordosis
    lungs in 205, 213
    pelvis and hip and effects of 146
lower limb (leg) 105–39
    alignment 138–9
    child
        in achondrodysplasia 431
        in survey for non-accidental injury
            429, 430
    fracture *see specific elements under* fracture
    length assessment 417–19
    positioning terminology 107
    recommended projections 106
    in rotation and abduction, hip/pelvis
        radiography with 147
lumbar vertebrae 164, 182–7
    levels/landmarks 166, 167
    myeloma 492
    paediatric 416
        in survey for non-accidental injury
            429
    sacralization of L5 182, 184
    trauma 164, 181, 185, 471
lumbarization of S1 182, 184
lumbosacral junction 164, 188–9
    transitional vertebrae 182, 184
luminescence, photostimulable *see*
        photostimulable luminescence
lunate dislocation 53, 58

lungs 198–213, 354–7
  anatomy/landmarks 204–5
  apices 212
  children
    neonatal 390–2
    post-neonatal 393–7
  general principles and radiological
    considerations 200–5
  oedema 220, 354
  positioning choices 198
  recommended projections 198
  upper anterior region 213
  ward radiography 354–7
    special care baby unit 365
  see also thorax
lying down see decubitus positions
lymph nodes, breast 438, 446
Lysholm skull unit 233

macroradiography 489–91
magnetic resonance imaging
  breast 447
  foreign body 472
    hazards of ferromagnetic materials 472,
      475
  shoulder 78
  skeletal survey 492
  skull base 246
magnification (image) 17
  dental panoramic radiography 319
  lungs 202
  mammography 459
  tomography 480, 484
  see also macroradiography
malignancy see cancer
malleolar fracture 115
mallet finger 47
mammography 435–63
  diagnostic requirements 440
  equipment 439
  exposure factors 440
  film
    identification 440
    processing 441
  good imaging performance and technique
    440–1
  image acquisition 440
  imaging parameters 440
  positioning terminology 437
  quality assurance 442
  radiation protection 435
  radiological considerations 444–7
  recommended projections 436
  see also breast
mammoscintigraphy 447
mandible 262, 271–3
  in C3/C7 vertebral radiography 173
  forensics 498
  periapical radiography in
    bisecting angle technique 298
    paralleling technique 302
    third molars 304
  projections (in dental radiography) 280
    lateral oblique 314–17
    occlusal 284, 308–9, 312–13
  trauma 262, 271, 272, 273
mandibular plane 327
masses, breast 445
Maissonneuve's fracture 125

mastoid air cells 252
mastoid process 250, 251, 252–3
maxilla
  on C1/C2 radiography, prominent 172
  periapical radiography in
    bisecting angle technique 298
    paralleling technique 301, 302
    third molars 305
  projections 280
    lateral oblique 314–15
    occlusal 307, 310–11
maxillary plane 327
maxillary sinuses/antra 260, 275, 276
  children 406
maxillofacial skeleton see facial bones; paranasal
  sinuses and specific bones
medial aspect (patient) 2, 107
  see also midline
medial rotation (internal rotation)
  arm, shoulder tendon calcification 92
  breast, for extended cranio-caudal view 452
  hip joint 147, 148
  knee joint 126
  lower limb 107
    insufficient 114
median sagittal (mid-sagittal) plane 3, 10, 11
  dental panoramic radiography, positioning
    errors 324
  skull 3, 230, 255, 256
    mandible 271, 272, 273
    temporomandibular joint 274
mediastinal mass, anterior 197, 211
medical exposure legislation see legal issues
mediolateral projection
  ankle joint 115
  oblique, breast, 45 degree 448–9
mental symphysis (symphysis menti) 272, 273,
  308
menton 327
mento-occipital projection, modified 264
mesenteric angiography 380
mesial tooth surface 284
metabolic disease, skeletal survey 492
metacarpal bones, fractures 40, 42, 45, 49
metal (incl. ferromagnetic) objects
  on dental panoramic radiography 322
  as foreign bodies 472
    swallowed by children 400
  MRI cautions 472, 475
metaphyseal fracture, non-accidental 430
metastases
  skeletal survey 493
  spinal 179, 493
metatarsal bone
  fifth
    fracture 115
    ossification 109
metatarsophalangeal sesamoid bones, first 113
metatarsus adductus 426
methicillin-resistant S. aureus 353
middle finger, lateral projection 46
midline occlusal projection 308
mid-sagittal plane see median sagittal plane
milliampere seconds 28
mobile equipment
  theatre radiography 368
    cholangiography 378
    dynamic hip screw insertion 374
  ward radiography 353

molars 281, 304–5
  in bisecting angle technique 298
  in paralleling technique 300, 301, 302
  third 304–5
    impacted 300
  see also bimolar projection
monitors
  digital imaging 26
  subjective contrast and 16
Monteggia fracture 60
mouth
  closed, TMJ radiography 274
  complete/full survey 289, 305
  floor, occlusal radiography 309, 313
  open
    in cervical spine radiography 170–2
    TMJ radiography 274
  see also extra-oral radiography; intra-oral
    radiography
movement(s)
  joint 6
    lower limb and foot 107
  subject, lung exposure times and 202
movement unsharpness 18, 20, 32
  abdominopelvic radiography 339
  macroradiography 490
  mammography 444
moving jaw technique 173
myeloma, skeletal survey 492, 493

nailing, intramedullary 373
nasal bones 270
nasal passages, foreign body 476
nasal spine, anterior and posterior 327
nasion 230, 327
nasopharynx (post-nasal space), children 406
National Radiological Protection Board, dose
  reference levels see dose
neck see cervical spine
necrotizing enterocolitis 399, 401
needle biopsy of breast, image-guided 460–1
neonates and babies
  chest radiography 390–2
  foot radiography 424, 425
  in incubators see incubators
  leg length assessment 417
  special care baby units 365, 387
  see also fetus
neoplasm see tumour
nephrolithotomy, percutaneous 377
nephrotomography 487
networking, digital imaging (DR) 25–6
newborns see neonates
nipples
  in mammography, in or not in profile 449,
    451, 452, 453, 454, 455, 456
  and nipple markers 199
Nøgaard projection 44
non-accidental injury see physical abuse; self-
  harm
nose see entries under nasal
nuclear medicine see radionuclide scans

object-to-film distance (FOD; OFD) 17
  shoulder 81
  trauma radiography 469, 470
  unsharpness and 20
object-to-focus distance (OFD),
  macroradiography 489

objective contrast *see* radiographic contrast
oblique lateral projection
  jaw 280
  subtalar joint 120, 122
oblique medial projection, subtalar joint 121
oblique mediolateral projection of breast, 45
    degree 448–9
oblique projection 8
  beam angulation in 9
  hand, child in skeletal survey for non-
    accidental injury 430
  humeral head/shoulder 89
  occlusal radiography
    mandible 313
    maxilla 310–11
  radiolunar joint (proximal) 67
  skull 235
  sternoclavicular joint 99
  wrist 58
  see also anterior oblique projection; antero-
    posterior oblique projection; dorsi-palmar
    oblique projection; dorsi-plantar oblique
    projection; lateral oblique projection;
    posterior oblique projection; postero-
    anterior oblique projection
observer and subjective contrast 15, 16
occipital bone
  in C1/C2 radiography 170, 171
  external protuberance (=inion) 230
occipito-frontal projections 234, 240–1, 257
  paranasal sinuses 277
occipito-mental projections 263–6
  30 degrees caudad 265
    modified reverse 266
  orbit, modified projection 269
    foreign body 477, 478
  paranasal sinuses 276
    children 406
occlusal plane 284
  positioning errors 324
occlusal radiography 280, 306–13
  mandible 284, 308–9, 312–13, 312–13
  radiological considerations 306
  recommended projections 306
  terminology 306
  uses 306
occlusal surface of tooth 284
ocular or orbital foreign body 269, 477–8
odontoid peg (dens) 171
oedema, pulmonary 220, 354
oesophagus 219
  foreign body 474
    children 400
  pH probe, children 391, 393, 395
olecranon process fracture 68
  child 422
opaque legends, facial bones 262
open reduction 372
operating theatre radiography 367–90
optic foramina 248
optical (photographic) density 12, 13
oral cavity *see* dental radiography; mouth
orbit 265, 269
  blowout fracture 406
  foreign body 269, 477–8
orbitale 327
orbito-meatal base line 230
  half-axial fronto-occipital 30 degrees caudad
    projection 243, 244

modified mento-occipital projection 264
modified occipito-mental projection 269
  foreign body 477
modified reverse occipito-metal 30 degrees
    caudad projection 266
occipito-frontal projections 240, 241
submento-vertical projection of jugulare
    foramina 249
orbito-meatal plane (Frankfort plane) 327
orthopaedic surgery 370–5
  non-trauma corrective 370
  trauma 371–4
orthopantomography *see* panoramic radiography
Osgood–Schlatter disease 128, 130
ossicles, accessory
  ankle/foot 109
  hand/wrist 45
ossification/ossification centres 423
  elbow 422
  fifth metatarsal bone 109
  multiple 384
osteoarthritis (OA), knee 129
osteophytosis, retropatellar joint 131
osteotomies 370
  leg length inequality 417
outlet projections (shoulder) 83–4

pacemaker
  permanent (implant) 216, 217, 218, 451
  temporary 356
PACS *see* Picture Archive and Communications
    System
padding, head 236
paddle projections of breast 458
  magnification technique 459
paediatrics *see* children
pain, rib trauma 220
palatal tooth surface 284
Palmer system 282
panoramic radiography/tomography
    (orthopantomography; rotational
    panoramic radiography) 280, 318–24
  cephalometric mode in 321, 325
  image formation and acquisition 318–23
  problems 323, 324
  uses 318
paralleling technique 289, 291, 300–4
paranasal sinuses 275–8, 406
  anatomy 260, 275
  children 406
  equipment 262
  patient preparation and immobilization 262
  recommended projections 262, 275
parasagittal planes, abdominopelvic cavity 332
parents of child 383
parietal fracture, child 403
  non-accidental 429, 503
pars interarticularis 187, 189
  defects 187
patella 130–5
  fracture 128, 130
pathology influencing subject contrast 14
pelvic cavity *see* abdominopelvic cavity
pelvis 142, 148–9, 156–8, 408–10
  anatomy and image appearances 143, 145,
    145–6
  child 408–10
    tilting (correction) 418
    tilting (uncorrected) 414

fracture 142, 155, 362
  in trauma
    forensic radiography 499
    radiographic lines in assessment of integrity
     145
  ward radiography 362
percutaneous foreign bodies 473
percutaneous nephrolithotomy 377
perforation, abdominal viscera 337, 341
  impending 359
periapical radiography 280, 295–305
  clinical indications 295
  film holding ± beam-holding instruments
    288, 300
  image geometry, optimization 291
pericardial pathology 217, 218
periodontal bone levels, beam angulation
    affecting 297
periodontal film-holding beam-alignment
    instruments 288
periodontal ligament 281
peripheral vascular procedures, emergency
    380
peritoneal cavity, free air 360
personnel/staff
  in forensic radiography, psychological trauma
    497
  in paediatric radiography 382
    required to hold baby 390
  in theatre radiography 368
Perthes' disease 409, 410
pes (talipes) deformations 424–7
petrous parts/ridges of temporal bone 250, 251,
    254, 263, 269, 276, 277
pH probe, oesophageal, in children 391, 393,
    395
phalangeal fractures
  fingers 47
    child, in survey for non-accidental injury
     430
  toes 112
pharynx 194–5
phleboliths, pelvic 347
phosphors, storage (digital imaging) 23
  dental radiography 287
photographic film *see* film
photographic unsharpness 19, 20
photostimulable luminescence 22
  in dental radiography 287
physical abuse (non-accidental injury) 496
  child *see* children
  elderly 496
Picture Archive and Communications System
    (PACS) 25
  components and workflow 27
  theatre radiography 369
pins 372
  femur/hip 150
pisiform 52
pituitary tumour 247
pixels 25
planes 3
  abdominopelvic cavity 332
  breast 437
  skull 3, 230, 255
    in cephalometry 327
  see also specific planes
plantar aspect, foot 107
plantarflexion 107

plaster of Paris
  acetabuloplasty, child 409
  ankle lateral radiograph through 116
  elbow axial radiograph through 64
  wrist PA radiograph through 57
plates 372
  femur/hip 150
pleural fluid/effusions 209, 213
  ward radiography 354, 355
    drain insertion 357
pneumonia 395, 396
pneumoperitoneum (free air in peritoneal
    cavity) 360
pneumothorax 207, 209
  neonatal 392
  ward radiography 355, 357
    drain insertion 357
  see also hydropneumothorax
pogonion 327
polyp, maxillary sinus 276
porion 327
portable equipment, ward radiography
    353
position, patient
  projections referring to 10–11
  terminology 3–6
    breast 437
    skull 234–5
  see also posture and specific positions
posterior oblique projection 8, 10, 11
  hip
    and acetabulum 155
    and upper third of femur 144, 151
  occlusal radiography of maxilla 311
  pelvis 156
  ribs (lower) 223
  spine
    cervical 176–7
    lumbar spine 187
    lumbosacral junction 189
    sacrum 190
  upper limbs
    fingers 46
    hands 44
  urinary tract 346, 347
posterior occlusal radiograph 309
posterior patient aspect 2
postero-anterior oblique projection
  knee joint 134
  mandible 273
  optic foramina 248
  sternoclavicular joint 99
postero-anterior projection 7, 11
  cephalometry 328
  clavicle 95
  hands
    both 43
    one 40, 42
  knee/patella 130
  lumbar vertebrae 183
  mandible 272
  sacro-iliac joints 159
  scaphoid 50
  scoliotic spine 411, 412–13
    Harrington Rod 415
  sternoclavicular joint 100
  thorax
    children 393, 394–5
    heart/aorta 216–17, 355

lungs 198, 199, 200, 201, 203, 206–7, 355,
    393, 394–5
  on ward 355
wrist 55, 56
post-mortem imaging (cadaver) 496
  dental radiography 498
  general radiography 499
  out of hours skeletal survey 503
  stillbirth 500–2
post-nasal space, children 406
postoperative radiography
  pelvis/lower limb 362
  thorax 357
posture
  hip/pelvis radiography 146
  shoulder radiography 78
  see also position
pregnancy
  fetal irradiation avoidance 35
    abdominopelvic cavity radiography 345
  pelvis at full-term 157
  teenage 386
premature infants, respiratory distress
    syndrome 365
premolars
  in bisecting angle technique 298
  in paralleling technique 301, 302
  unerupted maxillary, vertex occlusal
    radiograph 307
Pritchard Report 442
processing of image
  digital image 26
  film (=development) 16, 21
    dental radiography 290, 321
    mammography 441
    paediatric radiography 388
projections 7–11, 12
  definition of term 7, 12
  positioning for 4
  see also view and specific tissues and
    projections
pronation 6
prone (ventral decubitus) position 4
  abdomen, children 401
  elbow, spine 420
  knee joint/patella 133
prostheses see implants
prosthion 327
protection, radiation exposure 33–5
  abdominopelvic radiography 335,
    339, 360
    children 398, 399
    urinary tract radiography 345
  ankle joint radiography 117
  chest (incl. lung) radiography 203
    neonates 392
    post-neonatal children 393
  children (general aspects) 34, 382, 389
  dental radiography 290
  elbow radiography, child 421
  femoral shaft radiography 137
  forensic radiography 497
  hip/pelvis radiography 146, 149, 154, 362
    children 408, 409, 410
  knee joint radiography 131, 132
  lower limb radiography, children 417
  lumbosacral radiography 188, 207
  mammography 442
  shoulder radiography 78

skeletal survey for non-accidental injury
    (child) 429
skull radiography 236
  children 402
spinal radiography
  cervical 169, 172, 361
  child 411, 412
theatre radiography 369
tomography 485
upper limb radiography 39
  hands in posterior oblique projection 44
ward radiography 352, 360, 361, 362
psychological considerations
  children 383–4
  personnel in forensic radiography 497
pubic bone/pubis, fracture 148, 149
pubic symphysis 158
pyelography, retrograde 376

quality standards see image

radial scar 446
radiation
  dose see dose
  exposure and protection see exposure;
      protection
  risks 34
  scattered see scattered radiation
radiographic (objective) contrast 13, 15–16, 32
  shoulder 78
radiology information systems 25
radiolunar joint, proximal 67
radionuclide scans
  breast 447
  skeletal survey 492, 493
radio-opaque objects (patient's) in dental
    panoramic radiography 322
radiotherapy-related breast changes 446
radius
  distal 38
    dislocation 60
    fracture see fracture
  head/neck 66
    child 421, 422
    dislocation 422
    fracture 68, 421
  shaft, fracture 60
ramus, mandibular, lateral oblique 316–17
rectum, vibrator lodged in 476
reduction, open 372
referral criteria
  abdominopelvic radiography 334
    children 398
  children 382
    abdominal radiography 398
    chest problems in neonates 390
    hip/pelvis radiography 408
    skeletal survey for non-accidental injury 428
    skull radiography 402
  spine 416
    scoliosis 411
reflux disease, oesophageal pH probe in children
    391, 393, 395
renal imaging see kidney
reporting workstations 25
respiration (images acquired during) 199
  diaphragm movement 344
  sternum 226, 227
  see also expiration; inspiration

respiratory distress syndrome, neonatal 365
respiratory tract see airways and specific
    parts
retrograde pyelography 376
retromammary space 437
retropatellar joint osteophytosis 131
retroperitoneal disease 337
retrosternal thyroid 197
rheumatoid arthritis, skeletal survey 491
ribs 221, 222–5
    anatomy 204
    cervical 225
    fracture see fracture
    lower 221, 222–3
    upper 221, 224–5
        in clavicular fracture 97
rickets 423
    vitamin D-resistant 431
ring finger, lateral radiograph 46
Risser's sign 415
Rolando fracture 49
roots of teeth 281
    mandibular third molars 304
rotation 6
    ankle joint, over- and under- 115
    arm, shoulder tendon calcification 92
    head (in skull radiography) 241
    hip 147
    knee joint, over- and under- 127
    trunk, in chest X-ray 205, 207, 211, 227
    see also lateral rotation; medial rotation
rotational panoramic radiography see
    panoramic radiography
Royal College of Radiographers, quality
    assurance in mammography 443

sacralization of L5 182, 184
sacroiliac joints 142, 159–61
    fusion 493
    in lumbar projection 182
sacrum 159, 164, 190–1
    fracture 149, 191
    landmarks 166, 167
    lumbarization of S1 182, 184
    see also lumbosacral junction
safety consideration (radiation exposure)
    33–5
sagittal plane, median see median sagittal
    plane
salivary calculi 309, 313
salpingography 379
Salter–Harris III fracture of capitellum 422
scanning technology 23
scaphoid 38, 80–3
scapula 79, 101–2
    on chest PA X-ray 207
scar (breast)
    radial 446
    surgical 446
scattered/secondary radiation
    contrast and 16
    grids see grids
    macroradiography 491
    protection from 35
scintigraphy see radionuclide scans
scintillator detector 23
scleroderma, fingers 47
scoliosis 411–15
'Scottie dog' appearance 187

screens see intensifying screens
screws 372
    femur 150
    hip see hip screws
seborrheic wart, breast 444
secondary radiation see scattered radiation
secondary shadows in dental panoramic
    radiography 320
selenium, amorphous 23
self-harm, foreign body insertion 476
sella turcica 247, 251
    J-shaped 431
    midpoint (sella), in cephalometrics 327
semi-prone position, sternoclavicular joint 99
semi-recumbant/semi-erect position 4, 5, 11
    lungs 205
sesamoid bones
    first metatarsophalangeal 113
    tendon of medial head of gastrocnemius 130
set square system 282
sharpness and resolution 18–20, 32
    dental panoramic radiography 321
    lung radiography 100
    problems with see absorption unsharpness;
        geometrical unsharpness; movement
        unsharpness; photographic unsharpness
    soft tissue radiography 494
    tomography 485
Shenton's line 145
    disruption 149
shoulder 77–103
    basic projections 80–2
    in dental panoramic radiography, problems
        with 324
single exposure method, leg length assessment
    419
sinuses, paranasal see paranasal sinuses
sitting erect position
    abdominopelvic radiography 341
    trauma patient 467
skeletal survey
    for syndrome assessment 431
    trauma 471, 492
    non-accidental injury 428–30, 492, 503
skew-foot 427
skin folds
    chest-X ray 207
    mammography 444
skin lesions, breast 444
skull (cranium) 229–58, 402–5
    anatomical terminology 230
    cephalometric assessment see cephalometry
    children 236, 402–5
        survey for non-accidental injury 428, 429
    equipment 233
    forensic radiography 499
    image interpretation 230
    isocentric technique 255–7
    myeloma deposits 492
    non-isocentric technique 238–54
    non-isometric methods 238–54
    patient preparation 236
    planes see planes
    positioning terminology 234–5
    radiographic anatomy for positioning 231–2
    recommended technique 237
    stillborn fetus 502
    tomography 485
    see also facial bones

skull board 244
skull units 233
    basic position in isocentric skull technique
        256
    facial bone radiographs using, in intoxicated
        trauma patients 468
    submento-vertical projection 246
skyline projections, knee joint/patella 131
sleeping baby, chest radiography 390
small bowel
    atresia 399
    obstruction 341
        children 398, 399
        by foreign body 474
        ward radiography 358, 359
SN plane 327
SNA and SNB angle 327
soft tissues 494–5
    in chest-X-ray
        artefacts due to 205
        in large patients 207
    in dental radiography
        in oblique occlusal of maxilla 310
        in panoramic radiography, superimposition
            320
    radiography of 494–5
special care baby unit 365, 387
sphenoid sinuses 260, 275
spina bifida 412
spina cord
    compression 492
    tethering 416
spinal column see vertebral column
spinous processes 184
    as landmarks 177
splint, Thomas 362, 363
spondylolisthesis 187
spur, calcaneal 118
staff see personnel
standing see erect position
Staphylococcus aureus, methicillin-resistant 353
Stenver's projection 254
stereotactic techniques
    biopsy 460–1
    preoperative marker localization 461
sterile areas in theatre 369
sternal angle 181
sternal notch 181
sternoclavicular joint 79, 99–100
sternum 221, 226–8
    fracture 213, 220, 228
sthenic abdomen 333
stillbirth 500–2
stomach, outlet obstruction 336
stones see calculi
storage phosphors see phosphors
stress projections
    ankle joint 117
    knee joint 129
Stryker's projection 90
subclavian vein, pacemaker wire insertion 356
subject contrast 13, 14, 16, 32
    factors influencing 14
subjective contrast 13, 15, 32
    factors influencing 15, 16
subluxation
    acromioclavicular joint 94
    ankle joint 117
    atlantoaxial 169

subluxation (*contd*)
  knee joint 129
  sternoclavicular joint 100
submandibular duct 309, 313
submento-vertical projections 246
  jugular foramina 249
  temporal bones 251
    facial bones, modified projection 268
subphrenic abscess 343
subscapularis and its tendon 91
subspinale 327
subtalar joint 120–3
subtraction, bone, dual energy digital
        imaging of lungs 201
subtraction angiography 380
supero-inferior projection
  humeral neck 75
  patella/knee joint 132
  shoulder 81
supination 6
supine (dorsal decubitus) position 4, 11
  abdominopelvic cavity 338–9, 342
    children 401
    liver and diaphragm 343
    on ward 358, 360
  cervical spine 169–70, 177
    on ward 361
  chest incl. lungs 205, 209
    neonates 390–2
    post-neonatal children 396
    on ward 354, 355
  clavicle 96, 98
  elbow, child 420, 421
  glenohumeral joint 86
  skull 238, 246
    facial bones in lateral projection 267
    post-nasal space in children 406
  thoracic spine 182–3
supracondylar humeral fractures 69–71
  child 420
supramentale 327
suprapatellar bursa, effusion 128
supraspinatus and its tendon 78, 91
surgery 369–90
  breast, scar from 446
  leg length inequality 417
  radiography during 367–90
  radiography following *see* postoperative
      radiography
sutures (cranial) 404
swab left in chest 476
swimmers' projection 178
symphysis menti 272, 273, 308
symphysis pubis 158
syndrome assessment, skeletal survey
      431

talipes (pes) deformations 424–7
talocalcaneal (subtalar) joint 120–3
talocrural joint *see* ankle joint
talus in talipes equinovarus 424, 425,
      426, 427
tarsal coalition 426
tarsometatarsal (Lisfranc) joint, fracture
      dislocation 109
team work, trauma radiography 470
'teardrop' sign 145
teenagers *see* adolescents
teeth *see* tooth

temporal bones 250–1
  mastoid process 250, 251, 252–3
  petrous parts/ridges 250, 251, 254, 263, 269,
      276, 277
temporomandibular joint 274
  in dental panoramic radiography 321
tendinitis, supraspinatus 78
tendons, shoulder, calcification 91–3
tension band wiring 372
teres major and its tendon 91
terminology 2–11
  anatomical *see* anatomy
  dental radiography 206, 294
  positioning 3–6
theatre radiography 367–90
thenar eminence, foreign body 48, 49
thin-film transistor 23
Thomas splint 362, 363
Thompson's hip prosthesis 370
thoracic inlet 196–7
thoracic vertebrae 164, 179–81
  auto-tomography 181, 479
  levels/landmarks 166, 167
  paediatric 416
    in survey for non-accidental injury 429
  trauma 164, 471
  see also cervicothoracic junction
thorax (chest) 194–228, 354–7
  bones 220–8
  children 390–7
    asphyxiating thoracic dystrophy 431
    in survey for non-accidental injury 429
  drains *see* drains
  examination of X-ray 205
  identification of X-ray 203
  paediatric radiography 390–7
  swab left in 476
  trauma 220, 221
  ward radiography 353, 354–7
    special care baby unit 365
thumb 38, 48–9
  holding film for periapical radiography 295
thymus, children 396
thyroid gland, retrosternal 197
tibia 124
  external fixation 362, 372
  fracture *see* fracture
  hypoplasia 417
  osteotomy 370
  in skeletal survey for non-accidental injury
      430
tibiofibular joint, proximal 106, 125
tiling 23
tilting table, abdominopelvic radiography
      340
toes 106, 112–13
tomography (computed) *see* computed
      tomography
tomography (conventional) 479–88
  applications 486–8
  exposure factors 482, 486
  image quality 484–5
  inclined plane 481
  linear 482
    C3/C7 vertebrae 173
  panoramic *see* panoramic radiography
  principles 480–1
  procedure 486
  radiation protection 485

tube/film movement in, types of 482–4
  see also auto-tomography
tooth (teeth) 282–3
  anatomy/components 281
  anterior, positioning errors in dental
      panoramic radiography 324
  in bisecting angle technique 298
  in C1/C2 radiography 170, 171
  cephalogram showing, child 407
  deciduous/primary 281, 282, 283
  eruption 281
  forensics 498
  fragments in lip 310
  inhaled (following trauma) 475
  notation systems 282–3
  overlapping, in dental panoramic radiography
      320
  in paralleling technique 300, 301, 302
  permanent 281, 282, 283
  surfaces, terminology 284
  see also dental radiography *and specific teeth*
Townes projection 243–4
  reverse 245, 257
trabecular patterns, femoral neck 145
trachea 196–7, 488
  foreign body 475
  intubation *see* endotracheal tube
  tomography 488
traction 372
  femoral fracture, child 364
  spinal fracture dislocation 361
transpyloric plane 332
transtubercular plane 332
transverse plane
  body *see* axial plane
  breast 437
trauma/injury 371–4, 466–71
  acromioclavicular joint 94
  ankle joint 115
  facial bones 262, 267
    severely injured patient 266
  general aspects
    adapting technique 467
    assessment and monitoring of patient's
        condition 466, 468
    equipment considerations 468–70
    exposure factors 471
    planning examination 466
  glenohumeral joint 79, 86
  hip, radiographic lines in assessment of
      integrity 145
  non-accidental *see* physical abuse; self-harm
  pelvis *see* pelvis
  renal 337, 339
  skeletal survey *see* skeletal survey
  skull of child in 402, 429
  spinal
    cervical 164, 168, 169, 170, 171, 175, 176,
        177, 471
    cervicothoracic junction 178
    children 415
    lumbar 164, 181, 185, 471
    lumbosacral junction 164
    sacral 164
    thoracic 164, 471
  surgery 371–4
  thorax 220, 221
    ward radiography 354
  see also various types of trauma

trochanteric region, fracture 147
trolley, trauma patient 469, 470
tuberculosis, children 395
tumour
    lung 211, 212
    skull 246, 247, 248

ulna
    in deviation, radiograph of scaphoid in 51, 80
    distal 38
      dislocation 60
    fracture see fracture
ulnar groove 67
ultrasound
    breast 447
    foreign bodies 476
    intestinal obstruction 336
    shoulder 78
umbilical artery or vein catheter 392
upper limb (arm) 37–76
    child in survey for non-accidental injury 429
    projections
      positioning for 5
      recommended 38
    in shoulder radiography
      abduction for coracoid process
        demonstration 103
      rotation in tendon calcification 92
    table and patient position 39
ureter
    calculus 345
    in retrograde pyelography 376
urinary tract 345–7
    calculi 336, 345, 347
    interventional techniques 376–7
urography, intravenous 486, 487
uterine cavity 379

vagina, foreign body inserted in 476
valgus deformities 427
    hallux 111
    hindfoot 425, 426
valves (heart)
    calcification 217
    prosthetic 217
varus deformity
    forefoot 424
    hindfoot 426
vascular procedures, emergency 380
Velcro straps, head 236
vena cava, superior 214
    catheter wire in 357
venous pressure line, central 357
ventral decubitus position see prone position
ventricles 214
vertebral body
    cervical, injury 169
    lumbar 184
vertebral (spinal) column 163–92, 411–16
    in ATLS see Advanced Trauma and Life
        Support
    children 411–16
      in Jeune's syndrome 431
      in survey for non-accidental injury 429
    curves 165
    levels and landmarks 166–7
    metastases 179, 493
    myeloma 492
    positioning errors in dental panoramic
      radiography 324
    recommended projections 164
    ward radiography 363
vertex (skull) 230
vertex occlusal radiograph 284
    maxilla 307

vibrator lodged in rectum 476
view
    definition 12
    lung fields 204
viewing box
    paediatric radiography 388
    subjective contrast and 16
vitamin D-resistant rickets 431
Von Rosen projection 410

waiting area, children 383, 386
ward radiography 351–65
    general comments 352
    infection control 353
    radiation protection 352
wedge filter, soft tissue radiography 494
whiplash injury 175
wire(s)
    for fixation 372
    localization/marker, breast 461, 463
workstations
    acquisition 25
    reporting 25
wrist (carpus) 50–8
    dislocations see dislocations
    fracture 53

X-ray beam see beam
X-ray equipment see equipment
xiphisternal joint 181

zonography 484
Zsigmondy–Palmer system 282
zygapophyseal joint see facet joint
zygoma (incl. zygmomatic arch) 243,
    245, 268